MEDICAL PRACTICES
CONSTRUCTION AND
DESIGN MANUAL

GENERAL MEDICINE

OPHTHALMOLOGY

SURGERY

DERMATOLOGY

GASTROENTEROLOGY

OBSTETRICS

VASCULAR SURGERY

GYNAECOLOGY

OTOLARYNGOLOGY

INTERNAL MEDICINE

CARDIOLOGY

PAEDIATRICS AND YOUTH MEDICINE

COSMETIC SURGERY

ORAL AND MAXILLOFACIAL SURGERY

NATUROPATHY

NEUROSURGERY

NEUROLOGY

NUCLEAR MEDICINE

ORTHOPAEDICS

OSTEOPATHY

OTONEUROLOGY

PHYSIOTHERAPY

PLASTIC SURGERY

PSYCHIATRY

PSYCHOTHERAPY

RADIOLOGY

RADIOONCOLOGY

PAIN THERAPY

RADIOTHERAPY

UROLOGY

DENTISTRY

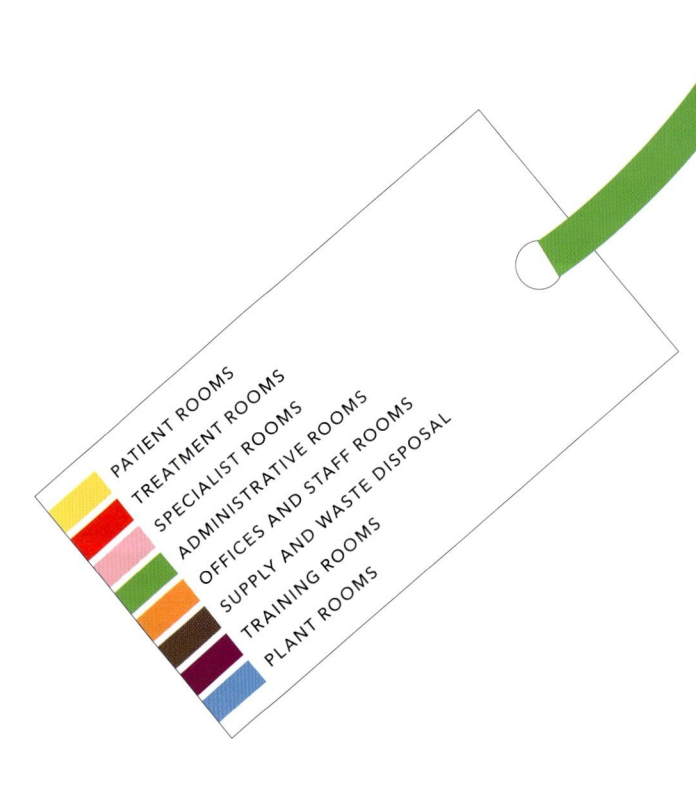

PATIENT ROOMS

TREATMENT ROOMS

SPECIALIST ROOMS

ADMINISTRATIVE ROOMS

OFFICES AND STAFF ROOMS

SUPPLY AND WASTE DISPOSAL

TRAINING ROOMS

PLANT ROOMS

MEDICAL PRACTICES
CONSTRUCTION AND DESIGN MANUAL

Edited by: Philipp Meuser
Scientific advisor: Prof. Franz Labryga

In memory of Dörte Becker †

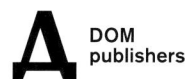

DOM publishers

CONTENT

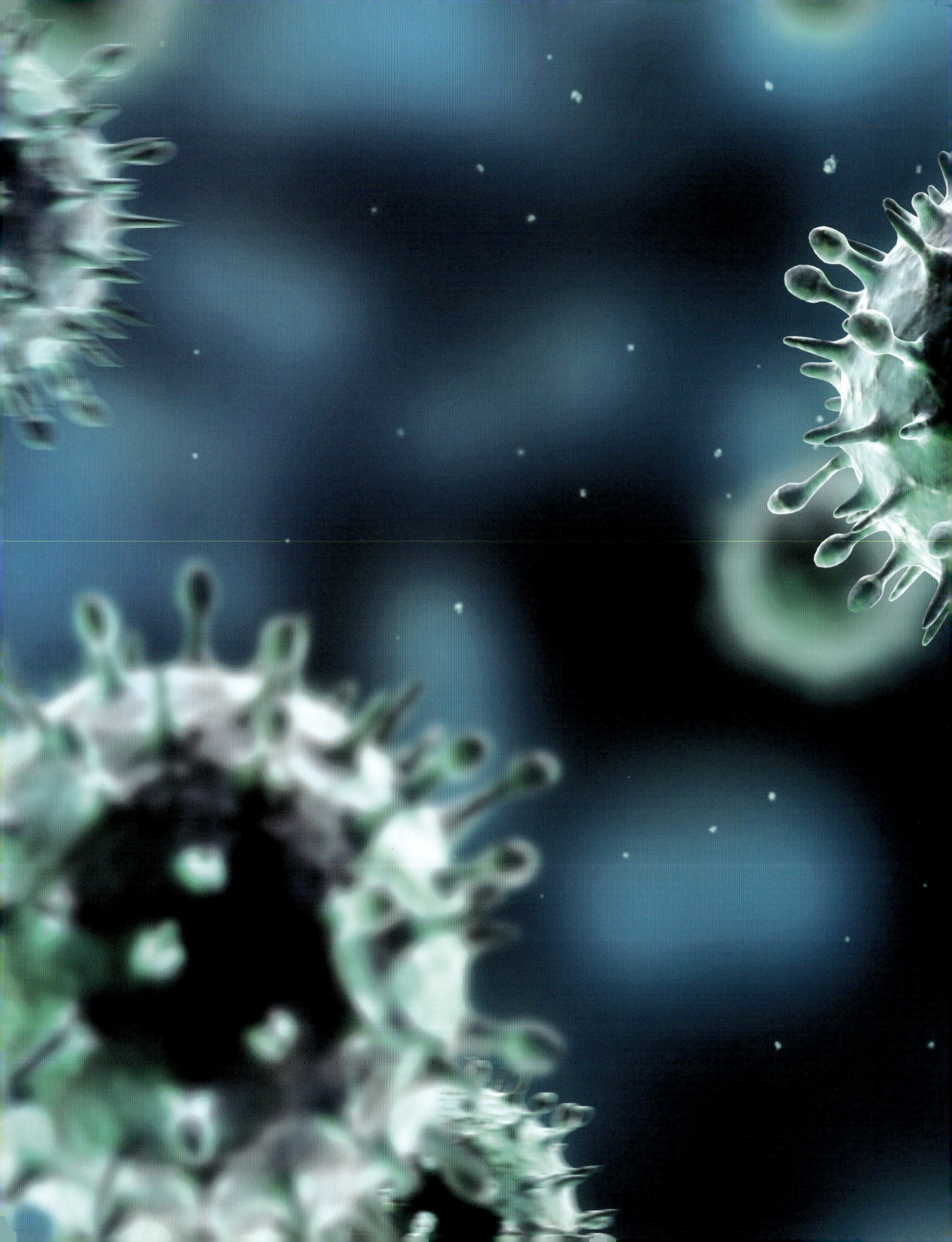

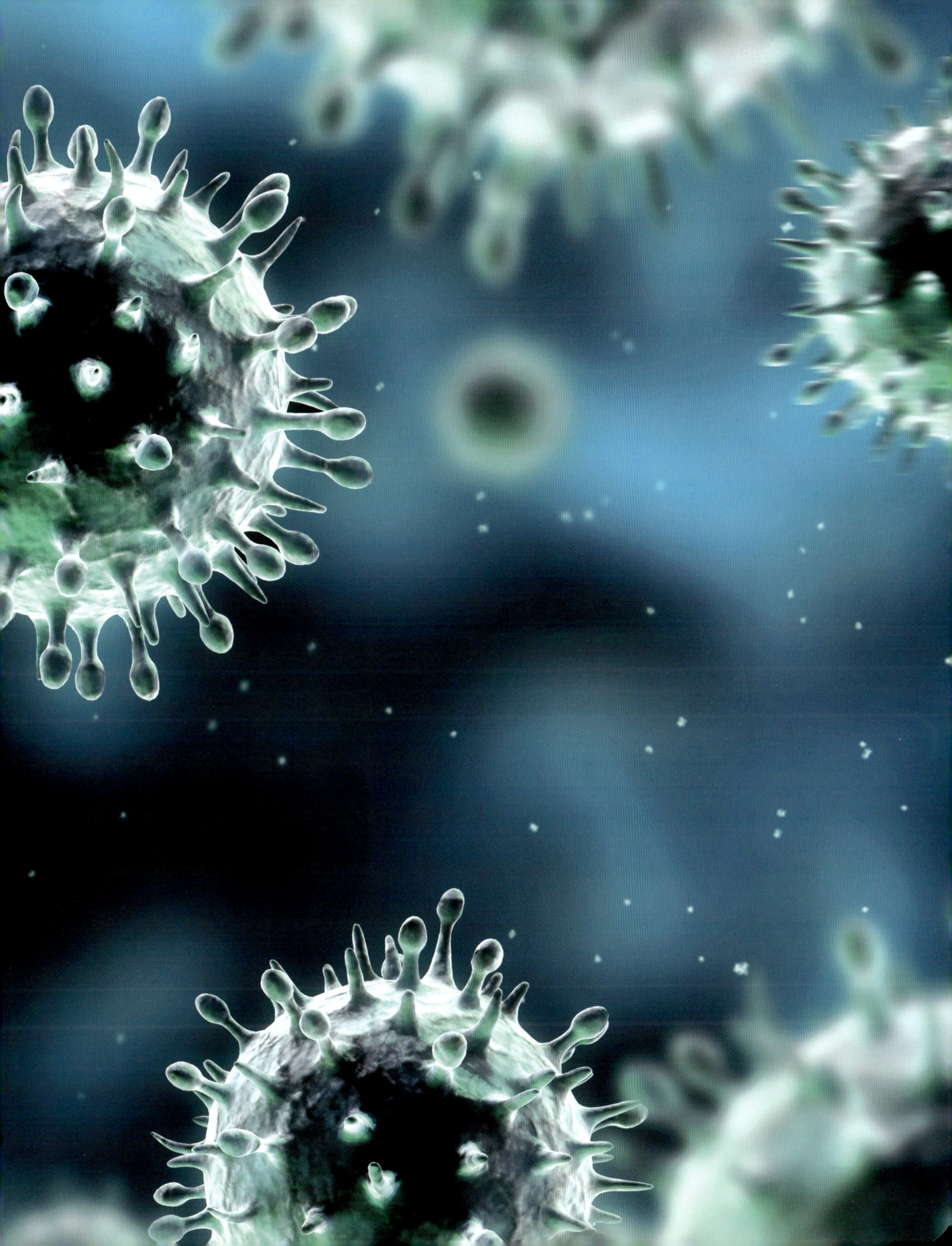

The German weekly magazine "Der Spiegel" dubbed him the "corpse manufacturer", producing human bodies as if on a serial assembly line and preparing them for the afterlife, by arranging them in ordinary, real-life poses as dancers, teachers, a rider astride the body of a horse prepared in the same way – just as if they had become fixed in the position of their final moments before death. In their second lives, these beings have taken on a different form and being turned inside out, displaying bones, tendons, muscles and internal organs.

The corpse cabinet of Dr. Gunther von Hagens, the well-known anatomist, is the result of a process he himself developed. Known as plastination, it was patented in 1977. It takes only a glance to understand that the exhibitions he has staged showcase human beings both as marvels and as models for creation. As medical man and director of the Institute of Plastination, Dr. von Hagens intends his highly provocative exhibitions to instruct the general public in the fascinating world of the "human body, its functions, diseases and changes" all within the context of health – a goal successfully achieved.

Since 2000, von Hagens has attracted some 30 million visitors to his exhibitions of post-mortal artefacts known around the globe as *Body Worlds*. In this, the media-savvy doctor paves the way. Even before health care reform was being publically debated in Germany, he set health education at the heart of this political initiative, whose implementation has altered the health care system in Germany like no other measure since 1945. It became the cornerstone of his thinking.

Awareness of one's personal health, prevention of illness and the quest for knowledge of how the body works have long been preoccupations of advanced cultures. But even though this line of thought is not new, Dr. Gunther von Hagens' museum-type displays are definitely a novel form of education. Such is his skill that he not only popularises medicine – he also markets his own genius as an inventor. But anatomist and Renaissance man von Hagens, who, with his hat, resembles the artist and marketing supremo Joseph Beuys, is also his own publicist: "Wherever there is a microphone or a camera, the taxidermist is immediately in evidence," writes "Der Spiegel". His consummate marketing skills exploit the modern media – with an internet presence, targeted media work and educationally outstanding exhibitions. The recipient of international patents and awards combining the roles of entrepreneur and adviser in the field of health care in a variety of different ways. Born in 1945 in Poland a self-proclaimed internationalist and intellectual adventurer, Dr. von Hagens combines the very characteristics essential to best promote his medical expertise in the health care market of the future. In this respect, too, he is a role model for his colleagues.

PHILIPP MEUSER

ARCHITECTURE AS A QUALITY FACTOR
INTRODUCTION

The privatisation of health

In Germany the drive for privatisation has turned health into a market subject to competition. The mere fact of being a doctor is simply not enough and by no means a guarantee of a state protected status or of automatic commercial success. Accredited medical associations insure around 135,000 GPs, specialists and therapists, most of them independent practitioners [figure for 2009]. Then there are approximately 24,000 non-medical practitioners and holistic therapists and providers of purely non-medicinal treatments centred on "wellness", all serving a vast and paying clientele. In recent years, these professional groups have radically changed public perception of the body, sickness and health. Anyone running a practice these days must not only succeed as a businessman but must also face the challenge of a fundamentally different attitude to quality of life. As regards the competition, it helps to have a strong personal profile, easily visible to everyone – and as for the change in outlook, the approach required is an ability to rethink one's orientation and adjust accordingly. Both personal profile and public perception affect the identity of the enterprise and the health of the doctor's business.

Health care reform their own contributions towards the cost of health care, has made people wary of consulting their doctor. The state approach means that people must assume at least some responsibility for their own sickness prevention. In the wake of such change, statutory health sickness schemes have followed with their own powerful publicity campaign to create a new image for their business. They are now called health insurance schemes or life insurance companies like DAK. This system has long since transformed the visitor to the doctor's surgery from "patient" [from the Latin "patiens" = sufferer, or someone who endures] to "client" [from Latin "cliens" = person to whom protection is due], that is customer. While it is true that the doctor is still the healer that he always has been, where nothing else is possible nowadays he tends to be cast in a new role, that of advisor seeking to advise his customers on matters of prevention. People who go to the doctor do not necessarily suffer from some acute illness. Today, patients are also motivated by prophylactic concerns, are health and beauty conscious or are simply looking for advice on how to find relief from the stresses of modern living.

This role of the doctor as health adviser is the end result of the health care reform and has never so far been taken into account in monetary terms. But it can only be a matter of time before the standard wording on drugs packaging "For the risks and side effects, consult your doctor or pharmacist' features in some different format as a service on the bill for the health insurance provider. Doctors are therefore subject to competition not only other doctors, but also in their role as businessmen vying for customers. For a doctor to stand out from his colleagues he must at the same time make himself visible to the customers. The solution is advertising. Doctors in Germany were not allowed to advertise until 13 July 2005, when the German Federal Constitutional Court, ruled on a constitutional suit contesting the prohibition on advertising brought by the Association of Statutory Health Insurance Physicians. The ruling overturned the ban and allows doctors a form of advertising which enables them to emphasise the image of and trust in doctors that patients have acquired through the services and care received. By law, doctors are now also permitted to publicise these aspects of their work by advertising in newspapers, magazines, on the internet and television. Even the size of the nameplate outside the practice is no longer specified.

In Germany, for doctors, this switch from a self-imposed ban on advertising presents both an opportunity and a challenge. Since not all his colleagues have the media savvy of a Gunther von Hagens, they need expert advice on how to project themselves. Moreover, 80 % of outpatient medical facilities are single-doctor practices with the remainder being largely two-doctor practices. Most doctors have total control of their business, shouldering all the risks and responsibilities including organisation of the practice – staffing, technology, finance, purchasing, marketing – at the same time as further training. They have no time to think about the next advertisement; besides, it

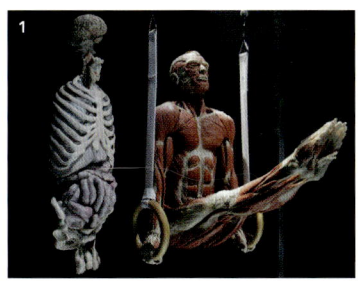 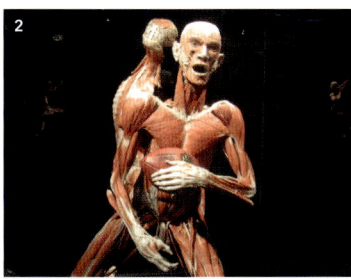 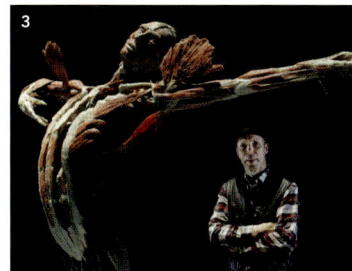

The popularisation of medicine:
Items on show in the *Body Worlds*
exhibition which has so far attracted over
30 million visitors around the world.
1 Ring gymnast with skeleton and
  intestines
2 Rugby player with ball
3 Gunther von Hagens behind a male
  exhibit

costs a vast amount to advertise in newspapers, magazines and as well on television.

However much the German associations of statutory physicians regulations are required to allow doctors to advertise, the remuneration system negotiated with the health insurance schemes conflicts sharply with all the rules of competition. This is because the system does not allow the "commercially particularly able, qualitatively good and popular doctors … to grow too strongly". Marketing experts Felix Cornelius and Wolfram Otto write that in consequence of the physicians' guild's code, "popular doctors don't become less popular because of it. But they no longer have any incentive to expand their practices." As a consequence of this switch, customers, that is patients, registered with less popular practices and who would like to change to another doctor, must accept longer waiting times; in the worst case scenarios, they have no opportunity to change practice at all because the popular doctors are not taking on any new customers. Ultimately, there is no financial incentive to extend consulting hours and the range of services. In short, the association of statutory physicians, guild system prevents payment for services that would clearly disadvantage those doctors with fewer patient visits. So the system effectively prevents doctors from advertising their services commercially and from using this facility to make themselves stand out from their colleagues. This means that the guild's code penalises the successful medical service providers and actually deprives the customers, that is the patients, of their right to choose their doctor freely.

Quality through brand creation and identity

One solution is to make quality visible through brand creation and identity. Nothing makes a service provider's self-image more effective and more cost efficiently visible over the long term, than a "corporate design' which answers the questions "Who am I? What am I? What do I have to offer?" And such a design is on business cards, the internet page and even through the design of the practice premises.

For these are the questions that the customer expects answers to, answers that he will consciously analyse for their meaning and on which he makes the decision as to whether or not he will even enter the premises, enter once and never again, or do so repeatedly. Naturally what is covered by the company's image must match its core values, including the attitude and appearance of the staff. This is vital because doctors all too easily forget that each visit by a patient to a practice constitutes an intrusion into the patient's privacy. After all, consulting a doctor is an intimate affair. It is a very personal matter, whether it is to do with the body, the mind or both. Essentially, this "advance payment' of trust is made intuitively by people who nowadays are self-assured and increasingly sceptical about health-related matters. The decision whether – if at all – to go to which doctor is made far away from the practice's front door. The appearance of the doctor's business card or homepage, which the patient will have consulted in advance, may well be decisive. Whatever feelings and expectations are aroused and whatever trust is engendered in the potential customer by these virtual visits, they need to be confirmed by the real environment of the practice: by the appearance, manner and conduct of the staff, even the architecture and design of the practice. It all comes down to the business's identity, which must chime with the character and service provision of the practice in terms of treatment, facilities and the very look of the building and with the customers themselves. The architecture and design serve to enhance the service provision, its quality and the practice's identity, which are experienced as a whole and viewed over the long term.

According to tradition, the architect of a medical practice has an obligation to fulfil as the creator of an artificial world of health. Artist, architect and polymath Leon Battista Alberti [1404–1472] provided expert advice for a healthy life in his "Della famiglia" [1434|1441]. In his work "De re aedificatoria" [1452], he described the climate, air, the locality and even the direction of the wind as essential influences affecting human well-being. "The environment provided by inhabited houses must be at the right temperature – even animals should feel at ease," he says there. The humanist Alberti concludes his holistic vision of cause and effect in a healthy environment with

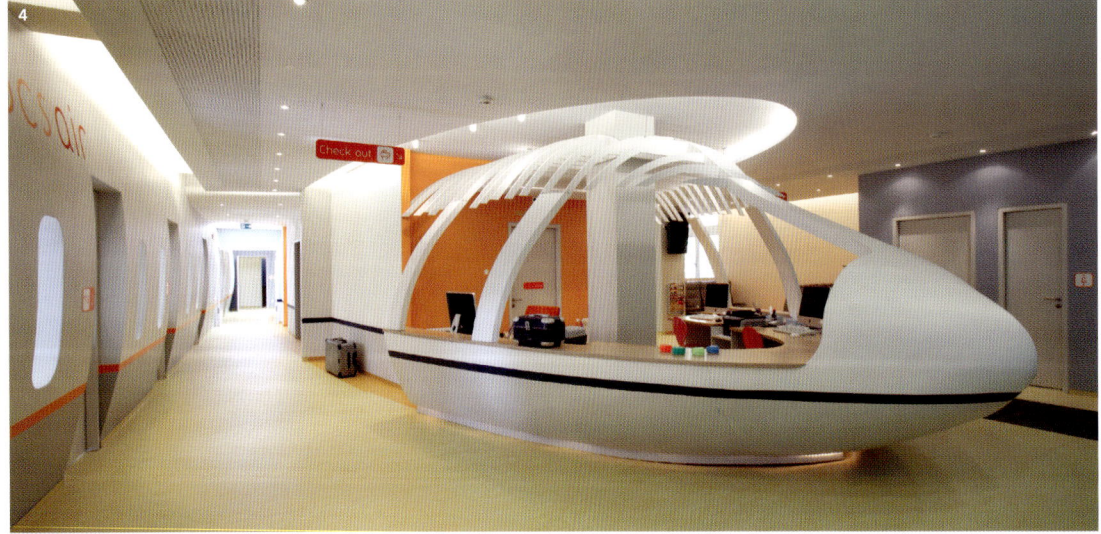

Dental practice "Kids Docs" in Berlin-Steglitz, Architects: planbar 3 [formerly BHZ planning office], colour design | guidance system: 3 für Formgebung, branding: metome.design
4 Reception area with a desk in the form of a plane cockpit
5 Treatment room with the child-friendly name "Elf room"

an apposite picture in which he depicts the town as a large house and the house as a tiny town. He goes in great detail into the minutiae hygiene technology in the water supply system. Not the only one to address architecture in practical and theoretical terms, Alberti was, alongside Andrea Palladio, one of the major scholars of his time. Knowledge was gained by taking a panoramic view of things and was further enhanced by referring back to ancient sources. Health and architecture are intimately connected together in advanced cultures. The right ambient temperature and atmosphere are part of a business's self-representation and the development of its unique brand. As already noted, this ranges from the business card, the headed notepaper and the internet presence to the design of the practice's premises.

A doctor's professional expertise is not the sole deciding factor in his commercial success. Such expertise tends to be perceived subjectively anyway and well ahead of any appointment. The intangible influences include the architecture of a practice, that is a practical room layout which reflects the practice's internal organisation. This knowledge acquired by architects and schooled in the humanist tradition is essential because they are able to integrate all the constituent elements, including an assessment of the doctor's clientele. They will be able to use exactly this knowledge to develop a finite corporate design in combination with other media-related brand markers as a single-source solution.

Marketing and branding

Since in Germany a doctor is one in over 135,000, to stand out, it is very important that he make visible the company's unique identity. An easy matter? Hardly. Yet the answers to the questions on a unique company identity are primarily linked to personality. The very first step is for a doctor to view his own medical practice as a business. Next it helps to imagine this company as a human being with a body, mind and soul. This is because a company identity, that is the corporate identity, can be compared with the identity of a person.

In order to run the company [that is practice] in a market-orientated fashion, it is important for the doctor to visualise the customers he already has or would like to attract in the future. The answers to such questions will determine everything that needs to be done to define the practice as a brand. It is precisely the customers who determine the practice's particular approach and profile and so also its corporate identity. The architecture of the practice, "hardware" as it were, is an essential ingredient in enabling visualisation of the company identity. Taken together with the media used to present the practice, the architecture creates harmonious and memorable picture of the practice. In sum, all the elements used in self-presentation, including the architecture should be unified in character in terms of form and colour and combine to make the practice's identity visible – and so you have the corporate design. An implicit logo which readily identifies the practice for everyone is extremely helpful here. This is all the more vital when the medical practice is part of a joint practice or a medical centre. The media-friendly corporate design as part of the company identity serves to ensure that a positive image of the practice is generated in the subconscious of the potential client well before they have been to the practice. Corporate design is what triggers a sense of recognition in someone entering the practice for the first time. And quite apart from the visual impression, the conduct of the staff, how they communicate, their professional expertise and even the internal organisation of the practice all have a decisive role to play. Patients as customers have a finely tuned sense for whether there is a match between the style – which renders the design [on every level] visible as "hardware" – and the staff, that is the "software" of the practice. To be sure there is no mismatch, it may well be helpful to have six to eight weeks' training in how to run the practice.

As well as the code of conduct, which makes palpable the special character of a medical practice, having a dress code for the staff makes it easier for the visitor to know who's who in the hierarchy. This is especially advisable in large or joint practices and in practices offering a wide range of services. Moreover, the actual location of the practice is important.

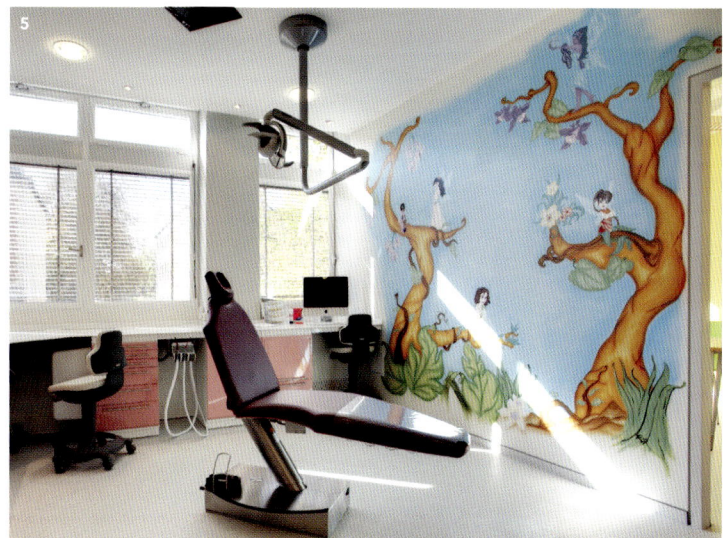

This starts with the area surrounding the building and the location of the practice within the building. It is at this point that it is especially important to consult the architect as qualified adviser.

"Tell me where you live and I'll tell you who you are!" This aphorism applies to the location of a company as well as, in this case, a medical practice. The impression given by the exterior influences the well-being of the visitor. It begins with the ring tone of the telephone, includes the typeface of the headed notepaper and extends right up to the architecture and design. If the choice of colours for the logo reflects the colour philosophy behind the practice's design that is definitely an advantage. Because it all comes down to the recognition effect.

Space and room planning

Architecture for medical practices generally means designs for the interior of a building. It rarely happens that the opening of a new practice involves the construction of a new purpose-built building or extension. Medical practices are generally located in residential, office or former factory buildings. This means that the design must accommodate the existing ground plan whether in the rented floor, office or residential unit. And this is were any problems can start – which can rapidly turn into a disaster before the ink is dry on the lease. So it is astonishing that the most time-consuming activity is walking to and fro, that is the distances covered every day in the practice. In general, the female auxiliary staff walk almost ten kilometres on an average day. Where work processes are made unnecessarily complicated, the layout of the premises generates additional costs if nothing else. And such instances are not rare, they are true of most cases. This is because nine out of ten practices are planned without architects and operate as outlined above. In other words, the poor design of nine out of ten practices can significantly distort the owner's balance sheet.

The remedy is a rational, architecturally designed layout achieved with a qualified planner – before the lease is signed.

Indeed, at the heart of any well-organised practice is a space and room design that has been properly thought through – and this means for the practice as a whole and each room individually.

But this can't be done until both doctor and architect know what services the doctor actually provides, who the doctor's customers are, now and in the future. All this dictates the choice of location, the design of the building, the details of the furnishings and fittings plus the specific needs in terms of floor space and the technical equipment to serve the rooms. During negotiations between landlord and tenant, the architect can be particularly helpful and valuable – for example with regard to the connection points needed for the service supply cables and lines, or issues and any consents needed from the authorities. A practice may be in a former apartment, but here too, the answers to the following questions are of crucial importance. Do the potential premises satisfy the building regulations? Can work place and hygiene regulations be complied with here? And, first and foremost, – is building consent necessary or will a change of use application have to be made?

The easiest way to settle all these points is to consult an experienced architect. He knows how to cast an expert's eye over the vision and expectations the doctor has of his practice, over the requirements and the site under consideration. As a qualified planner, taking into account the ground plan and standard of the potential premises, the technical requirements, the estimated building costs and the doctor's budget, the architect can judge whether the location being considered by the doctor is suitable or whether a conversion would be worthwhile.

The same applies to any structural work contemplated for an existing practice – in other words, would conversion be an option? If the reception desk is off to one side, if the distances are too great, if the staff keep getting in each other's way as they do their work and if that sort of fatal flaw is characteristic of the business, then a new practice design is needed. Even converting small medical practices into spacious, functioning healt care businesses provides ample scope for the skill and expertise of an architect.

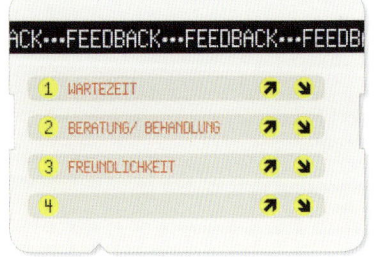
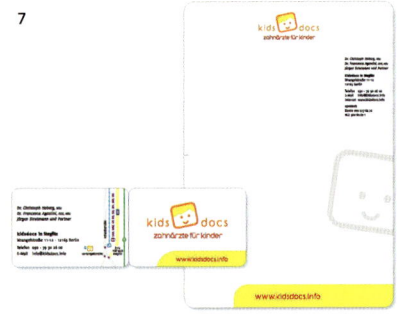
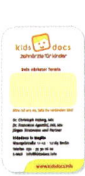

Dental practice "Kids Docs" in Berlin-Steglitz, Architects: planbar 3 [formerly BHZ planning office], colour design | guidance system: 3 für Formgebung, branding: metome.design
6 "Boarding card" for young patients
7 "Kids Docs" business equipment
8 Postcards

Space allocation

The structure of a medical practice can often say much more about a doctor's working methods than he would like or is even aware of. Clear workflows, rationally planned offices and the kind of benefits inherent in a peaceful atmosphere all depend largely on how the space is allocated. A well thought-out space allocation design will facilitate rational workflows, separate the work areas from the public areas and reflect the practice's workflows. This means everything, from reception to the treatment rooms, administration and even the waiting areas. The purpose of space allocation is clarity, in the form of a logical subdivision of available space for the different roles that make up the practice's workflow hierarchy. Allocating the practice's spaces in this way ensures that everything runs smoothly.

A well thought out-space design not only helps to cut down on walking distances and save time, and therefore reduce costs, but is also just as much an essential ingredient of the corporate identity as the choice of headed notepaper. The details of the practice's configurations express this identity non-verbally, that is visually. The space concept, taken as the template for the interior design, is also subject to the basic precept that the form must be fit for purpose. The reception area is the point from which the visitor should be able to grasp the layout of the practice. Reception should be sited at some central point. At the very least it should be clearly visible from the entrance and both welcome the visitor and be a credit to the practice – like a prestigious executive suite or a hotel lobby.

One should also bear in mind that the reception is more than just a place for visitors to report to. It is also the place for initial conversations, exchanging information, making arrangements and appointments for clients by staff. All important client details are forwarded from here straight to the next points in the system. If we compare the practice with human anatomy, then reception is to the practice as the heart is to the body. It is the point from which the whole of the practice's circulatory system is controlled and kept alive.

As regards the practice's other workflows, one could compare them with the reception desk in a hotel. It is as if the patient receives his "key" here, that is access to all the services available in the practice. Reception is the control point or heart of the practice. And just as the heart oversees the workings of the whole body, the practice's receptionist should be able to see all the doors so that she can keep the practice's workflows running smoothly. If the practice is logically structured, then the waiting rooms, treatment rooms and other rooms will all be grouped around the reception area. An alternative approach, however, is to have the rooms ranged along a corridor running from the reception lounge. In this case, the corridor also functions as guide to the practice's rooms. Space allocation permits of numerous variations. The point is to design workflows as effectively, and therefore as cost efficiently, as possible.

The watchword here is "rationalisation" which, according to Bruno Leo Friton, himself a doctor, applies to all measures taken together as a whole. According to Friton, such measures "are geared to designing a work process such that the greatest output is achieved with the least amount of effort. This is achieved by means of the configuration of a work place, observation of working patterns, fit-for-purpose preparation of a work process, simplification of the necessary work and elimination of superfluous work and by the design of special instruments and appliances." With reference to this precept, in 1961 Friton was already invoking the cultural philosopher Jacob Burckhardt and his optimistic description of a social authority: "I would wish that everything that can be mechanised would be mechanised as completely and as soon as possible so that the human spirit would have all the more power and leisure to do the rest."

With regard to health care reform, the *Deutsche Ärzteblatt* [the German Medical Association's journal] recently warned that the doctor with a stethoscope around his neck caring for his patients and wearing a white coat soiled with blood or other body fluids had been replaced by the doctor wearing a suit. Instead of a stethoscope around his neck, he'd be holding a time-and-motion chart in his hand and would most likely know the manual of process management by heart. Any marks on

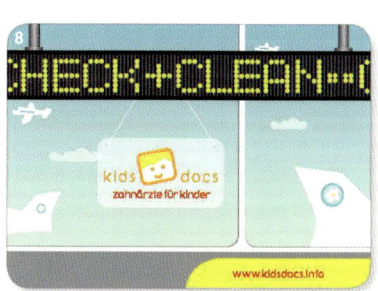
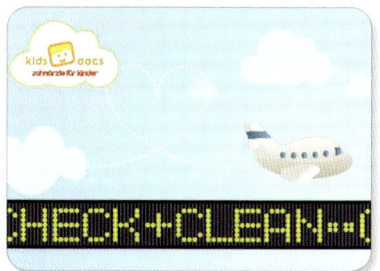
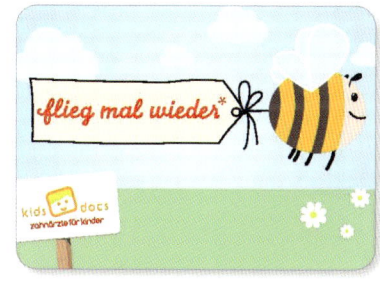
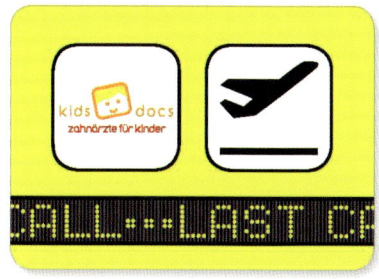
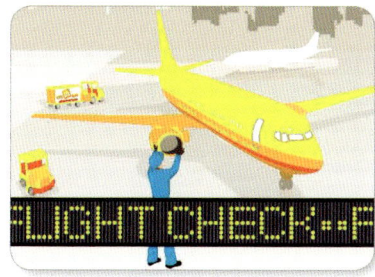
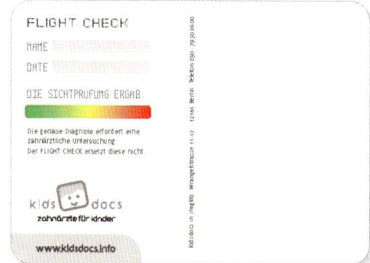

his clothes – if any – would be from the ink of his fountain pen or photocopier. Technology would be dictating to the human spirit and not the other way round. At least, everyone will have detected a pervasive hiatus , one which turns Friton's plausible statements on rationalisation into a template for Germany's medical practices.

The first thing a medical practice needs to install is an efficient intercom system. This type of technology does not need to be impersonal. The medium used to conduct a conversation does not define its character, rather, if anything does define it, it's the speakers themselves. The fact remains that a good intercom system saves two full working hours per day or at least two months' salary per year. It also makes no sense for the practice's staff to let patients into the waiting rooms themselves and then, having opened the door for them, to show them to the relevant treatment room. Neither auxiliary staff, nor doctors nor customers are small children. But it is supremely important and sensible to call the next patient from the reception area and tell him with a friendly smile where he is supposed to go. And that, of course, is only possible if the space allocation has been organised properly.

This involves locating the waiting area as far forward as possible in the practice, in the area to which the public has direct access. In doing so the public area is clearly demarcated from the working area and workflows are not disrupted. Sensible space allocation in harmony with

workflows also requires an interior design which functions as a non-verbal way finding system from floor to ceiling in terms of choice of materials, colour and lighting.

All this constitutes a "top-level cultural support system by means of technology" [Friton] because its implementation enables time to be spent in concentrating on the patient on learning from the patient and increasing scientific knowledge. Indeed, the medical vocation is still a craft. This preparatory work at the interface between theory and practice also means that the doctor and architect are excellent professional partners with shared goals service to their fellow human beings.

Interior design

Light, colour and the form of the materials for walls, floors, ceilings and furniture define the character of the medical practice. These elements should convey the company identity of a medical practice and at the same time harmonise with the professional bias of the doctor. It does not matter whether the practice is functional and cool with few nuances of colour, whether it is bright and transparent or has forceful design features. Nor does it matter whether it looks like an observatory or is defined by contrasts between old and new, or whether powerful organic forms and well accentuated photographic motifs or art predominate. The important thing is that the fittings can be seen to reflect a personality

as well to convey more than that. It is just the same when you first meet someone. The first ten seconds after entering a practice are crucial for the patient's feelings of liking or disliking the experience – and hence crucial for the success of the doctor. The first impression counts. And the first impression will be of the area surrounding the practice, the building in which it is housed, the doctor's nameplate, the ring tone and finally the reception area, the atmosphere.

In other words, we are dealing here with a combination of many factors which together exert an intuitive and unconscious effect. It is the same with a person. We do not register a person selectively. Instead, we take the person as a constellation of many features – how he moves, the type and colour of the clothes he is wearing and the surroundings we encounter him in. The intuitive overall impression creates an image in the mind that then determines whether we like him or not. In this connection, again, it is impossible to overemphasise that its architecture and design are indisputably at the heart of the corporate design of a medical practice.

This merging of several factors in the total experience determines perception and whether or not a client feels at ease in an environment. Even so, it is also true that it is impossible to please everyone. What one person finds unpleasant excites and stimulates another. It is a natural law that antipathy and sympathy determine whether something is attractive, to be kept at a distance or embraced. But it is also beyond dispute that the changing role

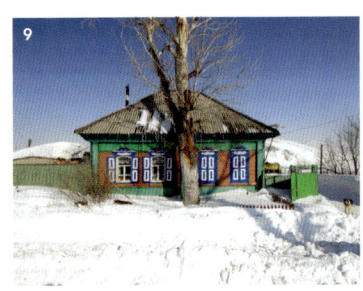

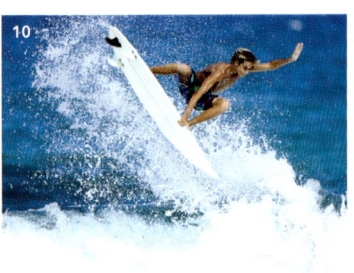

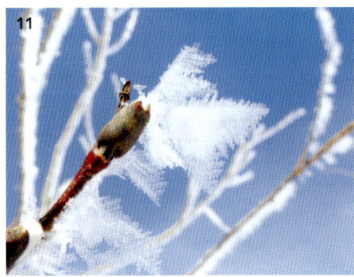

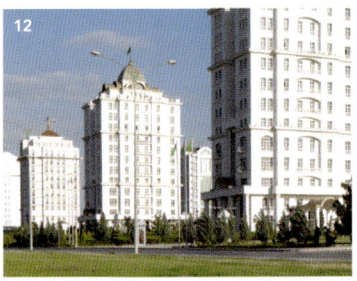

of the patient from someone who suffers and tolerates to someone in need of protection, has dawned on only a few doctors and been incorporated by them into the design of their premises. Only rarely in German treatment rooms and on the premises of therapists practising symptom-orientated academic medicine does one come across a practice with a contemporary, customer-centred design.

This is extremely unfortunate as the first impression also determines the tenor of the verbal messages. And in this way, the corporate design, the visual impression of the company's identity defined in human terms, continues to have its effect, as a form of recommendation, far beyond its own material limits. Recommendation by clients, however, is the most cost-efficient, effective and most enduring form of advertising for any businessman including doctors. Especially today. The design of the practice is therefore a factor in the doctor's self-presentation with a far-reaching effect as publicity.

For this commercial effect to occur, both form and function, as basic design factors, must be complemented by a relaxing and pleasant atmosphere for the client. Harmony is what drives everything. And it is significant that this harmony is generated by the combination of materials, form, colour and lighting.

If in doubt, remember that less is more when trying to get the message across to clients. This means that the choice of materials for the floor,

wall and ceiling together with the lighting and any pictorial subject matter have a substantial effect on mood. Light not only represents vitality but also underpins the whole image and the perception of things in one location.

So, to create a successful overall impression, it is absolutely essential to create a colour scheme that is implemented faithfully throughout the premises, from the furniture to the fittings. Here, both the practice's environment and the specialist bias of the doctor or the extremely unfortunate interests of a GP can influence design. Also, choices made for the design of the space, along with the surface areas, depend crucially on whether the practice is a single-doctor or joint practice or perhaps a medical centre accommodating doctors with different specialisms practising independently of one another. It may well be the case that a design leitmotiv is adopted to govern the colour, lighting, form and material scheme for the internet presence, business cards and architectural design. Although the medical services are configured at a particular location, it is important to express the individual character of the practice with everything — business cards, internet presence and design of the practice. In joint practices, the skill lies in making each individual doctor stand out visually from his colleagues.

Irrespective of the size and specialist bias of the practice, access to the building should be easy to see and find and free of obstructions.

Particularly, if the practice is sited in a residential or business block, it is important to have an obvious entrance area to distinguish the medical practice from its neighbours. A practice nameplate is not enough on its own. Instead, what is needed is a guidance and way finding system using visual prompts to guide the visitor from outside the practice into and throughout the practice. The basic elements of good architecture are colour, light and materials. In his standard work on the art of colour, published in 1961, the painter and art teacher Johannes Itten writes about the radiational power of colour. According to Itten, colours are "energies" which exert either a positive or negative influence on us, whether we are aware of it or not. We have the Catholic liberation theologian Dom Hélder Pessoa Câmara to thank for the following equally apposite insight about light: "Light transforms the things it falls on." For a professionally designed medical practice, this means giving due consideration to the effect of light entering from outside and the way colours and materials appear in artificial light – and making the appropriate choices. When using colours and materials, the way we combine them determines the quality of both the atmosphere in the rooms and the visitor guidance system. Not only floor and wall materials, but also colourful and eye-catching features and pictograms are simple resources to guide visitors as they move about the practice, or, in the case of a joint practice or medical centre, to draw attention at the same time to the variety of available services.

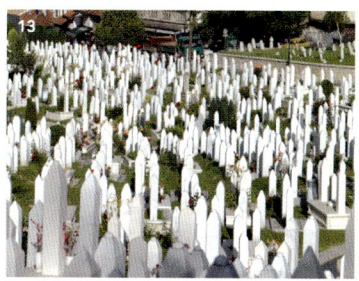
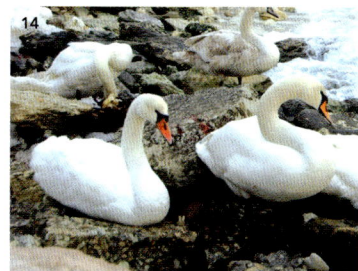
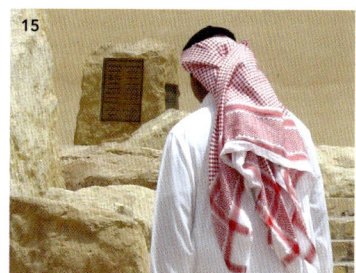

How colourful a "non-colour" can be:
White is the colour of ice and snow.
It is a symbol of purity and clarity,
serenity and innocence. It also works as
a symbol of inapproachability, sensitivity
and cool reserve.

9 Home in the Altai Mountains
10 Surfboarder in Hawaii
11 Crystals of ice on a flower bud
12 Marble palaces in Turkmenistan
13 Gravestones in Sarajevo
14 Swans on the Caspian Sea
15 Kaftan in Saudi Arabia

The more sparingly the resources are used, the greater the effect. The interior design should serve the purpose of a well functioning, non-verbal guidance system, complemented for example by a digital signage and way finding system, all of which are flexible and extremely easy.

Whatever specialist bias the health care business has, at its heart is always the reception area, as already stated. This is the visitor's point of arrival. First impressions are made here, impressions that decide whether the client feels secure, accepted and welcomed as a guest in the practice. Perhaps the patient even senses his fears, tensions, uncertainty and unease ebbing away when a friendly smile from the person at the reception desk, itself the centre of a soothing atmosphere, conveys the first sensations of healing. As in a hotel, the reception desk is the first point of call for communication and at the same time acts as a business card for the enterprise – in this case a medical practice – and the control centre for its internal operations. The visitor registers its appearance and activities subliminally and his unconscious begins to draw unseen conclusions about the whole enterprise. As regards customer relations, reception is the nerve centre of a practice.

The expression "Report here" should never be used, not in print nor as a verbal message. This expression, which smacks of the barracks and still leads a shadowy life in some official premises, should be avoided here at all costs.

A business such as a medical practice is no place to issue orders. This is a place where services are rendered. Here, the patient is king and not subject – and is always a guest. As terminology can change attitudes, it should be clear that the style and atmosphere of a practice's reception must match that of a five-star hotel in every respect. Bright, light, calm, relaxed and dependable – that is the impression to be created by the choice of materials and the lighting which should give the visitor an immediate grasp of where he is to go. As everone knows, the first impression isn't selective but general and takes in the whole space at once. A prominent, unobscured position for the reception desk is ideal. If reception is set at a slightly higher level, like a cockpit, this will also create the visual impression that the friendly staff has health care totally under control from here and throughout the practice.

Reception should be sited with a clear view of the consulting room and give clients enough room to move and avoid any feeling of being hemmed in to counteract the nervousness and apprehension that visitors to the doctor undoubtedly experience. Like this, the customer is able to gain an impression of his environment. This has a relaxing effect, breeds confidence and in the best cases dissipates fears and fosters a feeling of ease. In small practices, the spatial impression can be extended by arranging the reception area such that it looks out over some charming countryside view or an interesting

building. Otherwise, bright colours, a skilfully stage-managed lighting scheme and mirrors as well as bright materials – but only those that look light, all help to make the practice and reception look larger than they actually are. A wall covered with a photo reflecting the character of the practice or a mounted artwork can catch the eye and expand the dimensions of the practice – or at least divert attention and dispel nerves.

The combination of light and transparent materials and forms creates visions for the space. Round shapes make it easier, with little expense, to create a perception of depth, even in small practices, and so also reduce the sensation of being constricted. Round and undulating forms for the fittings and walls are relaxing and also generate a sense of well-being. Moreover, undulating wall surfaces can make it easier to find one's way around a medical practice. After hygiene, finding one's way around is the most important aspect of a practice. Both a rational room scheme and design features have a very important role to play. The interior design can be organic or associative. The shapes may refer to means of transportation such as a train, a ship, a car or a plane. The common feature of all these experience is a clear hierarchy and logical sequence of spaces. Creativity can be employed to objectify and reproduce this for the spatial design of a medical practice and gear it to the needs of the particular target group, making sure at the same time to find an original way to engender a positive atmosphere.

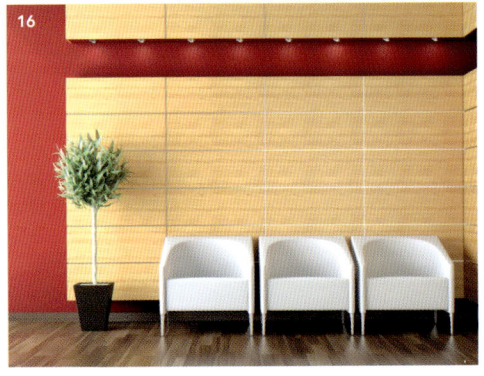
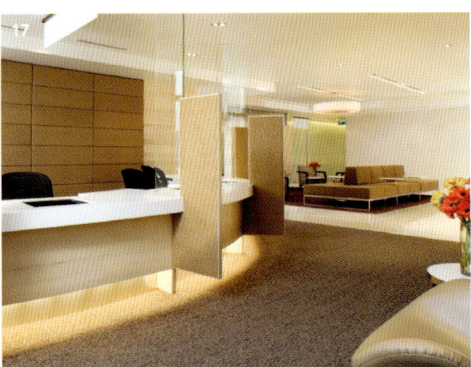
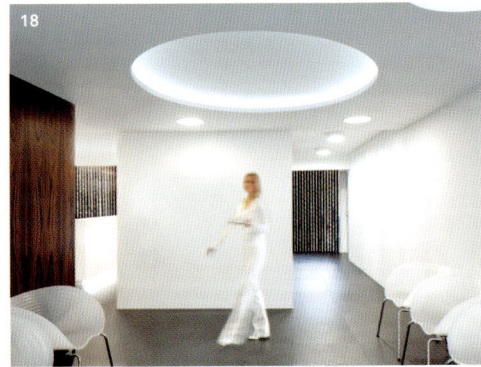

Waiting areas often serve the purpose of a business card for the company.
16 Executive suite in the USA
17 Customer consultation in a private bank
18 Practice in the Olympic village, Munich, Architect: Harald Stricker

Nor should one overlook the role of flooring as a guidance system. As well as real wood flooring and industrial-grade parquet, there have long been other options such as rubberised flooring or floor coverings which combine acoustic and visual advantages in that they look like textiles and have the comfortable, warm and calm feel of wall-to-wall carpeting without its disadvantages.

This type of flooring can be cut to whatever size you like and is easy to fit so that even round, flowing transitional spaces, for example between the working and waiting areas, can be marked out to great effect.

No one with an appointment at a company goes straight in to see the boss. A previous appointment may overrun or something may have happened to upset the scheduling. That is the normal state of affairs in a medical practice. You simply have to wait. And so there is a direct link between reception and a waiting room or – speaking generally – the waiting area or zone. On average, the time spent waiting in medical practices in Germany is 45 minutes. This means that the waiting area is where visiting patients spend more time out of the total time on a doctor's premises than anywhere else.

Whether or not a patient can stand this wait time will depend on whether the atmosphere is inviting and relaxing. To an extent, there needs to be something to take the patient's mind off the waiting – something which will differ from client to client. A practice which is geared mainly to children will highlight different aspects from one serving mainly older people. And a practice with a clientele spanning many generations ought to have different waiting areas geared to the different ages and tailored to their individual needs. The idea is to avoid conflict. Because one thing is clear – no matter how attractive the atmosphere of a medical practice, no one will ever associate it with the pleasures of going to a bar or staying in a hotel. After all, consulting a doctor is hardly a leisure time pursuit, but rather an unpleasant and unusual necessity. Germans are afraid of going to their doctor – they feel it in their bones, to varying degrees. A current survey conducted by Forsa, the public opinion research institute, on behalf of the Techniker Krankenkasse, the technicians' health insurance scheme, found that one in five people is afraid of going to the dentist.

This means that a place where a suspected or actual illness is diagnosed needs to be able to reduce fear and avoid tension. Waiting rooms are unsuitable for this because a waiting room gives the visitor the feeling of being shut out. Expressions such as waiting area or waiting zone convey a sense of openness. Interconnected rooms should also meet this need for openness. As soon as the patient enters the foyer of a practice, it should be made clear to him how free he is to make up his own mind about his visit. This greatly relaxes the patient's mood. Depending on the nature of the clientele, a combined bar and lounge feel can lighten the atmosphere for people as they wait. A play area for children designed so that a parent can either play with their children or have something to do while they wait would be a helpful addition. Apart from reading matter and something to drink, the choice of materials is important to create the right atmosphere.

Light is important in the waiting area. Subdued lighting creates a warm and comforting atmosphere. The other thing is colour. The positive energy emanating from both, achieved by the right choice of colours and the right technology, is put to the test in the waiting zone, as it stands in for the whole practice. The mood the patient feels here decides how things proceed from this point. Hygiene being the underlying theme of a practice's fixtures and fittings this implies the use of robust, elegant and natural materials. In this case, elegant also means resistant to rough handling. Nothing is worse than threadbare upholstery, scratched chairs or a worn floor. One recommendation would be to have comfortable armchairs suitable for reading. Where there is activity, robust wooden benches upholstered in some easy-to-care-for material would be more suitable.

Apart from the reception desk, the waiting area is the nerve centre of a doctor's practice. This is the place where a doctor's self-representation is expressed in the interior design and the decision is made whether the doctor gains the customer as a patient or loses him.

SOURCES

Becker, Dörte | Meuser, Philipp: Construction and Design Manual. Pharmacies. Berlin 2009.

Bergdolt, Klaus: Leib und Seele. Eine Kulturgeschichte des gesunden Lebens. Munich 1999.

Blech, Jörg: Der Leichenfabrikant. In: Der Spiegel 39 | 2002.

Damaschke, Sabine | Scheffer, Bernadette | Schossig, Elmar: Arztpraxen. Planungsgrundlagen und Architekturbeispiele. Leinfelden-Echterdingen 2003[2].

Feld, Michael: Es war einmal ... Der Arztberuf im Wandel. In: Deutsches Ärzteblatt 51.52 | 2003.

Fischer, Joachim | Meuser, Philipp: Construction and Design Manual. Accessible Architecture. Berlin 2009.

Itten, Johannes: Kunst der Farbe. Ravensburg 1961.

Kurow, Günther: Moderne Arztpraxis. Wege zu ihrer Rationalisierung. Berlin 1961.

Meuser, Philipp | Schirmer, Christoph: New Hospital Buildings in Germany. Berlin 2006.

Nickl-Weller, Christine [Ed.]: Health Care der Zukunft. Berlin 2007.

Thill, Klaus-Dieter: Marketing in der Arztpraxis. Cologne 2005.

Wolff, Reinhold: Rationelle Praxisorganisation. In: Beratungsservice für Ärzte. Vol. 2. Cologne 1998.

19 Joint dermatology practice in Hamburg-Reppenstedt, Architects: Seel Bobsin Partner

19

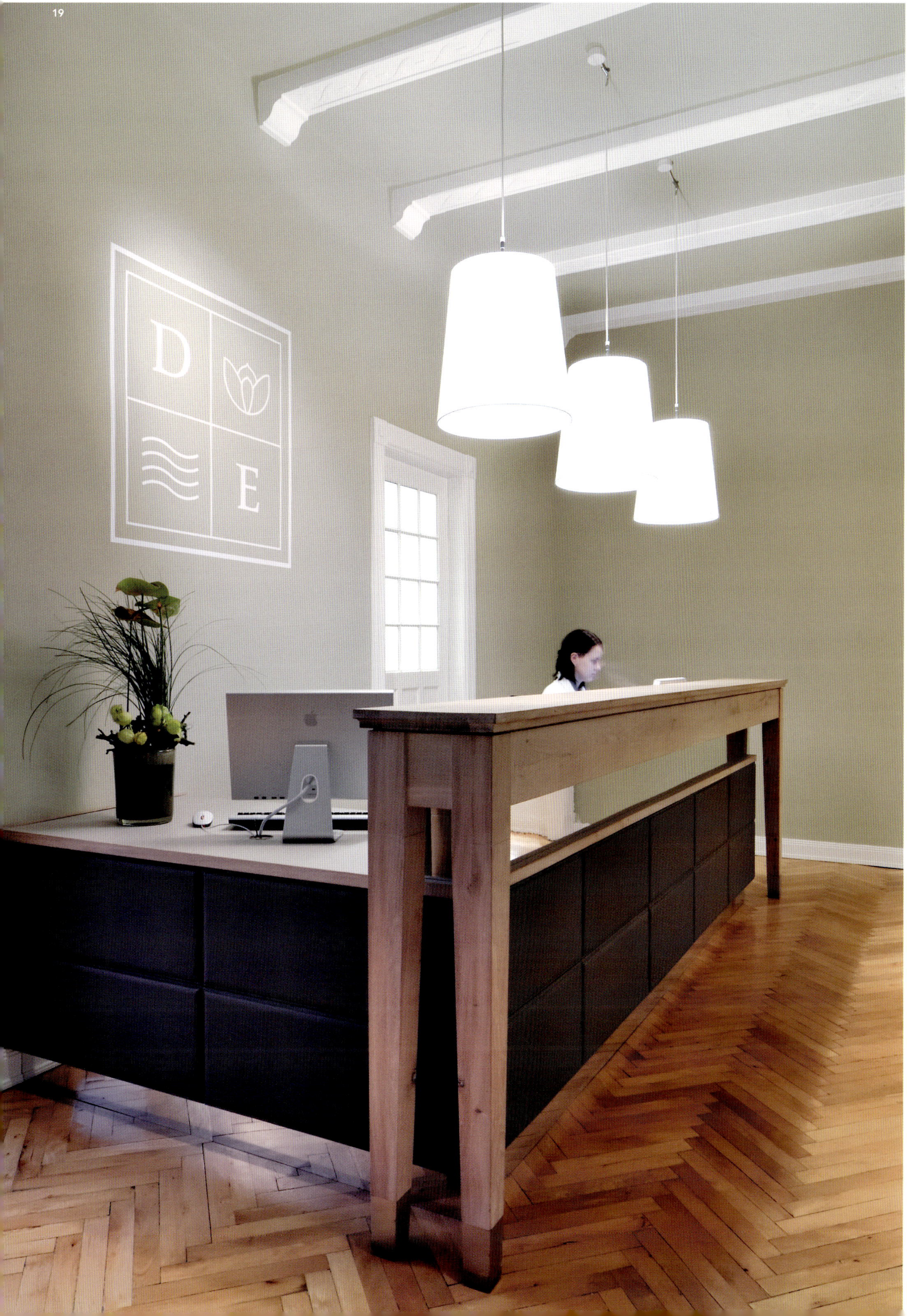

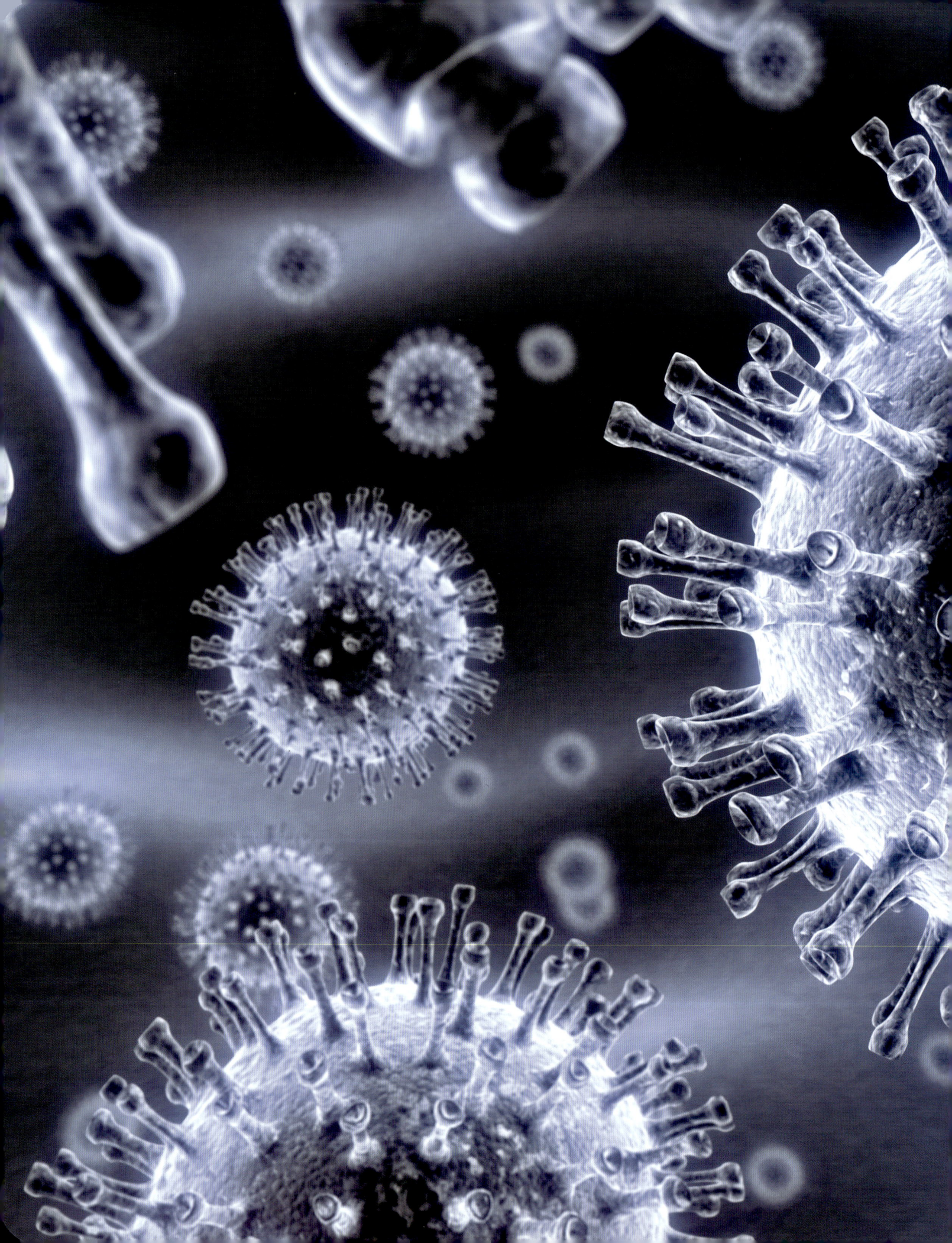

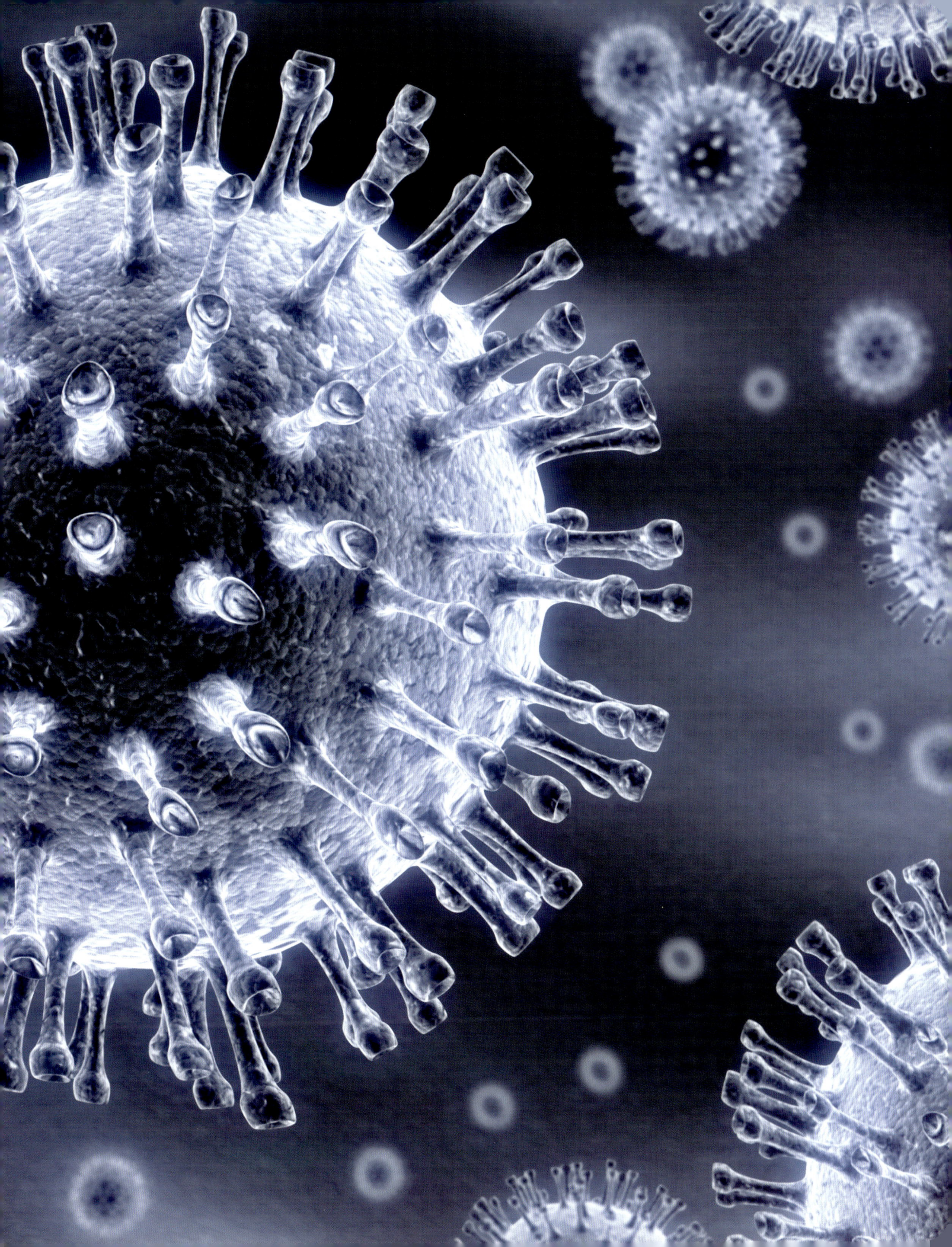

Anyone interested in planning medical practices or similar medical facilities must take a very broad view in order to grasp the extremely complex parameters and to draw the right conclusions so as to arrive at the best of all possible results.

UNDERLYING HEALTH CARE POLICY CONDITIONS

Medical care mandate

The German medical profession has a statutory care mandate. To meet this responsibility, there were, on 31 December 2008, 319,697 male and female doctors. Of these, 181,400 were involved in inpatient work and with authorities or corporations, and 138,300 worked in outpatient care. This last figure breaks down as follows: 119,800 doctors affiliated to a statutory health insurance scheme [including doctors in partnerships], 12,600 doctors and practice assistants in employment and 5,900 doctors in private practice. The figure for affiliated doctors is made up of 58,500 practitioners and 61,300 specialist doctors [Fig. 1][1].

In 2007, a total of 662,000 people were employed in German medical practices. Non-medical employees includes male and female medical assistants, nurses, medical technical staff, and employees in social and other professions; approximately 79 %[2] of the non-medical employees were women.

GENERAL PRACTITIONERS | Nowadays the first port of call for patients with medical problems is still the general practitioner. Between the GP and the patient there is normally a relationship of trust and consequently he often fulfils the role of a family doctor.

The general practitioner usually works on a self-employed basis [a registered doctor]; sometimes he is employed as a doctor. He is generally designated professionally as a doctor specialising in general medicine or also in internal medicine. In complex cases, he refers patients for diagnosis and treatment to an appropriately trained specialist physician.

General practitioners usually work in their own practice but if the patient is seriously ill, the doctor will visit him at home. A relatively recent innovation, there is also the concept of a "general practitioner in the hospital" who accompanies his patient, even in the clinic, as a sort of pilot. He will also provide care both before and after treatment, that is during the whole course of the illness.

SPECIALIST DOCTORS | If a doctor has decided to follow a particular branch of medicine, has completed several years of continuous training in his subject and has graduated with an appropriate specialist qualification, he may be known in Germany as a specialist [Fig. 2].

Qualification recognition is the prerogative of the Medical Councils or is subject to the medical profession laws of the German Länder and

FRANZ LABRYGA

PRINCIPLES OF PLANNING
MEDICAL PRACTICES

the continuous training codes of the different regional Medical Councils.

USE OF THE DOCTOR'S SERVICES | In Germany, many people need to consult their doctor relatively often: approximately 18 times per year. Compared with this, Norwegians only go to their doctor three times a year [3].

INTEGRATED CARE | It is useful, when planning facilities for outpatient care, to familiarise oneself with a new cross-sector care strategy, which has been developing for some time and which aims to foster improvements in the quality of patient care. It implies stronger links between general practitioners and specialists, hospitals and other institutions.

A variety of health care reforms has laid the foundations for this evolution. It involves reaching joint-working agreements which are intended to facilitate cooperation between various institutions in a newly emerging care scenario and to avoid unnecessary costs.

RESOURCE SPENDING | In the year 2006, over EUR 245 billion spent on health care in Germany [4]. Analysis of the various types of service shows that doctors accounted for the main expense. They examine and treat, they prescribe, they place orders and so essentially control the extent to which health care services are being used [Fig. 3]. Analysis of the health care expenditure

of the different institutions is also instructive. Such analysis clearly shows that the expenditure of the outpatient facilities – at approximately EUR 120 billion – is some EUR 30 billion higher than that of the inpatient and partly inpatient facilities [Fig. 4].

A good indicator of the value of health is expenditure. In 2008, it amounted to EUR 2,970, that is 10.6 % of GDP [gross domestic product]. In Europe, only France [11.0 %] and Switzerland [11.3 %] spend more, though the highest expenditure is in the United States [15.3 %].

International comparative studies, which include additional efficiency indicators, show that Germany is roughly in the middle.

RESULTS OF SURVEYS | The increasing significance of medical care is reflected in the growing number of scientific studies. They often supply important indicators on the efficacy of health care policy measures, reveal important connections and produce relevant data for decision-making. Some examples [see below] should make this clear:

A study by the Institute for Quality and Efficiency in Health care shows that a doctor in Germany currently spends an average of 7.8 minutes per patient; the equivalent figures for the UK are 11.1 minutes and for the USA 19 minutes. It is quite clear that simple conversations between patient and doctor are inadequately remunerated. Financially speaking it is only worth treating a

patient if equipment as costly as is technically possible is used for diagnostics and therapy.

According to the results of the Ernst & Young 2009 Health Barometer, 85 % of Germans give health care in their region a positive rating; 90 % of those questioned rated the medical care provided by general practitioners as "good or very good"; whereas specialist doctors scored 88 % and doctors in hospitals 84 %.

The results of the survey make it clear that patients like a "familiar face and individual care". In future, health care approval will tend to decline because of the increasing rise in costs. Patients do not want "high-tech medicine tailored to cost efficiency"[5].

Federal Medical Councils

At the head of the medical self-regulatory system in Germany is the Federal Medical Council acting as an umbrella organisation for the 17 German Medical Councils.

It takes an "active part in forming opinion on health care policy issues in society and develops perspectives for a health care and social policy that addresses the concerns of citizens and emphasises personal responsibility".[1]

The continued training code has direct consequences for the planning of medical practices because it defines the designations of specialist doctors, main areas of interest [specialisations within a specialised field] and additional designations. The head office of the Federal Medical Council is in Germany's capital Berlin.

Association of Statutory Health Insurance Physicians in Germany

The Federal Association of Statutory Health Insurance Physicians is the umbrella organisation which covers all such existing Associations [German acronym – KV] in each of the German Länder. Under § 75 [1] of the Social Code V6, it is the responsibility of this body to guarantee the medical care of insured persons by affiliated doctors.

Registered doctors and psychotherapists, employed doctors and authorised hospital doctors ensure the "right of patients to adequate, fit-for-purpose and economic care having due regard to the generally accepted state of medical knowledge."[7]

The Associations of Statutory Physicians rule on licences to practise and needs planning. If needs are already covered, a licence will only be granted if an existing practice is taken over.

Health insurance schemes

In Germany the cost of medical care is borne largely by two types of insurance schemes, as set out below:

STATUTORY HEALTH INSURANCE [SHI – GESETZLICHE KRANKENVERSICHERUNG – GKV] | This was launched by Bismarck. Today, approximately 87 % of all insured people belong to this scheme.[2] Social Code V limits the available scope of services to those that are "economic, adequate, necessary and fit-for-purpose". Following the solidarity principle, all those insured pay the same, irrespective of whether they are healthy or sick, young or old.

PRIVATE HEALTH INSURANCE [PHI – PRIVATE KRANKENVERSICHERUNG – PKV] | After the launch of SHI, private enterprises created PHI for those on higher incomes. A number of different companies provide these services. Approximately 13 % of insured persons belong to PHI schemes[2]. Each insured person is charged a separate amount under the cost reimbursement principle that reflects their age, sex, state of health and individual requirements.

The Institute for Quality and Efficiency in Health care

Like many of today's social developments, medical care also relies on the support and findings of scientific research. 2004 saw the foundation of the "technically independent, incorporated, scientific Institute for Quality and Efficiency in Health care" [Institut für Qualität und Wirtschaftlichkeit im Gesundheitswesen]. Its headquarters are in Cologne and it is enshrined in Social Code V. It operates under a mandate from the Federal Ministry of Health and the Joint Federal Committee.

Its main remit is to improve the quality of patient care. Other tasks are the evaluation of the cost-benefit ratio of drugs, assessment of guidelines for the treatment of important illnesses and provision of information on the efficiency and quality of health care services.

The institute sees itself as the advanced guard for evidence-based medicine [EBM] which aligns diagnosis and therapeutic measures with the current state of medical knowledge and where, in specific cases, the experience of the doctor is also taken into account[8].

The institute is fully funded by the public health care system. It is to be expected that the institute and its work make a considerable contribution to the most beneficial allocation of the rising costs of health care.

LAWS, REGULATIONS AND OTHER PROVISIONS

When planning medical practices it is useful to know the most important provisions governing this very complex area of work; such knowledge may actually lead to the development of facilities ideally suited to their functions.

Social Code

Social law in Germany is set out in the Social Code. So far the Code comprises twelve volumes the fifth of which deals with the organisation, mandatory insurance and services of the statutory health insurance schemes and their legal relations with

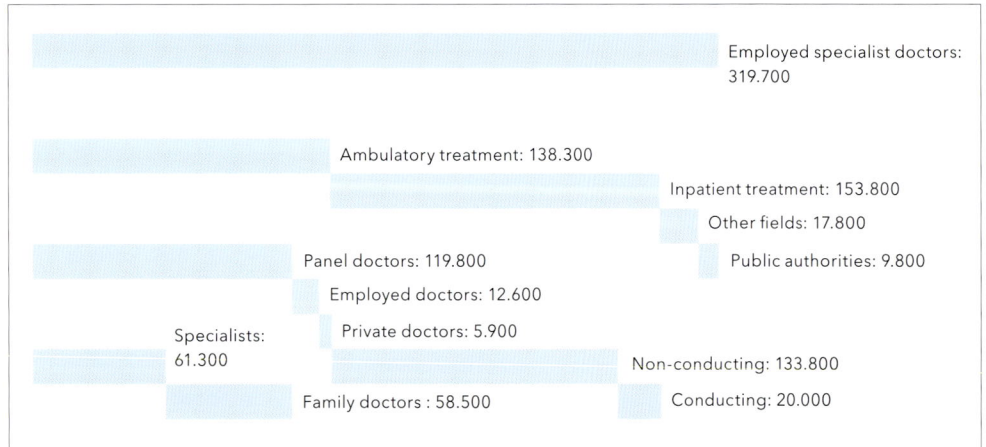

Employed specialist doctors: 319.700

Ambulatory treatment: 138.300

Inpatient treatment: 153.800

Other fields: 17.800

Panel doctors: 119.800

Public authorities: 9.800

Employed doctors: 12.600

Private doctors: 5.900

Specialists: 61.300

Non-conducting: 133.800

Family doctors : 58.500

Conducting: 20.000

doctors, dentists and pharmacists.[6] Outpatient care under the health insurance scheme is regulated in § 71 whereas § 77 lays down the main task of the Associations of Statutory Physicians as meeting the responsibilities assigned to them by Social Code volume V.

SHI [German – GKV] Modernisation Act

In 2003, reform of the German health care system was initiated by the Act on the Modernisation of Statutory Health Insurance[9]. Its main purpose is to reduce the contributions made to statutory health insurance . The following rules need mentioning:

– The provision of a general practitioner system as the first point of call for patients who are then referred to the relevant specialist doctors, should lead to better care.

– Subject to financial sanctions, a duty to undertake continued training will be incumbent on doctors.

– An independent institute will be created to evaluate the quality and economic efficiency of the treatment of certain illnesses.

– The ban by which pharmacists are prevented from owning more than one pharmacy will be lifted. In future, up to three branch pharmacies will be permitted in addition to the main pharmacy.

Affiliated Physicians Amendment Act

Since 2007 the effect of this Act has been to relax the conditions under which registered

doctors practise. This Act allows a doctor to network with other medical practices, medical care centres and even hospitals so that patients with particular diseases can be cared for jointly.[10] The Act is intended to cut out bottlenecks in outpatient care, especially in the former East Germany.

Hospital Funding Reform Act

The financial situation of hospitals has seriously deteriorated in recent years. The same is also true of the clinical medical practices under consideration here. The reason is the inexorable rise of staffing and equipment costs. This is further fuelled by the growing reluctance of the Länder to meet their statutory obligation, as enshrined in the Hospital Funding Act [German acronym – KHG][11], to fund hospital investment. This has led to a situation in which the supporting authorities have had to fund part of the necessary investments from the resources for patient care, a purpose for which they are not intended.

The Hospital Funding Reform Act[12] , passed by the Federal Parliament in the Spring of 2009, is supposed to improve the financial situation of hospitals. It seek to lay down a stable financial foundation giving hospitals a long-term financial perspective. The intention is to create a modern system of investment funding based on performance-related fixed sum investments for necessary building work. This will be in addition to investments for wage and salary increases.

Other provisions

Nowadays, standards are laid down for the delivery of quality in outpatient medicine. This means that medical practices are supervised and inspected like state authorities. The Association of Statutory Health Insurance Physicians has provided an overview of the statutory apparatus entitled "Supervision and Inspection of Medical Practices by Authorities"[13]. Other than that, the following acts, regulations and guidelines should be followed:

– Protection against Infection Act
  § 16 Action by responsibility authorities
  § 36 Maintenance of hygiene to prevent infection
– Medical Devices Act
  § 26 Carrying out supervision
– Medical Devices Operator Regulation
  § 6 Safety checks
– Medical Devices Safety Scheme Regulation
  § 3 Mandatory reporting
– Hazardous Substance Regulation
  §20 Official exceptions, orders and empowerments
– Biosubstance Regulation
  § 16 Notification of the authority
– Health and Safety at Work Act
  § 21 Responsible authorities; Co-operation with accident insurance funding bodies
– Youth Employment Protection Act
  § 51 Supervisory authority, inspection law and reporting obligations
–Maternity Protection Act
  § 20 Supervisory authority

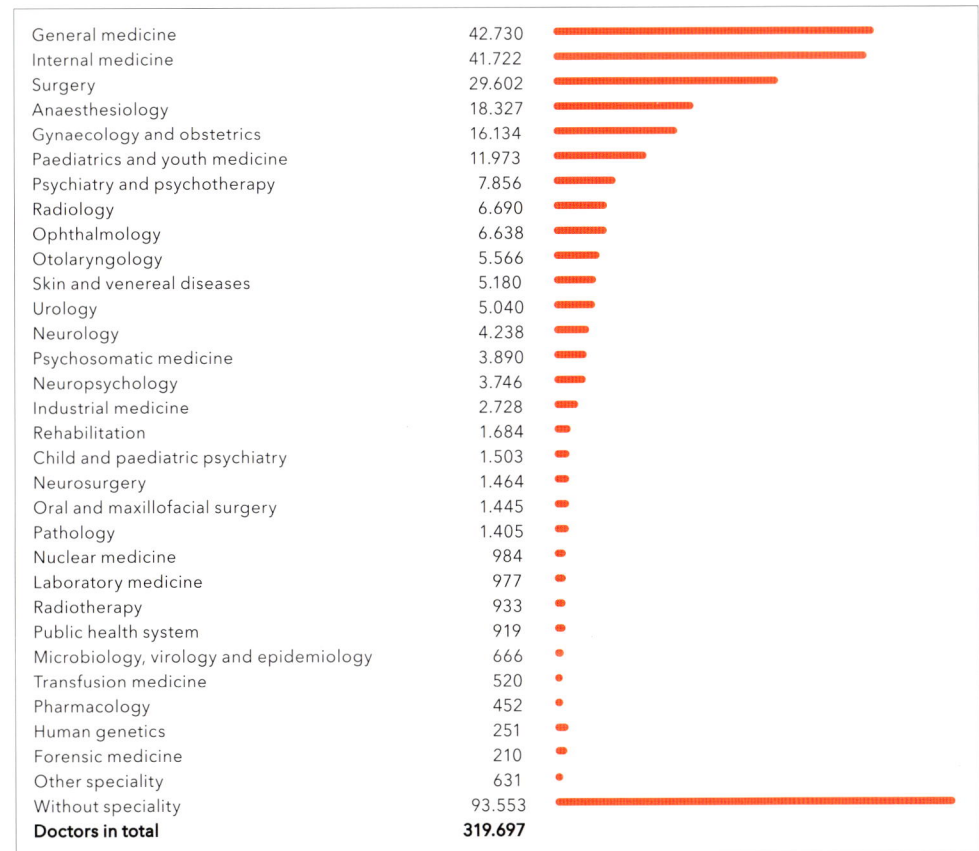

General medicine	42.730	
Internal medicine	41.722	
Surgery	29.602	
Anaesthesiology	18.327	
Gynaecology and obstetrics	16.134	
Paediatrics and youth medicine	11.973	
Psychiatry and psychotherapy	7.856	
Radiology	6.690	
Ophthalmology	6.638	
Otolaryngology	5.566	
Skin and venereal diseases	5.180	
Urology	5.040	
Neurology	4.238	
Psychosomatic medicine	3.890	
Neuropsychology	3.746	
Industrial medicine	2.728	
Rehabilitation	1.684	
Child and paediatric psychiatry	1.503	
Neurosurgery	1.464	
Oral and maxillofacial surgery	1.445	
Pathology	1.405	
Nuclear medicine	984	
Laboratory medicine	977	
Radiotherapy	933	
Public health system	919	
Microbiology, virology and epidemiology	666	
Transfusion medicine	520	
Pharmacology	452	
Human genetics	251	
Forensic medicine	210	
Other speciality	631	
Without speciality	93.553	
Doctors in total	**319.697**	

- X-ray Regulation
  § 17 Quality assurance in different medical and dental facilities
- Health care Services Act
  § 11 Supervision of health care facilities
- Radiation Protection Regulation
- Provisions of the Occupational Health and Safety Association
- Recommendations of the Commission for Hospital Hygiene and Infection Prevention
- DIN provisions, for example DIN EN 554, DIN EN 285 and DIN EN 13060.

TYPES OF MEDICAL PRACTICES

Over the past ten years, developments in health care policy, in medicine and in the labour market have led to medical activities being carried out in a variety of forms.

Doctors have adapted their practices to new demands by increasing the size of their usable floor space. Some doctors practising independently have decided to run their practices together with one or more other colleagues.

Financial imperatives and the standards set by the state have resulted in practices with quite different characters. The underlying conditions in which doctors work are subject to constant and increasing changes and this has resulted in numerous different types of specialist doctor practices and special forms.

Subdivision according to size
[taking single-doctor practices as an example]

In order to bring a little order into what may seem a rather confused picture and gain an initial overview, it would seem helpful to subdivide medical practices according to the size of their usable floor space. The subdivisions adopted below for small, medium and large single-doctor practices are taken from the properties showcased in this book.

Subdivision into three sizes gives us the opportunity to develop standard functional and spatial allocation plans suitable for the description and illustration of examples and allows comparisons within the different size groups.

SMALL SINGLE-DOCTOR PRACTICE | Small medical practices have a usable floor space of up to 125 square metres. Medical work should not be carried out in premises which are too small or have too few rooms. From 100 square metres upwards, they contain the rooms necessary for efficient operation; the surface area should be no smaller than this.

MEDIUM-SIZED SINGLE-DOCTOR PRACTICE | Medium-sized single-doctor practices always have a usable floor space of between 126 square metres and 174 square metres. They are furnished and fitted out and will have the necessary rooms at the required size.

LARGE SINGLE-DOCTOR PRACTICE | Over 176 square metres, large single-doctor practices are regarded as being generously equipped practices with adequate usable floor spaces.

Subdivision into specialist areas

The original single-doctor practice was the province of the general practitioner who served and helped patients from his catchment area with all their health and hospital problems.

Subsequent developments in medicine have led to continued training for doctors who have specialised in certain medical areas.

GENERAL PRACTITIONER PRACTICE | The general practitioner fulfils an essential task, providing basic care for people especially in thinly populated and rural areas. He normally works in the fields of general or internal medicine and may also have a recognised specialist qualification.

SPECIALIST DOCTOR PRACTICE | The regional Medical Councils are responsible for the definition and remits of the specialist areas and their demarcation from each other. The register of the Federal Continuous Training Code of the Federal Medical Councils [as amended on 23 March 2008] provides the basis for the planning of specialist doctor practices[14]. It provides recommendations for the regional Medical Councils. No distinction is drawn in this register between areas and specialist doctor competences – both allow a specialist doctor practice

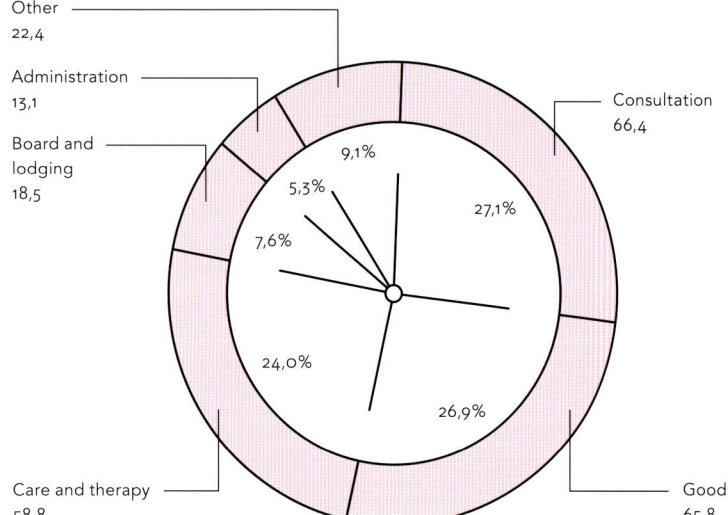

Other
22,4

Administration
13,1

Board and
lodging
18,5

Care and therapy
58,8

Consultation
66,4

9,1%

5,3%

7,6%

27,1%

24,0%

26,9%

Goods
65,8

3 Health care expenditure of the different services in Germany, 2006
(in total EUR 245 billion Euro)

to be set up the following disciplines:
- Anaesthesiology
- Anatomy
- Occupational medicine
- Ophthalmology
- Biochemistry
- General surgery
- Vascular surgery
- Cardiac surgery
- Paediatric surgery
- Orthopaedics and accident surgery
- Plastic and cosmetic surgery
- Thoracic surgery
- Internal surgery
- Gynaecology and obstetrics
- Ear, nose and throat medicine
- Speech and childhood hearing impairments
- Skin and sexual diseases
- Human genetics
- Hygiene and environmental medicine
- Internal and general medicine
- Internal medicine
- Internal medicine and angiology
- Internal medicine and endocrinology and diabetes
- Internal medicine and gastroenterology
- Internal medicine and haematology and oncology
- Internal medicine and cardiology
- Internal medicine and nephrology
- Internal medicine and pneumology
- Internal medicine and rheumatology

- Paediatric and adolescent medicine
- Paediatric and adolescent psychiatry and psychotherapy
- Laboratory medicine
- Microbiology, virology and infectious disease epidemiology
- Maxillofacial surgery
- Neurosurgery
- Neurology
- Neuropathology
- Nuclear medicine
- Public health care
- Pathology
- Pharmacology
- Pharmacology and toxicology
- Physical and rehabilitation medicine
- Physiology
- Psychiatry and psychotherapy
- Psychosomatic medicine and psychotherapy
- Radiology
- Forensic medicine
- Radiotherapy
- Transfusion medicine
- Urology.

In addition to the specialist medical areas, the Continuous Training Code currently includes a further 46 extra training options, among which are for example: acupuncture, allergology, diabetes, geriatrics, homoeopathy, intensive care, laboratory diagnostics, natural healing methods, emergency medicine, palliative care,

physiotherapy and also balneology, sports medicine and tropical medicine.

Subdivision according to number of practices

As well as the option of enlarging a single-doctor practice by adding more usable floor space, a further option, and one taken with increasing frequency today, especially for financial reasons, is to expand by adding on further medical practices.

TWO-DOCTOR PRACTICE | The two doctors in a two-doctor practice have the choice of working as a professional team [also joint practice or partnership] in the same specialist field or, deliberately, in two different fields.

Working in the same specialist field has the particular advantage that each can stand in for the other when one is taking continuous training or is on holiday or sick and, of course, if one is pregnant or is on maternity | paternity leave. Working in the same specialist field allows the highest possible degree of synergy because the doctors will use the same staff, the same rooms and equipment. However, offering different specialist fields is of particular benefit to patients because this expands the range of available services and may allow for further specialist treatment in the same practice. Specialists in two different fields working together broaden the range of diagnostic and treatment options. The use of staff, the same rooms and appliances by two professionals make a two-doctor practice more cost-effective.

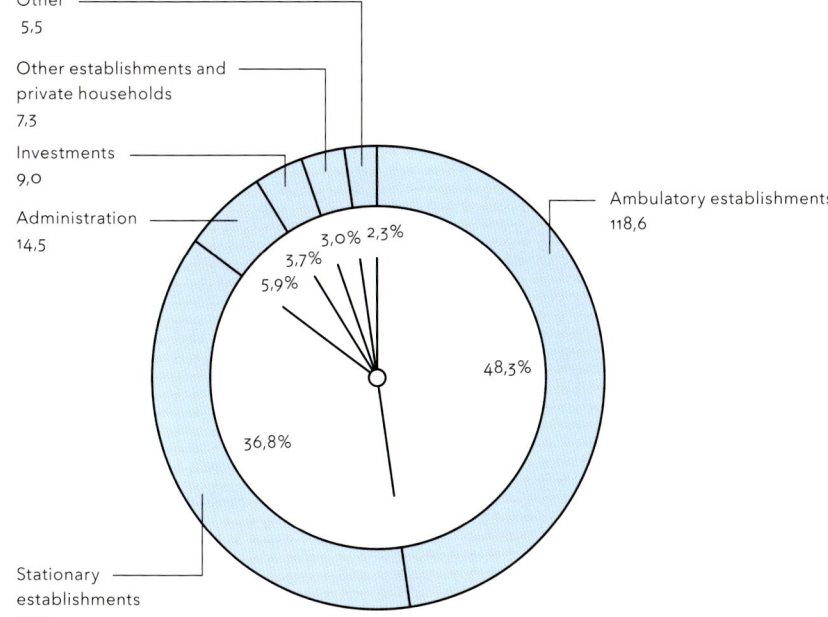

Other
5,5

Other establishments and private households
7,3

Investments
9,0

Administration
14,5

Ambulatory establishments
118,6

3,0% 2,3%
3,7%
5,9%
48,3%
36,8%

Stationary establishments
90,1

4 Health care expenditure of the different institutions in Germany, 2006
(in total EUR 245 billion Euro)

MULTI-DOCTOR PRACTICE | The advantages cited above of a two-doctor practice are increased if there are more than two specialist doctors. So far there is no discernible upper limit on the number of doctors that can work together. Combinations of up to approximately 40 medical practices working together deliver a perfectly efficient patient care service.

Subdivision into business models

Naturally, commercial aspects play a major role in the running of medical practices. This is especially true of patient accounting systems and the sharing out of the income from the facilities.

JOINT PRACTICE | In a business described as a joint practice with two or more specialist doctor practices, the principle is that they should be regarded as a single commercial entity. This co-operation model is a commercial and organisational merger to enable the joint practice of a profession. The Federal Medical Council's latest term for this is "professional community".

PRACTICE COMMUNITY | A practice community uses the same rooms, yet the practices remain independent of each other from a legal point of view – so there is no joint accounting system.

APPLIANCE SHARING SCHEME | In an appliance sharing scheme, a special way of sharing the use of expensive medical appliances; the actual use of the appliances is paid for under a jointly agreed accounting system.

MEDICAL CENTRE | One could take as the model here antique shops grouped together in the same street and offering customers as broad a range of items for sale as possible without any individual shop feeling threatened by competition from the others. A medical centre is similar, generally with doctors specialising in different fields, often situated in a multi-storey building. The doctors advertise their presence with an attractive sign that makes a deeper impression on patients than it would if they practised alone. Frequently, they are able to assist each other and there may be the joint use of ancillary facilities, for example a health-oriented café. A pharmacist and other health care facilities are glad to have premises there, too, either in the medical centre itself or nearby.

OUTPATIENTS CLINIC | The concept of cross-disciplinary practices in which to some extent the use of staff, rooms and medical equipment is shared, is not an invention of the former German Democratic Republic, but was rather the way in which most outpatient care was organised. Patients attending outpatient clinics can be referred to other practices in the same building and can continue to be treated there without having to travel long distances and with little loss of time. However, because of their size, outpatients clinics are only financially viable in central locations so that, in fact, many patients do have to travel very long distances. A further disadvantage occurs when employed doctors are not sufficiently involved in the clinic's turnover. After German reunification, doctors remained in the old buildings. Single-doctor practices emerged that regrouped under the roof of a medical centre.

Today, there are still outpatients clinics in most of the former socialist states, though there are some in Sweden, too. In South Africa, there are even mobile outpatients clinics.

MULTI-DOCTOR PRACTICE WITH CLINIC | As distinct from the multi-doctor practice already described, in which there is only outpatient care, in this sort of practice complemented by a clinic, patients can also be cared for after invasive inpatient treatment. This primarily applies to practices that perform operations.

An inpatient stay lasts in general from one to three days. The functional and spatial allocation plan usually required for inpatient care does not apply here. All that is needed are wards [with two beds or preferably one bed and a bathroom] and the side rooms for care-related purposes. The essential feature is the assured delivery of care, even at night. If a longer inpatient stay is needed, the patient ought to be moved to the inpatient department of a hospital.

The type of joint practice described here with its similarities to a clinic is often designated as a practice clinic. However, the term is sometimes used for practices that can only provide patients with a room and couch on which to lie down for a few hours post-operatively.

HOSPITAL OUTPATIENTS DEPARTMENT | In years gone by, the Germany health care industry made a sharp distinction between outpatient and in-patient care. The care of outpatients lies in the hands of the registered doctors and inpatient care was the province of the hospital. Only hospitals with a teaching remit were allowed to provide care for outpatients as well because that was the only way of ensuring that medical students received a broad enough training. In these institutions the term outpatient clinic is still in use today.

As a consequence of the developments set out above, hospitals generally have a "medical service" which is in charge of examining and treating hospital patients.

The lifting of the distinction described above means that the "medical service" can also treat outpatients in hospitals. German hospital outpatient departments can now also be run in direct co-operation with registered doctors.

MEDICAL CARE CENTRE | On January 2004, the Statutory Health Insurance Modernisation Act came into force. This Act licensed medical care centres to provide care by affiliated doctors for patients insured under the statutory and private health insurance schemes. A medical care centre [MCC, German acronym – MVZ] is a cross-disciplinary facility run by a doctor and in which doctors work either as owners or employees. A MCC can be set up by pharmacists, preventive medicine and rehabilitation organisations and hospitals, not only by doctors and psychotherapists, provided they are involved in the medical care of insured patients by virtue of a licence, authority or contract.

For patients, it is important to be aware that they are not entitled to personal treatment by one of the doctors in the MCC.

HEALTH CENTRE | The breakdown of the rigid distinction between outpatient and inpatient examinations and treatment has lent wings to the imagination of service providers and led to the creation of an institution called the health centre. This can deliver all the health care services for the population – almost without limitation.

In the health centre, a full, networked health care service is available for statutory health scheme and private patients. The integration in an electronic network of the medical staff can prevent long waiting times, save unnecessary duplicated examinations and enable doctors to discuss treatment methods and the prescription of drugs. There is practically no limit to the ways in which different health care institutions can co-operate and provide "integrated care". Many patients wish to have all health facilities grouped together in one place. As examples of how to satisfy this requirement, health information desks, sports medicine facilities, a pharmacy or a health care product sales outlet can be added as extra features.

SPECIAL FACILITIES FOR THE PROVISION OF MEDICAL CARE | Quite apart from the medical care facilities and institutions discussed above, there are numerous other special medical service provisions, for example:
– Obstetric clinic
– Rehabilitation centre
– Day clinic
– Drug outpatients department
– Geriatric centre – Hospice.

OPERATIONAL DATA

Before planning ideas for the rigid of outpatient care can be implemented, it is essential to discuss how the institution is to be run. This requires a vision or a corporate strategy – architects speak of business objective planning. This will form the basis for subsequent concept planning and conversion into the actual building. [See below for illustrations of important operational aspects relevant for the planning of medical practices.]

Business objectives
In their definitive book "Unternehmen Arztpraxis"[15], Schurr, Kunhardt and Dumont present a detailed

analysis of many of the business aspects of a medical practice concept that need to be addressed:

Once the individual objectives have been worked out, a business process management scheme needs to be developed, which will enable the individual objectives to be measured. This makes it possible to evaluate and compare alternatives, the result of which will be informed decisions.

Catchment area

The population profile of the catchment area and the type of patients have an importance for the commercial development of the practice which cannot be overstated. Successful medical practices take account of such data and use them to tailor their publicity strategy.

The size of the catchment area supplying the majority of the patients is a good indicator of the prominence and importance of a medical practice. Quite a number of medical practices have an extensive catchment area because their location, for example within a rural area, is relatively sparsely populated.

If patients have to travel long distances to the medical practice, either on foot, by public transport or by car, the doctors need to think about what welcoming facilities they can offer them. Things to consider are places to rest, especially for old and handicapped patients, and refreshments, for instance a mineral water dispenser.

Location

The criteria that apply to the choice of a good home also apply to medical practices. The first three main criteria are location, location and location. For this reason, it is of paramount importance to make a thorough analysis of the location before drawing up customised plans in order to discover the most appropriate place for the future medical practice. The following criteria can be helpful:
– places with a high number of passers-by, perhaps in main thoroughfares, pedestrian zones or in buildings where the passers-by are constantly changing, such as department stores or shopping centres, railways stations and airports;
– places in or near other health care facilities. The best places are hospitals, health businesses or centres, gym and physiotherapy practices, care support points and podiatry practices, cosmetic studios and wellness centres.

The following are not helpful:
– locations too close to existing medical practices, unless patient numbers make this competition acceptable and unless this competitive situation turns out to be advantageous;
– locations not easily accessible by the local transport. In general, locations further than 200 metres from a public transport stop are not acceptable.

General and specialist doctor' services
Volume V of the Social Code contains a breakdown of medical services. The main groups are the following:
– Services to prevent illness and exacerbation of existing illness
– Services to aid the early detection of illness
– Services for the treatment of illness
– Services for medical rehabilitation.

The services are delivered by general practitioners and specialist doctors. The above breakdown does not take into account the location in which services are delivered. Following the lifting of the former strict demarcations between outpatient and inpatient care, all medical services can in principle be delivered anywhere. This applies, for example, even to operations and the technically expensive services of nuclear medicine. Increasingly, there are doctors who provide their services both in medical practices and in facilities intended mainly for inpatient care.

Special doctors' services
In Germany, the financial situation of registered doctors has become significantly harsher and this has forced them to keep their range of service under constant review and to expand it. Imagination and creativity have led to the creation of numerous new services to help enhance the appeal of the practice concerned. There are many fields in which medical practices have become decidedly proactive:

EXPANSION OF THE RANGE OF SERVICES |
– Following continuous training opportunities in fields which have a strong appeal for patients, for example acupuncture, natural healing methods, allergology, diabetology, geriatrics, sleep medicine and sports medicine.
– Provision of individual health care services. Consideration needs to be given to the sorts of patients willing, in the future, to pay for such services out of their own pockets.
– Stronger networking with company doctors.

EXERCISE OF HEALTH CARE TASKS |
– Information and education campaigns
– Prophylactic measures
– Early detection of illness.

EXPANSION OF SERVICES |
– Information by email
– Supply of medication to patients' homes
– Collection of cost estimates from hospitals
– Acceptance of orders by telephone, fax and email
– Organisation of self-help groups
– Setting up health-oriented cafés

RUNNING COURSES AND SEMINARS |
– Courses on healthy eating
– Lectures on particular disease profiles, for example diabetes
– Readings on subjects around health promotion
– Seminars on dietetics and healthy eating
– Provision of informative brochures.
The planner ought to be aware of the type and scope of any special services since these activities have consequences for the type and number of rooms and their use.

Operational organisation:
TREATMENT AREAS | The treatment areas laid down in the medical practice's objectives need to be kept under constant review because they can vary with the changing health care policy standards. Schurr, Kunhardt and Dumont have collected the factors which determine the treatment areas[15]:
– Training conditions
– Previous and planned medical concept
– Patient demand
– Competing services in the region
– Fixtures and fittings in the practice
– Legal situation
– Financial situation of the medical practice and practice owner

- Cooperation opportunities or co-operation necessities
- Medical innovations

TREATMENT PATHWAYS | The subject of the development and application of treatment pathways, which are also termed guidelines or standards, is increasingly the object of intense debate at specialist medical congresses. The call for evidence-based medicine [EBM], which is to be as internationally valid as possible, is intensifying, even in relation to quality assurance for medical services, nowadays universally regarded as essential.

Treatment pathways have the following important characteristics:
- Description of the objective of a treatment
- References to other treatment pathways or sources of EBM
- Aids for decision-making
- Instructions for doctors' conduct
- Support of the process-oriented programme
- Overview of the required personnel and physical resources
- Information source for all patients.

After application of the treatment pathway, maintaining a detailed record should help keep the individual elements of the pathway developing.

QUALITY ASSURANCE | Improvement and assurance of the quality of the medical activities is one of the key roles of patient-driven, need-driven and commercial care. Transparency about the quality of treatment results and a good degree of quality in patient care are the main goals of quality assurance.

The Social Code [§ 135a and § 137][6] is the legal basis for quality assurance. Numerous institutions work in the field of quality assurance, for example the Medical Councils, the Associations of Statutory Physicians, the Joint Federal Committee, the Institute for Quality and Efficiency in Health care, the hospital companies and the medical service providers of the health insurance schemes.

QUALITY MANAGEMENT | The standard of quality necessary in medical care institutions is achieved through a range of measures. These include optimum work process design, improvement of communication structures, increased patient and staff satisfaction, measures to raise patient safety, development of joint care formats and quality indicators, and the setting up of quality control systems as well as the fitting out and design of work rooms so as to be fit for purpose.

All activities, which are grouped together under the general heading of "Quality Management" [QM], nowadays form a part of business management. Continuous medical training is one of the core tasks. For example, Medical Council seminars promulgate the principles of QM. For outpatient care, the Medical Centre for Quality in Medicine published the QMA Compendium. Its third edition appeared in 2008.[16]

Among the features it contains are quality management benchmarks for practice, quality criteria and quality indicators, a perspective for the future of quality management in outpatient medical care and, finally, a patient questionnaire [equally useful for architects] for assessment of outpatient care.

USE OF STAFF | The success of a practice depends entirely on the professional expertise of the staff. This is why special attention should be given to staff selection. Staff management is no minor matter. Here, the practice's management has to decide between authoritarian, laissez-faire and democratic management styles.[15] Finally, there needs to be a good working atmosphere in the practice that gives every member of staff the feeling of being safe, accepted and having room to develop.

The type and especially the number of staff members are determining factors which relate to the size of the work space, staff rest room and changing room areas.

USE OF EDP | It is no longer possible to run a medical practice efficiently without using any computers. In any case, before suitable hardware and software are selected, professional advice should be taken if at all possible. Once the choices are made, they will have a major influence on the quality of all work activities, that means for example, appointment management, accounting, documentation, quality assurance, communication and market research.[15]

Problems arise when different software systems need to work together and when data are exchanged between different integrated care locations. According to estimates, 70 % of all transactions are still in paper form.[15] The paperless medical practice simplifies data processing, but special care must be paid to data protection and data security. A 30-year retention period is recommended for treatment data, so thought must be given to finding suitable storage locations.

The Statutory Health Insurance Modernisation Act has created a new requirement in connection with the launch of the electronic health record card; it is intended to contribute transparency and quality in treatment and to improve efficiency. Here, the patient can decide which of his data is to be stored.

WASTE DISPOSAL | The Federal Ministry for the Environment has issued strict rules for disposal. Waste generated in medical practices is generally collected at regular intervals by waste disposal companies. Special attention must be paid to hazardous substances, including drugs and organic and inorganic chemicals and anaesthetics that can no longer be used. Disposal of these is governed by the Narcotics Act. A special regulation governs out-of-date drugs.

Practice logo

A carefully selected logo accurately reflecting the spirit and philosophy of the medical practice can make a definite contribution to the success of the business. A good logo must meet five requirements; it must be:[15]
– Easily recognisable
– Easily understood
– Unmistakable
– Memorable
– Reproducible.
The logo should not be limited to the symbol itself – in other words, it is helpful to repeat the colour and forms in the design of printed matter, whether it is notepaper, receipts, brochures or notices. The logo is rendered particularly memorable if its colours and forms are used in the design of the practice's rooms.

Operating costs

Finally, all the thinking about operational matters that has gone into the organisation of a patient-friendly and dynamic medical practice ultimately has the aim of keeping operating costs within economically acceptable limits.

STAFFING COSTS | These can account for up to two thirds of the overheads. This is why careful thought should be devoted to using staff efficiently. Efficient staffing ratios are dependent on having streamlined the medical practice's essential work processes as rationally as possible.

MATERIALS COSTS | These are composed mainly of funding costs, depreciation, publicity costs, vehicle and travel costs, office and administration costs, insurance, rents and utilities costs. A good operating result is dependent on cutting out any wastage in these areas.

Supervision of medical practices by the authorities

A variety of laws and regulations lays down measures to ensure that quality standards for medical care are met. Examples of these are the Protection against Infection Act, the recommendations of the Robert Koch Institute Commission for Hospital Hygiene and the Prevention of Infection, the Medical Devices Act, the Health and Safety at Work Act and the provisions of the Occupational Health and Safety Association. Different institutions are tasked with supervisory roles, especially the health care offices as bodies within the public health care service. They conduct inspections with or without prior notice. If deficiencies are detected, fines are normally imposed immediately, though in particularly serious instances, restrictions may be imposed on the practice's activities or the practice may even be closed. In 2005, the Association of Statutory Health Insurance Physicians published a special paper entitled "Supervision and Inspection of Medical Practices by Authorities"[15]. Among the reports included are accounts of the numerous statutory bases and methods for inspecting medical practices subject to the procedures of Joint Self-Government. The publication's appendices contain helpful examples of checklists for medical practice inspections.

CONSTRUCTION DATA

Once the details of the practice's proposed operations have been worked out, construction data can be calculated and collated. Both data packages form the basis for further action and decisions on the design and form of a medical practice.

Town-planning conditions

SITE | If a new building is planned, points to consider when choosing the site include the size and any existing conditions impinging on development potential as well as cost per square metres. A far-sighted property developer will seek to acquire a site large enough to allow extensions later so that the practice can grow if necessary.

TRANSPORTATION LINKS | Good transportation links are very important for a medical practice if it is to thrive. This is particularly true of customers who come on foot and also for those using public transport who need the nearest stop to be close.

MONUMENT PROTECTION | A medical practice subject to a protection order because it is an old building of outstanding architectural merit is something to be treasured by both the owner and his clients, which is why people like going to such buildings. The authorities generally impose strict conditions on such buildings making it very difficult to make alterations with the result that the practice frequently has to accept a degree of functional inconvenience.

Measures intended to maintain the substance of the building can also be very expensive. Sometimes, consolation comes in the form of financial support from public funds and occasionally even from sponsors keen to maintain the historical heritage.

Usable floor space

Apart from the area accessible to vehicles, the floor area and technical function area, the usable floor space is the most important type of area defined in DIN 27717 for the subdivision of the total floor area of a building. Unlike the other three types of areas, the usable floor space provides information on the particular remit of the project. This is the most important parameter of a ground plan for medical practices.

Since size is one of the key distinguishing features of medical practices, the usable floor spaces are used to differentiate between them. Evaluation of the usable floor spaces of the examples cited in this book and analysis of the existing developmental trends lead to the following main classifications for medical practices:

SINGLE-DOCTOR PRACTICES |
– Small single-doctor practices:
 usable floor space of up to 125 sqm
– Medium-sized single-doctor practices: usable floor space of between 126 sqm and 175 sqm
– Large single-doctor practices:
 usable floor space over 175 sqm

MULTI-DOCTOR PRACTICES |
– Small multi-doctor practices:
 usable floor space of up to 200 sqm
– Medium-sized multi-doctor practices: usable floor space of between 201 sqm and 400 sqm
– Large multi-doctor practices:
 usable floor space over 400 sqm

Functional and spatial allocation plans

The functional and spatial allocation plans define the usable floor space. Other areas only become apparent at the design phase. Details of rooms are given in terms of number, type and size in square metres. The light exposure required by the rooms should be stated, using the following symbols:
O   Natural daylight necessary
◉   Natural daylight desirable
●   Natural daylight unnecessary

DIN 13080 "Division of Hospitals into Functional Areas and Functional Sections"[18], a standard which has been applied successfully for over 20 years in hospital planning both in Germany and beyond its borders, contains a recommendation for the subdivisions of functional and spatial allocation plans. According to the above standard, the rooms should be subdivided into four groups:
– Main rooms
– Ancillary rooms

– Communication rooms
– Staff rooms.

It is left to the discretion of the function and space planner whether to subdivide the spaces according to his functional and spatial allocation plan or to choose the mode of subdivision in terms of function groups described in the following section; the latter makes it possible to have major differences between the rooms. For this reason, this book will focus on function groups.

Subdivision into function groups

A variety of different types of rooms can be incorporated into the plans for a medical practice. To reduce the large number of different rooms, some with similar purposes have been grouped under a single heading.

It has proved useful for planning purposes to assign the approximately 80 different types of rooms left over after nomenclature standardisation to particular room units.

Because, unlike in hospitals, the room units in medical practices are relatively small, the classificatory term "function group" is used here. As in DIN 1308018 , colours are used additionally. These make it considerably easier both to grasp the organisation of the ground plan and to analyse and compare plans. Not every medical practice will use the eight function groups illustrated briefly below. However, they are representative, depending on the type and size of the practice and its service profile.

PATIENT ROOMS | Every medical practice works primarily for the benefit of its patients. Accordingly, all the rooms and equipment should be planned with this in mind. Bearing in mind the need to have rooms with different functions, rooms can be reserved primarily for the use of patients – for example, a reception room, waiting room with a children's play corner, consultation room, changing cubicles, patient transfer hatchway, recovery room and sickroom. Special attention should be given to these patient rooms at design stage. This is the point where sensitive patients pick up on how they are valued by the practice. In the ground plans the patient room function group is marked in yellow.

EXAMINATION AND TREATMENT ROOMS | The rooms in which the basic medical services are carried out constitute the "production area" of the business. These are the rooms used for doctor-patient consultations, for taking patient histories, initial examinations and blood samples: the general examination and treatment rooms, even those that double as consultation rooms, individual examination rooms, individual treatment rooms and the necessary laboratory rooms with different specialised uses, for example, as a urine lab or a lab analysing blood samples. This function group is marked below in red.

SPECIALIST MEDICAL ROOMS | The "production areas" of a medical practice also consist of the rooms destined for specialist examinations and treatments. They comprise their own function group, which is the one with the most variety because the rooms are of such different types. They are not so different in size – there is a much greater difference in the way they are equipped.

There are approximately 70 specialist fields catered for in the Continuous Training Codes across the Länder and this is reflected in the number and type of specialist examination and treatment rooms. Also, most specialist fields require extra rooms specific to their field. This function group is coloured pink.

ADMINISTRATION ROOMS | This relatively small function group covers the rooms required for the administration of the medical practice. Key features are an office or even several offices, designed to fulfil different administrative roles, an administration department or, in large medical practices, several such offices for the different specialist fields. Administration rooms are shown in the ground plans in green.

SERVICE AND STAFF ROOMS | Service, recovery, changing and sanitary areas intended for the staff constitute their own function group. It is useful to locate the rooms together in a quiet section of the practice.

In a medical practice that attaches importance to social compact issues, these rooms will be given the necessary special attention. Provision of recovery and rest rooms and table tennis rooms will definitely remain the exception. Some larger practices will have service rooms for particular groups of staff. These rooms are marked in orange.

SUPPLY AND DISPOSAL ROOMS | The rooms required to meet the supply and disposal needs of medical practices include primarily the sterile and unsterile work rooms, stores and equipment rooms, a cleaner's room and a disposal room. The supply and waste disposal rooms are coloured brown.

TRAINING AND TEACHING ROOMS | Rarely, rooms are provided for various staff and patient training options. These will be lecture, teaching and seminar rooms, which may also be multi-purpose rooms which can be reserved for future developments. These rooms are marked in violet.

TECHNICAL SERVICE ROOMS | The blue marking in the ground plans identifies the rooms for technical equipment, such as, for example, the control rooms for X-ray, CT and MRI scanning equipment, EDP rooms, development rooms, rooms to house heating and air-conditioning plant and mechanical service rooms.

Important individual rooms

Of the approximately 80 standard rooms in a medical practice, some are largely destined to everyday purposes. These are the rooms in the administration, service and social room function groups, some of the supply and disposal rooms and the training and teaching rooms. Some indications of special types will suffice.

Some of the individual rooms typical of medical practices need to be looked at in closer detail here. The order in which the rooms are presented follows the sequence of function groups described in the previous section. In general it is true that these rooms do not necessarily have to be usable floor spaces completely enclosed by walls; they are often open or half open areas to create an overall impression of the greatest transparency.

RECEPTION ROOM | Just as a well designed business card gives an indication of the nature of the owner, the reception area also conveys an initial impression of the whole medical practice. Natural daylight immediately by the entrance is highly desirable. Here there should at least be some preferably daylight exposure to create a soothing ambiance, a generous subdivision of the space, suitable, well designed furniture and, most important, an understanding, friendly person who listens to requests patiently, gives accurate information and can accompany the patient into the waiting room.

WAITING ROOM | It would be best for patients if the practice could manage without a waiting room. Unfortunately, however, even the best organisations have been unable to arrange for patients' appointments to be kept so promptly that waiting times and therefore a waiting room prove unnecessary. Crowded waiting rooms are not generally a sign of a well run appointment system.

The following factors should be taken into account as regards the size of the waiting room: the number of doctors, the practice's hours of business, the average duration of treatments, the type of appointment system and average number of patients without appointments and emergency cases. The last group can ruin any scheduling system, no matter how precise. In any case, care should be taken that the number of waiting patients per doctor never exceeds five, otherwise, as patients arrive, they get the feeling of being part of a mass production system. This is why large practices have discovered the benefit of having a second waiting room which, ideally, should be in the immediate vicinity of the reception desk. This can also be used for patients at risk of infection. Mineral water should be available for patients in the waiting room. Having a range of current magazines makes the waiting time seem shorter and these should reflect the interests of patients. A clock and leafy plants also add to the feeling of wellbeing.

CHILDREN'S PLAY AREA | Since parents increasingly have to bring their small children with them to the medical practice, suitable toys should be available in the waiting room. It is helpful to set up the playing area in a corner because this keeps the children in one part of the waiting room where it is easier to keep an eye on them.

CONSULTATION ROOM | For a first consultation with the doctor or for longer, detailed discussions [perhaps with several relatives], large medical practices have found it beneficial to a special meeting room, which should be exposed to natural light if at all possible. This option frees up the doctor's examination and treatment room [consultation room]. It should be furnished with a group of four to six chairs arranged together. There should be a supply of fresh water.

CHANGING CUBICLE | Provision for changing cubicles needs to be arranged in consultation with the doctor in charge. They can be in the form of a curtained off space or a separate cubicle and should be located outside the examination and treatment rooms, even outside some specialist medical rooms. These cubicles should have enough space to enable handicapped people to change, if necessary with a helper. Cubicles satisfy the wish for privacy.

PATIENT TRANSFER HATCHWAY | Some treatments require special protection against contamination. For these, the construction will need to make provision for a patient transfer passage. This applies mainly to invasive procedures carried out in an operating theatre. Patients enter the passage either on foot or lying down and are then transferred to an operating trolley or a mobile operating table. The route goes into the operating theatre via a holding area and then, after the operation, back into the patient transfer area. Now that outpatient operations are permitted in properly equipped specialist medical practices, there are more and more practices carrying out such work. The rule enshrined in the Robert Koch Institute guideline is crucial here, that is that outpatient operations must meet the same hygiene standards as for inpatient operations.[19]

RECOVERY ROOM | Peace and quiet may be necessary and beneficial for patients immediately after exhausting examinations or treatments. A simple room with a couch and somewhere to sit for an accompanying person is enough to meet this need. However, if a recovery room also has a soothing picture, some leafy plants and fresh water, then it becomes something more – an oasis of peace.

SINGLE-BED ROOM | Specialist practices with a clinic section have rooms, in addition to those necessary for outpatient care, that are available for a patient requiring an inpatient stay.

The single-bed room is a place for a post-operative patient who cannot leave the practice on the same day or has to stay for observation, care and nighttime treatment. Essentially, the sickbays of a specialist medical practice do not differ from those of a hospital because the patients have the same needs. The only difference is that the length of stay in a specialist medical practice is considerably shorter than in a hospital.

A single-bed room should contain a bed [adjustable if at all possible], a bedside table with a drawer, a wardrobe, a table with two seats [one of which should be particularly comfortable], a television, telephone and an internet connection point for a computer. The sickbay should have an en suite bathroom complete with a wash basin, shower and lavatory. Relatively few practices go to the expense of having the larger areas needed for handicapped patients and the more costly equipment in the bathroom.

TWO-BED ROOM | Some patients prefer a two-bed room because they appreciate having someone with them for company, someone who can summon immediate help in an emergency. Otherwise, the requirements for two-bed rooms are the same as for a single-bed room. Having the same space around them and the same furniture, they present economic advantages. From the point of view of the staff, they are easier to take care of. This however should not be taken as reason for dispensing with the single-bed room, which in many cases is urgently needed.

EXAMINATION AND TREATMENT ROOM | The core of a medical practice is the general examination and treatment room. This is where the main activities of the practice take place – diagnosis and treatment involving the main "players", the patient and the doctor.

The examination and treatment room generally doubles as the doctor's working and consulting room where patient and doctor meet for initial consultations, the taking of patient histories and for conducting basic examinations. These lead to the specialist medical rooms where the specialist diagnostic and treatment procedures are carried out.

The furniture of the usual examination and treatment room will consist of the doctor's desk and an examination couch. In addition, there will be a variety of cupboards and shelves for instruments and books and some appliances, for example, scales to measure weight and equipment to record physical dimensions. Depending on the doctor's personal inclinations, the room should radiate warmth, which may be objective, sober or homely. The doctor should pay special attention to this at design stage.

CONSULTATION ROOM | Some larger medical practices have a separate consultation room in addition to the examination and treatment room. It is an advantage if diagnostic and therapeutic procedures – which of course are commonly associated with small – can be conducted away from the doctor-patient consultation. As the space has no medical or technical equipment, the consultation room can take on a homely, almost private character. Sound insulation materials need to be considered when fitting out the room to ensure that the confidential nature of the consultation is not breached. The room should have adequate space to move around, comfortable seating, carefully chosen lighting etc.

LABORATORY | Diagnostic examinations of the blood and other body fluids involve the taking of samples. This is generally carried out in a screened off part of the laboratory or in a small adjacent room with a hatch. Depending on the available appliances, the analyses are carried out in the same laboratory or in a central laboratory. Numerous regulations govern the construction and fitting out of laboratories. The priority regulations to adhere to will be the Construction Code of the particular federal Land, the fire protection regulations and DIN 12924, section 420. These regulations govern, for example, the minimum size [12 square metres], require that walls, ceilings and floors are constructed of fire-resistant materials, specify a second escape route, an exhaust vent with a suction unit for work with flammable liquids and at least one fire extinguisher. Other requirements include good lighting, light that displays true colours, both natural and mechanical ventilation and surfaces that are easy to clean.

SPECIALIST EXAMINATION AND TREATMENT ROOM | Most medical practices are specialist practices with a specific medical remit; they have the space and appliances needed for that specialist field. Depending on the specialist field, there will be separate rooms for examination and for treatment and also rooms in which both are possible. The following are some examples of specialist examination fields: allergies, audiometry, blood pressure, computer tomography, echocardiography, electrocardiography, endoscopy, gynaecology, hearing tests, pulmonary function, magnetic resonance imaging [MRI], mammography, psychiatry, X-ray diagnostics, sonography and ultrasound. Examples of specialist treatments are: acupuncture, surgery, dermatology, dental hygiene, ergotherapy, infusions, inhalations, gymnastics, maxillary orthopaedics, cosmetics, laser treatment, massage, oral hygiene, nuclear medicine, prophylaxis, shock therapy, first aid and dentistry. Each of the necessary rooms will have its own ideal design in terms of size and equipment. For this reason, it is not possible to give a detailed description of the examination and treatment rooms in this account of the general fundamentals of planning. The specialist architect or specialist planner will need to work out the appropriate solution with the specialist doctor.

Since flexibility of use is desirable, the rooms in the planning examples contained in this text are assumed to have a standard usable floor space of 14 square metres. Where the specialist examination and treatment room is also used as the doctor's consultation room, the usable floor space increases to 22 square metres.

PREPARATION ROOM | Before major interventions, operations or some complex diagnostic procedures, patient preparation time is needed. In larger medical practices a preparation room should be available for this. The siting of the room is determined by its main use. Its dimensions should be the same as those of the specialist examination and treatment rooms. In emergencies, this room can also be used for other purposes.

INTERVENTION ROOM | Most medical practices, generally those constituted as multi-doctor practices with a clinic but also health centres and hospitals contain their own intervention area in which patients with life-threatening symptoms are examined and treated. The room should be in the immediate vicinity of the entrance and it should have sufficient space to move about in and be well lit and ventilated.

When operations are performed in the practice, the intervention room can also function as a preparation room or a holding area. The route from here to the operating unit should be as short and straight as possible.

OPERATING THEATRE | The fact that more and more outpatient operations are being performed in medical practices does not mean that such practices require the same spatial configurations as are usual in hospitals. Nevertheless, certain basic criteria must be met to ensure that medical interventions are performed under the proper conditions and especially that adherence to hygiene standards is guaranteed. The operating theatre must be located in a quiet area, screened off from the rest of the practice. The patient reaches this area via a patient transfer passage or, if applicable, via a holding area. Post-operatively, the patient is generally taken while still recumbent to a post-anaesthesia care unit, adjacent if at all possible, and he will remain here until he has fully regained consciousness. After that and depending on the severity of the intervention, he will stay in a single-bed or two-bed room for one or two days on average. The operating theatre should measure at least 36 square metres and, where feasible, be lit by natural daylight. Whether the room is ventilated – or better, air-conditioned – depends on the type of operation and also on the financial means of the operator. That applies also to the installation of a laminar flow unit.

POST-ANAESTHESIA CARE UNIT | After operations in which the patient has been anaesthetised, he should spend approximately two to five hours during the recovery period in a post-anaesthesia care unit. Here he will be subject to close observation and medical care. The post-anaesthesia care unit should have windows. As they come to, patients generally find it a wonderful experience to see natural daylight or even the sun. The number of beds in each case [at least two] depends on the number, type and duration of the operations. The post-anaesthesia care unit should be suitably fitted out with the necessary media and monitoring units.

ADMINISTRATION DEPARTMENT | To cope with the growing volume of secretarial duties, it may be useful, in large multi-doctor practices and hospitals, to set up one or several administration departments. The administration department supports the manager or managers of the unit and handles tasks which have to do with external relations, ordering, accounting, bookkeeping, prescription processing and correspondence.

Obviously, the number of staff working in the administration department depends on the volume of work.

OFFICE | As an alternative or as an addition to the administration department, a separate office – or in larger medical practices two such offices – is a practical means of ensuring that the mounting load [despite EDP] of administrative work is carried out undisturbed. This keeps files from heaping up in the rooms intended for medical duties.

The office should be in the vicinity of the reception area, be lit by natural daylight and appropriately furnished. A medical practice generates files that must be stored. Sufficient space for such storage [allowing for the years to come] needs to be included in the plans unless a separate archiving room is available. In large medical practices, separate offices can be included for essential administrative duties, for example for accounting and the correspondence service, which will also be responsible for writing medical reports.

ARCHIVE | An archive is useful in large medical practices to accommodate the swelling flood of files. This room can also house a photocopier, and any ladders, chairs and spare equipment that may be necessary.

STUDY ROOM | In major practices, but especially in hospital outpatient departments, study rooms can aid the performance of the organisation because this is the place for undisturbed, concentrated and creative work. Such rooms need not occupy a great deal of space. The important thing is that they are individually well designed. Study rooms are for medical directors, senior physicians, nurses and midwives.

STAFF CHANGING ROOM | According to the Work Place Regulation[21], each member of staff is entitled to and must have an individual cloakroom facility and a locker in which to keep valuables. However, small single-sex changing cubicles are preferable to meet the personal needs and hygiene standards of employees. A shower with direct access to the changing area is desirable. After all, a medical establishment has a particular duty to respect the hygiene and wellbeing of its staff.

STAFF REST ROOM | § 29 of the Work Place Regulation[21] lays down that employers with a staff of over ten must provide an easily accessible room for break periods. In a medical practice, this should be the rule even if there are fewer than ten employees because eating at the work place is inconsistent with maintaining hygiene standards. A fitted pantry will do in most cases. In larger medical practices this can become a separate room. A view out on to a green area would serve the needs of staff for relaxation particularly well.

STAFF LAVATORY | Under the Work Place Regulation, workforces of more than five are entitled to separate single-sex lavatory facilities. These must be for the exclusive use of the staff.

STERILISATION ROOM | There are various ways of organising the supply of sterile material for a medical practice. In any case, a storage facility for sterile material is essential. This must be available for disposable materials and goods sterilised outside the practice and, where applicable, for goods sterilised in the practice itself.

If sterile goods are supplied from an external source, only storage space is essential, but additional work surfaces are useful for handling materials. However, if the materials are sterilised in the practice, whatever the quantity, a sterilisation room with the required appliances is essential. For hygiene reasons, unclean work before sterilisation in a sterilisation room must be carried out in a sterilisation room – unclean, whereas work after sterilisation should be carried out in a sterilisation room – clean.

WORK ROOM – CLEAN | In almost every medical establishment, lots of tasks must be carried out in a clean environment. In general, the staff use the examination and treatment room for this. However, the situation cannot be regarded as ideal with regard to hygiene. Better would be a separate room which is reserved solely for clean work. The room can be kept small. It requires a work surface with a water tap and shelves.

WORK ROOM – UNCLEAN | By way of contrast, the above remarks on the work room – clean are valid for this work room. On closer inspection, there is a stronger justification for setting up this room.

STORE | In Germany, it has long been the practice of suppliers of medical and office goods to deliver immediately on receipt of an order, ideally on the same day, so that goods no longer need to be kept in storage for long periods. However, there is still a need for medical practices to keep a small stock of materials on the premises. A properly constructed and managed store only needs a small area. Its size depends on that of the practice itself and its purchasing policy.

APPLIANCE ROOM | In general, medical and technical appliances are kept in the examination and in the treatment rooms when in use. An appliance room can be useful in case a newly acquired piece of equipment should fail or to store equipment used only on an occasional basis.

CLEANER'S ROOM | Many medical practices have not provided space for a cleaner's room. As a result, a cleaning trolley stands in a corner of a corridor, a vacuum cleaner is stowed in a cupboard not intended for this and cleaning materials are kept in various places. This situation is not acceptable if an efficient cleaning service is to operate. In the eyes of patients, this is a clear sign that the ground plan has been inadequately designed.

DISPOSAL ROOM | In future, it may well be that the waste of an affluent society won't be so highly valued – even so, the sorting of medical practice waste into different categories is a major priority for reasons of hygiene. A small room specifically set aside to accommodate different types of waste makes it unlikely that a medical practice's waste will pose any risks.

SEMINAR ROOM | Despite there being now almost far too much in the way of media contact, the direct exchange of information between doctor and patient will not lose its importance. In a large medical practice, a seminar room with information materials and a technical medical library provides good opportunities for face to face discussions, lectures with slide shows and any type of further training, also for ancillary staff. One should not forget that a practice enhances its image by having such a facility.

MULTI-PURPOSE ROOM | Taking the longer view, it makes good sense to have a spare area with no specific intended purpose. Medical developments happen so quickly – anything can suddenly create the need for space. New medical standards can emerge overnight and require a rethinking of a previous strategy – with space implications. Such new developments cannot be accommodated completely but a room of this type can help get round many a bottleneck.

TECHNICAL ROOM | Often no attention is paid to the need for a utility room, the room in which all the utility supply services enter the premises. This feature may be omitted at design stage for lack of space and because there is inadequate coordination of the various technical work elements. However such a room makes sense for servicing work.

Structural characteristics
A range of quantity data is needed to make an assessment of a design in addition to any statement on quality-related characteristics.

GROSS FLOOR AREA | According to DIN 27717, the GFA in square metres is the sum of the floor areas of all the ground plans of the building project. By relation to the usable floor spaces, which have been discussed above, this value gives an indication of the compactness of the building solution.

GROSS CUBIC VOLUME | Also according to DIN 27717, the GCV in square metres is the volume of the body of the building enclosed by all the external boundary lines.

CONSTRUCTION COSTS | DIN 276 provides the framework for calculating the construction costs of building engineering[22]. The cost groups in question are 300 Structure – Construction designs and 400 Structure – Technical plant. Because it is desirable to be able to make comparisons the costs should always include VAT. The construction costs per cubic metre of gross cubic volume are often quoted as a value for purposes of comparison.

TOTAL COSTS | DIN 27622 also applies here, specifically cost groups 200 to 700. These are total costs including VAT. The cost of the site itself is not included as it can vary enormously because it is dependent on local circumstances.

The total costs are also known as investment costs. Together with the operating costs they are the most important criteria for decision-making on new buildings, extensions or conversions for a medical practice. The characteristic value of the total costs per square metre of usable floor space is a particularly potent figure.

Parties involved in planning

In view of the many aspects to be considered with regard to building work for the health care business, it is useful to form a planning support committee. This committee advises on all matters relating to planning and construction and attempts to find efficient solutions that all can agree on if possible.

The main players in this group are the client, as an investor with no background in the subject, and | or the user[s] and manager[s] of the medical practice. The practice planners take on the coordinating and controlling responsibilities. In general, these are independent architects or interior designers, increasingly also representatives of construction companies specialising in building medical practices. If the client does not introduce a specialist customer, than the doctor managing or designated to manage the business must be a member of the planning team, backed up by a member of the medical staff. It is important that all questions on operational procedures, on the functional and spatial allocation plan, and on the execution planning are discussed in detail with these specialist individuals closely involved in the day to day running of the practice. The effort made here is worthwhile if it helps prevent constructional and organisational errors. Because the main business of the medical practice is the delivery of services to patients, it can only be beneficial to have their approval of the planning decisions. Therefore it

is a good idea to find at least one interested patient to follow the planning procedure through with criticism and input. The results of a questionnaire conducted among the patients can be included here, either instead of or in addition to those of a single interested patient. It may be useful to invite representatives of the supervisory authorities to attend meetings of the planning committee.

ELEMENTS OF THE DESIGN

Conventional architecture firms are not normally commissioned to design medical practices. Experienced architects and facility planners have often specialised for years in design commissions of this sort. Thus, often the client will have to deal with architects for whom such a commission is their first and constitutes a challenge. Especially for these architects, the following suggestions should give ideas for the design. They are also suitable for potential clients and operators since they give an overview of the planning process.

Functions

Observation of the daily routine in a medical practice often makes clear that there are various inadequacies and opportunities for improvement. For this reason, it is worthwhile making a thorough analysis of the functional procedures and the relations between functions that this

reveals before the planned construction work to ensure that operations are as smooth and effective as possible. The following illustrations will consider some aspects of design planning.

FUNCTIONAL RELATIONS BETWEEN THE FUNCTION GROUPS | Among the first things to consider at design stage is how to clarify the relations between the function groups. The matrix of functional relations [Fig. 5] will bring these out sharply. Three function groups lie at the heart of a medical practice: patient rooms, examination and treatment rooms and specialist medical rooms. The other functions are grouped around this core, depending on the size and service structure of the medical practices.

Note should be taken of the strength of the relations between functions.

FUNCTIONALLY POSITIVE ARRANGEMENT OF THE FUNCTION GROUPS IN TWO-STOREY OR THREE-STOREY MEDICAL PRACTICES | If there are several floors, movements between the different floors will necessarily create extra work. Here, it makes a difference if the distances covered are via an easily accessible lift or have to be walked up and down narrow angled staircases or even spiral staircases.

The picture of the scheme [Fig. 6] shows an appropriate layout for the function groups for small, medium-sized and large practices spread over two or three floors. Always immediately adjacent are patient rooms, examination and treatment rooms and specialist medical rooms. If the rooms in the basement have sufficient natural daylight, the service and staff rooms can be located here. It is more convenient to have the supply and disposal rooms close to the examination and treatment rooms and specialist medical rooms. Alternatively, the upper floor can be used for the function group of the service and staff rooms.

INDIVIDUAL FUNCTIONS | Essentially, the rooms of a particular function group should be located as close together as possible. After all, this was the rationale behind setting up the function groups in this way.

There are standards to be met by a sequence of operational functions which require close relations between function groups, for example between patient rooms and specialist medical rooms. There are some relations within function groups that should be adhered to – for example between reception | waiting room and operating theatre and post-anaesthesia care unit.

FORMING ZONES IN THE GROUND PLANS | The form of the ground plan of a medical practice depends largely on how the available floor space is divided up in what is generally an existing building. If there is any choice in the way the floor space is allocated or if a detached medical practice building is being planned, it is appropriate to think about zoning the ground plan [Fig. 7]. The type of zoning determines the type of construction the medical practice will have. The concern here is the arrangement of the rooms as a patient entering the premises will see them.

A distinction is made between one-, two- and three-zone premises. The individual room zones can be directly adjacent to each other, but they can also be separated by corridors. In a one-zone ground plan, all the rooms are grouped together. In a two-zone plan the rooms are arranged one behind the other. The rooms in a three-zone ground plan are ranged even further back. In principle, these planning variants apply for small, medium-sized and large medical practices in one-, two- and three-storey buildings. Three storeys are not an option for small practices.

The zoning style and the number of storeys are determining factors for the efficiency of a ground plan of a medical practice. In general, it is true that single-storey, two and three-zone premises provide the best conditions to patients. Patients in such premises are not faced with having to move from storey to storey, an important consideration, and such practices are very compact, irrespective of their size.

Also, the typology of the building and energy consumption profile are further advantages. A measure of the compactness is the extent of vertical external surfaces [U]. This feature has the smallest values by far in the two recommended premise types.

Environmental conditions

With regard to the increased incidence of allergies and sensitivities among patients and staff, it is important, even in medical practices, to think seriously about measures for a healthier environment. This involves thinking critically about choice of site, decisions on materials for construction and equipment and about environmentally friendly measures for running the medical practice.

SITE SELECTION | It is best to avoid, if at all possible, being in the immediate vicinity of a petrol station, a dry cleaner's or industrial premises that release chemicals into the air, and having car parks close to the entrance.

CHOICE OF MATERIALS FOR CONSTRUCTION AND EQUIPMENT | Essentially, materials with a low gas emission potential should be selected. Hard surfaces are preferable because they present a less likelihood of deposits of harmful substances forming on them. Preferred media are tiles, stone, terrazzo, hard wood and linoleum as floor coverings, rough-textured wallpaper and curtains.

ENVIRONMENTALLY FRIENDLY OPERATIONAL MEASURES[23] | The following are some of numerous actions that can achieve environmental improvement in medical practices:
– Selection of suitable disinfectants [for example, without phenol]
– Strict avoidance of cleaning materials containing

	Patient rooms	Examination and treatment rooms	Specialist rooms	Administrative rooms	Offices and staff rooms	Supply and waste disposal rooms	Training rooms	Plant rooms
Patient rooms		1	1	2	3	4	2	4
Examination and treatment rooms	1		1	3	2	2	3	3
Specialist rooms	1	1		3	2	2	3	2
Administrative rooms	2	3	3		3	3	2	4
Offices and staff rooms	3	2	2	3		3	3	3
Supply and waste disposal rooms	4	2	2	3	3		4	3
Training rooms	2	3	3	2	3	4		4
Plant rooms	4	3	2	4	3	3	4	

1 – Various functional relations

2 – Certain functional relations

3 – A few functional relations

4 – No functional relations

5 Matrix of the functional relations between the function groups

chemicals, of sprays, perfumes, ether oils, cigarette smoke and pesticides
– As far as possible, minimisation of electric smog [for patients who react to electric and electromagnetic fields]
– Air quality improvement [especially for hypersensitive patients]
– No daily newspapers in waiting rooms because of their high solvent content
– For sensitive patients, avoidance of cut flower because of pesticide contamination and leafy plants because of potential mould in the growing medium. A desirable homely effect can also be created with art works and objects made of safe materials.

Hygiene standards

In facilities for outpatient examination and treatment, care must be taken to ensure that patients and staff are protected against infectious pathogens. The guidelines for hospital hygiene and infection prevention of the Robert Koch Institute in Berlin set out the standard requirements for the prevention and containment of infections. Particularly relevant is the appendix entitled "Hygiene Requirements for the Functional and Constructional Design of Hospital Facilities for the Care of Outpatients'.[24] Even the rules for hospital outpatient departments, suitably adapted for medical practices and other outpatient care facilities, are definitely relevant, for example:
– If major diagnostic and therapeutic facilities

are available, waiting room separation is preferable.
– Several patients should not be examined and treated at the same time in the same room.
– A separate waiting room should be provided for patients suspected of having an infection.
The guideline's requirements may well seem extravagant, but considering the growing worldwide hazard presented by new viral infections, they ought to take on increasing significance.

Natural light

In recent decades, the desire for natural light in rooms has grown significantly. Essentially, rooms in which people work for lengthy periods and rooms in which staff spend time must be lit by natural daylight. The German Länder have different regulations specifying the operative times. Solutions in which as far as possible all work and rest rooms have some natural daylight are regarded as forward-looking. With regard to the suggestions in the functional and spatial allocation plans about natural daylight, architects are enjoined to find ways, even with technical aids, that allow people working in medical practices to natural light as possible.

Way finding

The increasing overload of stimuli that people are exposed to is certainly responsible for the fact that some people, particularly senior citizens, have problems finding their way around

buildings. Even the entrance often presents a psychological barrier. The pathway through a medical practice can seem like the entrance to a maze. Routes indicated by lighting and coloured markings on ceilings and walls, and the choice of materials and flooring can be of assistance here. But locating the built-in and moveable furnishings in clear and obvious positions helps as well.

Technical equipment

The sources of standards to be met by technical equipment are quoted in the chapter entitled "Laws, Regulations and other Provisions". For reasons of space, illustrations of technical equipment can only be referred to briefly here:

STATICS | If renovation work is to be undertaken, the planner must work with the existing structural characteristics for reasons of economy. For new buildings, the planner should design for statics that create the largest possible bearing distances. They create spacious areas not divided up by intrusive walls or supports and enable design freedom and flexible changes .

VENTILATION | The medical practice should appeal to the senses in many ways, with fragrant aromas for example, but care should be taken to ensure these are not overpowering because people's sensitivity to smell differs markedly. This is why it is necessary to install a ventilation unit that is effective and easy to control, one which creates a

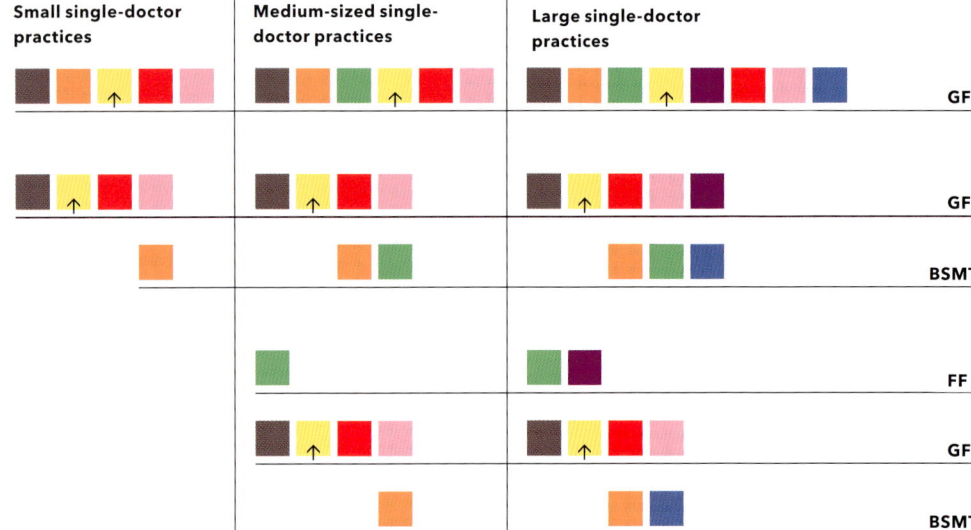

6 Arrangement of the function groups in one-, two- and three-story buildings

neutral atmosphere comparable with clean outside air. The time may come when further research is going to produce fragrances which can be used in ventilation units to generate a health-enhancing effect.

HEATING, COOLING, AIR HUMIDITY AND FILTERING | The Work Place Regulation[21] stipulates that work rooms should have a minimum temperature of 21 °C and a maximum temperature of 25 °C. This creates a pleasant ambient temperature for patients as well. For comfort, an agreeable degree of coolness and a pleasant level of air humidity are needed on hot days because dry air has a negative effect on the airways. Finally, filtration of incoming air is desirable for people suffering from allergies. Conventional heating systems, cooling appliances, air humidifiers and filters are available as solutions for these needs.

AIR CONDITIONING | The requirements cited in the foregoing section are all met by a modern air conditioning system. The decision to install such a system in new buildings must be made when planning starts; installing such facilities later is more costly. A good air conditioning system has the advantage of delivering an ambient atmosphere that can be adjusted at any time without draughts and disruptive noise. There will be no need for space for radiators. It is important to check in good time if the investment and operating costs can be kept within acceptable limits.

ACOUSTICS | Noise abatement is one of today's paramount concerns in the field of environmental protection. The Construction Codes of the Länder stipulate insulation to prevent noise carrying in buildings. DIN 410925 contains requirements to be met by rooms and components and the Work Place Regulation[21] governs noise levels in work and staff rooms. The requirements can be met by separating construction components, choosing the right floorings that reduce structure-borne and airborne noise, by installing ceilings with acoustic properties and noise-absorbing wall cladding and through the design of facilities and equipment and the use of noise-insulating doors. All this is highly desirable, especially with regard to the need to maintain patient privacy.

LIGHTING | Planning lighting equipment is a difficult task for planners because the field is so complicated. This should be undertaken by a qualified specialist because it is so important for the overall appearance of the medical practice. The chapter "Elements of the Design" deals with the requirements for exterior and interior lighting.

PROTECTION AGAINST BURGLARY | There is a heightened risk of burglary in medical practices, not only because of the material value of medical and office equipment but because of the lure presented by drugs on the premises. This risk cannot be eliminated completely but the use of

technology can reduce it considerably. Roller shutters and grilles are the principal means used. Also used are high-resistance safety glass and motion detectors that trigger lighting and acoustic warnings. Video monitoring systems have proved effective because they can help identify culprits. A radio link to nearby police stations can lead to early arrests. These also serve as strong deterrents.

FIRE PROTECTION | The Construction Codes of the Länder, the Work Place Regulation[21], DIN 410226, the Occupational Health and Safety Office and the Occupational Health and Safety Associations all attach great importance to preventing fires in medical practices, particularly in laboratories. There are requirements for the fire resistance classification of load-bearing and non load-bearing parts of buildings and the fire resistant properties of building materials. The length and number of escape routes are also laid down.

Special features of renovations

The fact that facilities and the substance of the building have become worn is the reasons for renovation work. Another reason is generally the need to make better use of the areas and spaces and to improve operational procedures. Recently, minor or major work can result from changes to technical equipment, for example the installation of a new lighting system, new heating, ventilation, cooling and filtration plant or even whole air conditioning systems.

One room zone

60 m × 6 m   U = 132 m

2 × 30 m × 6 m   U = 144 m

3 × 15 m × 8 m   U = 138 m

Two room zones

30 m × 12 m   U = 84 m

2 × 15 m × 12 m   U = 108 m

3 × 10 m × 12 m   U = 132 m

Three room zones

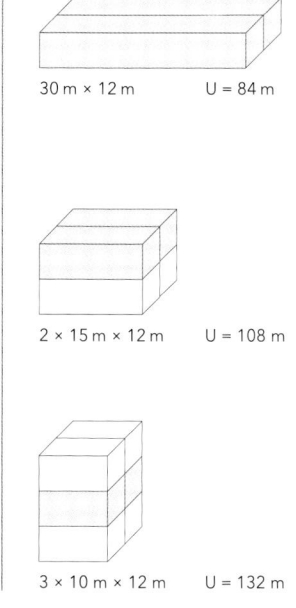
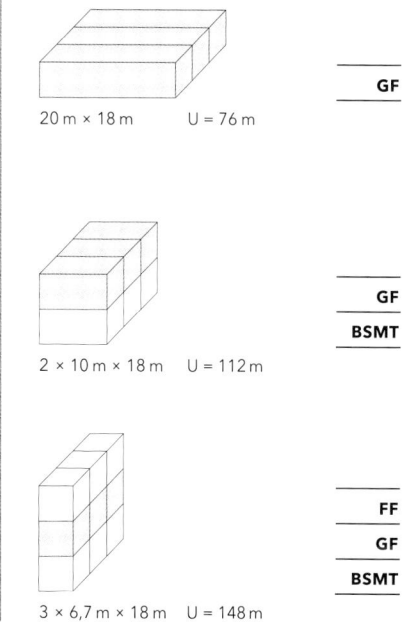

20 m × 18 m   U = 76 m   GF

2 × 10 m × 18 m   U = 112 m   GF / BSMT

3 × 6,7 m × 18 m   U = 148 m   FF / GF / BSMT

7   Schemes for one-, two- and three-story medical practices with one to three room zones. The verticals are exaggerated in height for reasons of clarity. The converted room is the same size in all schemes. U means extent of the external areas in metres.

Whereas the erection of a new building is only subject to the need to finish by a fixed date, renovations, including extensions and conversions, are associated with significantly greater difficulties. Temporary closure of the medical practice certainly guarantees the quickest progress for building work. Generally, however, this route is not taken for commercial reasons so that the building work must proceed while the business is running. Dustproof partitioning will be necessary to protect patients and staff alike, but also mainly for hygiene reasons. It should at the same time help reduce building noise. Normally, it is also necessary to move some facilities or to clear some function groups. In such cases, careful advance consideration should be given to ways in which the necessary operations of the practice can continue during the individual phases of building work. Renovations entail inconvenience to everyone affected by them. Hence, it is advisable to apologise to the people concerned in good time.

STANDARD FUNCTIONAL AND SPATIAL ALLOCATION PLANS, FUNCTION SCHEMES AND STANDARD GROUND PLANS FOR SINGLE-DOCTOR PRACTICES

The functional and spatial allocation plans, function schemes and ground plans described below for small, medium-sized and large single-doctor and multi-doctor practices are intended to clarify, by means of a standard example, the basics of operation and construction. In this case, standard means a sample or model of minimum expense allowing for a functional and efficient solution.

The subdivision explained in the section entitled "Subdivision into Function Groups" applies to functional and spatial allocation plans. These plans also contain a suggestion for light exposure [see section entitled "Functional and Spatial Allocation Plans"]. Distinctions are made between individual rooms [functional elements] and rooms that need to be immediately adjacent [function units] which, taken together, always form function groups. The plan code prefixes [PCP – German acronym PKZ] identify the function groups and then in succession the function units and functional elements.

The function schemes show all the rooms and the functional relations. The different sized squares chosen to symbolise the rooms give an indication of the size of the usable floor spaces.

Conversion of the function scheme into a ground plan presupposes a ground plan format into which the individual rooms of the functional and spatial allocation plan must be fitted. This task can be compared to a jigsaw puzzle because the individual components need to be cut to size taking due account of the available area and of the functional and [potential] structural engineering demands. So it is understandable that with respect to a given functional and spatial allocation plan, minor "off-cuts" occur or occasionally a small area remains which can then be used as a box room or a technical room.

The standard ground plans are not intended to serve as templates for designs. They represent, as an example in the deliberately selected one-storey format, only a visualisation of the functional and spatial allocation plans. [The one-storey format has been chosen because it cuts out stairs and lifts and is therefore compact.] The standard ground plans are therefore evidence of feasibility and a guide in the initial planning considerations. Designs remain the province of the architects, interior designers and other medical practice planners, who work together creatively with the doctors and their colleagues to produce individual solutions.

Standards for a small single-doctor practice

In Germany, the number of small medical practices [up to 125 square metres usable floor space] out of the total number of such practices is showing definite signs of shrinking. This is with regard to the further development of outpatient care and also to the growing medical options and the raised expectations of patients. Taking commercial aspects into account, there is an accelerating trend towards larger medical practices, generally in the form of two-doctor or multi-doctor practices, because they benefit from the available synergies, giving a greater chance of survival. However, small single-doctor practices, especially those in rural and thinly populated areas, retain their raison d'être.

FUNCTIONAL AND SPATIAL ALLOCATION PLANS AND FUNCTION SCHEMES | The functional and spatial allocation plan presented as an example [Fig. 8], at 100 square metres, lies in the lower range of benchmarks cited in the chapter entitled "Functional and Spatial Allocation Plans" where these benchmarks for small single-doctor practices range upwards to 125 square metres. In cases where the areas quoted here are not available some rooms must be reduced in size or abandoned. It may also be possible to combine some functions, for example the staff rest room and changing cubicle or work room – unclean area and cleaner's room, in order to save a few square metres of usable floor space. However, in this, the functional and spatial allocation plan approaches a lower limit, below which it is no longer certain that a practice can be run on commercially sound lines. The function scheme emphasises the desirable direct relationship between the reception area and the waiting area, the adjacent site of the examination and treatment rooms and the specialist medical rooms and the combination of the service and staff rooms [Fig. 9].

GROUND PLAN | The choice of a rectangle with two room zones for the schematic ground plan of the medical practice results from the view that the premises should feature a large measure of compactness and efficiency [Figs. 10 and 11]. The rooms are ranged along two sides of a straight central corridor so that they all receive natural daylight. The function groups of the patient rooms and the supply and disposal rooms are on the side of the entrance. On the opposite side are the examination and treatment rooms, the specialist medical rooms and the service and staff rooms. In a good position almost in the middle of the corridor there is a wind trap through which patients pass into the reception area, the adjacent waiting area and, immediately opposite, the examination and treatment room. An advantage of this ground plan solution is that the rooms are easy to find and reach. The directly adjacent location of the reception and waiting areas makes it possible to see the patients.

Standards for a medium-sized single-doctor practice

The design principles which apply for small single-doctor practices also apply for the medium-sized version, with some modifications.

FUNCTIONAL AND SPATIAL ALLOCATION PLAN AND FUNCTION SCHEME | In addition to the larger size and different room types, the functional and spatial allocation plan for the small single-doctor practice has here been extended with an additional small examination room and an office [Fig. 12]. With 150 square metres of usable floor space, it occupies the middle zone of the benchmarks [125 square metres to 175 square metres] and has the size of medical practices frequently encountered today. Compared with the small single-doctor practice, all the function groups in the function scheme have been extended and furthermore the function group "Administration Rooms" is represented by one room located in the vicinity of the reception areas [Fig. 13].

GROUND PLAN | The only change in the room plan, compared with a single-doctor practice, is the addition of an office opposite the reception area and the enlargement of the room group "Examination Rooms". [Figs. 14 and 15].

Standards for a large single-doctor practice

The previously selected layout can be retained for large single-doctor practices.

FUNCTIONAL AND SPATIAL ALLOCATION PLAN AND FUNCTION SCHEME | Compared with the foregoing detailed description of single-doctor practices, some rooms have been enlarged further. Additional features are an examination and treatment room, a children's play corner and a room from the function group "Training and Teaching Rooms", which can be used as a multi-purpose or spare room [Fig. 16].

The size [200 square metres usable floor space] is somewhat above the benchmark for large single-doctor practices, which start at 175 square metres. There are numerous single-doctor practices in this size range. Their usable floor space rises to about 250 square metres.

PCP	FUNCTION GROUP FUNCTION UNIT FUNCTIONAL ELEMENT	LIGHT EXPOSURE	USABLE FLOOR IN SQM
1	**Patient rooms**		**30**
1.1	Reception room	○	10
1.2	Waiting room with cloakroom	○	18
1.3	Patient lavatory [L + G]		
1.3.1	Anteroom	●	1
1.3.2	Lavatory	●	1
2	**Examination and treatment rooms**		**34**
2.1	Examination and treatment room [Consultation room]	○	22
2.2	Laboratory	○	12
3	**Specialist medical rooms**		**8**
3.1	Examination room – Electrocardiography	●	8
5	**Offices and staff rooms**		**16**
5.1	Staff rest room with pantry	○	8
5.2	Staff changing facilities with shower	◐	6
5.3	Staff lavatory [L + G]		
5.3.1	Anteroom	●	1
5.3.2	Lavatory	●	1
6	**Supply and waste disposal rooms**		**12**
6.1	Work room – Unclean	○	4
6.2	Stores	●	4
6.3	Cleaner's room	●	4

Usable floor of a small single-doctor practice   **100**

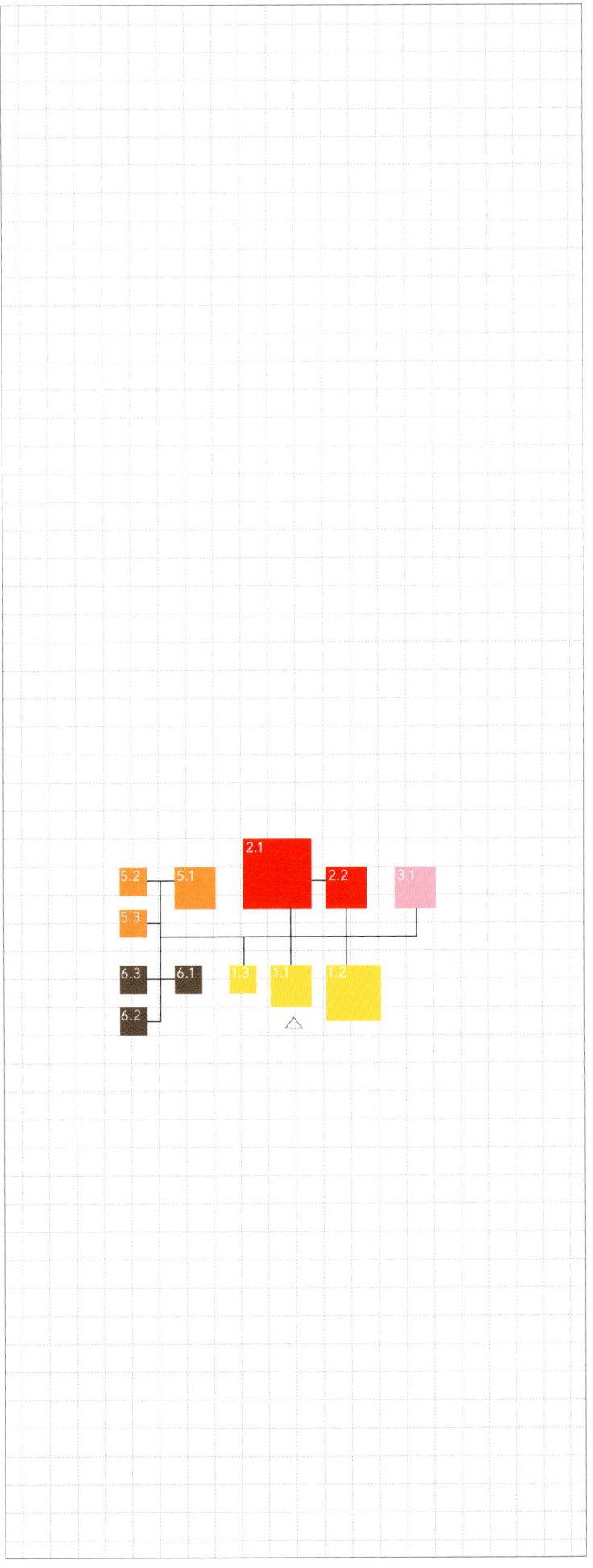

The function group "Patient Rooms" has received an additional room with the function of children's play corner directly adjacent to the waiting area. Also, the function group "Examination and Treatment Rooms" has been enlarged by an additional examination room. A multi-purpose room can be added to it, connected by a sliding door if possible. This functional and spatial allocation plan also has a technical room added to it [Fig. 17].

GROUND PLAN | The central corridor solution with two room zones gives a large single-doctor practice sufficient development potential, even if more rooms have been added. Whatever the case, small dead end corridors must be added. It is essential to be aware at planning stage that the inward facing rooms that this will create will have to do without natural daylight [Figs. 18 and 19].

STANDARD FUNCTIONAL AND SPATIAL ALLOCATION PLANS, FUNCTION SCHEMES AND STANDARD GROUND PLANS FOR MULTI-DOCTOR PRACTICES

Standards for a small multi-doctor practice
As there is an increasing trend towards two-doctor and multi-doctor practices providing outpatient care, this type of practice will be described in greater detail with the aid of a few examples.

The small multi-doctor practice is the most economic user of space.

FUNCTIONAL AND SPATIAL ALLOCATION PLAN AND FUNCTION SCHEME | The smallest workable size for a multi-doctor practice is around 150 square metres of usable floor space [Fig. 20]. For the standard example, 200 square metres has been chosen. This means that small multi-doctor practices have roughly the same space needs as large single-doctor practices.

The essential difference from single-doctor practices is in the form adopted here of a joint practice, that is in the interactions between at least three specialist fields whose managers each have their own examination and treatment rooms, using them also as consultation rooms; all the other rooms of the practice are being run jointly.

As regards the basic structure, the main change is to the function group "Examination and Treatment Rooms". The specialist medical rooms replace several additional individual rooms. The examination and treatment rooms are not only used as consultation rooms, but also take on a specialist character, that is they contain the medical and technical facilities necessary to provide specialist medical services. The room allocation deducible from the function scheme corresponds largely to that of a large single-doctor practice. Only the general examination and treatment rooms are replaced by specialist medical rooms. In the small multi-doctor practice there is no space for a children's play corner, a multi-purpose room and technical room [Fig. 21].

GROUND PLAN | The layout of a small multi-doctor practice is similar to that of the large single-doctor practice [Figs. 22 and 23]. On the side opposite the entrance area, the available space allows the creation of a laboratory and X-ray room. These rooms are transferred to the entrance side and are accessible via the dead end corridor. All the rooms of the efficient rectangular ground plan receive natural daylight.

Standards for a medium-sized multi-doctor practice
Medium-sized multi-doctor practices are quite common. Obviously, their size is suitable for the duties they have to perform and synergy effects work particularly well.

FUNCTIONAL AND SPATIAL ALLOCATION PLAN AND FUNCTION SCHEME | The benchmarks for the usable floor spaces amount to between 250 and 400 square metres. [Fig. 24]. The example chosen here is that of a medium-sized multi-doctor practice with 300 square metres of usable floor space which has rooms for five identical or different specialist fields. It should be noted that with different specialist fields, depending on the field, there will be an additional specialist examination and treatment room of one type or another.

With this in mind, the 300 square metres of usable floor space must be regarded as the lower limit for a medium-sized multi-doctor practice with five specialist fields.

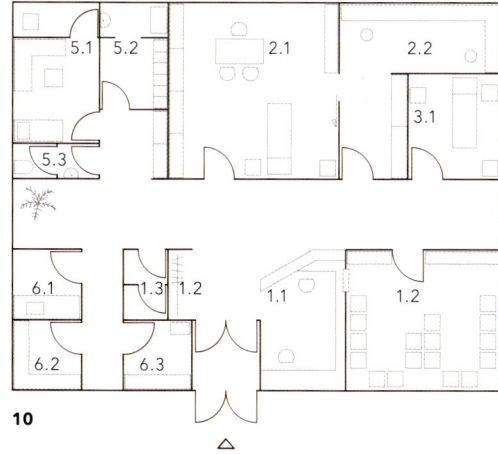

10

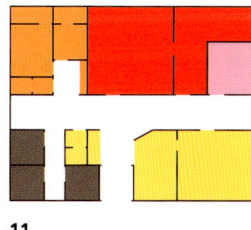

11

8 Example of a functional and spatial allocation plan for a small single-doctor practice
9 Function scheme of a small single-doctor practice
10 Standard ground plan of a small single-doctor practice, scale 1:200
11 Colour scheme for the ground plan of a small single-doctor practice, scale 1:400

PCP	FUNCTION GROUP FUNCTION UNIT FUNCTIONAL ELEMENT	LIGHT EXPOSURE	USABLE FLOOR IN SQM
1	**Patient rooms**		**40**
1.1	Reception room	○	14
1.2	Waiting room with cloakroom	○	22
1.3	Patient lavatory [L]		
1.3.1	Anteroom	●	1
1.3.2	Lavatory	●	1
1.4	Patient lavatory [G]		
1.4.1	Anteroom	●	1
1.4.2	Lavatory	●	1
2	**Examination and treatment rooms**		**42**
2.1	Examination and treatment room [Consultation room]	○	22
2.2	Examination room and changing facilities	○	8
2.3	Laboratory	○	12
3	**Specialist medical rooms**		**8**
3.1	Examination room – Ultrasound	●	8
4	**Administration rooms**		**10**
4.1	Office	○	10
5	**Offices and staff rooms**		**32**
5.1	Staff rest room with pantry	○	12
5.2	Staff changing facilities – L		
5.2.1	Changing facilities	◓	8
5.2.2	Shower	●	2
5.3	Staff changing facilities – G		
5.3.1	Changing facilities	◓	4
5.3.2	Shower	●	2
5.4	Staff lavatory [L]		
5.4.1	Anteroom	●	1
5.4.2	Lavatory	●	1
5.5	Staff lavatory [G]		
5.5.1	Anteroom	●	1
5.5.2	Lavatory	●	1
6	**Supply and waste disposal rooms**		**18**
6.1	Work room – Unclean	○	6
6.2	Stores	●	8
6.3	Cleaner's room	●	4

Usable floor of a medium-sized single-doctor practice 150

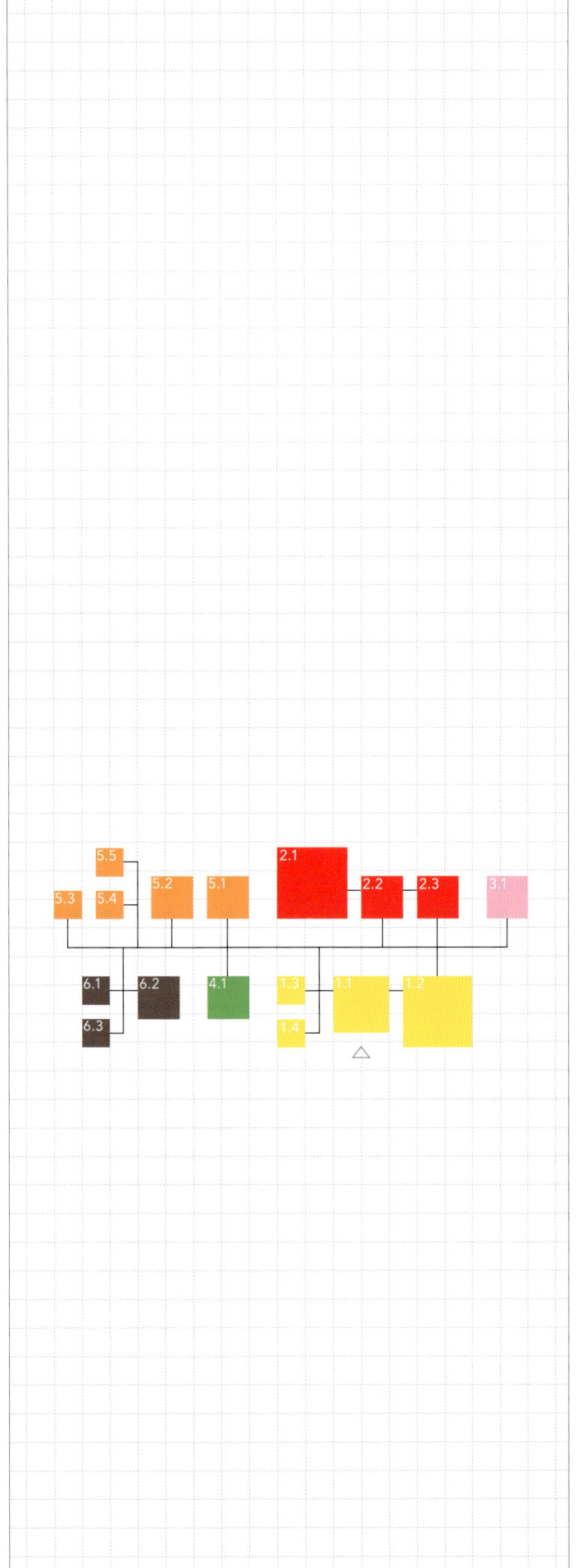

The function scheme for the medium-sized multi-doctor practice includes additional rooms for the function groups Specialist Medical Rooms and Supply and Disposal Rooms. In addition there will also be a multi-purpose room and a technical room [Fig. 25].

GROUND PLAN | Retention of the previous ground plan structure shows that the limits of this form have been reached. A central corridor should not extend any further. A longer corridor is unacceptable, not only because of the long distances but also for design reasons [Figs. 26 and 27]. The alternative ground plan developed specifically for the medium-sized multi-doctor practice contains the same rooms, but needs 10 % more floor area after deducting the inner courtyard. The reason for the introduction of the inner courtyard in this schematic ground plan is the need to light all the practice rooms with natural daylight. Even so, the inner courtyard increases the overall quality of the design [Figs. 28 and 29].

Unlike the initial scheme, in which natural daylight penetrates the building both via the ends of corridors designed to allow the passage of light and via the central reception and waiting area, the alternative scheme seems to be flooded with light via the ends of four corridors designed to allow the passage of light, the similarly light-filled reception and waiting area and the inner courtyard [Fig. 30].

A comparison of the distances to be walked shows, for example, that the distances between the furthest apart specialist medical rooms, measured from the middle of the door walls, are more or less the same [16.0 metres and 16.5 metres]. The central location of the staff rooms means that these distances are acceptable. Even if some distances should be a little longer, they would not pose a problem, as they would be balanced by the enhanced experience of the alternative.

Standards for a large multi-doctor practice
Recent developments in health care policy tend to concentrate outpatient care increasingly in large high-performance and economically efficient centres. The large multi-doctor practice is one of the first facilities of this type. Additionally, in Germany, hospital outpatient departments, medical centres, diagnostic centres, medical care centres and health centres have also sprung up. Essentially, these are also large multi-doctor practices but follow a different care approach.

FUNCTIONAL AND SPATIAL ALLOCATION PLAN AND FUNCTION SCHEME | The group of Multi-Doctor Practices begins at over 400 square metres of usable floor space. There is practically no upper space limit because these projects also include large medical buildings which can house up to 40 practices and more. Assuming an average minimum size of 60 square metres for a specialist

medical practice, then the medical centre referred to above would have at least 2,400 square metres of usable floor space. The example chosen here has seven specialist medical practices with a usable floor space of 500 square metres [Fig. 31]. In comparison with the medium-sized multi-doctor practice, four specialist examination and treatment rooms have been added. The available space for the remaining rooms has been expanded and given different uses.

With regard to the function groups Patients, Specialist Medical Rooms, Administration Rooms, and Service and Staff Rooms and compared with the previous model, the function scheme for large multi-doctor practices shows that some individual rooms have been enlarged and given different uses, whereas the remaining function groups have merely been given more usable floor space. The linear arrangement of the related function groups displays a high degree of clarity and order. As for the supply and disposal rooms, the sterilisation rooms are, for functional reasons, situated in the vicinity of the specialist medical rooms [Fig. 32].

GROUND PLAN | The structure of the ground plan is the same as that of the medium-sized multi-doctor practice variant [Figs. 33 and 34]. Because of the enlargement and different uses of some rooms, the office and the multi-purpose room must be accommodated by the inner courtyard. The two connections for the examination and treatment rooms have been lengthened by the addition of some

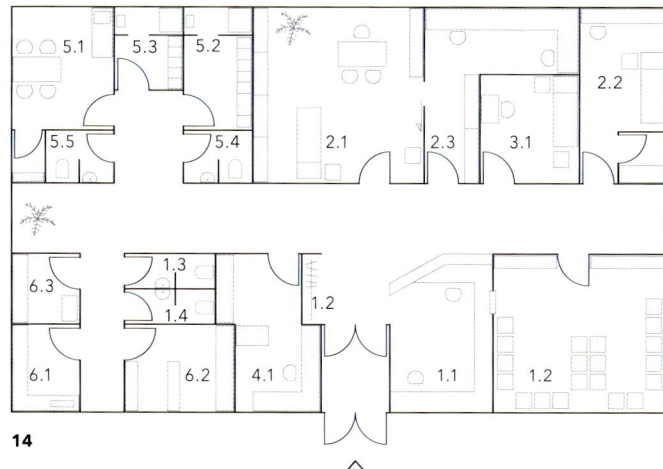

14

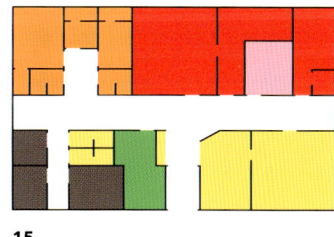

15

12 Example of a functional and spatial allocation plan for a medium-sized single-doctor practice
13 Function scheme of a medium-sized single-doctor practice
14 Standard ground plan of a medium-sized single-doctor practice, scale 1:200
15 Colour scheme for the ground plan of a medium-size single-doctor practice, scale 1:400

PCP	FUNCTION GROUP FUNCTION UNIT FUNCTIONAL ELEMENT	LIGHT EXPOSURE	USABLE FLOOR IN SQM
1	**Patient rooms**		**50**
1.1	Reception room	○	16
1.2	Waiting room with cloakroom	○	26
1.3	Play room	○	4
1.4	Patient lavatory [L]		
1.4.1	Anteroom	●	1
1.4.2	Lavatory	●	1
1.5	Patient lavatory [G]		
1.5.1	Anteroom	●	1
1.5.2	Lavatory	●	1
2	**Examination and treatment rooms**		**50**
2.1	Examination and treatment room [Consultation room]	○	22
2.2	Examination room	○	8
2.3	Examination room	○	8
2.4	Laboratory	○	12
3	**Specialist medical rooms**		**8**
3.1	Examination room – Electrocardiography and Ultrasound	●	8
4	**Administration rooms**		**12**
4.1	Office	○	12
5	**Offices and staff rooms**		**40**
5.1	Staff rest room with pantry	○	16
5.2	Staff changing facilities – L		
5.2.1	Changing facilities	◉	10
5.2.2	Shower	●	2
5.3	Staff changing facilities – G		
5.3.1	Changing facilities	◉	6
5.3.2	Shower	●	2
5.4	Staff lavatory [L]		
5.4.1	Anteroom	●	1
5.4.2	Lavatory	●	1
5.5	Staff lavatory [G]		
5.5.1	Anteroom	●	1
5.5.2	Lavatory	●	1
6	**Supply and waste disposal rooms**		**20**
6.1	Work room – Unclean	○	6
6.2	Stores	●	10
6.3	Cleaner's room	●	4
7	**Training rooms**		**18**
7.1	Multi-purpose room [Extension]	○	18
8	**Plant rooms**		**2**
8.1	Technical room	●	2
	Usable floor a large single-doctor practice		**200**

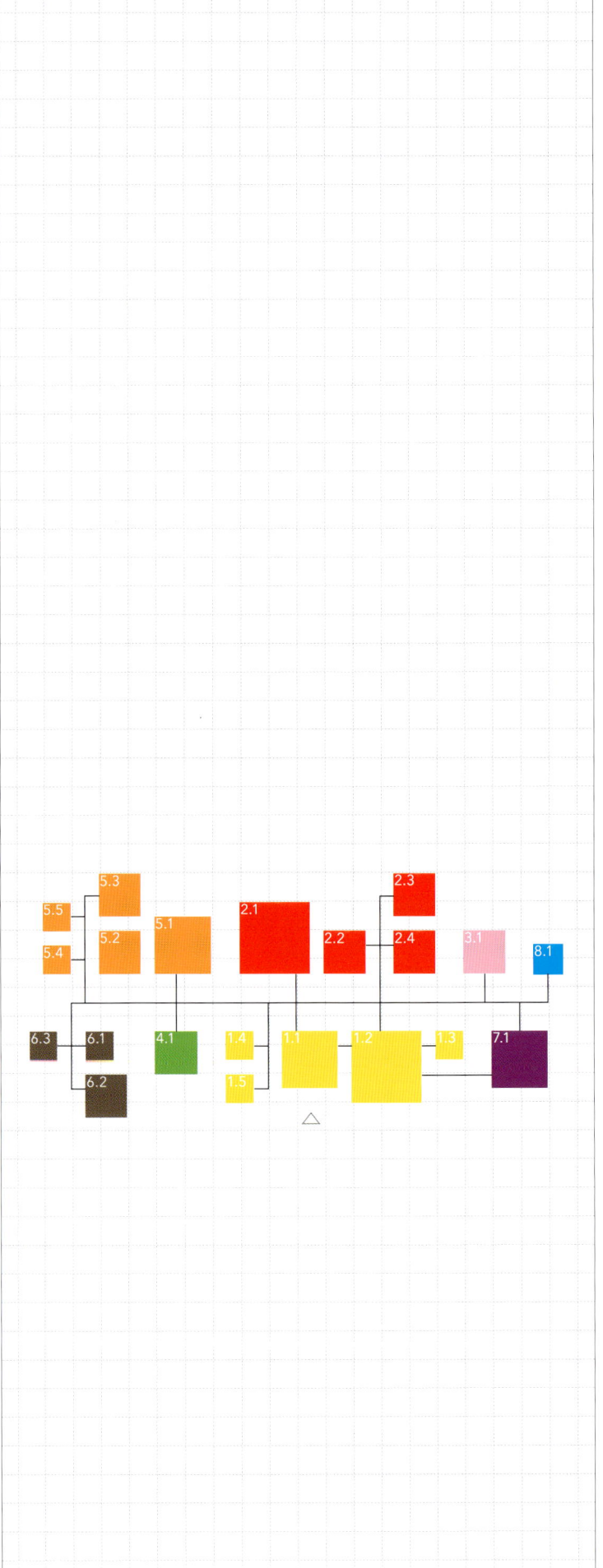

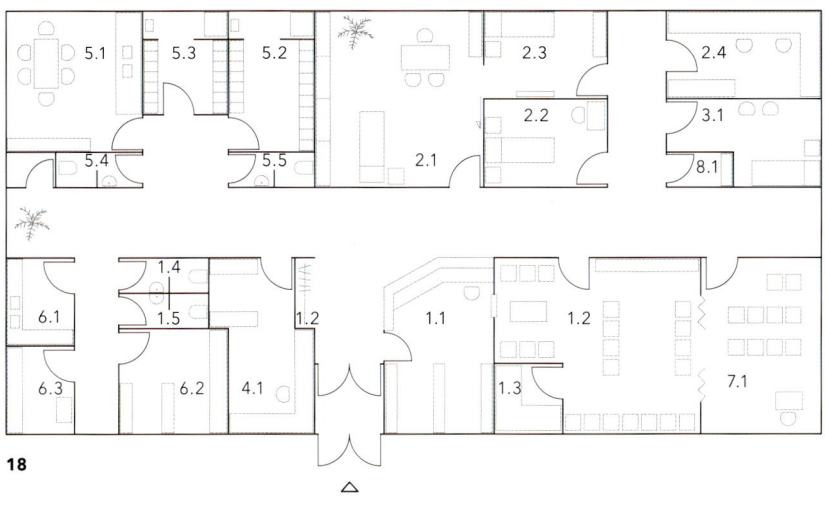

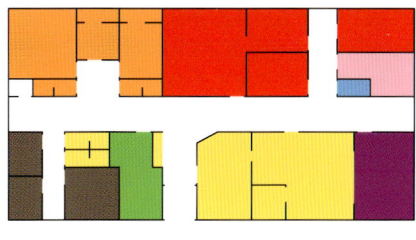

18

19

PCP	FUNCTION GROUP FUNCTION UNIT FUNCTIONAL ELEMENT	LIGHT EXPOSURE	USABLE FLOOR IN SQM
1	**Patient rooms**		**46**
1.1	Reception room	○	16
1.2	Waiting room with cloakroom	○	26
1.3	Patient lavatory [L]		
1.3.1	Anteroom	●	1
1.3.2	Lavatory	●	1
1.4	Patient lavatory [G]		
1.4.1	Anteroom	●	1
1.4.2	Lavatory	●	1
2	**Examination and treatment rooms**		**12**
2.1	Laboratory	○	12
3	**Specialist medical rooms**		**74**
3.1	Examination and treatment room [Consultation room] – Mouth, jaw and facial surgery 1	○	22
3.2	Examination and treatment room [Consultation room] – Mouth, jaw and facial surgery 2	○	22
3.3	Examination and treatment room [Consultation room] – Mouth, jaw and facial surgery 3	○	22
3.4	Examination room – X-ray	●	8
4	**Administration rooms**		**12**
4.1	Office	○	12
5	**Offices and staff rooms**		**40**
5.1	Staff rest room with pantry	○	16
5.2	Staff changing facilities – L		
5.2.1	Changing facilities	◉	10
5.2.2	Shower	●	2
5.3	Staff changing facilities – G		
5.3.1	Changing facilities	◉	6
5.3.2	Shower	●	2
5.4	Staff lavatory [L]		
5.4.1	Anteroom	●	1
5.4.2	Lavatory	●	1
5.5	Staff lavatory [G]		
5.5.1	Anteroom	●	1
5.5.2	Lavatory	●	1
6	**Supply and waste disposal rooms**		**16**
6.1	Work room – Unclean	○	6
6.2	Stores	●	6
6.3	Cleaner's room	●	4

Usable floor of a small multi-doctor practice   **200**

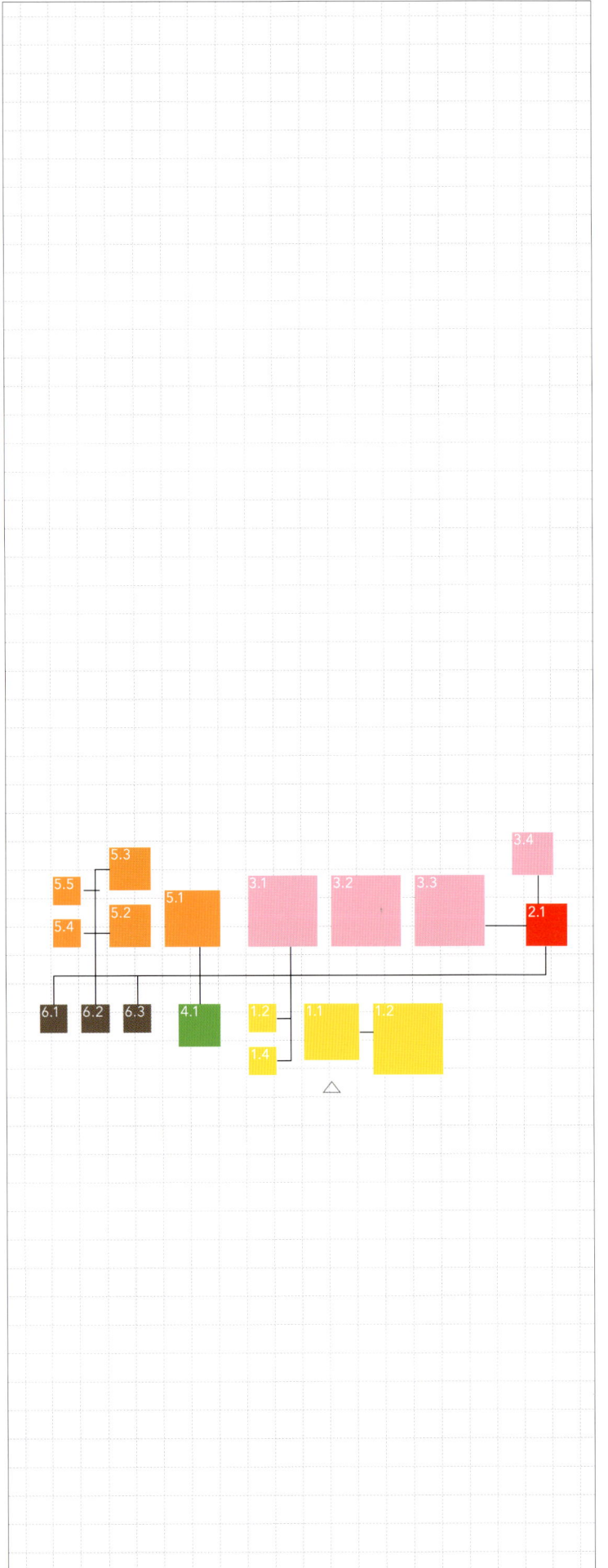

specialist medical rooms. The ground plan incorporates the area of an almost equilateral rectangle, which gives the building geometry an ideal shape. Once again, however, this shows that the limits for this form have been reached. The second ground plan level should be considered for even bigger premises. The administration, service and staff rooms should be shifted first of all to this level. All of the rooms of the 500 square metres multi-doctor practice receive natural daylight with the exception of some ancillary rooms.

NOTES ON THE FUNCTIONAL AND SPATIAL ALLOCATION PLANS FOR SELECTED FACILITIES

Specialist medical practices

The highly diffuse nature of specialist medical fields and the effect this has on the design and layout of medical practices demands wide-ranging specialist knowledge. However, the architect can only acquire this know-how if he works closely with the doctors involved. The present author had the opportunity of working with doctors in this way, resulting in a planning manual for hospitals and care homes.[27] The listed suggestions include some that are applicable to hospital outpatient departments. Suitably adapted, they apply also to specialist medical practices.

Some years ago, Damaschke, Scheffer and Schossig published a book which examined in detail the different functional and spatial allocation plans of numerous medical practices. It also presented examples and illustrated functional, spatial and design aspects.[28] Now considered as a classic text, Teut and Nedeljkov's book "The Group Practice" [1973] also takes in experience gained in the German Democratic Republic. It provides information on technical planning principles, minimum space needs and functional interrelations.[29]

OPHTHALMOLOGICAL SPECIALIST MEDICAL PRACTICE | Among the range of services provided here, the key areas are electrophysiological diagnostics, visual field diagnostics, laser therapy, eye training and ultrasound diagnostics. If operating facilities are available, resections and treatments for such disorders as cataracts, and drooping eyelids can be carried out.

Depending on the range of services provided, the main rooms are: examination room, eye training room, visual field checking room, laser coagulation room, sonography room, a room for fluorescence angiography and a room for electroretinography [dark room].

SURGICAL SPECIALIST MEDICAL PRACTICE | The following are some of the key areas with regard to examination and treatment: general surgical diagnostics and therapy, obesity treatment and follow-up care, hand examination and treatment, emergency examination and treatment, rectal examinations and treatments, soft-laser treatment, tumour follow up care, thyroid examination and treatment [nuclear medicine diagnostics and therapy related disciplines]. A separate room for rectal examinations should be provided in addition to general examination and treatment rooms. It is useful to site this room near to diagnostic facilities, for example radiology and endoscopy units and an operating unit.

ORTHOPAEDIC SPECIALIST MEDICAL PRACTICE | Listed here are some of the services delivered: examination and treatment of ailments of the feet, hips, knee, shoulders and spinal column, orthopaedic diseases of newborn babies and the delivery of oncological orthopaedics. The main rooms needed are examination and treatment rooms and rooms for ultrasound, plaster of Paris casts and infusions, and a recovery room is also needed as an extra. The waiting room must have comfortable armchairs with arm rests and armchairs with raised seats [for patients with sitting supports]. It is helpful if the medical practice is sited near to X-ray diagnostics and physical diagnostics facilities.

UROLOGICAL SPECIALIST MEDICAL PRACTICE | Among the range of services provided here are diagnostics and therapy for general urological ailments, fertility problems and endocrinology of the aging male, incontinence, also neurological diagnostics, stoma aftercare, pre-operative diagnostics and post-operative care for those suffering from tumors.

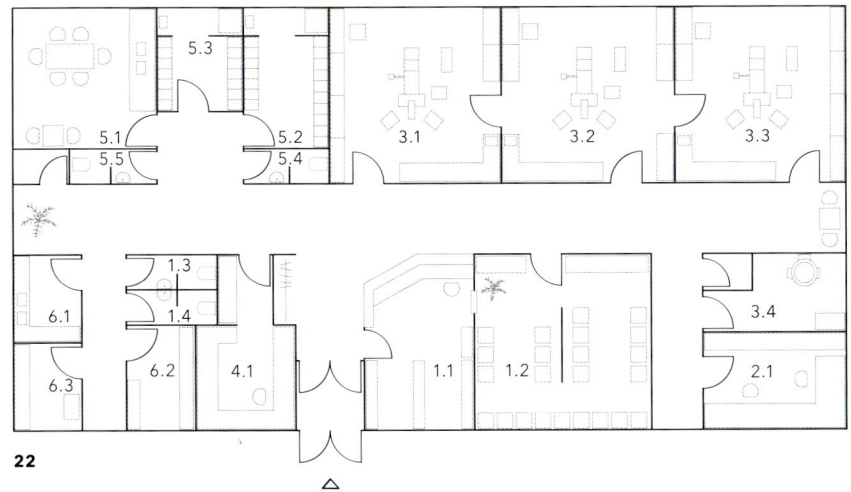

22

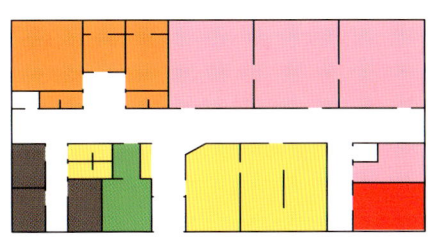

23

PCP	FUNCTION GROUP FUNCTION UNIT FUNCTIONAL ELEMENT	LIGHT EXPOSURE	USABLE FLOOR IN SQM
1	**Patient rooms**		**54**
1.1	Reception room	O	20
1.2	Waiting room with cloakroom	O	26
1.3	Play room	O	4
1.4	Patient lavatory [L]		
1.4.1	Anteroom	●	1
1.4.2	Lavatory	●	1
1.5	Patient lavatory [G]		
1.5.1	Anteroom	●	1
1.5.2	Lavatory	●	1
2	**Examination and treatment rooms**		**12**
2.1	Laboratory	O	12
3	**Specialist medical rooms**		**118**
3.1	Examination and treatment room [Consultation room] – Gynaecology and obstetrics	O	22
3.2	Examination and treatment room [Consultation room] – Urology	O	22
3.3	Examination and treatment room [Consultation room] – Ophthalmology	O	22
3.4	Examination and treatment room [Consultation room] – Otolaryngology	O	22
3.5	Examination and treatment room [Consultation room] – Skin and venereal diseases	O	22
3.6	Examination room – X-ray	●	8
4	**Administration rooms**		**14**
4.1	Office	O	14
5	**Offices and staff rooms**		**42**
5.1	Staff rest room with pantry	O	18
5.2	Staff changing facilities – L		
5.2.1	Changing facilities	◉	10
5.2.2	Shower	●	2
5.3	Staff changing facilities – G		
5.3.1	Changing facilities	◉	6
5.3.2	Shower	●	2
5.4	Staff lavatory [L]		
5.4.1	Anteroom	●	1
5.4.2	Lavatory	●	1
5.5	Staff lavatory [G]		
5.5.1	Anteroom	●	1
5.5.2	Lavatory	●	1
6	**Supply and waste disposal rooms**		**38**
6.1	Sterilisation		
6.1.1	Sterilisation room	O	8
6.1.2	Stores – Sterile goods	●	6
6.2	Work room – Clean	O	6
6.3	Work room – Unclean	O	6
6.4	Stores	●	8
6.5	Cleaner's room	●	4
7	**Training rooms**		**18**
7.1	Multi-purpose room [Extension]	O	18
8	**Plant rooms**		**4**
8.1	Terminal compartment	●	4
	Usable floor of a medium-sized multi-doctor practice		**300**

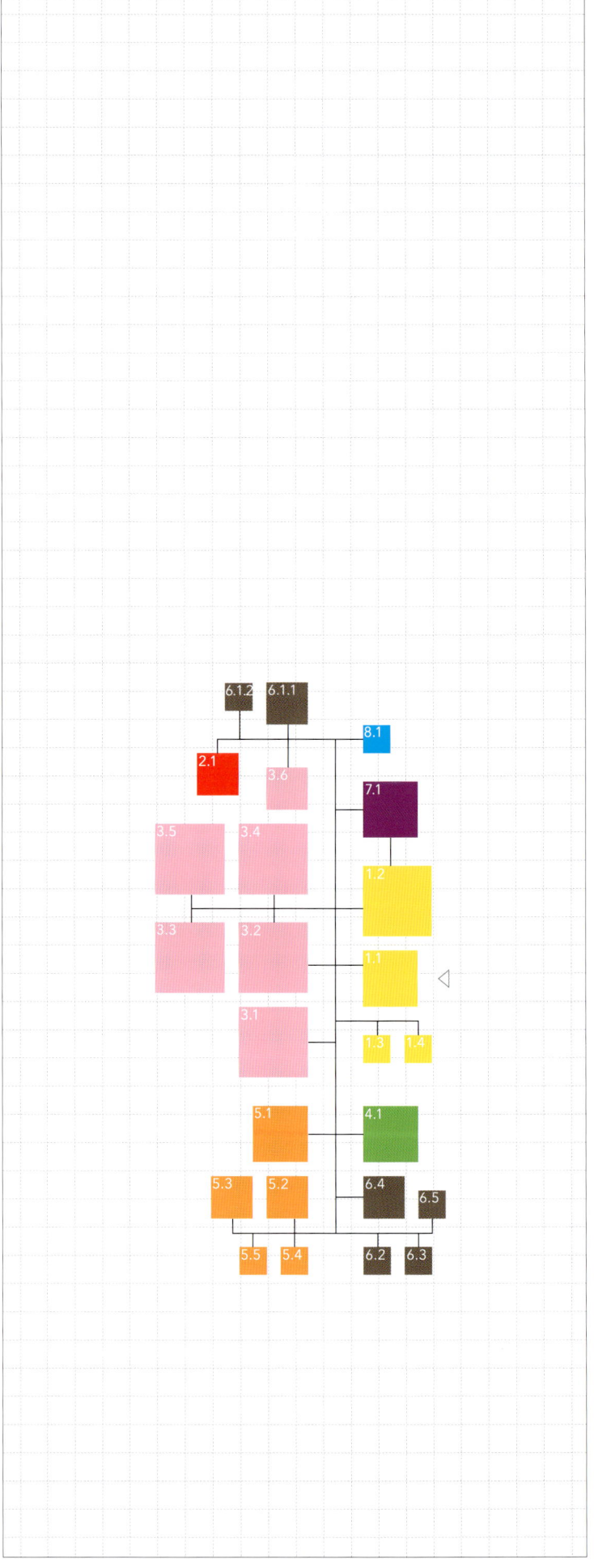

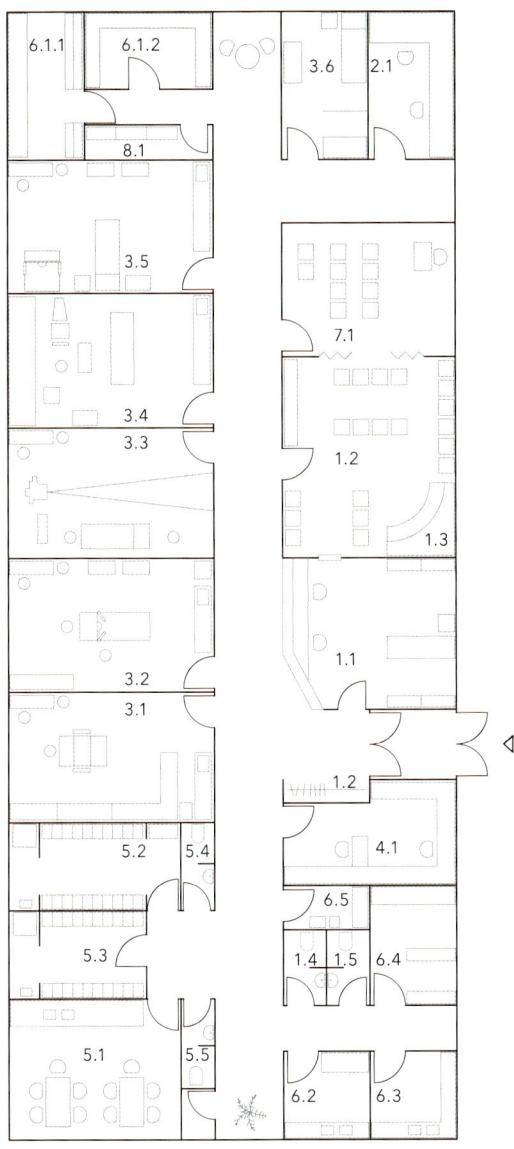

26

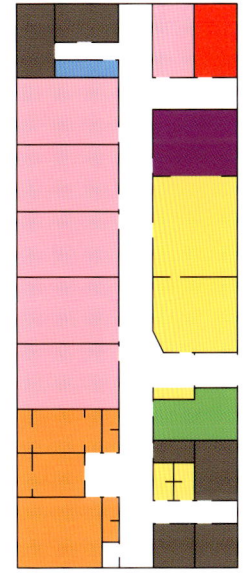

27

24 Example of a functional and spatial
allocation plan for a medium-sized multi-
doctor practice
25 Function scheme of a medium-sized
multi-doctor practice
26 Standard ground plan of a medium-
sized multi-doctor practice, variant 1,
scale 1:200
27 Colour scheme for the ground plan of
a medium-size multi-doctor practice,
variant 1, scale 1:400

PCP	FUNCTION GROUP FUNCTION UNIT FUNCTIONAL ELEMENT	LIGHT EXPOSURE	USABLE FLOOR IN SQM
1	**Patient rooms**		**54**
1.1	Reception room	O	20
1.2	Waiting room with cloakroom	O	26
1.3	Play room	O	4
1.4	Patient lavatory [L]		
1.4.1	Anteroom	●	1
1.4.2	Lavatory	●	1
1.5	Patient lavatory [G]		
1.5.1	Anteroom	●	1
1.5.2	Lavatory	●	1
2	**Examination and treatment rooms**		**12**
2.1	Laboratory	O	12
3	**Specialist medical rooms**		**118**
3.1	Examination and treatment room [Consultation room] – Gynaecology and obstetrics	O	22
3.2	Examination and treatment room [Consultation room] – Urology	O	22
3.3	Examination and treatment room [Consultation room] – Ophthalmology	O	22
3.4	Examination and treatment room [Consultation room] – Otolaryngology	O	22
3.5	Examination and treatment room [Consultation room] – Skin and venereal diseases	O	22
3.6	Examination room – X-ray	●	8
4	**Administration rooms**		**14**
4.1	Office	O	14
5	**Offices and staff rooms**		**42**
5.1	Staff rest room with pantry	O	18
5.2	Staff changing facilities – L		
5.2.1	Changing facilities	◉	10
5.2.2	Shower	●	2
5.3	Staff changing facilities – G		
5.3.1	Changing facilities	◉	6
5.3.2	Shower	●	2
5.4	Staff lavatory [L]		
5.4.1	Anteroom	●	1
5.4.2	Lavatory	●	1
5.5	Staff lavatory [G]		
5.5.1	Anteroom	●	1
5.5.2	Lavatory	●	1
6	**Supply and waste disposal rooms**		**38**
6.1	Sterilisation		
6.1.1	Sterilisation room	O	8
6.1.2	Stores – Sterile goods	●	6
6.2	Work room – Clean	O	6
6.3	Work room – Unclean	O	6
6.4	Stores	●	8
6.5	Cleaner's room	●	4
7	**Training rooms**		**18**
7.1	Multi-purpose room [Extension]	O	18
8	**Plant rooms**		**4**
8.1	Terminal compartment	●	4
	Usable floor of a medium-sized multi-doctor practice		**300**

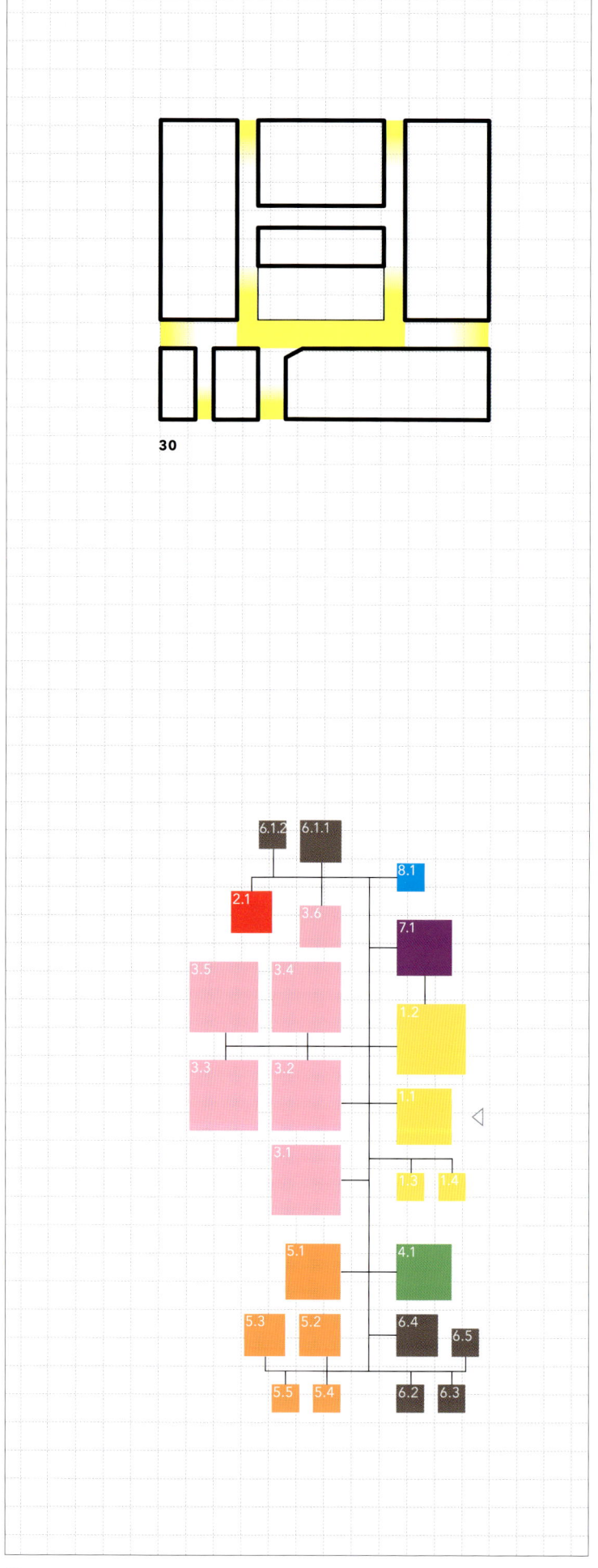

30

Among the main rooms needed are examination and treatment rooms for cytoscopic examinations, a room for urodynamics and, if applicable, a lithotripsy room. Ancillary facilities needed are an instrument preparation room and a wash room. It is useful to be close to X-ray diagnostic and laboratory medicine facilities.

ORAL AND MAXILLOFACIAL SURGERY SPECIALIST MEDICAL PRACTICE | The following are some of the key areas with regard to examination and treatment: acute and pain therapy with infiltration, trepanation, incision, drainage including tooth extraction, acute treatments for wounds, surgery with local anaesthesia, specific diagnostic procedures [for example ultrasound, model analysis, face bow, laser scanning], plate treatment for patients with cleft lips, jaws and palates, radiological diagnostics [panoramic X-ray and X-ray micro images] and dental laboratory work.

The main rooms needed are examination and treatment rooms with facilities for ultrasound and laser, X-ray room, a planning room [for X-ray assessment, model measurement, and operations planning], an operation unit with a laboratory for plaster of Paris and plastics processing. One of the ancillary rooms should be an appliance | instrument preparation room. It is helpful to be close to the X-ray diagnostic and laboratory medicine facilities.

Short distances to the related specialist fields of ear, nose and throat medicine, plastic surgery and possible ophthalmology are also useful.

Other facilities:

HOSPITAL OUTPATIENT DEPARTMENTS | Subject to the categories of DIN 13080, in Germany every hospital has the functional category 1.02 Medical Service, which covers all outpatient departments as part categories.[18] Since every hospital has a different medical service profile, the number and type of outpatient departments must be ascertained in each case. The content of the individual outpatient departments is determined by their main rooms. In addition, there are the first-line communication, ancillary and staff rooms, which are arranged centrally, part centrally or non-centrally, always depending on the need and organisation format.
– The first-line communication rooms include the registration point, medical records office, waiting rooms for ambulant or non-ambulant patients, toilets and the disposal room.
– The ancillary rooms include work rooms – clean and unclean, stores – medical goods and laundry, appliance room and cleaner's room
– The staff rooms include the medical director's study [head of staff – physician], administration department, senior physician's study, wash rooms for doctors and staff, meeting room plus library, standby emergency room, changing cubicles and lavatories for staff and if necessary a

study room for managerial nursing staff in the specialist field and study room for technicians.

As hospital outpatient departments examine and treat ambulant inpatients, inpatients occupying beds and ambulant patients arriving from admissions, a good deal of thought needs to be devoted to the siting of facilities in the hospital. Compared with normal medical practices, there is a need here for wider corridors and doors, larger waiting rooms and changing cubicles for inpatients transported on stretchers or mobile beds. In particular, however, the main rooms for examinations and treatments must be of adequate dimensions to allow for appropriately sized usable floor spaces.

MEDICAL CARE CENTRE | In 2008, there were already over 1,100 medical care centres in Germany[7]. There is an increasing trend towards building more medical care centres because more and more doctors are looking to work in this sort of centre. No standard can be devised for this functional and spatial allocation plan because the individual facilities have quite different characteristics depending on their location, range of services, size and organisation. Each medical care centre contains numerous specialist medical practices and a range of more or less jointly used functional units for diagnosis and therapy – for example, a laboratory, X-ray diagnostics and endoscopy units, physiotherapy and a unit for outpatient operations. Medical care centres exclusively treat outpatients.

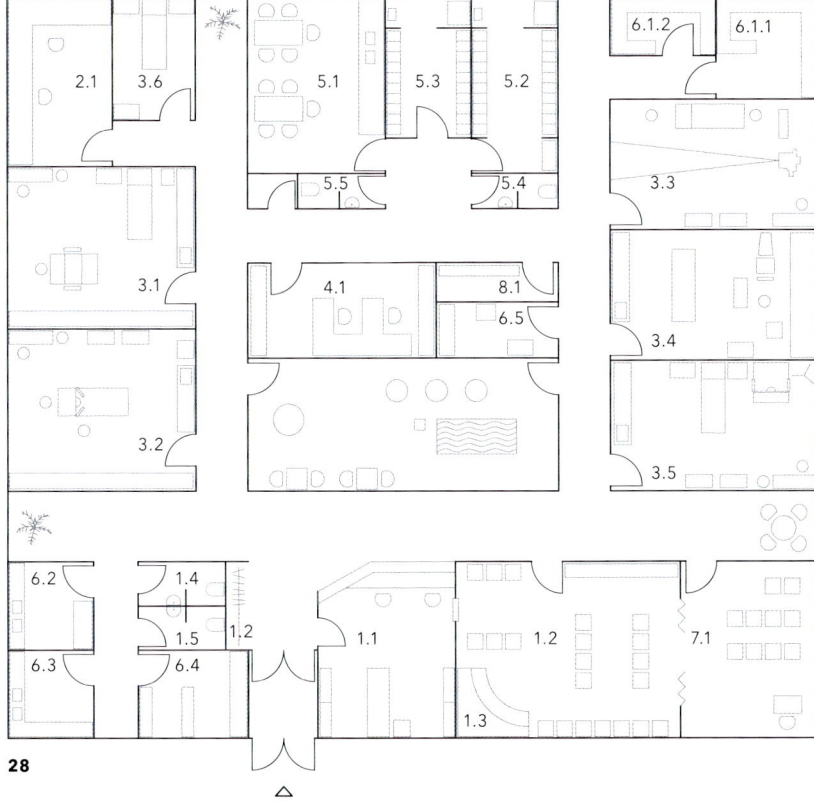

28

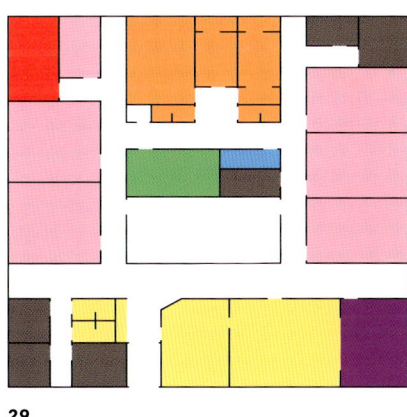

29

24 Example of a functional and spatial allocation plan for a medium-sized multi-doctor practice
25 Function scheme of a medium-sized multi-doctor practice
28 Standard ground plan of a medium-sized multi-doctor practice, variant 2, scale 1:200 [as the functional and spatial allocation plan [Fig. 16], but as underground section]
29 Colour scheme for the ground plan [Fig. 18], variant 2, scale 1:400
30 Scheme of the underground section with possible incidence of light

PCP	FUNCTION GROUP FUNCTION UNIT FUNCTIONAL ELEMENT	LIGHT EXPOSURE	USABLE FLOOR IN SQM
1	**Patient rooms**		**102**
1.1	Reception room	O	20
1.2	Waiting rooms		
1.2.1	Waiting room 1	O	28
1.2.2	Waiting room 2	O	14
1.2.3	Play room	O	6
1.2.4	Cloakroom	●	4
1.3	Meeting room	O	10
1.4	Hygiene room	◉	6
1.5	Patient lavatory [L]		
1.5.1	Anteroom	●	2
1.5.2	Lavatory	●	2
1.6	Patient lavatory [G]		
1.6.1	Anteroom	●	2
1.6.2	Lavatory	●	2
1.7	Lavatory for handicapped persons	●	6
2	**Examination and treatment rooms**		**14**
2.1	Laboratory	O	14
3	**Specialist medical rooms**		**194**
3.1	Examination and treatment room [Consultation room] – Mouth, jaw and facial surgery 1	O	22
3.2	Examination and treatment room [Consultation room] – Mouth, jaw and facial surgery 2	O	22
3.3	Examination and treatment room [Consultation room] – Neurology	O	22
3.4	Examination and treatment room [Consultation room] – Ear, nose and throat medicine	O	22
3.5	Examination and treatment room [Consultation room] – Urology	O	22
3.6	Examination and treatment room [Consultation room] – Gynaecology and obstetrics	O	22
3.7	Examination and treatment room [Consultation room] – Paediatrics and youth medicine	O	22
3.8	Examination room – X-ray	●	12
3.9	Examination room – Electrocardiography	O	14
3.10	Examination room – Ultrasound	O	14
4	**Administration rooms**		**32**
4.1	Office		
4.1.1	Office – Prescription processing	O	16
4.1.2	Office – Bookkeeping	O	16
5	**Offices and staff rooms**		**64**
5.1.1	Staff rest room	O	26
5.1.2	Pantry	O	8
5.2	Staff changing facilities – L		
5.2.1	Changing facilities	●	12
5.2.2	Shower	●	2
5.3	Staff changing facilities – G		
5.3.1	Changing facilities	●	6
5.3.2	Shower	●	2
5.4	Staff lavatory [L]		
5.4.1	Anteroom	●	2
5.4.2	Lavatory	●	2
5.5	Staff lavatory [G]		
5.5.1	Anteroom	●	2
5.5.2	Lavatory	●	2
6	**Supply and waste disposal rooms**		**54**
6.1	Sterilisation		
6.1.1	Sterilisation room	O	14
6.1.2	Stores – Sterile goods	◉	8
6.2	Work room – Clean	O	6
6.3	Work room – Unclean	O	6
6.4	Stores	●	16
6.5	Cleaner's room	●	4
7	**Training rooms**		**32**
7.1	Multi-purpose room [Extension]	O	32
8	**Plant rooms**		**6**
8.1	Technical room	●	6
	Usable floor of a large multi-doctor practice		**500**

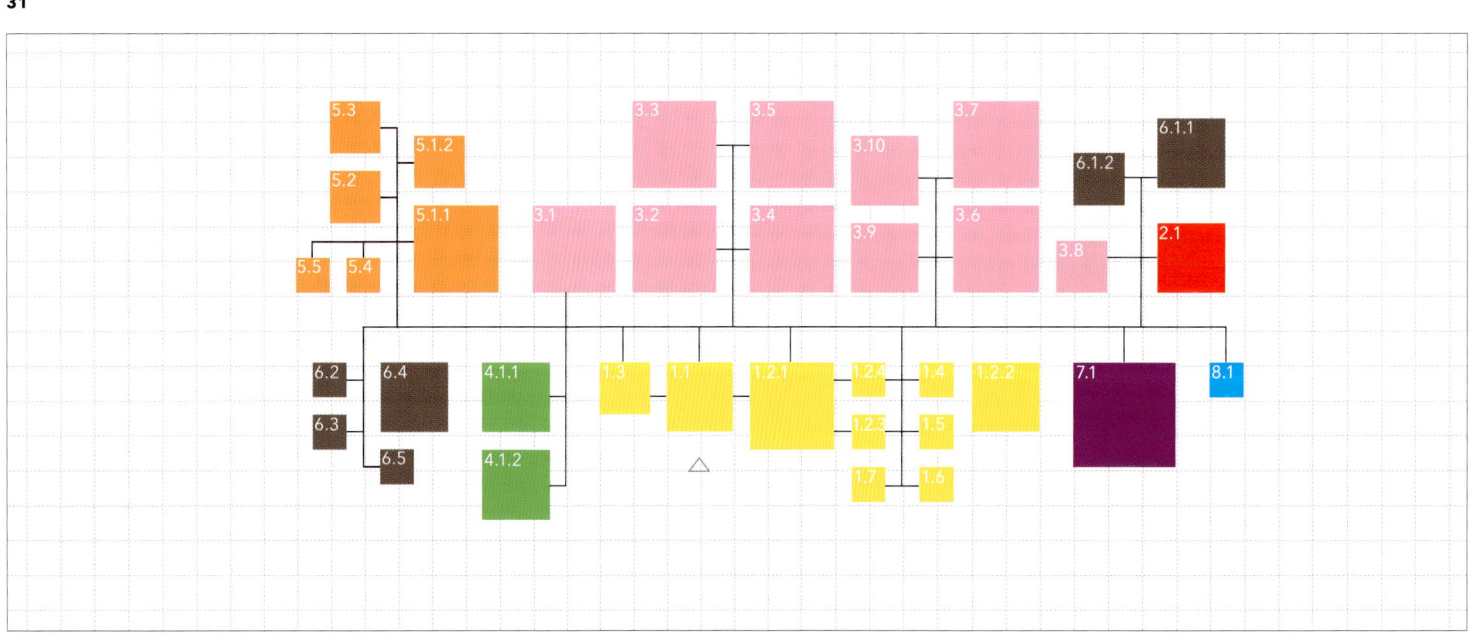

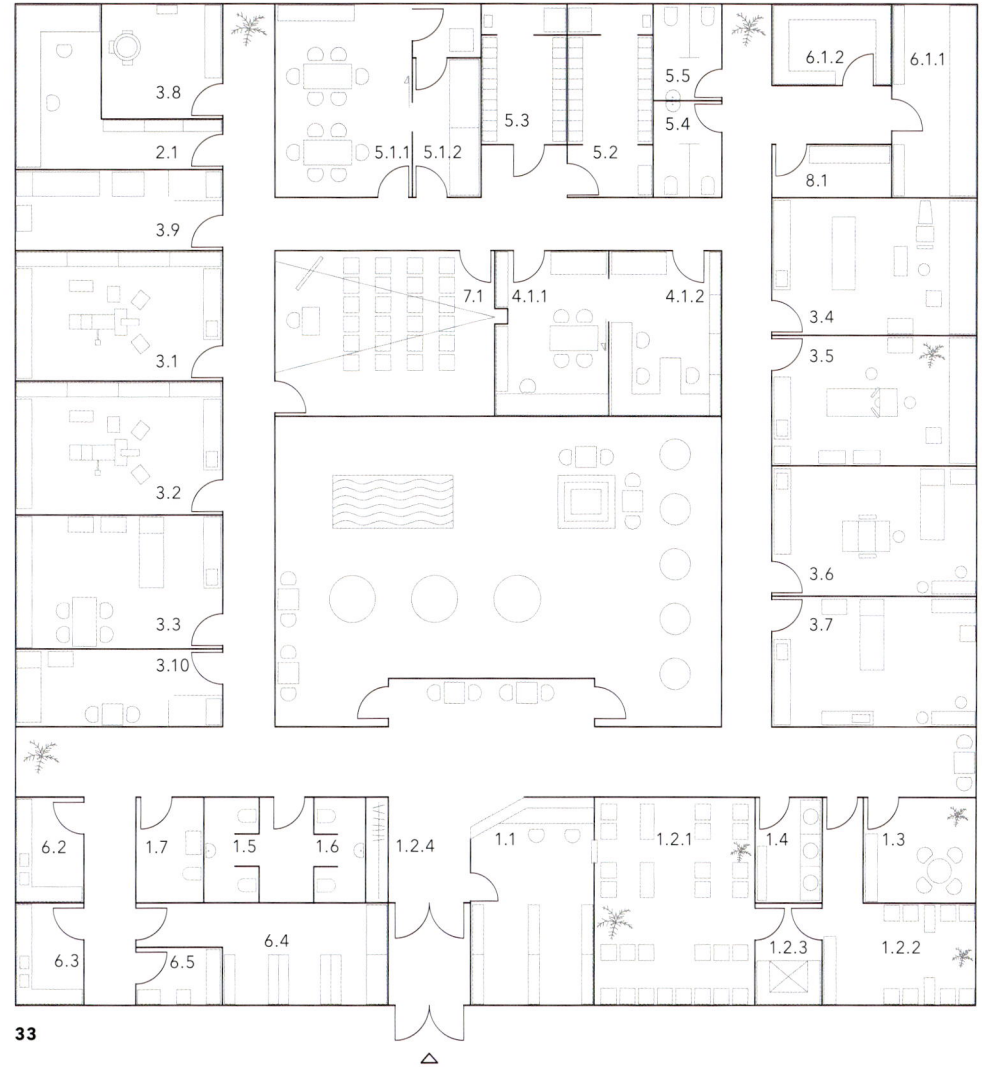

33

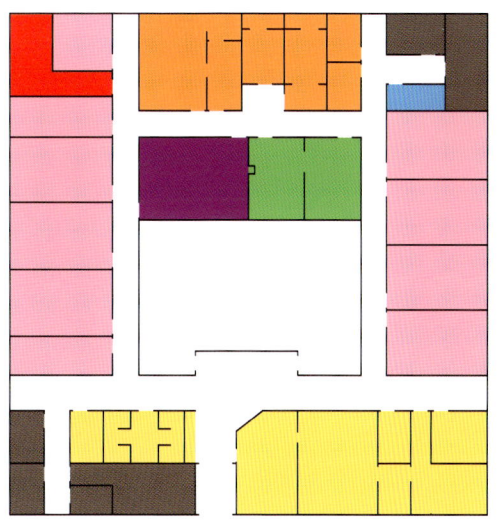

34

31 Example of a functional and spatial allocation plan for a large multi-doctor practice

32 Function scheme of a large multi-doctor practice

33 Standard ground plan of a large multi-doctor practice, scale 1:200

34 Colour scheme for the ground plan of a large multi-doctor practice, scale 1:400

DESIGN FEATURES

External architecture

The appearance of many buildings indicates what purposes they serve. Since medical practices can be important in life, some sort of means of recognition would certainly be helpful. Designers should consider it part of their remit to devise suitable architectural features that would serve as a means of easy identification.

BODY OF THE BUILDING | Medical practices frequently occupy parts of multi-storey buildings which may be residential or commercial blocks or even medical centres. In such cases, the medical practice generally has to fit in with the existing external architecture.

Often, however, medical practices are also designed as separate buildings. In such cases an independent architectural design is possible. The forms of such structures, generally to a maximum of three storeys high, can attract patients and indicate that their visit will be an interesting one. In general there are no limits to the imagination and formal language of the architects. It is a good tip, however, to ensure that, despite the desire to place a somewhat individual stamp on the building, the architecture of the medical practice is in keeping with the landscape and the surrounding buildings. Or as Mies van der Rohe's said: Less is more.

FRONT ELEVATION | Depending on whether the medical practice forms part of a larger building or has the building to itself, the front elevation can display a variety of different features. In the former case, it is often only possible to attach some lighting features showing the name of the medical practice. In the latter case, the scope for design is considerably greater because of the open and closed walls, and through using expressive materials, a variety of colours and light and shade. Here, too, one should guard against producing an excess of sensory impressions which after all are incompatible with the serious character of a medical practice.

ENTRANCE | Patients approaching a medical practice are often not in the best of health and so the main entrance to the practice should be clearly recognisable as such from some distance – as it should also be for the handicapped and those unfamiliar with the locality. It is often useful to include one or two secondary entrances as well to shorten the distances patients need to cover. Other helpful features would be an invitingly designed entrance and lighting to identify the building during the hours of darkness. Automatic doors and a lack of barriers make access easier for patients with wheelchairs and prams. Easy-to-read opening hours information should be displayed in the entrance area. Subject to the Industrial Code, the name of the owner can be displayed as well.

EXTERNAL LIGHTING | External lighting should help patients find their way. It should emphasise the entrance in particular. The intensity of the lighting should be in keeping with the ambient lighting to avoid any possibility of dazzle.

Interior design

Any planner will be aware that spread out in front of him is the whole wide field of architectural design for the interiors of medical practices. Taking his experience as the starting point, he must approach his work with creativity, a solid awareness of quality and knowledge of the effect of hard and soft forms, bright and muted colours, light and shade. He must also use his knowledge of materials paying attention to every single detail.

MATERIALS AND SURFACES | The facilities can be designed with natural surfaces displaying their own natural colouring combined with artificial surfaces in a wide variety of colours. Care should be taken with the whole concept to ensure that hardwearing and easy-to-clean materials are selected.

Because of the demand for hygiene, appliances should be made of durable and hard-wearing materials. Walls can be varied as follows: generally, plastering is sufficient – they can be painted white or in colours or they can be papered. Washable wall coverings should be used for operational and sanitary rooms. Ceilings are usually lowered to accommodate the technical fittings for lighting, ventilation and air conditioning. As such fittings need to be accessible for servicing, ceilings are generally made of panels. These are also often used because they have excellent acoustic properties. So far there have been only a few examples of ceilings used as a showground for highly imaginative designs. Any decision on flooring needs to be made after consideration of a range of aspects. These include the intended effect of the surface within the design concept as a whole, especially the dimensions of the existing substrate [in the case of conversions], the robustness, sound insulation properties, anti-slip properties, ease of cleaning – and crucially its cost-efficiency. Flooring to be laid in the entrance area should include a large enough foot mat, built in and flush with the floor surface.

FURNITURE AND FITTINGS | The ambitious aim of a medical practice planner should be to create an individual character for the practice, especially easy to achieve with well chosen features. Reliance solely on mass produced furniture is less apt to produce this effect, but individually produced designer pieces are often out of reach of the budget. This is an area where the planner must work with sensitivity to select a coherent blend. All the fitting and furnishing components should fuse together into an overarching design concept that expresses the image desired by the medical practice.

Small but important details are places to deposit bags and fittings to hold the walking aids of patients so that they can discuss their medical histories unencumbered.

INTERIOR LIGHTING | Suitably adapted, the principles discussed for the exterior also apply to the interior. Light accompanies patients as soon as they enter and makes it easier for them to find their way. Accent lighting highlights pathways and room notices. It is important to ensure that the lighting brings out the true colours and is warm enough to create a welcoming atmosphere. There will be places where the angle of the lighting will be important – to avoid creating disturbing shadows. Choices for the work rooms should strive for sufficient lighting intensities, lack of dazzle, avoidance of reflections in screens, low energy needs and low rated heat input. The minimum requirements of DIN 5035 and the provisions of the Work Place Directive apply.[21]

COLOURS | Colours are crucial for the appearance of all surfaces and impact psychologically on patients and staff alike. According to Frieling, colours can have the following effects: calming, aggressive, oppressive, encouraging, alienating, soft, alarming, stimulating, warming, eye-directing, constricting, reassuring, pleasant, irritating, distracting, cold, awareness arousing, heightening, cooling, deepening, illuminating, communicative, activating, lightweight, covering, cherishing and recuperative.[31] The right amount of colour can therefore aid way finding in the space, alter proportions and raise moods. Too many bright colours are inadvisable because they generally only generate a short-term effect. The surfaces of facilities, appliances, walls, ceilings and floors, always visible and also generally accessible to the senses through touch, are the main objects that can have design roles and create challenges.

PLANTS | The competent hygienists hold different views on the use of plants in medical establishments. There are rooms in particular need of protection from infection and harmful substances where plants have no place [see the chapter entitled "Environmental Conditions"] and there are rooms where there are no objections for reasons of hygiene against plants. Most of the rooms in medical practices fall into this group. Magnificently coloured flowers and leafy plants exert a refreshing and revitalising effect on patients and staff alike. Particularly, patients coming to the practice for the first time will register the friendly atmosphere the plants help create.

ART | The way a medical practice or some other medical care facility is decorated with artworks can in fact make a clear and memorable statement about the philosophy and spirit of the establishment. There are countless possibilities – so there is no risk of being boring and repetitive. And no artwork once selected has to be on show for ever: variatio delectat. Depending on the means of the operator, modestly priced photos and prints [ideally in clip-in picture frames] can be used to decorate the rooms of the practice – as well as valuable paintings and sculptures. One idea would be to work with art students or famous artists who are generally happy to use the walls of such rooms as display areas for their work.

Careful attention should be paid to artwork selection because it is intended to appeal to a sensitive group of people. So particularly colourful and friendly subjects are definitely to be preferred to sombre scenarios. Schiller's words from the prologue to Wallenstein are worth repeating here: "Life is serious, art serene."

PLANNING AND BUILDING STAGES

Preparatory work
After the initial bright idea to expand, convert or renovate the existing medical practice or to build a new one, the client must assemble a number of basic facts with the main parties involved. No more than brief details are needed for the following tips because these tasks must, of necessity, be taken on by specialist planners with as much experience and expertise as possible.

LOCATION ANALYSIS | As already mentioned in the chapter entitled Location, the choice of location must never be left to chance, whether a new building is being planned, or an extension of an existing practice or even a move to new premises

or the taking over of another practice. Instead, before any planning decision, the determining factors of the location must be analysed with great care. Other important factors are the distances to existing competing medical practices and medical centres and other medical facilities, the transportation situation and links to public transport and parking facilities, population density, the probable incidence of passers-by, the size of possible target groups [families, singles, senior citizens], work and educational opportunities and also cultural and leisure amenities. Not least, the choice of the right location is also dependent on the rent and property prices in the region as well as on one's own financial resources. There may be a choice of locations. Much experience is needed to make the necessary evaluation and weigh up the many facts to be considered and then recommend a priority solution. Such matters are best left to an experienced specialist whose skills will pay for themselves.

OBJECTIVE PLANNING | Objective planning has been recommended for years by specialist groups because of the large number of flawed decisions made in construction. The principles of construction and operation can be worked out with these people [the location analysis discussed above can also form part of this process]. Before conversion work, a target-performance comparison is carried out and schematic

variants are developed for achieving the objectives before the solution to be implemented can be proposed. This will be after the evaluative analysis made in the light of the probable investment and operating costs. Objective planning procedures should also reflect the future developments of the medical practice and possible options for any alterations and the associated extensions. Annex 4 to DIN 13080 "Concepts and Analysis for Objective Planning for General Hospitals"[18] contains helpful hints which naturally apply to medical practices.

SCHEDULING | As well as the ideas emerging from objective planning on the estimated planning process timeframe, a major element in planning in a specific building project is precise scheduling. All phases are subdivided into precise periods and dates for completion are set. An essential feature of effective scheduling is ongoing monitoring and, if necessary, updating. Under the motto "time is money", significant extra costs, which work overruns always entail, can be avoided if a building project is completed on time. This applies particularly to renovations and conversions carried out while business continues. Such situations generally cause disruption and inconvenience that customers and staff alike must tolerate, but they should not be allowed to continue a day longer than absolutely necessary.

FUNCTIONAL AND SPATIAL ALLOCATION PLANNING | Once the basic decisions have been taken on the medical practice being planned, the next essential step is the creation of a functional and spatial allocation plan. Here, too, specialised planners need to be called in, if possible, who will carry out this task right at the start of the whole project. They operate jointly with the manager[s] of the medical practice and designated colleagues. See the chapter on Construction Data for tips on the formal breakdown and the necessary tasks.

Care should be taken to ensure that each room with its required usable floor space is listed in the functional and spatial allocation plan. The best approach at this point is to prepare rough sketches for critical spaces to show evidence of the given usable floor space values. In a good functional and spatial allocation plan no room is forgotten [not even the cleaner's room]. An appropriate area is reserved for the rooms to be developed and no unnecessary areas are required because these not only raise construction costs but also the running costs for the whole life of the practice.

COST PLANNING AND FUNDING | The investment costs incurred through building work are always of concern to the client, but especially at the beginning of the planning process. If at all possible, the client wants to have a clear understanding of the costs at an early stage so that he can make decisions with some confidence. Once he knows the cost frame he has the opportunity,

for example, of opting for the right alternative among the drafts and a standard for the basic features.

A specific empirically established value for the costs per square metres of usable floor space, obtained by making costs analyses of comparable medical practices, will allow an estimate of the total costs to be made. This value needs to be understood as having limitations and must be modified by taking into account local and temporal conditions or different standards. For conversions and renovations, the process described can be applied only to a very limited degree because of the very different characteristics that are possible. This is precisely the point that needs the years of experience of specialist planners.

In Germany medical institutions administered by public authorities, which today are only rarely able to meet their statutory duty to promote investment, have been beset by problems for decades. This backlog of delayed investment has now reached the two-figure billion Euro mark. Since there is scarcely any hope of improvement in the short or long term, new investment models are being developed, for example in the form of public private partnerships [PPP]. These offer a variety of options for the public and private sectors to work together.

In the new Hospital Funding Reform Act[12] the legislation envisages a reform of public investment funding and in § 10 intends to develop

standard investment assessment criteria to apply across Germany so as better to calculate the investment needs of the individual Länder.

Planning services

In the fee code for architects [HOAI][52] § 15 sets out the services to be supplied by contractors. The work fields specified are: new buildings, new equipment, reconstructions, extensions, conversions, modernisations, enlargements to create more space, maintenance and repairs. The services break down into nine service engineering groups in terms of basic services and specialised services; most important of them are treated briefly here.

PREPLANNING | Essential services are analysis of basics, the production of a planning concept including examination of possible alternatives, clarification and illustration of the essential town planning, design, functional, technical, building, commercial and energy efficiency parameters, preliminary negotiations with authorities and a cost estimate subject to DIN 27622. Special services include, for example, the creation of a funding plan and a building work and operating cost benefit analysis.

DESIGN PLANNING | The basic services of design planning comprise first and foremost the design drawings to a scale of 1:100 and for the enlargements to create more space at a scale of 1:50 and 1:20, negotiations with authorities and others involved in planning as specialists as to the design's fitness for approval and a cost calculation subject to DIN 27622.

EXECUTION PLANNING | This phase includes the execution, detail and structural drawings at scales of 1:50 to 1:1, including the materials specifications. These plans are of major importance for medical practices because they determine the organisation of the details.

SITE COORDINATION AND MONITORING | After delivery of the basic services outlined here – Preparation and Involvement in Contract Award, the job of site coordination and monitoring is to review the site to ascertain whether it conforms with the building consent and all relevant provisions regarding the details of the design. The basic services of this phase also encompass the creation of a schedule, the cost statement subject to DIN 27622, the application for official inspection and approval and supervision of the elimination of any defects detected.

COMMISSIONING | Although this is not part of the HOAI service profile, it can be useful to plan the commissioning. This is especially desirable when building work is carried out while the business remains in operation to ensure a prudent, smooth-running transition to the new start. An opening ceremony, with a speech, drinks and small gifts is effective publicity. The author of this text would be delighted to be invited!

SOURCES

1 www.bundesaerztekammer.de

2 www.gbe-bund.de

3 Kuhrt, N.: Gut behandelt. In: ZEIT WISSEN 2009. Number 4. Pages 14–26.

4 Robert Koch-Institut [Ed.]. Böhm, K. | Müller, M.: Ausgaben und Finanzierung des Gesundheitswesens. Heft 45 der Gesundheitsberichterstattung. Berlin 2009. www.gbe-bund.de

5 Gemeinschaft fachärztlicher Berufsverbände. Menzel, H. [Ed.]: Viele Deutsche beklagen Verschlechterung der Gesundheitsversorgung. Facharzt Aktuell 03 | 2009.

6 Sozialgesetzbuch [SGB]. Fünftes Buch [V]. Gesetz of 20.12.1988. BGBL. I. Page 2.477.

7 Kassenärztliche Bundesvereinigung: Aufgaben der Kassenärztlichen Vereinigungen. http://www.kbv.de/wir_ueber_uns/107.html

8 Institut für Qualität und Wirtschaftlichkeit im Gesundheitswesen: Über uns. www.iqwig.de/ueber-uns,21html

9 GKV-Modernisierungsgesetz of 14.11.2003. BGBL. I. 2003. Number 55. Page 2.110 ff.

10 Vertragsarztrechtsänderungsgesetz of 22.12.2006. BGBL. Page 3.439.

11 Krankenhausfinanzierungsgesetz of 10.4.1991. BGBL. I. Page 886.

12 Krankenhausfinanzierungsreformgesetz [KHRG] of 17.3.2009. BGBL. I. Page 534.

13 Kassenärztliche Bundesvereinigung: Überwachungen und Begehungen von Arztpraxen durch Behörden. Berlin 2005.

14 Bundesärztekammer: [Muster-] Richtlinien über den Inhalt der Weiterbildung of 28.3.2008.

15 Schurr, M. | Kunhardt, H. | Dumont, M.: Unternehmen Arztpraxis – Ihr Erfolgsmanagement. Heidelberg 2008.

16 Ärztliches Zentrum für Qualität in der Medizin: Kompendium Q-M-A. Qualitätsmanagement in der ambulanten Versorgung. Cologne 2008³.

17 DIN 277-1: 2005-02. Grundflächen und Rauminhalte von Bauwerken im Hochbau – Part 1: Begriffe, Ermittlungsgrundlagen | DIN 277-2: 2005-02. Grundflächen und Rauminhalte von Bauwerken im Hochbau – Part 2: Gliederung der Netto-Grundfläche [Nutzflächen, Technische Funktionsflächen und Verkehrsflächen] | DIN 277-3: 2005-04. Grundflächen und Rauminhalte von Bauwerken im Hochbau – Part 3: Mengen und Bezugseinheiten.

18 DIN 13080: 2003-07. Gliederung des Krankenhauses in Funktionsbereiche und Funktionsstellen | Beiblatt 1: 2003-07. Gliederung des Krankenhauses in Funktionsbereiche und Funktionsstellen – Hinweise zur Anwendung für Allgemeine Krankenhäuser | Beiblatt 2: 2003-07. Gliederung des Krankenhauses in Funktionsbereiche und Funktionsstellen – Hinweise zur Anwendung für Hochschul- und Universitätskliniken | Beiblatt 3: 1999-10. Gliederung des Krankenhauses in Funktionsbereiche und Funktionsstellen – Formblatt zur Ermittlung von Flächen im Krankenhaus | Beiblatt 4: 2004-07. Gliederung des Krankenhauses in Funktionsbereiche und Funktionsstellen – Begriffe und Gliederung der Zielplanung für Allgemeine Krankenhäuser.

19 Robert Koch-Institut: Anforderungen der Hygiene beim ambulanten Operieren in Krankenhaus und Praxis. Bundesgesundheitsblatt 1994. Number 5.

20 DIN 12924-4: 1994-01. Laboreinrichtungen. Abzüge, Abzüge in Apotheken, Hauptmaße.

21 Verordnung über Arbeitsstätten [Arbeitsstättenverordnung – ArbStättV]. Bundesgesetzblatt I. Page 1.595.

22 DIN 276-1: 2006-11. Kosten im Bauwesen – Part 1: Hochbau.

23 Müller, S. K. – Chemical Sensitivity Network [CSN]: Umweltbedingungen in der Arztpraxis des 21. Jahrhunderts – Gesünder für Arzt und Patient. www.csn-deutschland.de

24 Robert Koch-Institut: Anforderungen der Hygiene an die funktionelle und bauliche Gestaltung von Krankenhauseinrichtungen für die Versorgung ambulanter Patienten. Bundesgesundheitsblatt 1980. Number 11. Page 164–165.

25 DIN 4109: 1989-11. Schallschutz im Hochbau. Anforderungen und Nachweise [vorgesehener Ersatz durch DIN 4109-1: 2006-10].

26 DIN 4102-1: 1998-05. Brandverhalten von Baustoffen und Bauteilen – Part 1: Baustoffe, Begriffe, Anforderungen und Prüfungen.

27 Wiener Krankenanstaltenverbund [Ed.]. Aumayr, J. | Herbek, S. | Kastl, J. | Labryga, F. | Mejstrik, W. | Staudinger, Ch.: Planungshandbuch für Krankenhäuser und Pflegeheime. Vienna 2003.

28 Damaschke, S. | Scheffer, B. | Schossig, E.: Arztpraxen, Planungsgrundlagen und Architekturbeispiele. Leinfelden-Echterdingen 2003².

29 Teut, A. | Nedeljkov, G.: Die Gruppenpraxis. Düsseldorf 1973.

30 DIN 5035-8: 2007-07. Beleuchtung mit künstlichem Licht – Part 8: Arbeitsplatzleuchten.

31 Frieling, H.: Farbe am Arbeitsplatz. Munich 1992.

32 Honorarordnung für Architekten und Ingenieure in der ab 1.1.1996 gültigen Fassung. Stuttgart | Berlin | Cologne 1995. Revision on 18.8.2009.

PROJECTS

GENERAL MEDICINE

OPHTHALMOLOGY

SURGERY

DERMATOLOGY

GASTROENTEROLOGY

OBSTETRICS

VASCULAR SURGERY

GYNAECOLOGY

OTOLARYNGOLOGY

INTERNAL MEDICINE

CARDIOLOGY

PAEDIATRICS AND YOUTH MEDICINE

COSMETIC SURGERY

ORAL AND MAXILLOFACIAL SURGERY

NATUROPATHY

NEUROSURGERY

NEUROLOGY

NUCLEAR MEDICINE

ORTHOPAEDICS

OSTEOPATHY

OTONEUROLOGY

PHYSIOTHERAPY

PLASTIC SURGERY

PSYCHIATRY

PSYCHOTHERAPY

RADIOLOGY

RADIOONCOLOGY

PAIN THERAPY

RADIOTHERAPY

UROLOGY

DENTISTRY

The unusual shape of the "silver tower", a former hotel dating back to the 1970s, with its striking oval façade and rounded windows provided the template for the practice conversion.

Over one entire floor, the previous haphazard room structure was broken up and divided into several zones. In the centre is the new, transparent foyer, which extends between two treatment areas. Flush, amorphously shaped ceiling lights guide the patient from the entrance to reception and the waiting area. High-gloss white walls divide the open floor plan into separate areas, without hemming it in. The reflective surfaces visually extend the room – the flush inset pigeonholes, the visitor's coat-rack and the X-ray storage room do not detract from the overall impression of openness. All superfluous fittings have been removed, the bearing structure has been pared right down and the fire doors concealed. Dark furniture stands on the light grey rubber floor; the glossy varnished reception desk and the low waiting area tables are curved. The colour fluctuates between dark blue and petrol green depending on the angle of view. The twelfth floor of the "Silver Tower" affords stunning views over the city; light curtains can be drawn if necessary.

BHEND.KLAMMER   **ORTHOPAEDICS AT ROSENBERG**
ST. GALLEN | CH

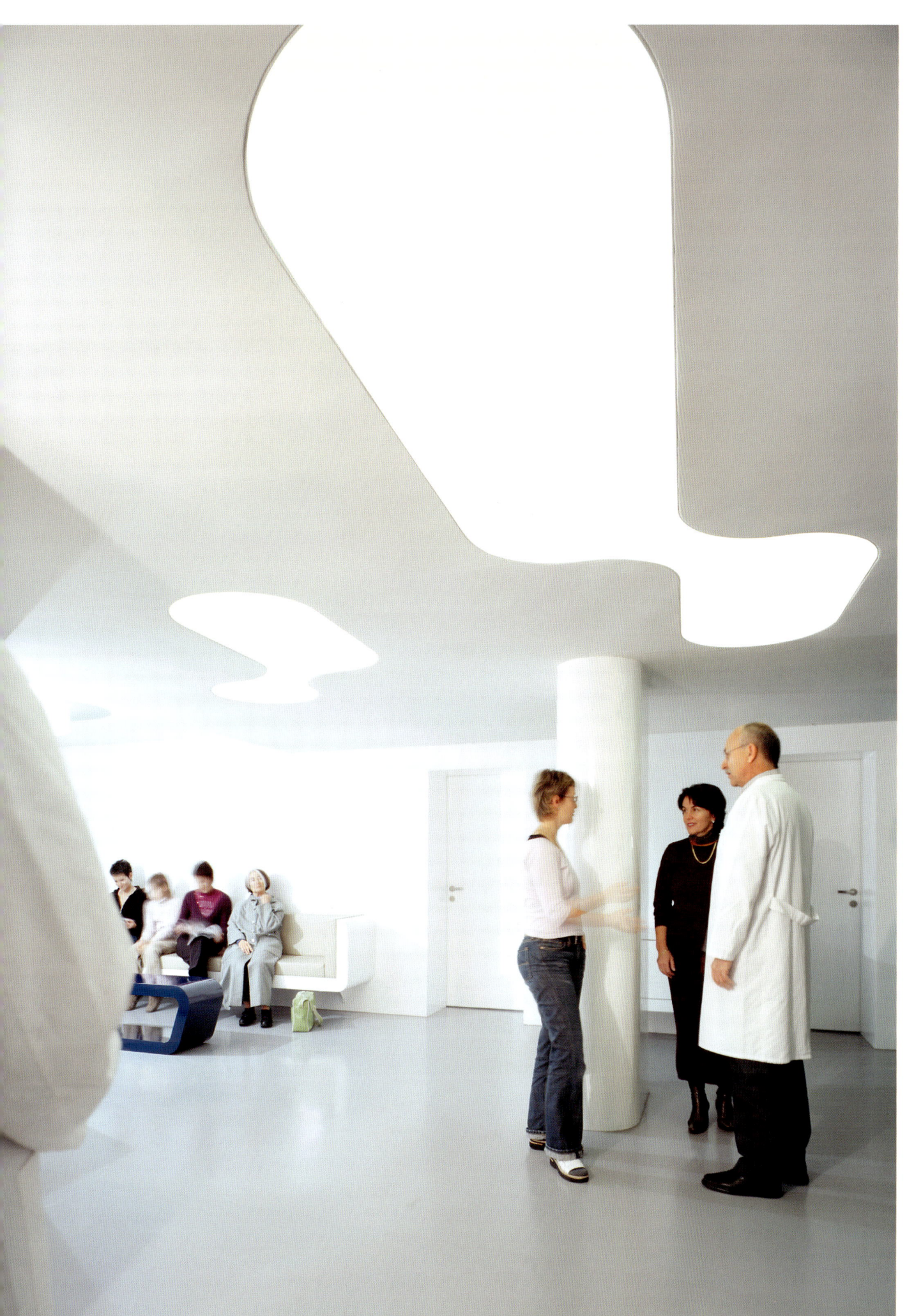

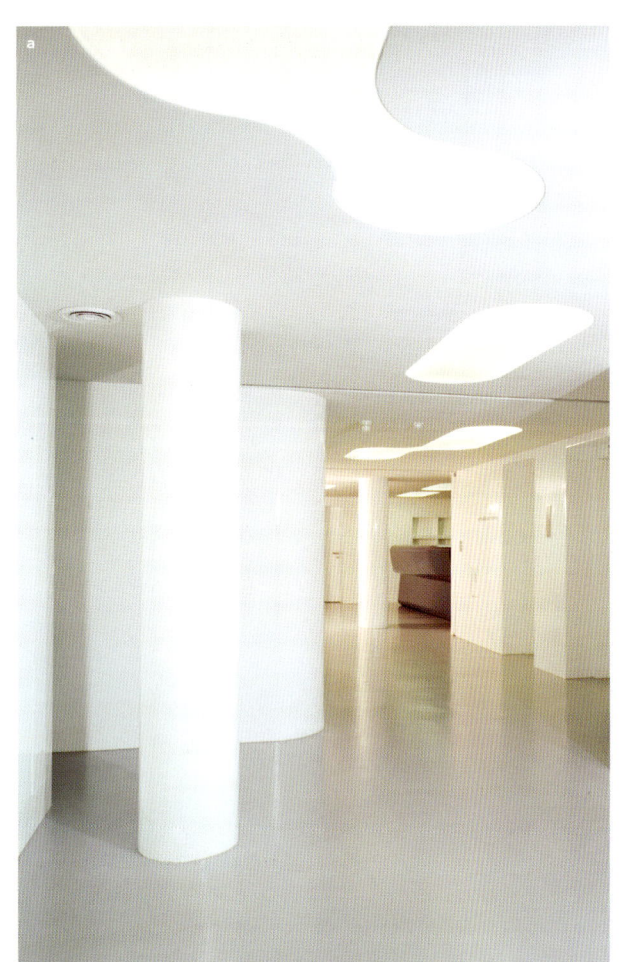

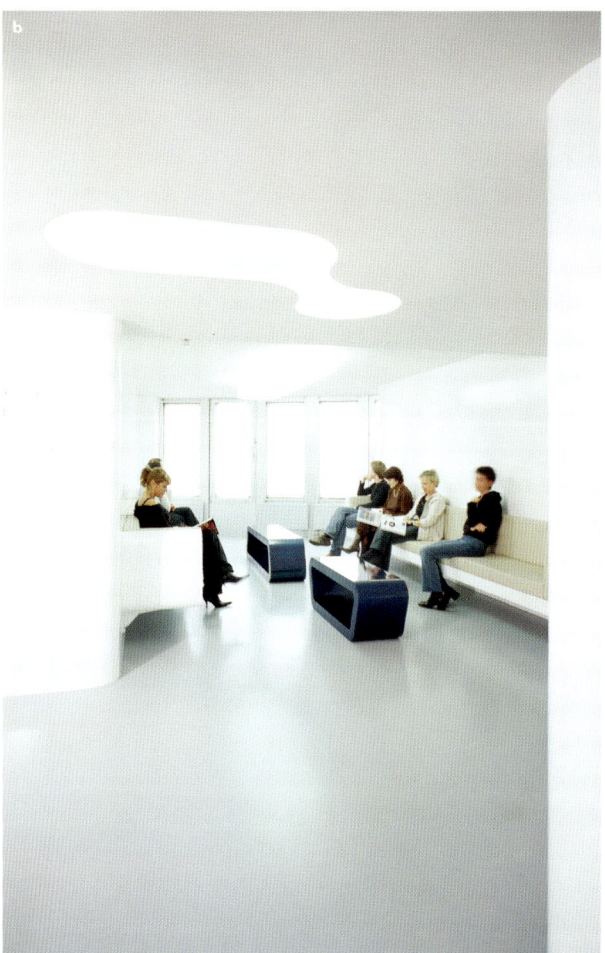

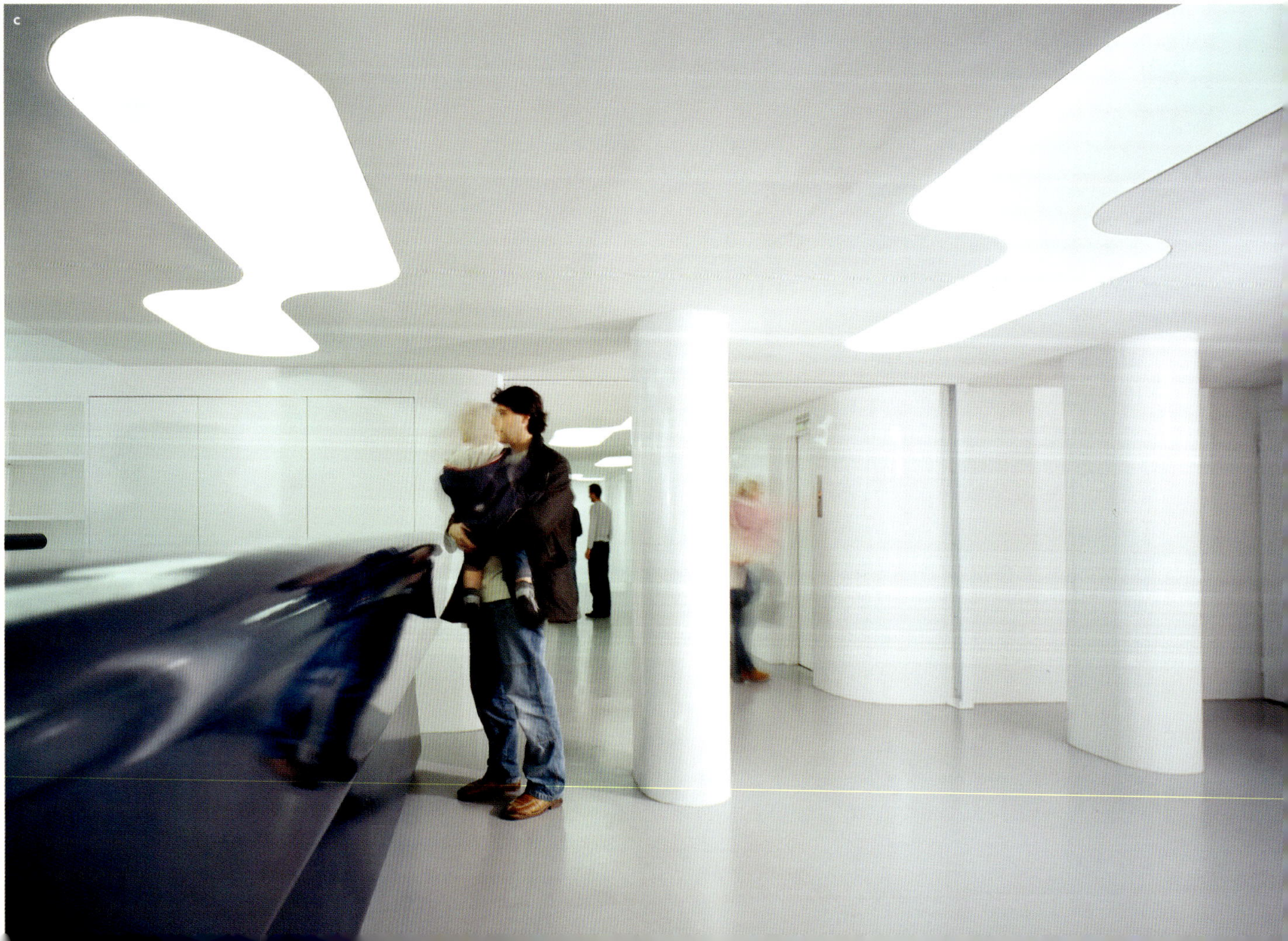

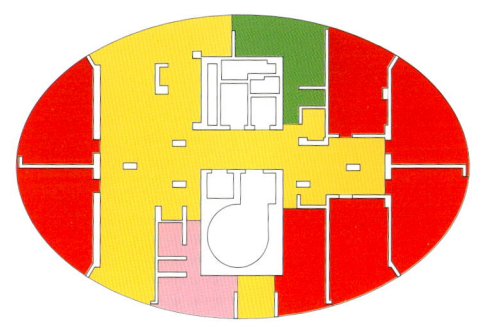

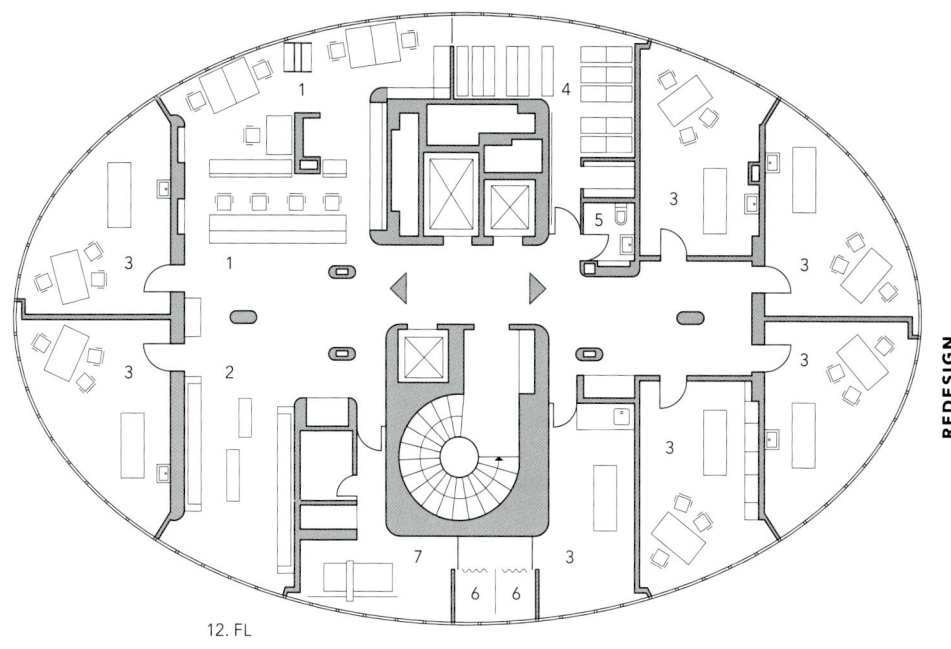

12. FL

**Client	Operator**	Orthopaedics at Rosenberg
Planning time	2003 – 2004
Construction time	07 2004 – 08 2004
Usable floor space	291 sqm
Gross cubic capacity	1,460 cbm
Total cost	600,000 EUR

a During conversion superfluous fittings were removed and the bearing structure pared right down.

b The open floor plan is broken up into individual areas by high-gloss white walls.

c The varnished reception desk, petrol green | dark blue depending on the angle of view, contrasts with the light grey rubber floor.

Diagrammatic plans, to scale 1:400
Floor plans, to scale 1:200

Floor plan layout

1 Reception	**4** Filing room	**6** Changing cubicle
2 Waiting area	**5** Patient toilet	**7** Examination X-ray
3 Treatment room		

Usable floor spaces

Patient rooms	**yellow**	121 sqm	42 %
Examination			
Treatment rooms	**red**	134 sqm	46 %
Specialist rooms	**pink**	17 sqm	6 %
Administrative rooms	**green**	19 sqm	6 %
Total		291 sqm	100 %

Performance data

Outpatients per year	10,000
Number and type of services per year	X-rays [6,500]
Clinic opening hours	5 days	50 hours
Waiting time [with	without appointment]	10 – 20 min.	45 min.
Number of staff	15
Clinic planning advice	Further expansion of reception and waiting area

Keen to extend the range of services it offers, the Cologne Cosmetic Dentistry Clinic has added on a prophylaxis area and a laboratory. These rooms are directly adjacent to the existing clinic, but have their own separate entrance, reception and waiting area.

Although the design of the prophylaxis area contrasts with that of the existing practice rooms, it harmonises with them in terms of colour. The gleaming, almost clinical white chosen by the architects as a healing colour predominates in both clinic and prophylaxis area. Yellow and green light panels provide strong colour accents. The design focus is on the open-plan reception and waiting area with its unostentatious white reception desk positioned in front of the ceiling-high window façade. Natural light shines in through the large panes to illuminate the bright and cheerful waiting area opposite. Large pendulum lights and bench seating in dark upholstery create a welcoming and relaxing environment. The range of services on offer includes a dental shop, which is housed in the lockable, discreetly lit wall cupboard behind the desk.

BRANDHERM +KRUMREY

PROPHYLAXIS CLINIC
COLOGNE | G

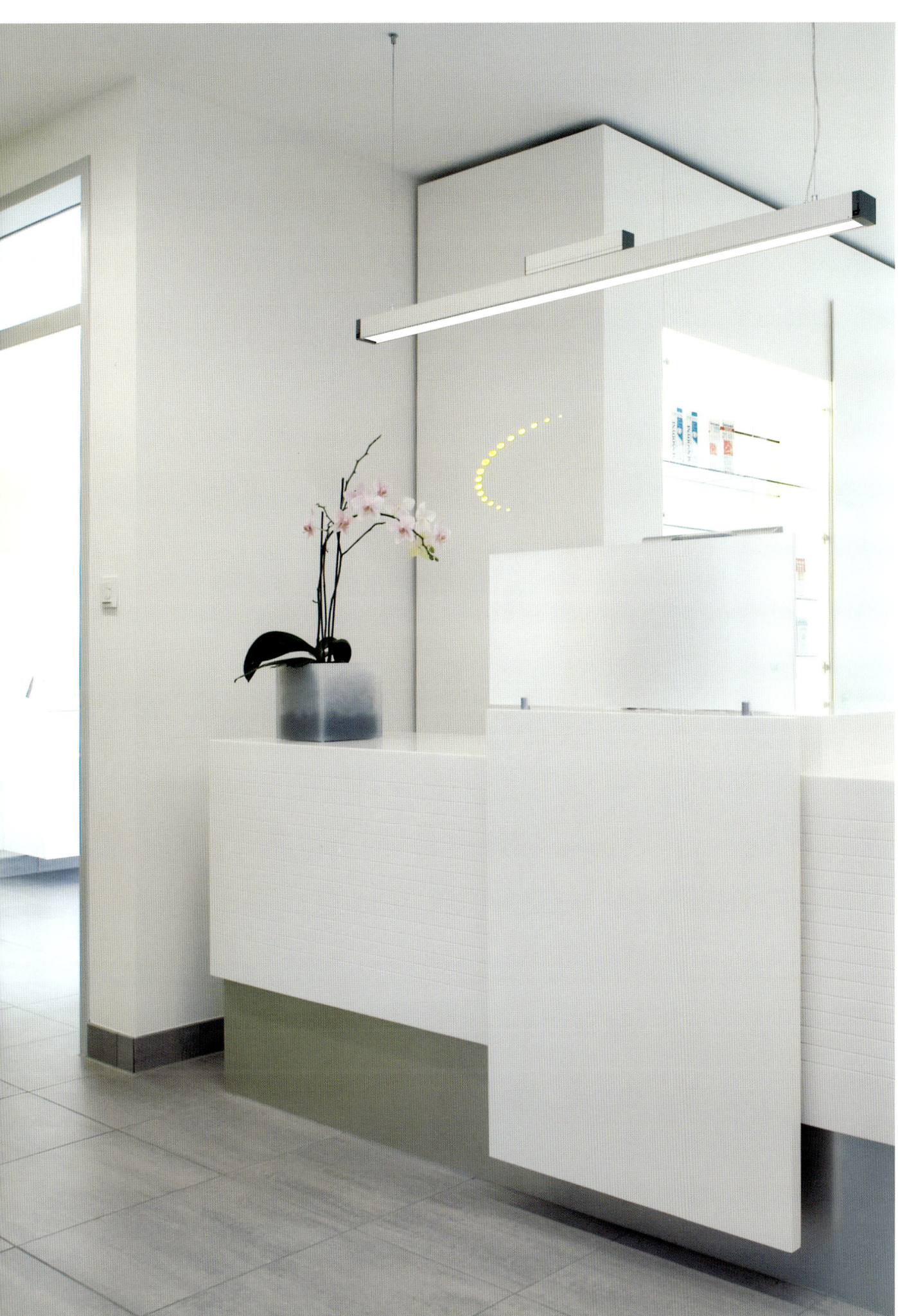

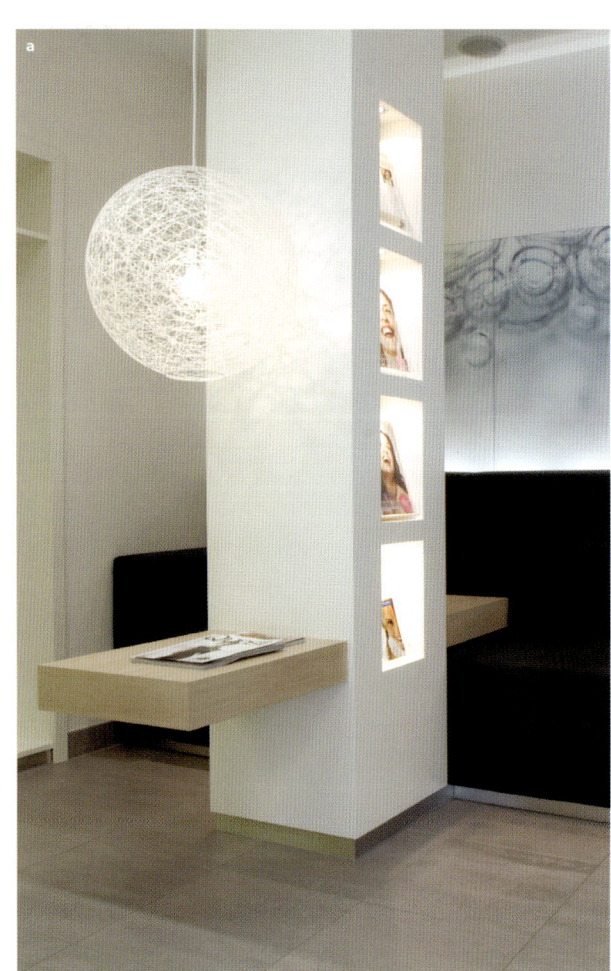

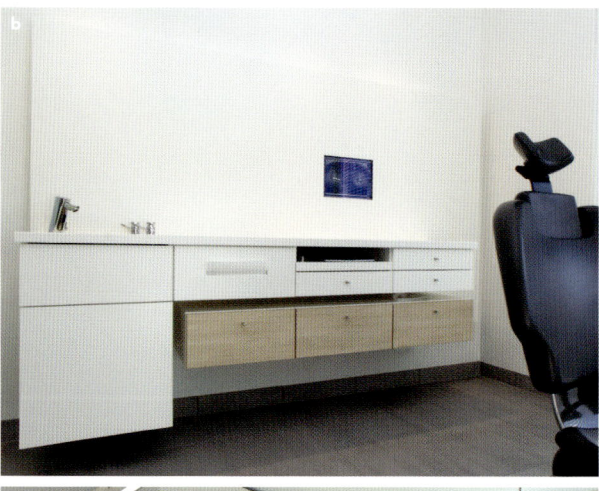

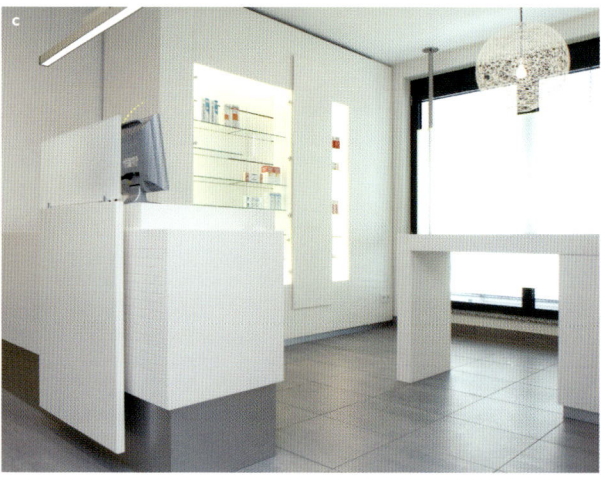

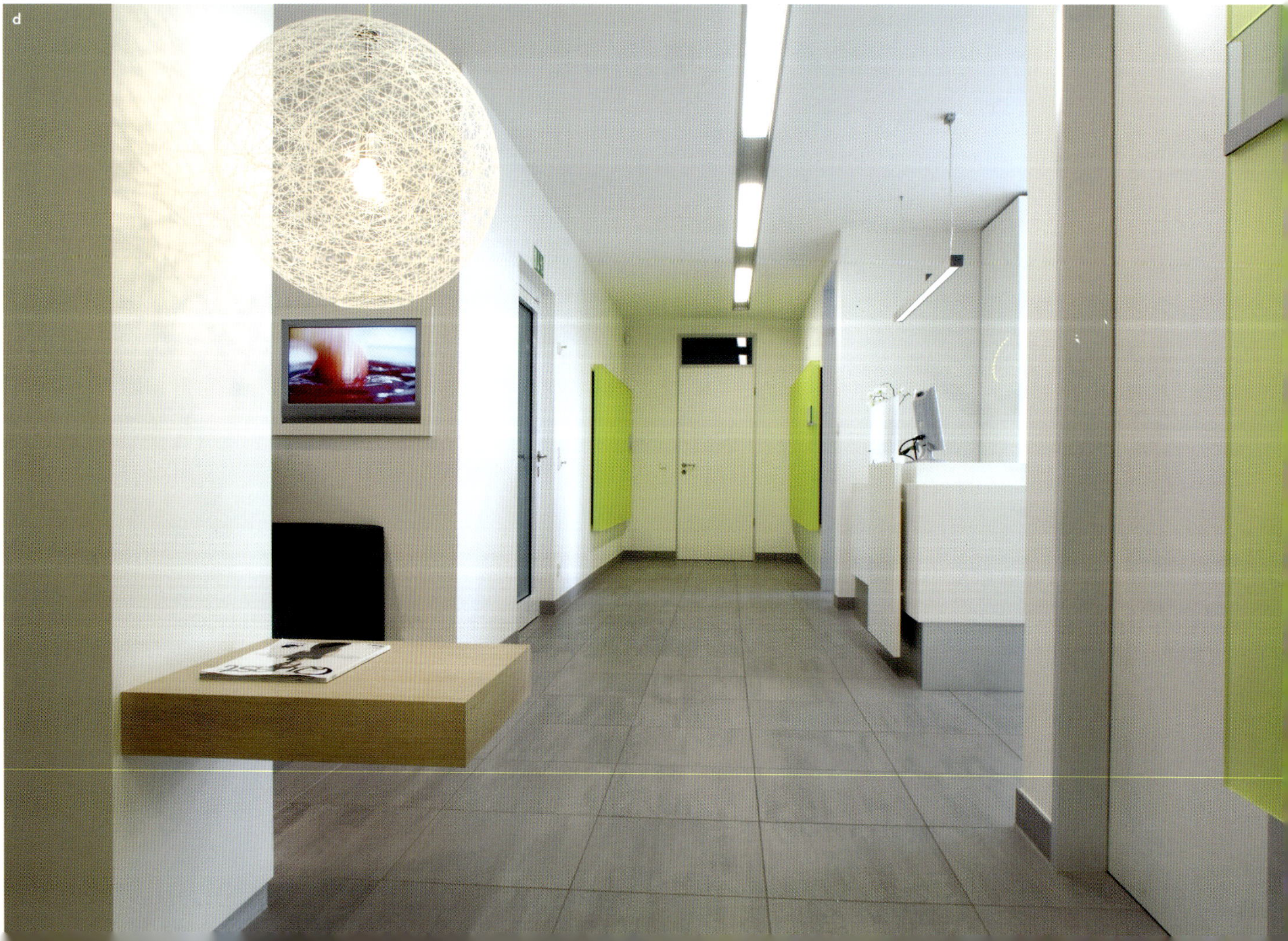

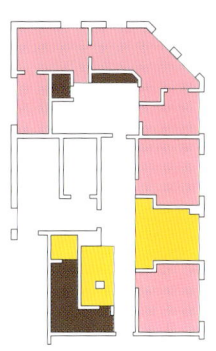
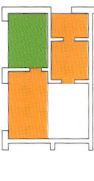

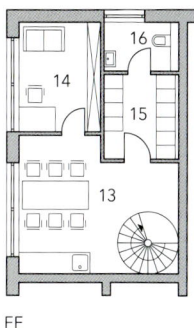

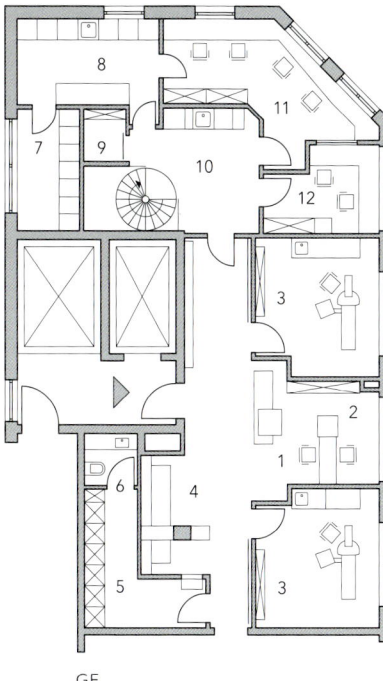

FF

GF

Client | Operator   Dr. Daniel Förster-Marenbach
    Dr. Maike Marenbach
Construction time   2006
Usable floor space   124 sqm
Gross cubic capacity   400 cbm

a   The waiting area with comfortable bench seating in dark upholstery invites patients to relax.
b   The shining white chosen as a healing colour makes the treatment rooms bright and welcoming.
c   A small dental shop behind the reception desk supplements the range of services offered by the prophylaxis clinic.
d   Brilliant yellow light panels provide strong colour accents in the foyer.

Diagrammatic plans, to scale 1:400
Floor plans, to scale 1:200

Floor plan layout

1 Reception	**6** Patient toilet	**13** Staff lounge
2 Consultation room prevention	**7** Cast room	**14** Office and store room
3 Treatment room prevention	**8** Plaster room	**15** Staff changing cubicle
4 Waiting area	**9** Cleaning room	**16** Staff toilet
5 Store room	**10** Sterilisation room	
	11 Plant room	
	12 Ceramic room	

The prophylaxis annex has its own suite of room, concentrated along one corridor with extensions. A separate rear corridor section houses the sterilisation room, which would benefit from being more firmly screened off. A spiral staircase leads to the upper floor and to the administrative and staff rooms.

Usable floor spaces

Patient rooms	**yellow**	21 sqm	17 %
Specialist rooms	**pink**	67 sqm	54 %
Administrative rooms	**green**	7 sqm	6 %
Offices	Staff rooms	**orange**	17 sqm	14 %
Supply	Waste disposal	**brown**	12 sqm	9 %
Total		124 sqm	100 %

Performance data

Outpatients per year	1,500
Clinic opening hours	4 days prophylaxis
	5 days laboratory
Waiting time	5 – 10 min.
Type and number of staff	2 – 3 technicians
	1 – 2 dental hygienists

Think positive! This uplifting motto provided the inspiration for the conversion of the existing premises of the Cologne Specialist Clinic. The reception and waiting area, which does not benefit from natural light, has been transformed into a "thoroughly feel-good environment". This Centre for Radio-Oncology is normally the preserve of seriously ill, mainly male patients. During their time at the clinic they need to feel that they are in good hands, well cared for and, if possible, should not be kept waiting for treatment. On this basis, the small waiting area located in a brightly lit corner is adequate. A light wall with a floral photo motif creates a relaxed atmosphere, while in the foyer a large backlit photo wall creates an impression of floodlit space. The materials are a study in contrasts: high gloss versus matt, translucent versus opaque colour.

A distinctive technical feature of the practice is the ten-tonne X-ray protection room with its ultra-modern equipment. During radiation therapy patients have to spend several minutes alone in this room; its bright splash of colour is therefore intended to be especially attractive.

BRANDHERM +KRUMREY

CENTRE FOR RADIO-ONCOLOGY
COLOGNE | G

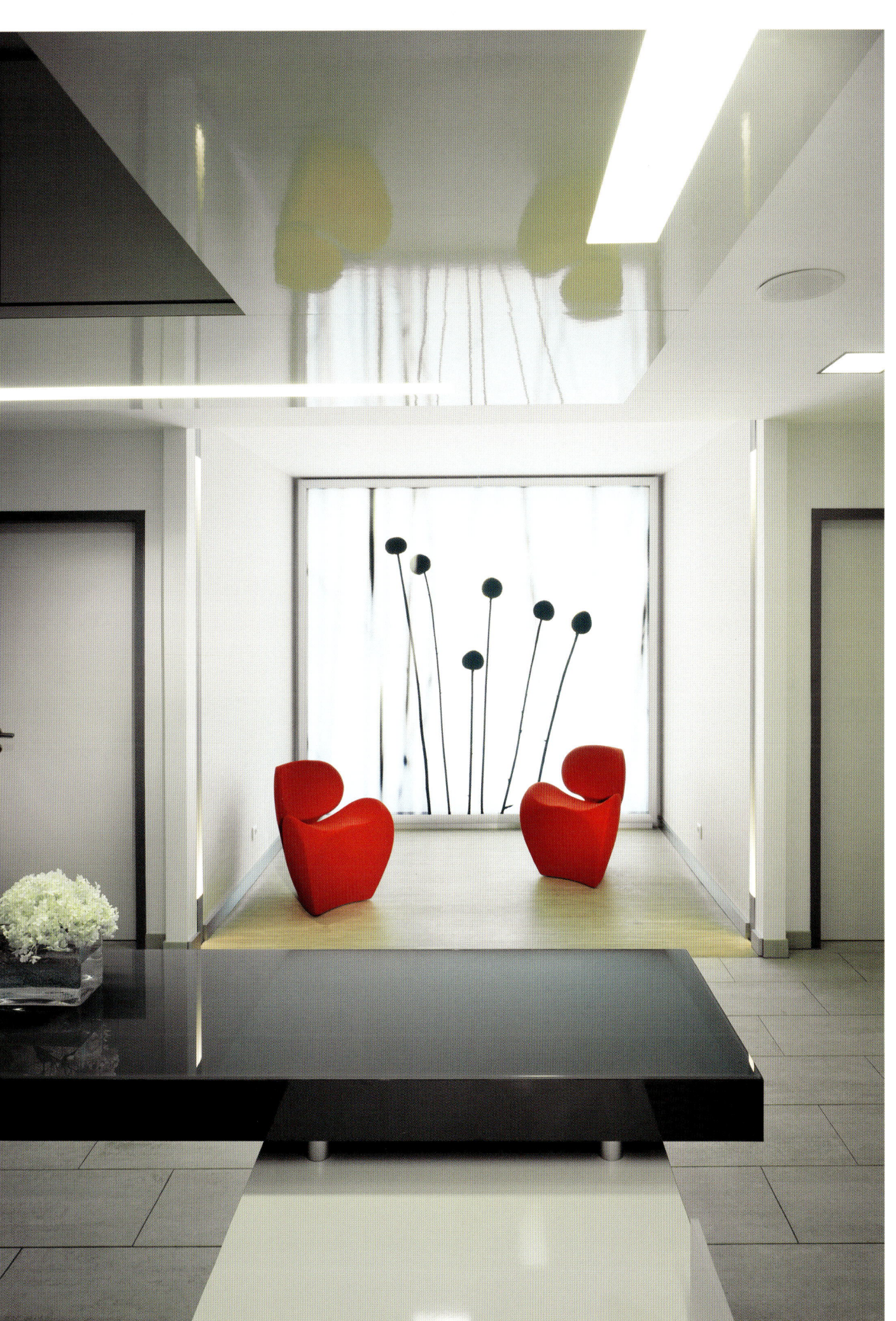

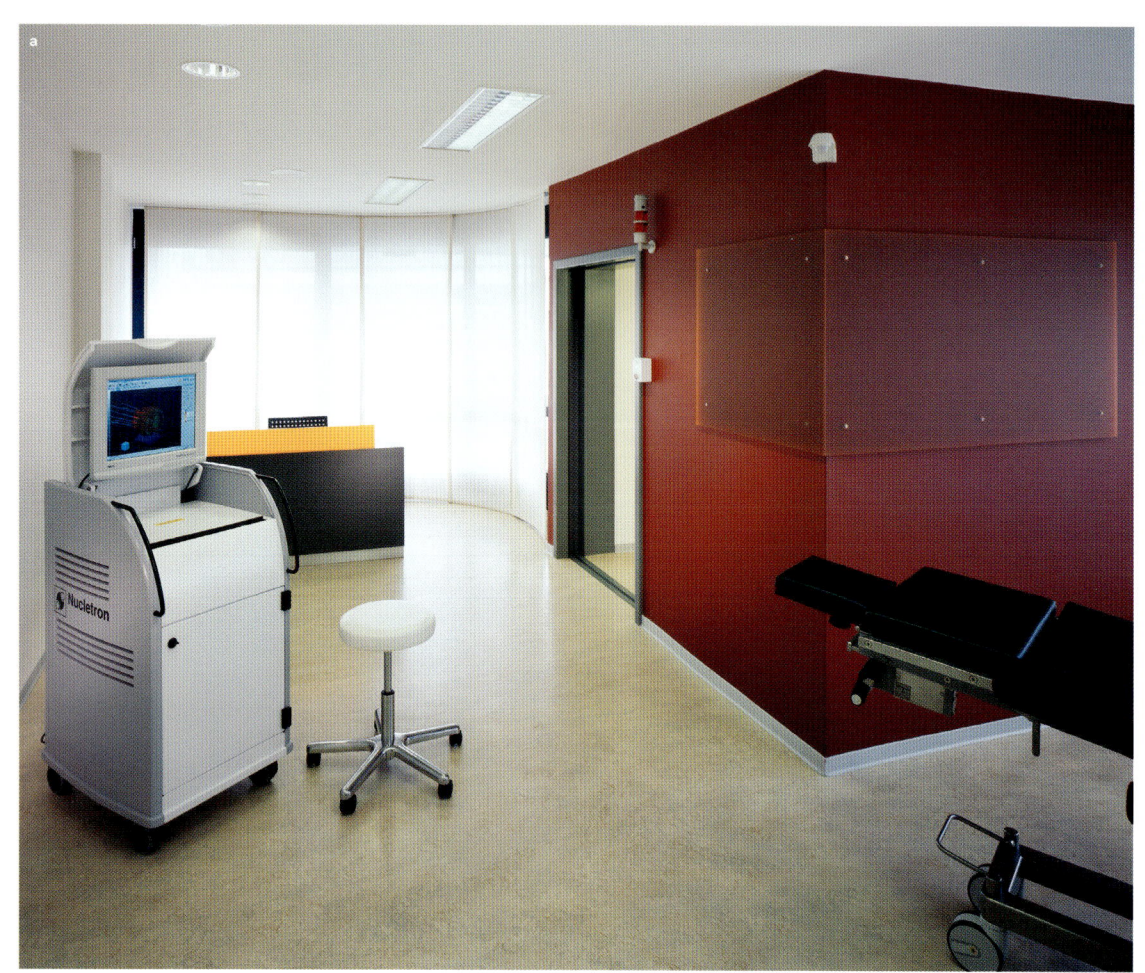

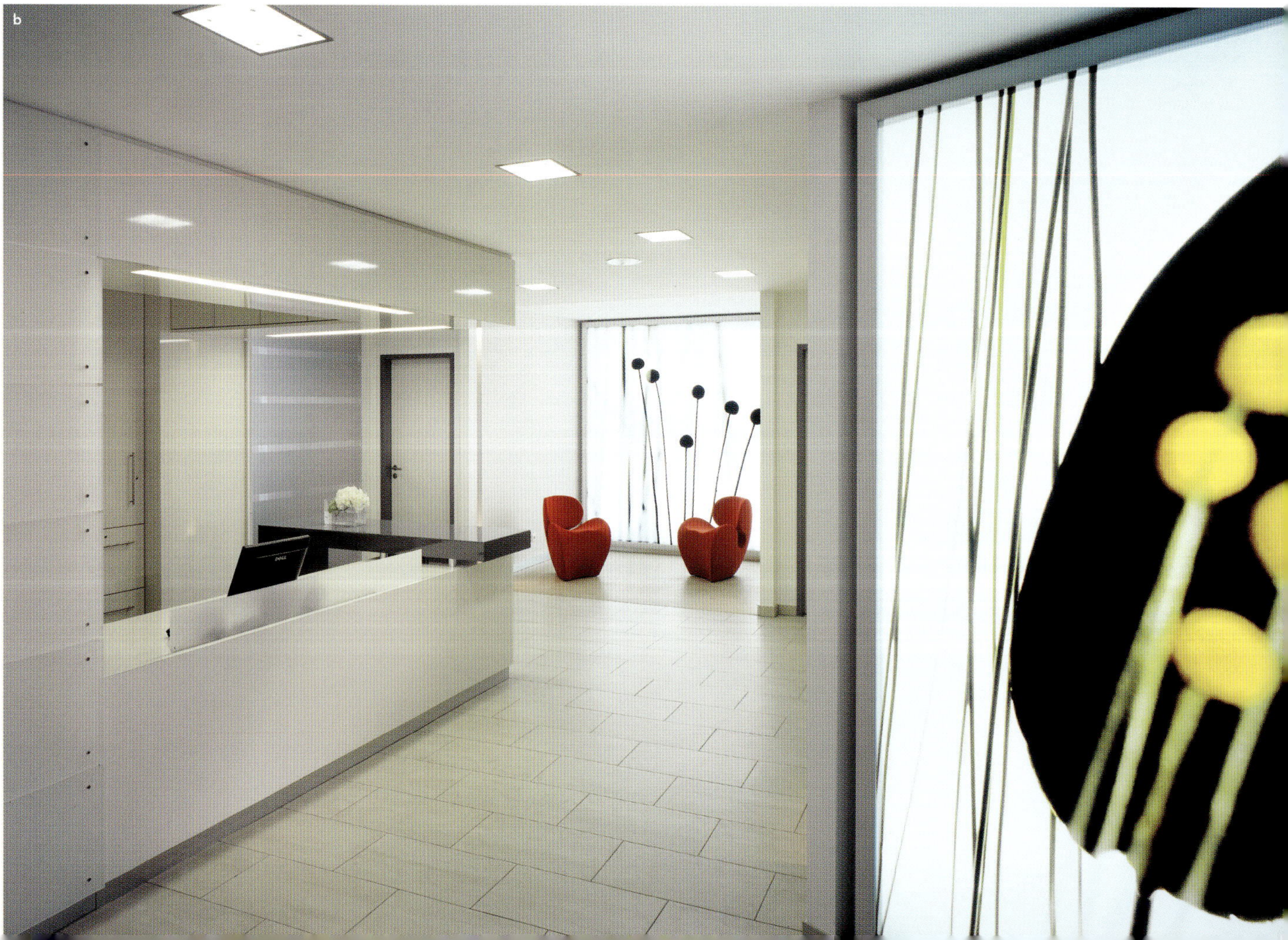

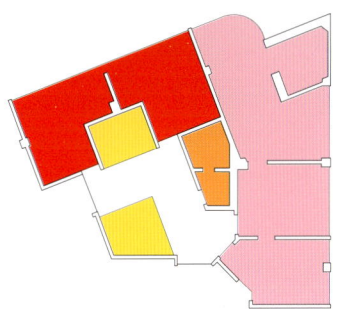

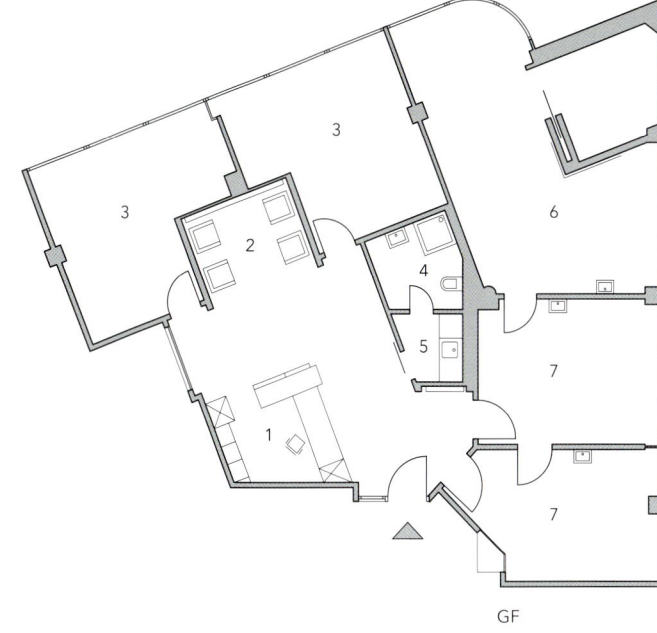

GF

Client	Dr. Gregor Spira
	Jürgen Metz
Operator	Dr. Gregor Spira
	Dr. Carsten Weise
Construction time	02 2003 – 04 2003
Usable floor space	165 sqm
	Redesign [in part]
	42 sqm

a The X-ray protection room behind the red
wall is equipped with an ultra-modern
system.
b The large backlit photo wall in the foyer
creates the impression of a floodlit space.

Diagrammatic plans, to scale 1:400
Floor plans, to scale 1:200

Floor plan layout

1	Reception	**4**	Staff toilet and	**6**	Radiotherapy
2	Waiting area		shower	**7**	Examination and
3	Consultation room	**5**	Small kitchen		recovery room

From the entrance to the triangular floor plan of the partnership practice,
patients proceed into a large room, past the reception desk, with its
unobstructed sight lines into the waiting area. On the other two sides of
the triangle, the consultation, examination and recovery rooms, some of
them interconnected, benefit from full natural light. A patient toilet, staff
lounge, administrative office, storage and cleaning facilities would be useful
additions.

Usable floor spaces

Patient rooms	**yellow**	19 sqm	12 %
Examination |			
Treatment rooms	**red**	48 sqm	29 %
Specialist rooms	**pink**	89 sqm	54 %
Offices | Staff rooms	**orange**	9 sqm	5 %
Total		165 sqm	100 %

Performance data

Outpatients per year	470 – 550
Inpatients per year	400
	[1,200 nursing days]
Number and type of services per year	LDR [170], HDR [500]
Clinic opening hours	5 days | 40 hours
Waiting time	10 – 45 hours
Type and number of staff	2 specialists
	3 part-time staff

Close to the Allgäu mountains! The surrounding mountain scenery is reflected in the interior design of this new dental practice: backlit friezes provide decorative light sources in the waiting area and even the dominant colour, blue, references the nearby mountains. The colour palette – varying shades of blue contrasting with orange – was chosen specifically for its psychological effect: calming and relaxing, cooling and therapeutic. People often dread a visit to the dentist, and the interior concept is intended to allay their fears. Cool, soothing blue is counterbalanced by a warm cheerful orange, reinforcing the healing effect. Dark oak parquet flooring leads patients through the public areas.

The upper floor of the gutted mansion in the centre of Marktoberdorf, which dates back to 1723, houses a cuboid sterilisation room, around which the treatment rooms are arranged. Glass doors backed by translucent film printed with poetry create a feeling of space and transparency, at the same time entertaining and relaxing the patients.

KLAUS R. BÜRGER   **DENTAL CLINIC**
MARKTOBERDORF | G

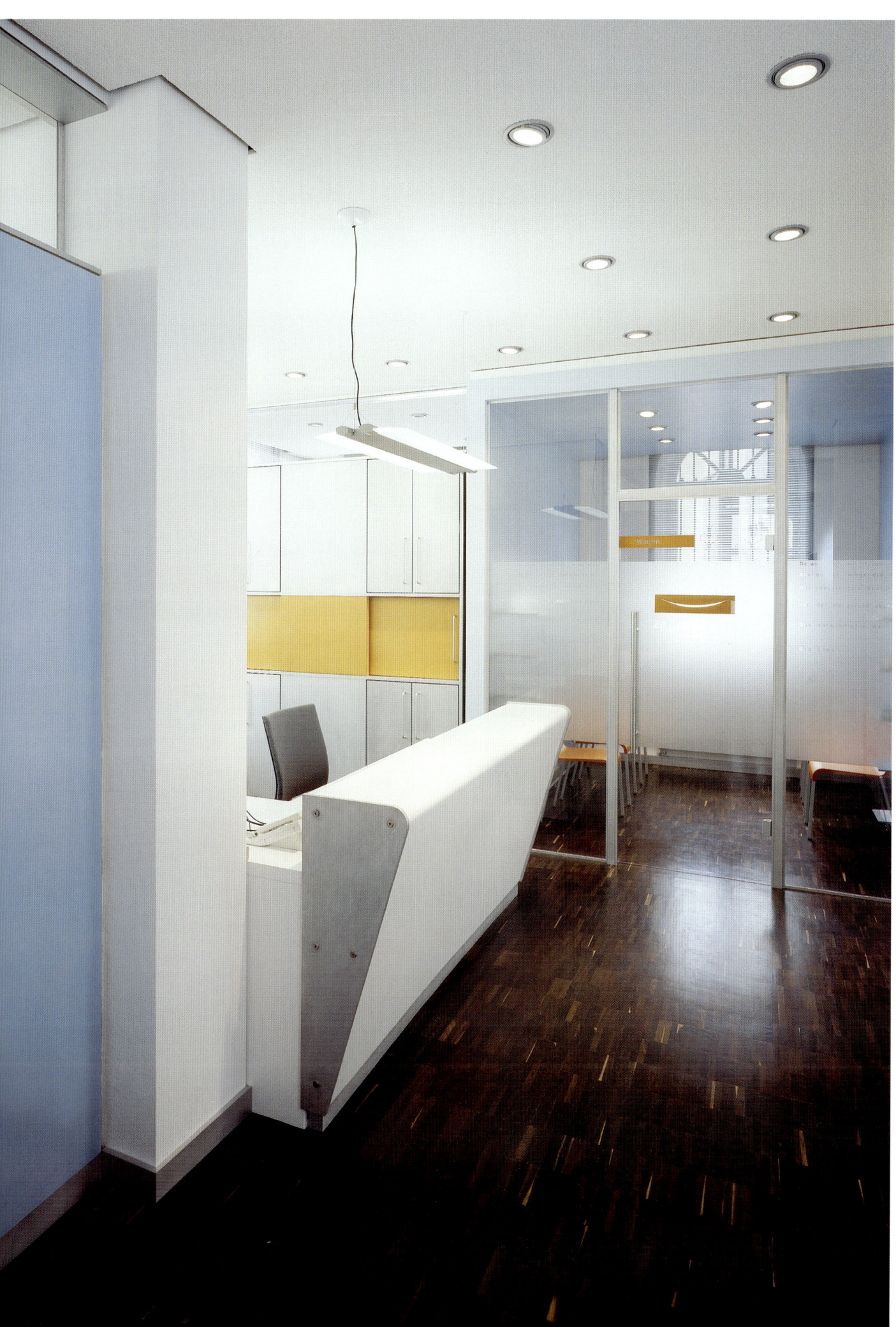

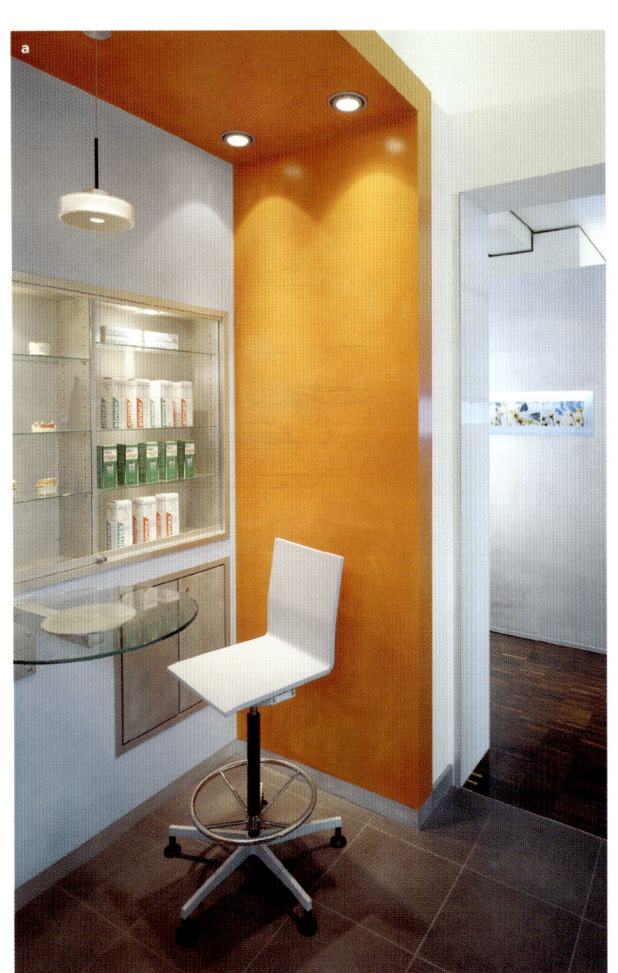

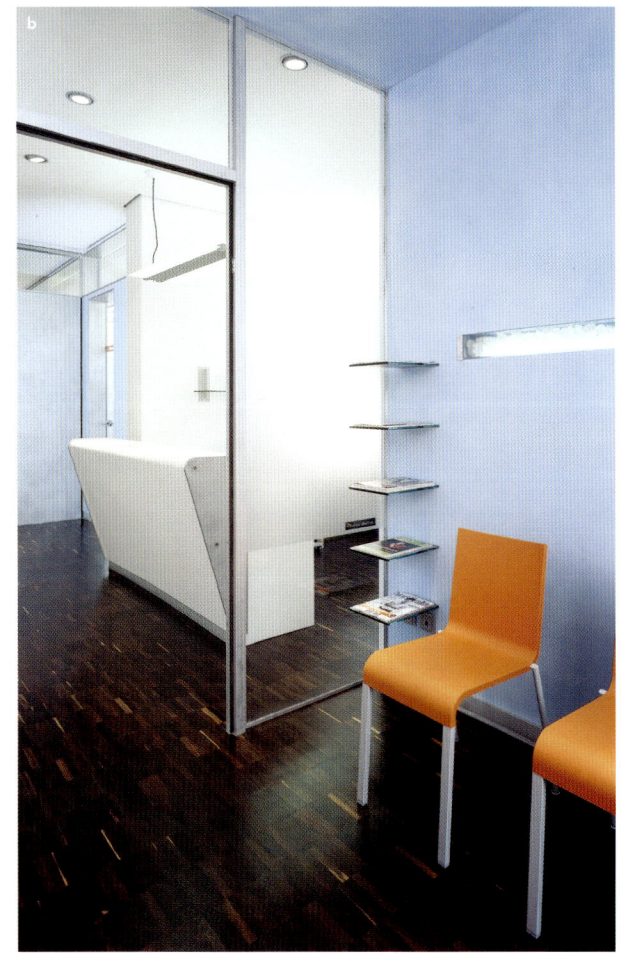

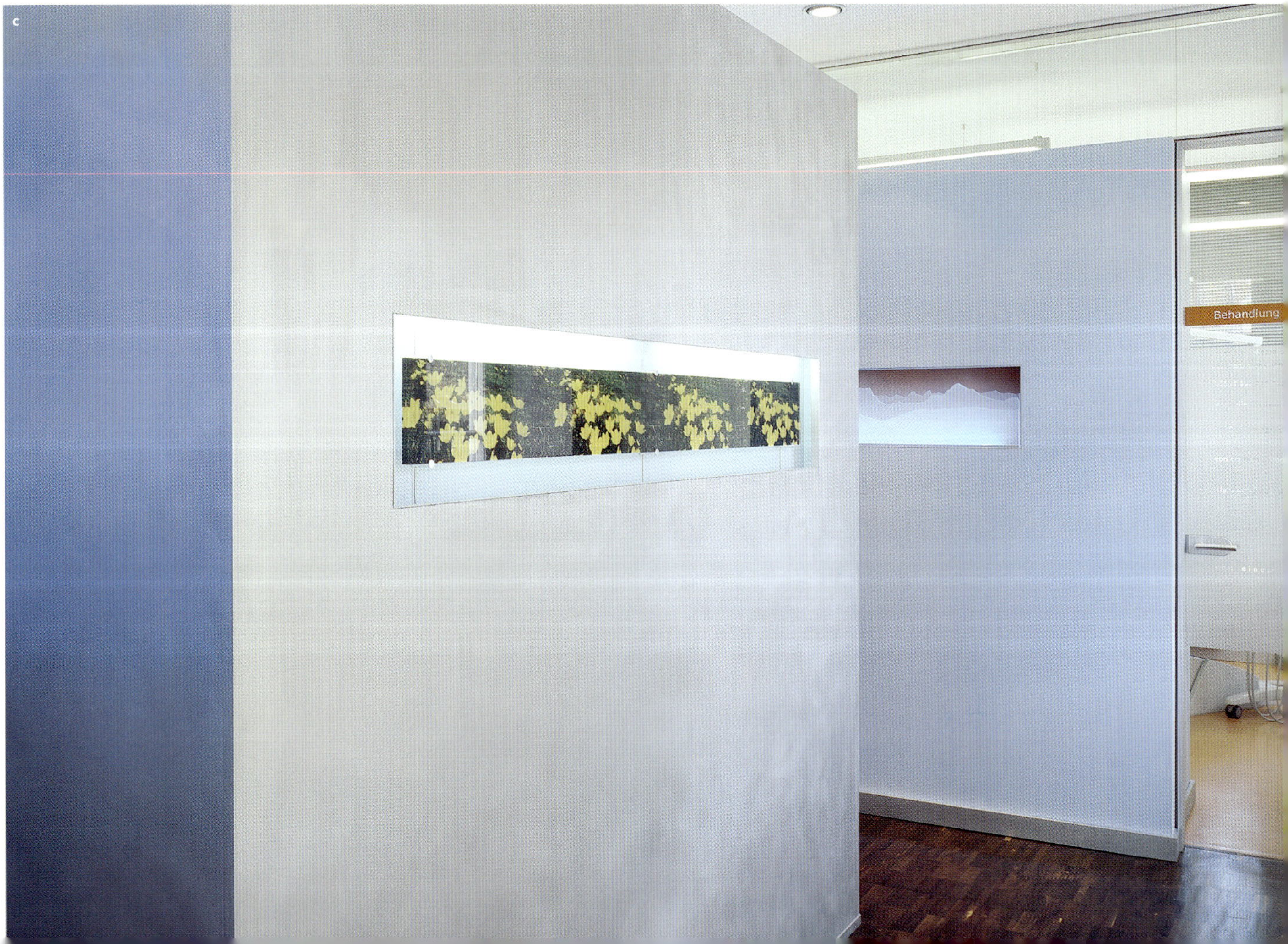

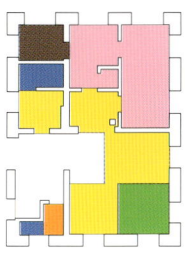
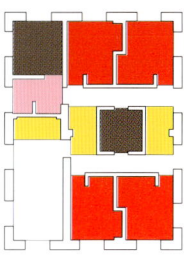
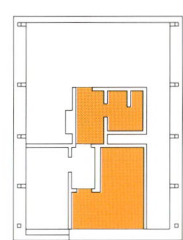

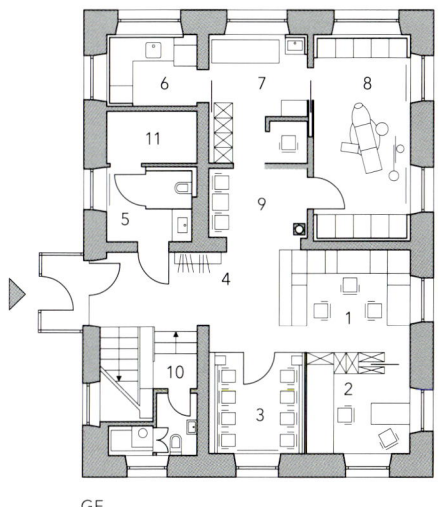
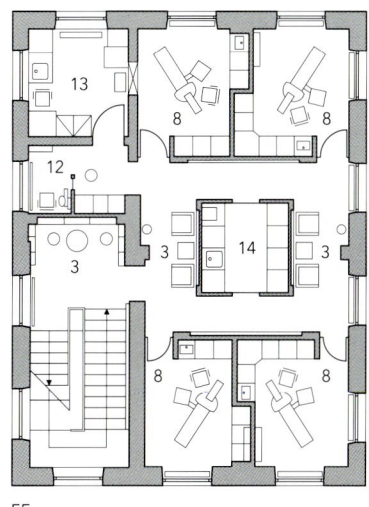
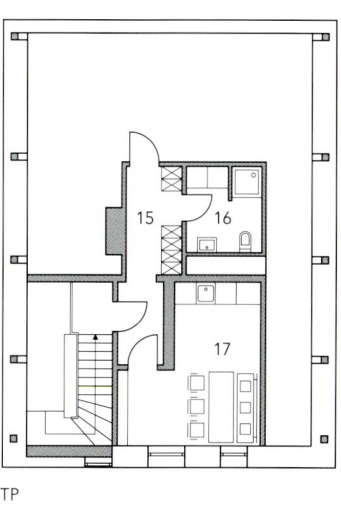

GF   FF   TP

Client | Operator   Dr. Johann Karg
                         Dr. Volker Baumeister
Planning time   11 2004 – 03 2005
Construction time   01 2005 – 03 2005
Usable floor space   181 sqm

a Predominant cool blue is counterbalanced
   by a warm cheerful orange; dark oak parquet
   flooring leads the patient through the public
   areas.
b Glass doors create a sense of openness and
   transparency; poetry printed on translucent
   film helps to relax patients.
c The walls are decorated with backlit friezes of
   mountain landscapes and floral motifs.

Diagrammatic plans, to scale 1:400
Floor plans, to scale 1:200

Floor plan layout

1	Reception	8	Treatment room	15	Staff changing
2	Office	9	Information		cubicle
3	Waiting area	10	Staff toilet	16	Staff toilet and
4	Coat-rack	11	Boiler room		shower
5	Patient toilet	12	Examination X-ray	17	Staff lounge
6	Workroom	13	Store room		
7	Recovery room	14	Sterilisation room		

Careful thought has gone into the layout of the rooms of this partnership
clinic, which are spread over three floors of the rectangular floor plan. Every
square metre has been put to good use, including the corridors and even the
stair-heads. All the rooms needing natural light have windows. Reception,
waiting area and office adjoin one another. Appropriately, only the staff rooms
are located on the attic floor.

Usable floor spaces

Patient rooms	yellow	43 sqm	24 %
Examination			
Treatment rooms	red	42 sqm	23 %
Specialist rooms	pink	33 sqm	18 %
Administrative rooms	green	9 sqm	5 %
Offices	Staff rooms	orange	28 sqm	15 %
Supply	Waste disposal	brown	21 sqm	12 %
Plant rooms	blue	5 sqm	3 %
Total		181 sqm	100 %

On the extensive Zurich Clinic site, the Cardiovascular Centre is housed in a former office building. It includes several examination and treatment rooms for the use of general practitioners in the neighbouring clinic, which also performs operations.

The clinic conversion retained the existing structures and facilities, focusing the design concept on the defining central aisle. The sleek and stylish look incorporates high-grade materials such as brass and wood veneers. Individual treatment rooms line one side of the long central aisle, with various side-rooms opposite, including two waiting area alcoves. The wall panels of back-painted glass and the wood veneer of the partition walls to the consultation rooms, with a bold grain and reddish sheen ["Red Gum"], accentuate the room structure. Reflective glass and ceiling material with a shiny finish help to create an illusion of width in what is a narrow corridor. Skylights along the upper edge of the partition walls provide natural lighting. The angular reception desk, with mountings, baseboards and edge trims made of smooth varnished brass, lends the foyer an air of understated opulence in which the clinic's wealthy clientele will feel at home.

**CONEX_
ARCHITEKTEN
UEBERWASSER
ARCHITEKTUR**

CARDIOVASCULAR CLINIC
ZURICH | CH

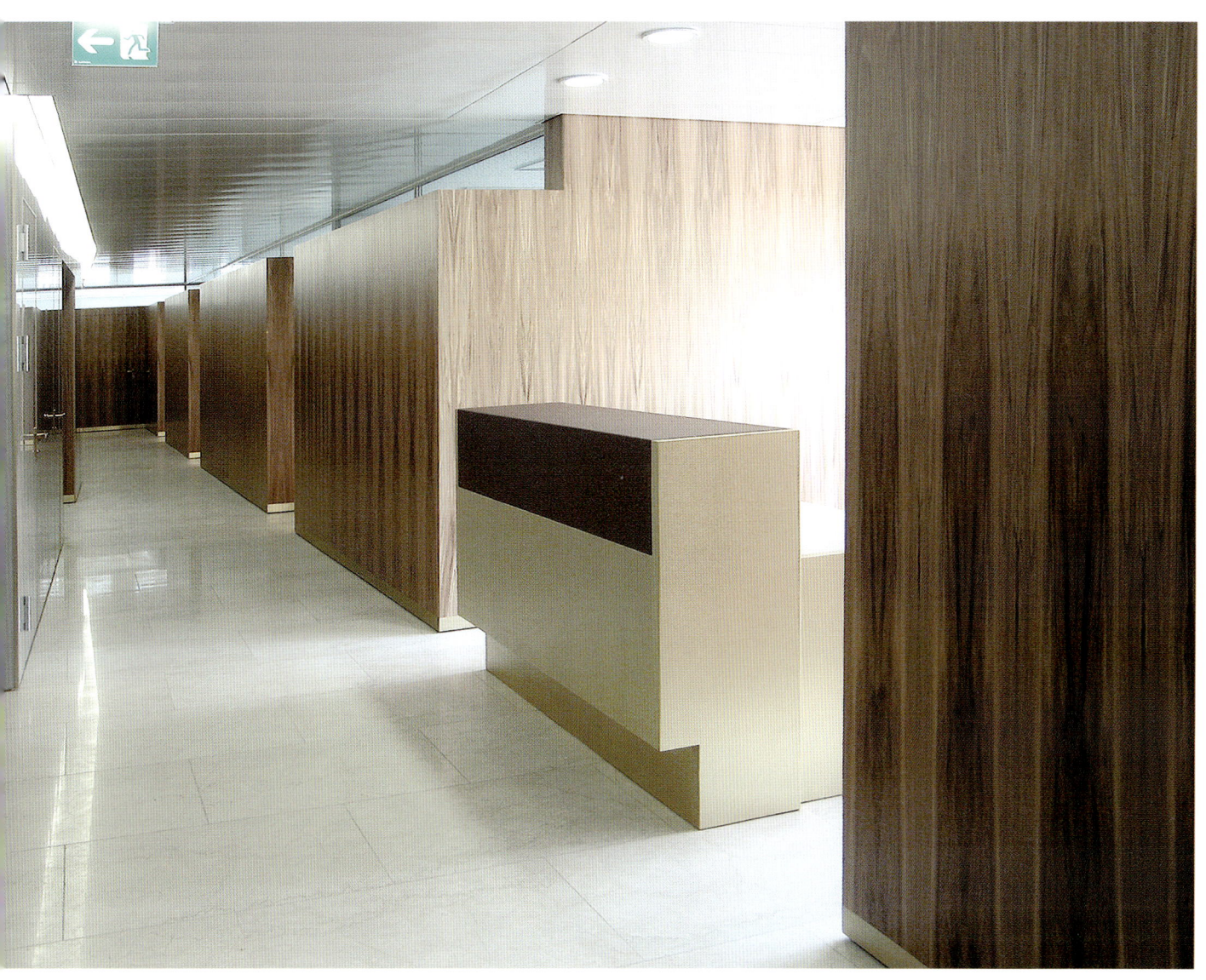

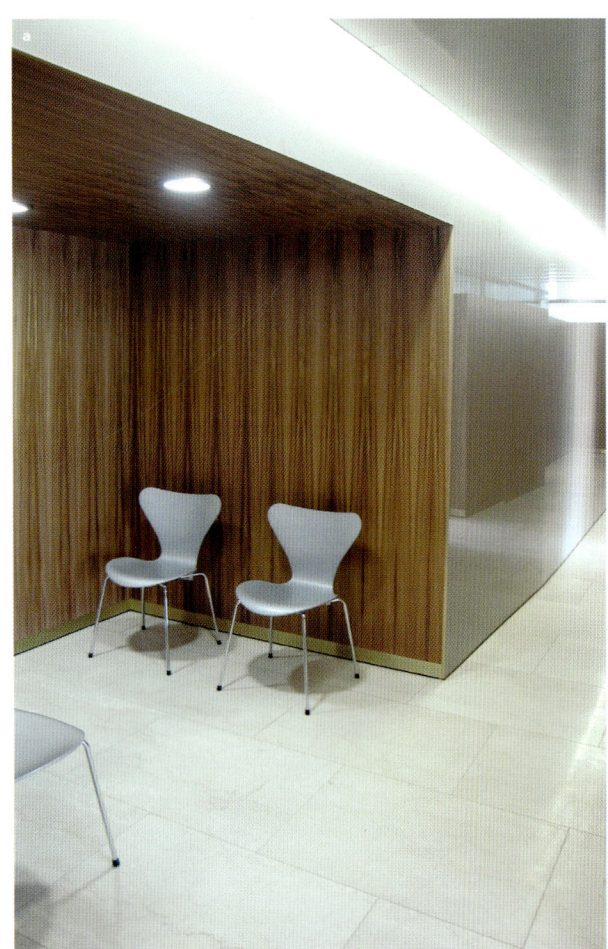

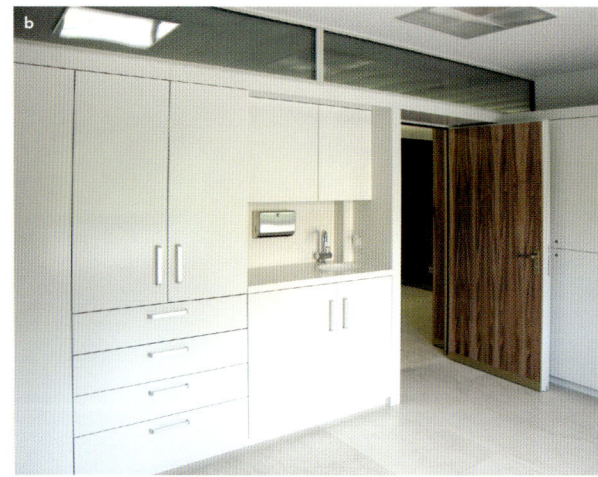

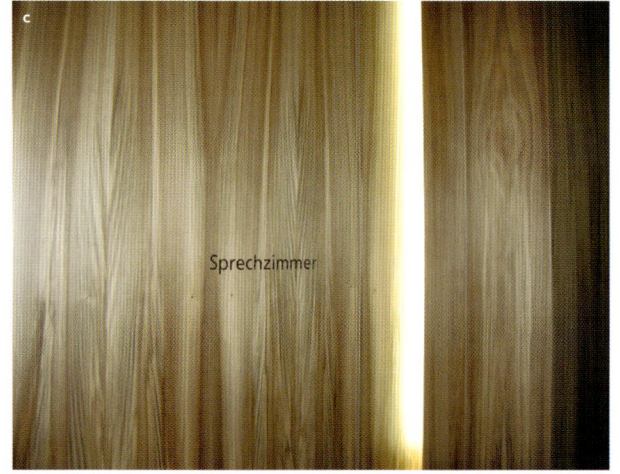

Sprechzimmer

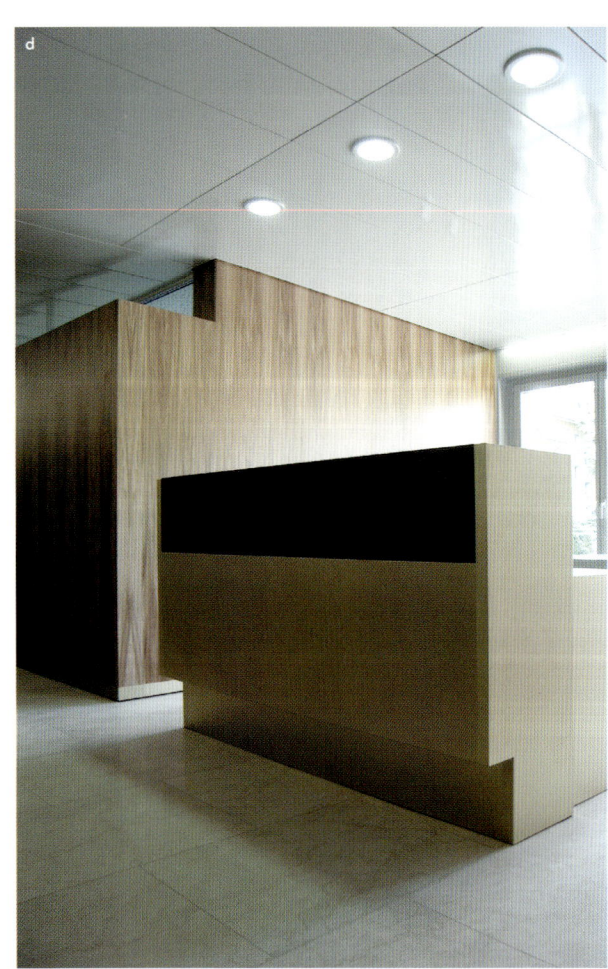

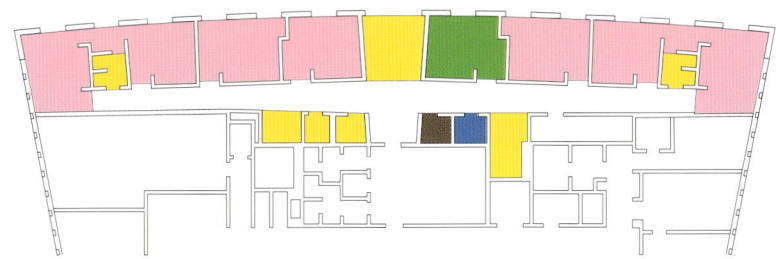

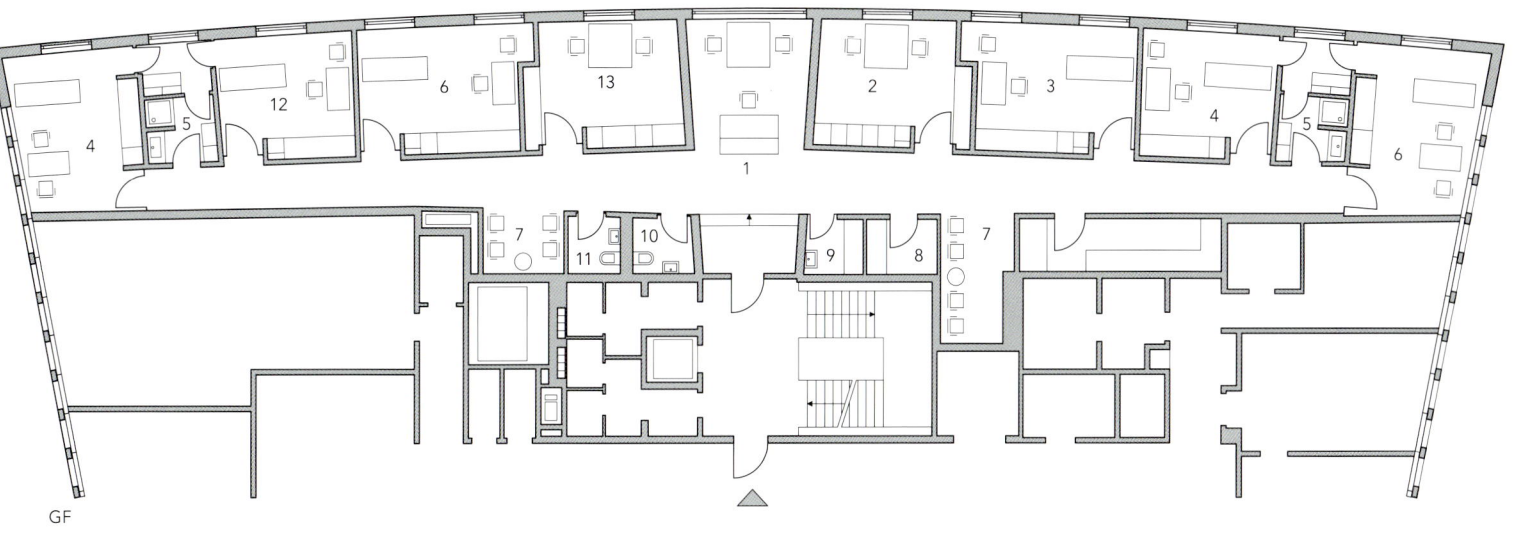

GF

Client	Cardiovascular Clinic
Operator	Cardiovascular Clinic
Construction time	2007
Gross floor area	295 sqm
Usable floor space	174 sqm
Construction cost	1.24 million EUR

a Treatment rooms line one side of the long central aisle, with side-rooms including the two waiting area alcoves opposite.

b The skylights at the top of the partition walls allow natural light to penetrate the central aisle.

c High-grade materials including brass and wood veneer create a sleek and stylish look.

d Wall panels of back-painted glass and boldly grained wood veneer accentuate the room structure.

Diagrammatic plans, to scale 1:400
Floor plans, to scale 1:200

Floor plan layout

1	Reception	**5**	Patient toilet and shower	**9**	Cleaning room
2	Administrative office			**10**	Patient toilet G
3	Examination pacemaker	**6**	Examination echocardiography	**11**	Patient toilet L
4	Examination ergometry	**7**	Waiting area	**12**	Examination electrocardiogram
		8	Installations room	**13**	Holter analysis

The floor plan usually found in an office building is not necessarily suited to a cardiovascular centre. There are long passageways. The waiting areas, positioned off-centre, have no contact with the reception room in the middle of the building. Apart from the waiting area, all the main practice rooms benefit from natural light. The addition of staff rooms would be beneficial.

Usable floor spaces

Patient rooms	**yellow**	37 sqm	21 %
Specialist rooms	**pink**	116 sqm	67 %
Administrative rooms	**green**	15 sqm	8 %
Supply	Waste disposal	**brown**	3 sqm	2 %
Plant rooms	**blue**	3 sqm	2 %
Total		174 sqm	100 %

The group practice of the ENT doctor and his wife, a qualified psychotherapist, extends over three floors in an open-plan studio house. The conversion has retained the openness of the rooms and the view through to the private garden, which the architects achieved by using ceiling height glass partition walls and an inspired lighting concept. On the garden side the extension has an impressive glass façade, while the street façade is broken only by small windows. Direct halogen lighting and indirect light from fluorescent lamps, combined with minimalist building materials – wood, aluminium and satinised acrylic glass – create a warm and light atmosphere in the practice rooms. In the basement, which receives minimal natural light, the smooth cast floor is a gleaming mood-lifting orange. The other rooms also play with colour – shades of green, yellow and orange give each one a different feel.

The practice's three storeys are connected by a spiral staircase. On the top floor, an indirectly lit, translucent curtain over the round stairwell serves as a room divider.

**COSSMANN_
DE BRUYN**

ENT AND PSYCHOTHERAPY CLINIC
DÜSSELDORF | G

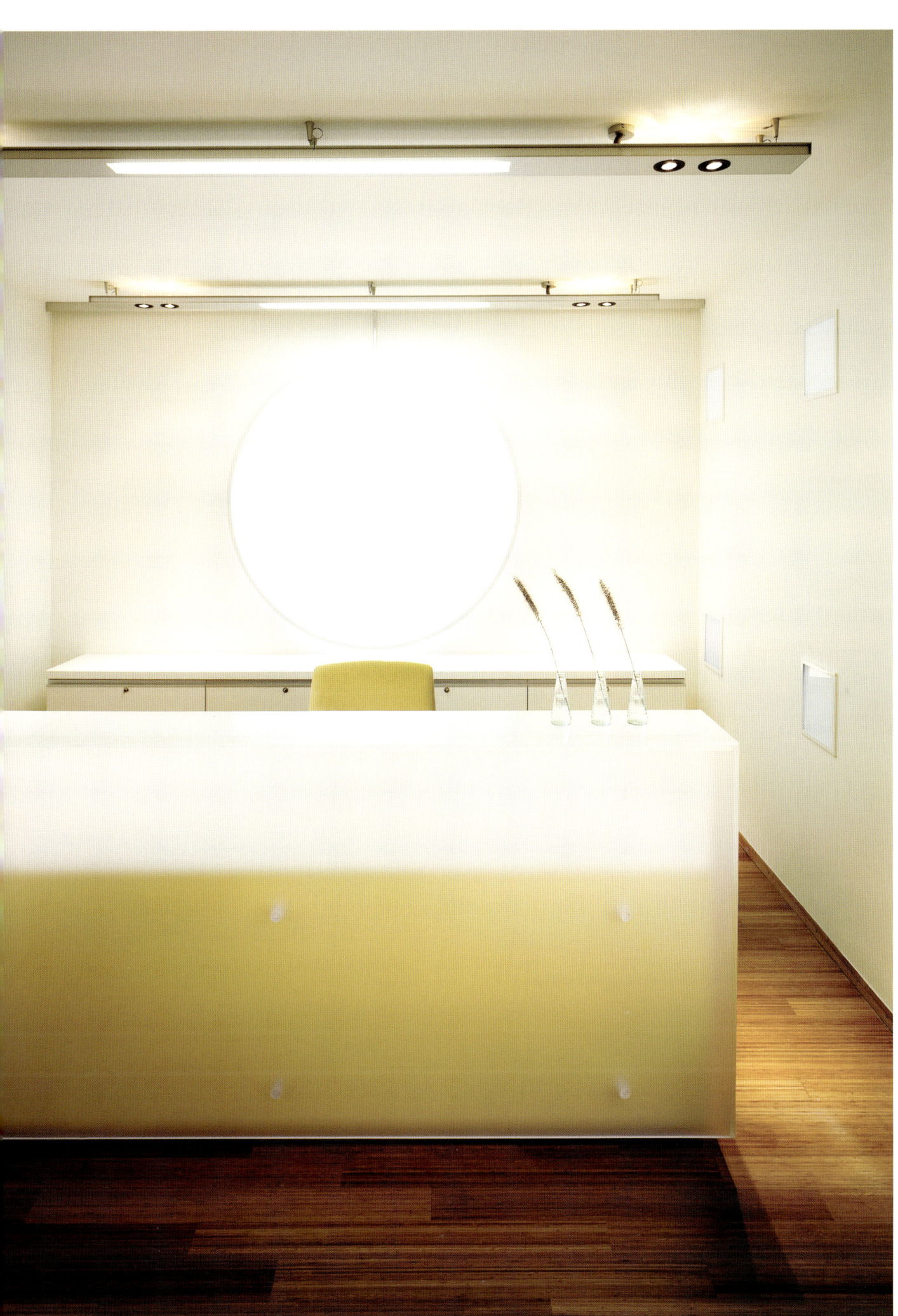

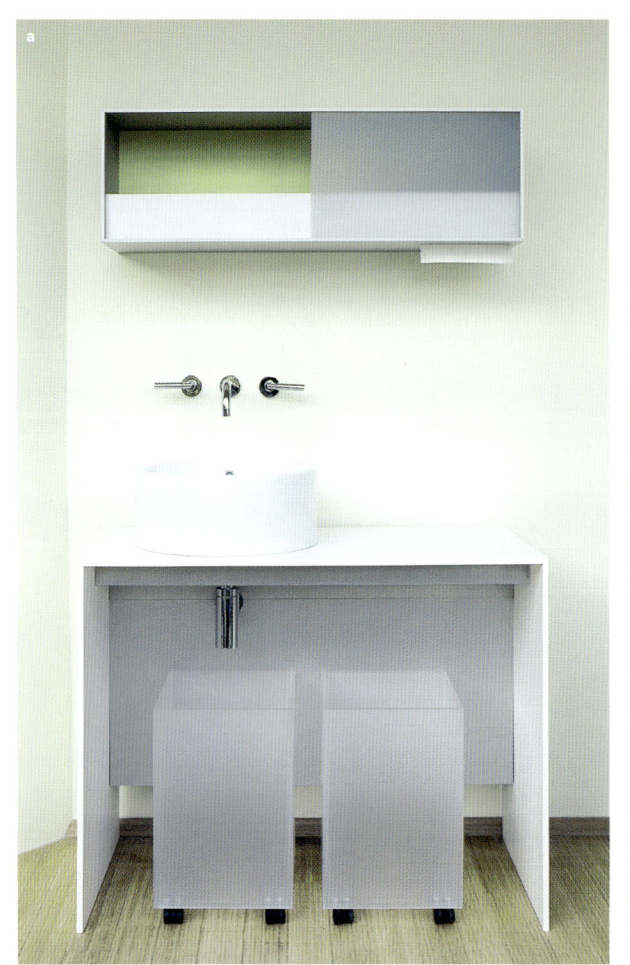

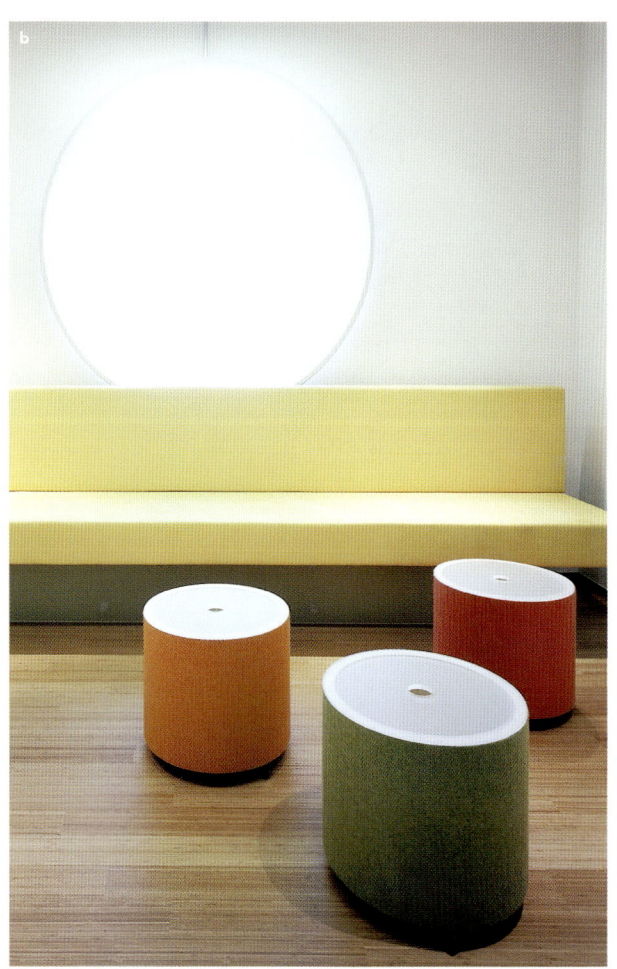

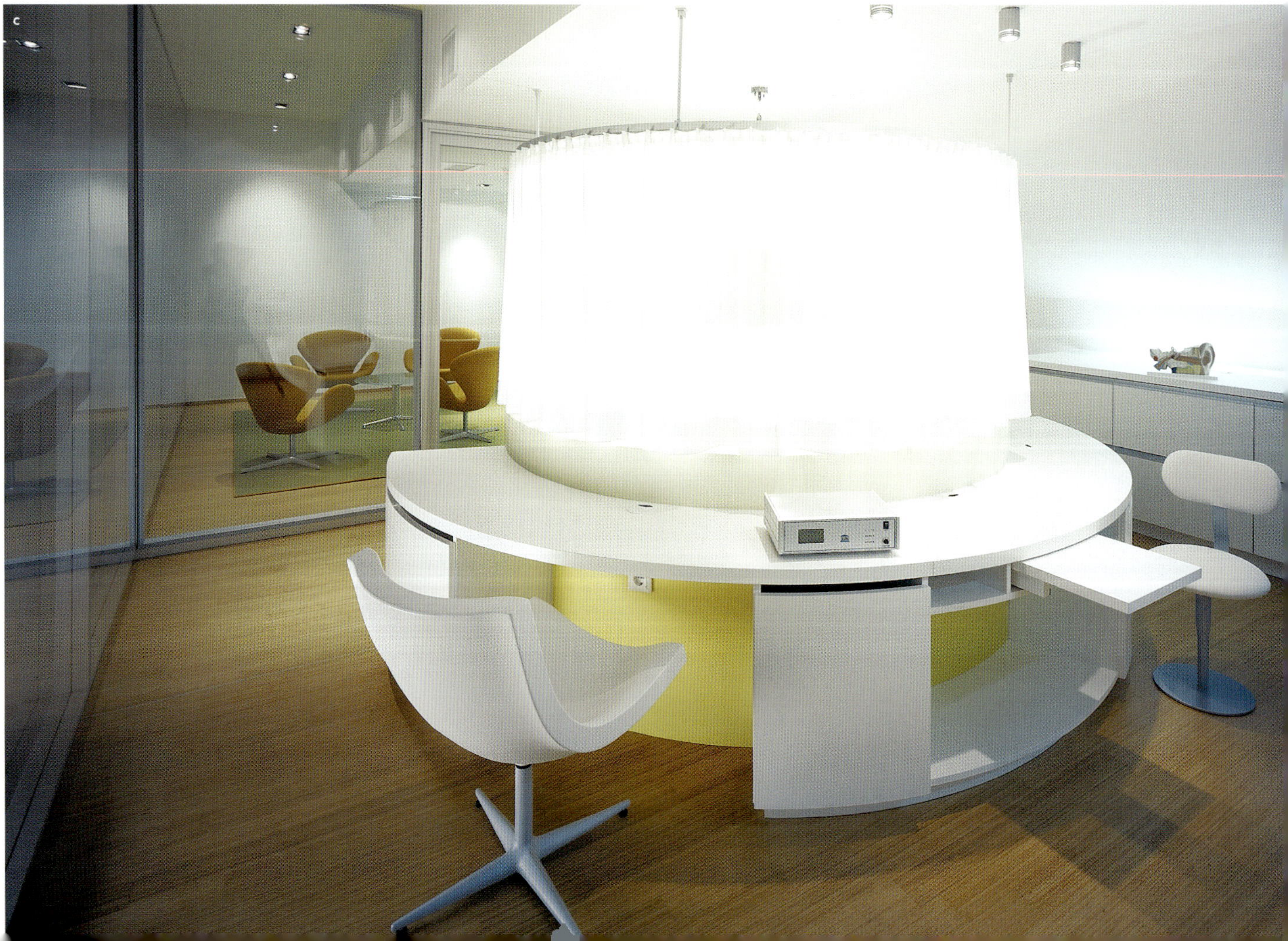

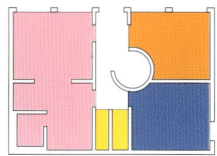
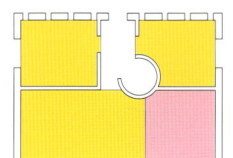
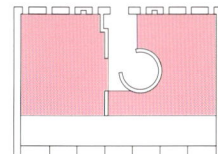

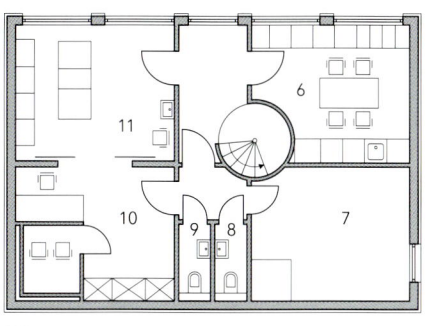

BSMT

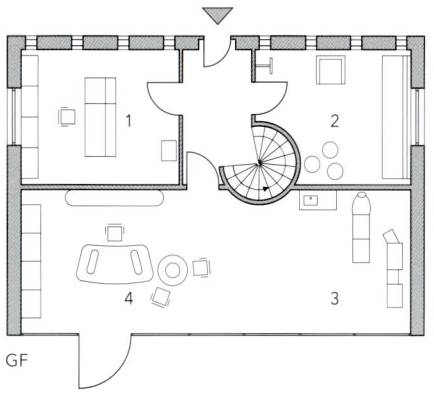

GF

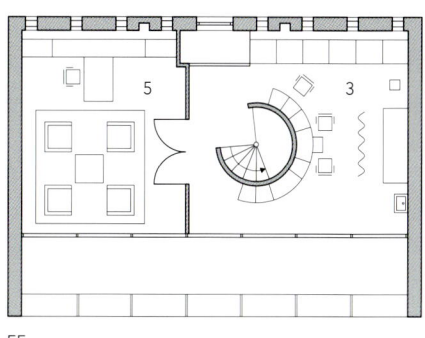

FF

Client	Dr. Claus Birken
Operator	Dr. Claus Birken
	Heike Kupka
Construction time	2003
Usable floor space	204 sqm

a The treatment room is defined by simple a functionality.

b Minimalist building materials – aluminium, wood and satinised acrylic glass – give the waiting area a warm and airy atmosphere.

c The translucent curtain over the round stair-well on the top floor serves as a room divider.

Diagrammatic plans, to scale 1:400
Floor plans, to scale 1:200

Floor plan layout

1	Reception		psychotherapy	**9**	Toilet L
2	Waiting area	**6**	Staff changing	**10**	Examination
3	Treatment room		cubicle		audiometry
4	Consultation room	**7**	Installations room	**11**	Organic resonance
5	Treatment room	**8**	Toilet G		

The resulting floor plan, for all three levels with only small corridor areas, is clearly divided. All rooms except one examination room benefit from natural light. The vertical connection in the shape of a spiral staircase may prove problematic for disabled and older patients and should perhaps be adapted.

Usable floor spaces

Patient rooms	**yellow**	65 sqm	32 %
Specialist rooms	**pink**	106 sqm	52 %
Offices | Staff rooms	**orange**	16 sqm	8 %
Plant rooms	**blue**	17 sqm	8 %
Total		204 sqm	100 %

"Diving in another world." Submersion in an underwater world, fluidity, glistening surfaces and a flowing continuum of rooms were the concepts that underpinned the design of this practice. Patients should feel that they have stepped through an invisible mirror, leaving their world behind and diving into a new one – strange and yet oddly familiar. "Go with the flow – don't stop!"

This new practice, the creation of a young gastroenterologist, occupies part of a health centre. The layout of this spacious environment is designed to uplift and relax. From the moment they enter the open-plan entrance area – foyer, reception and waiting area flow seamlessly together – patients are made to feel at ease. The fibreboard and walnut seating elements are upholstered in silver-coated foam; walls and furniture are in various shades of blue and white, reinforcing the impression of a fantasy underwater world. Fish motifs play on the lines "Move like a jellyfish" from the song "Bubble Toes" by Jack Johnson, the inspiration behind the design. In the long corridor, on either side of which are treatment rooms and side-rooms, key words in yellow and orange stand out on the light walls. The floor covering is a smooth silk-matt, light blue epoxy resin, adding to the surreal, dreamlike effect produced by the practice rooms.

REGINA DAHMEN-INGENHOVEN

GASTROENTEROLOGY
REMSCHEID | G

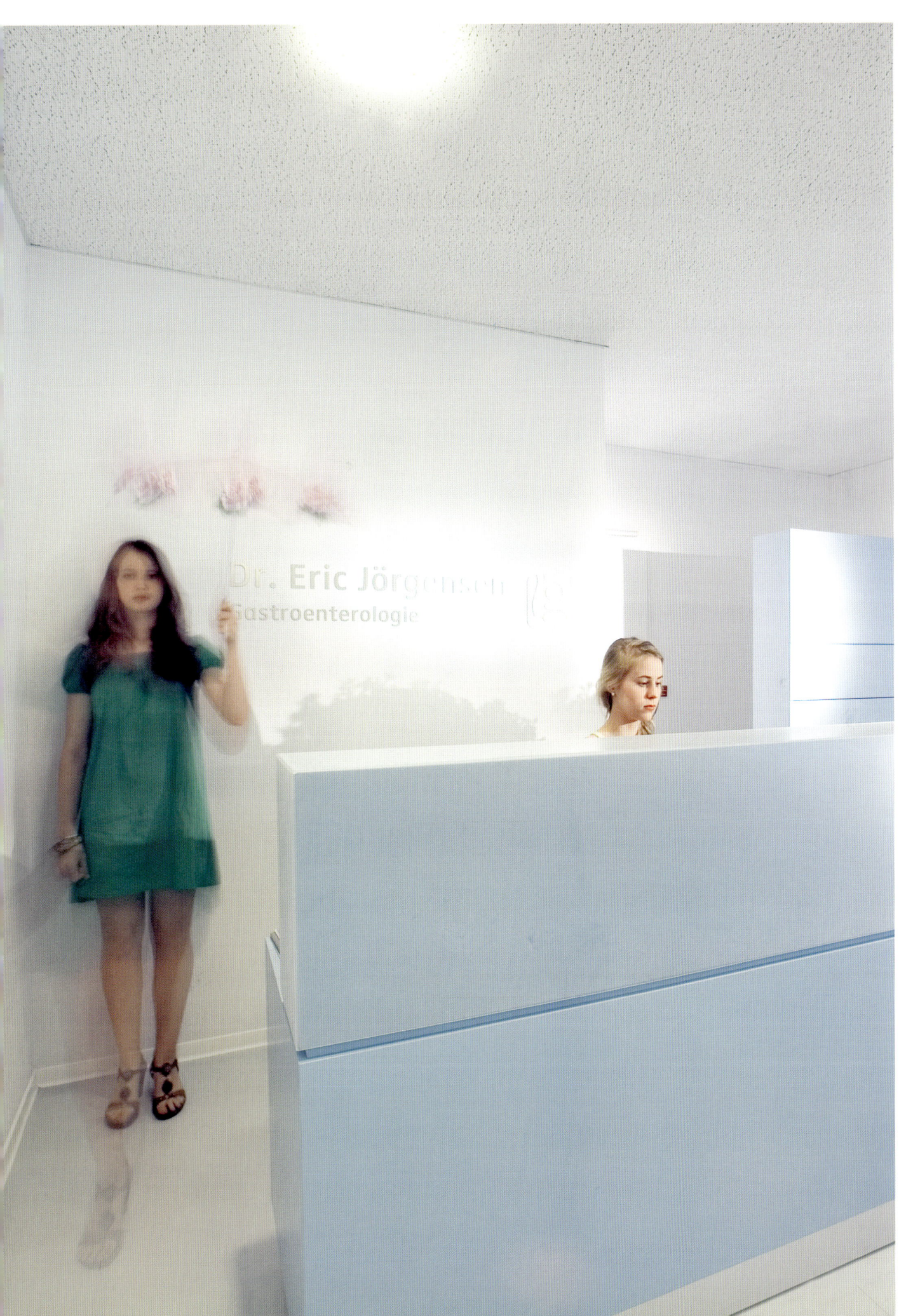

Dr. Eric Jörgensen
Gastroenterologie

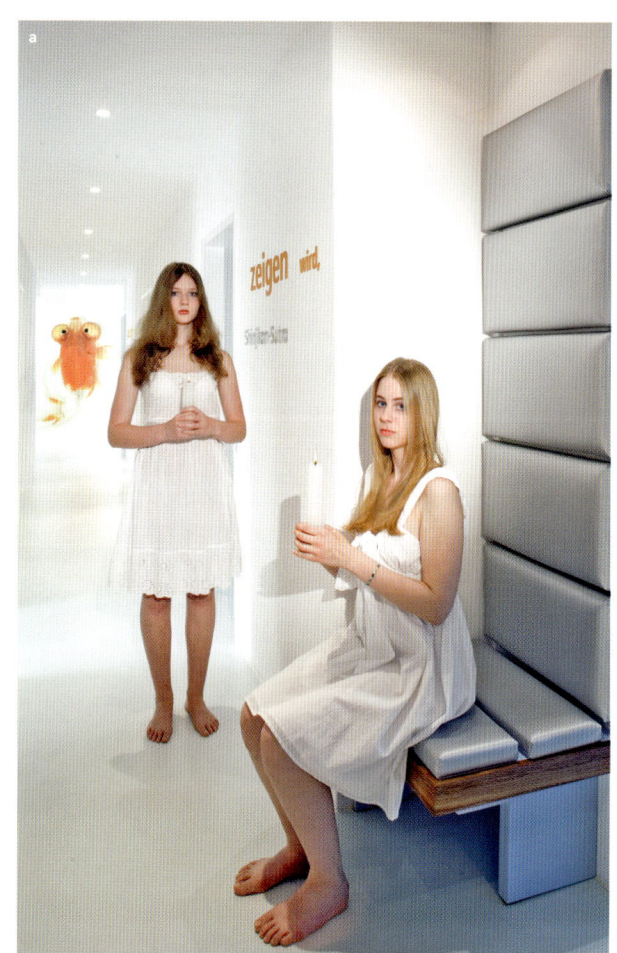

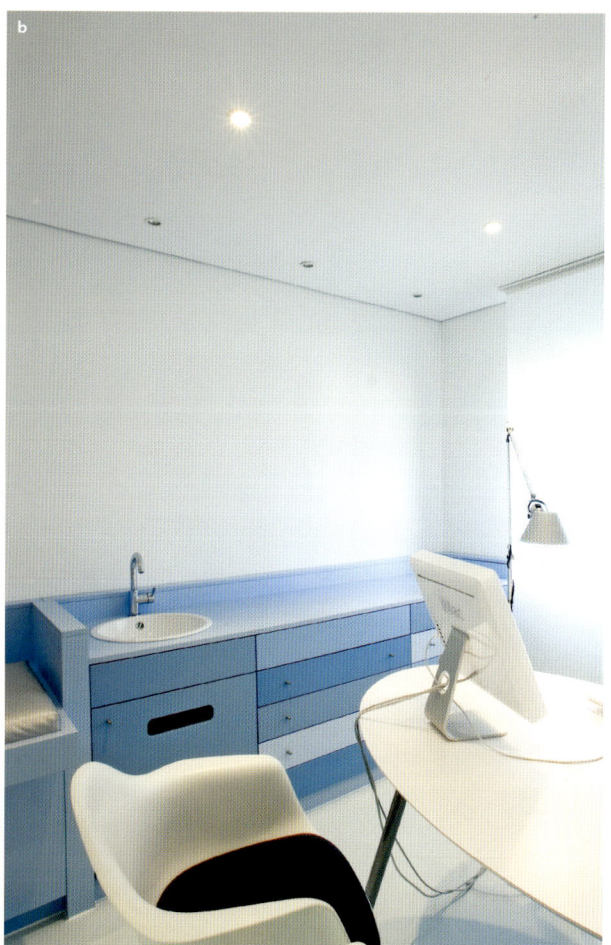

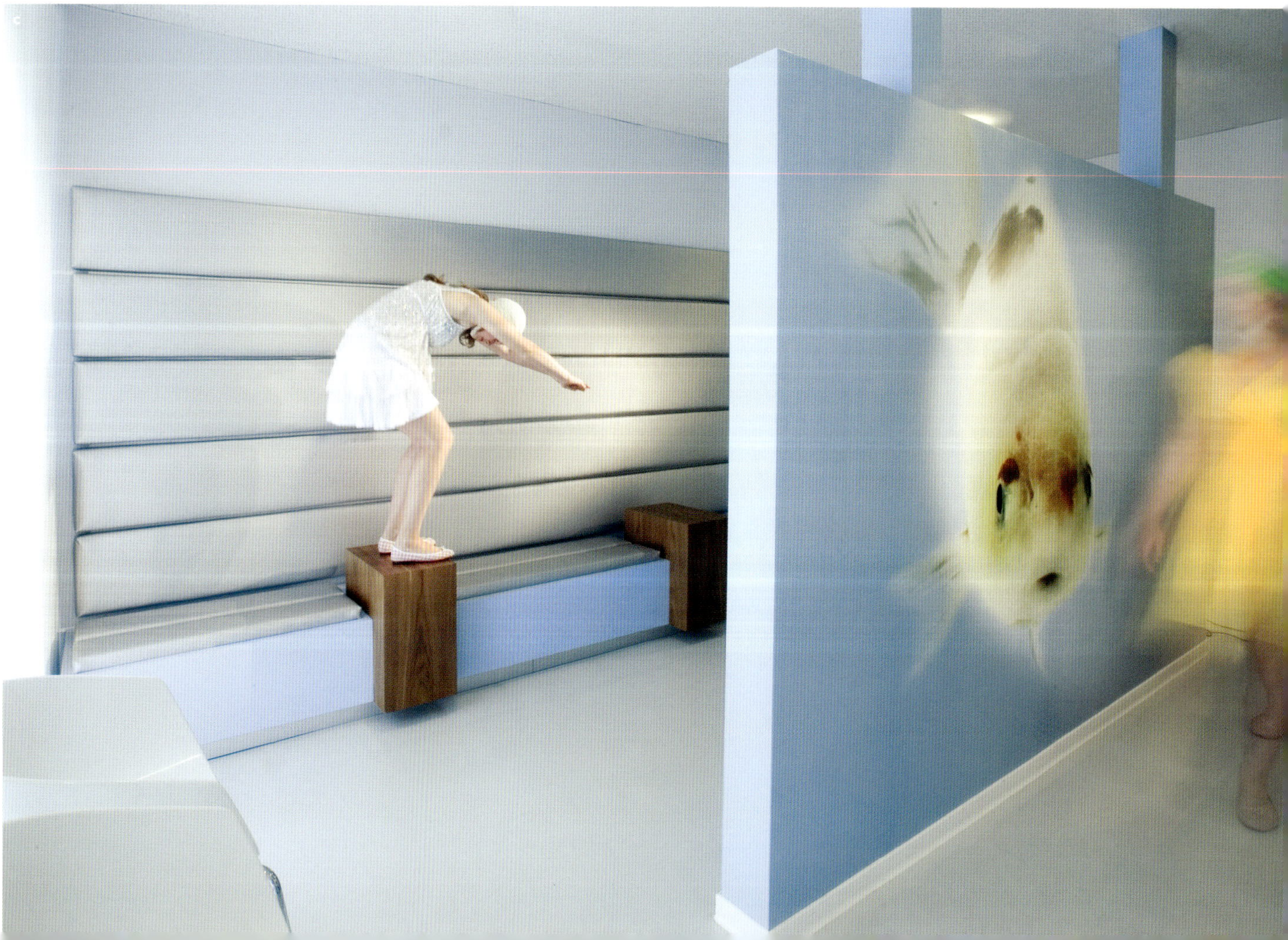

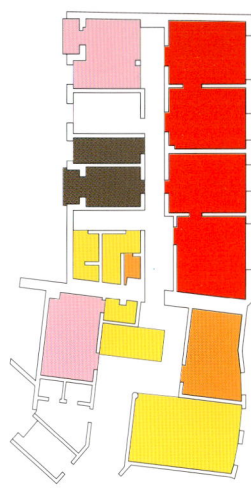

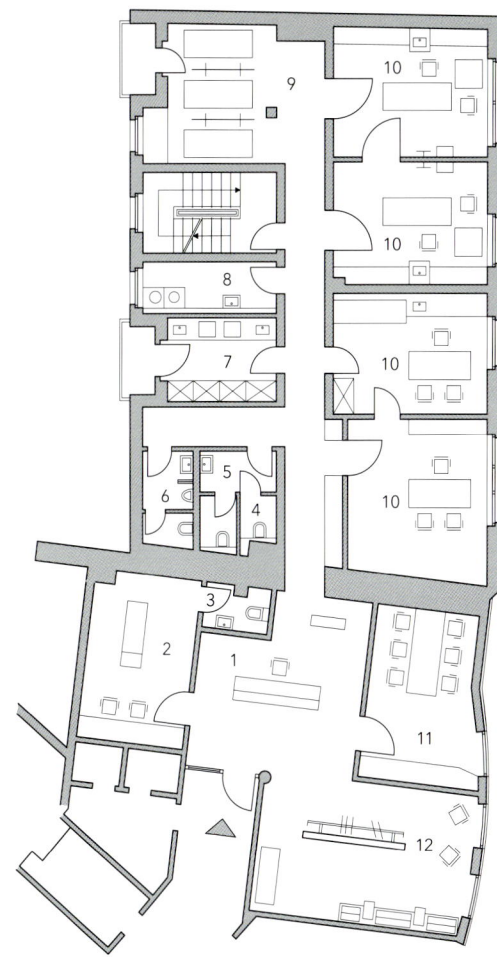

GF

Client	Dr. Eric Jörgensen
Operator	Dr. Eric Jörgensen
	Ingomar Scheller
Planning time	07 2007 – 08 2007
Construction time	10 2007 – 12 2007
Usable floor space	172 sqm
Construction cost	50,000 EUR

a In the long corridor, on either side of which are treatment rooms and side-rooms, key words in yellow and orange stand out on the light walls.

b Walls and furniture are in various shades of blue and white.

c The floor covering is a smooth, silk-matt, adding to the surreal, dream-like effect produced by the practice rooms.

Diagrammatic plans, to scale 1:400
Floor plans, to scale 1:200

Floor plan layout

1	Reception	**5**	Patient toilet L	**9**	Recovery room
2	Examination ultrasound	**6**	Patient toilet G	**10**	Examination
3	Patient toilet	**7**	Store room laundry	**11**	Staff lounge
4	Staff toilet	**8**	Workroom laundry	**12**	Waiting area

The rooms in this partnership practice, accessed by a spacious foyer and a straight corridor, have a functional layout which facilitates patient care. Reception and waiting area adjoin each other. Apart from one examination room, all rooms needing natural light have windows. The practice would benefit from the addition of an office for administrative tasks and dedicated space for storage and cleaning.

Usable floor spaces

Patient rooms	**yellow**	42 sqm	25 %
Examination | Treatment rooms	**red**	67 sqm	39 %
Specialist rooms	**pink**	31 sqm	18 %
Offices | Staff rooms	**orange**	16 sqm	9 %
Supply | Waste disposal	**brown**	16 sqm	9 %
Total		172 sqm	100 %

Performance data

Outpatients per year	8,000 – 9,000
Number and type of services per year	Intestinoscopy
	Capsule endoscopy
	Colonoscopy
Clinic opening hours	5 days | 56 hours
Waiting time [with | without appointment]	0 – 30 min. | 0 – 60 min.
Type and number of staff	3 doctors
	8 clerical staff
	2 trainees
Clinic planning advice	Budget for potential extension

Green as a lemongrass Spritzer, blue as a tingly Refresher sweet and orange as the peel of ripe fruit. This is the pleasing effect produced by the dental practice in Düsseldorf city centre. The open-plan interior, modelled on a club, bar and lounge, gives the small practice a spacious feel and is key to its welcoming atmosphere. Furniture and reception desk are dotted around like islands in the room, providing a fluid transition to the other areas of the practice. White walls, finely striped oak parquet flooring and colourful accents such as the architect designed orange upholstered waiting bench create a soothing environment, which allows patients temporarily to forget their everyday cares and anxieties. Behind an aquamarine blue, clear PEP wall are three treatment rooms. The ultra-transparent acrylic glass honeycomb panels originally came from the technical laboratory of ski manufacturer Blizzard. The striking green X-ray box uses the latest X-ray technology, a radiation gun resembling a hairdryer. The patient sits on a softly upholstered "X-ray throne".

The guiding principle is to distract the patient from the "torture" associated with a visit to the dentist. The doctor hopes that patients will come to him not only because they have toothache, but also because of the aesthetic ambiance.

REGINA DAHMEN-INGENHOVEN

"LOUNGE DENTAL" DENTAL PRACTICE
DÜSSELDORF | G

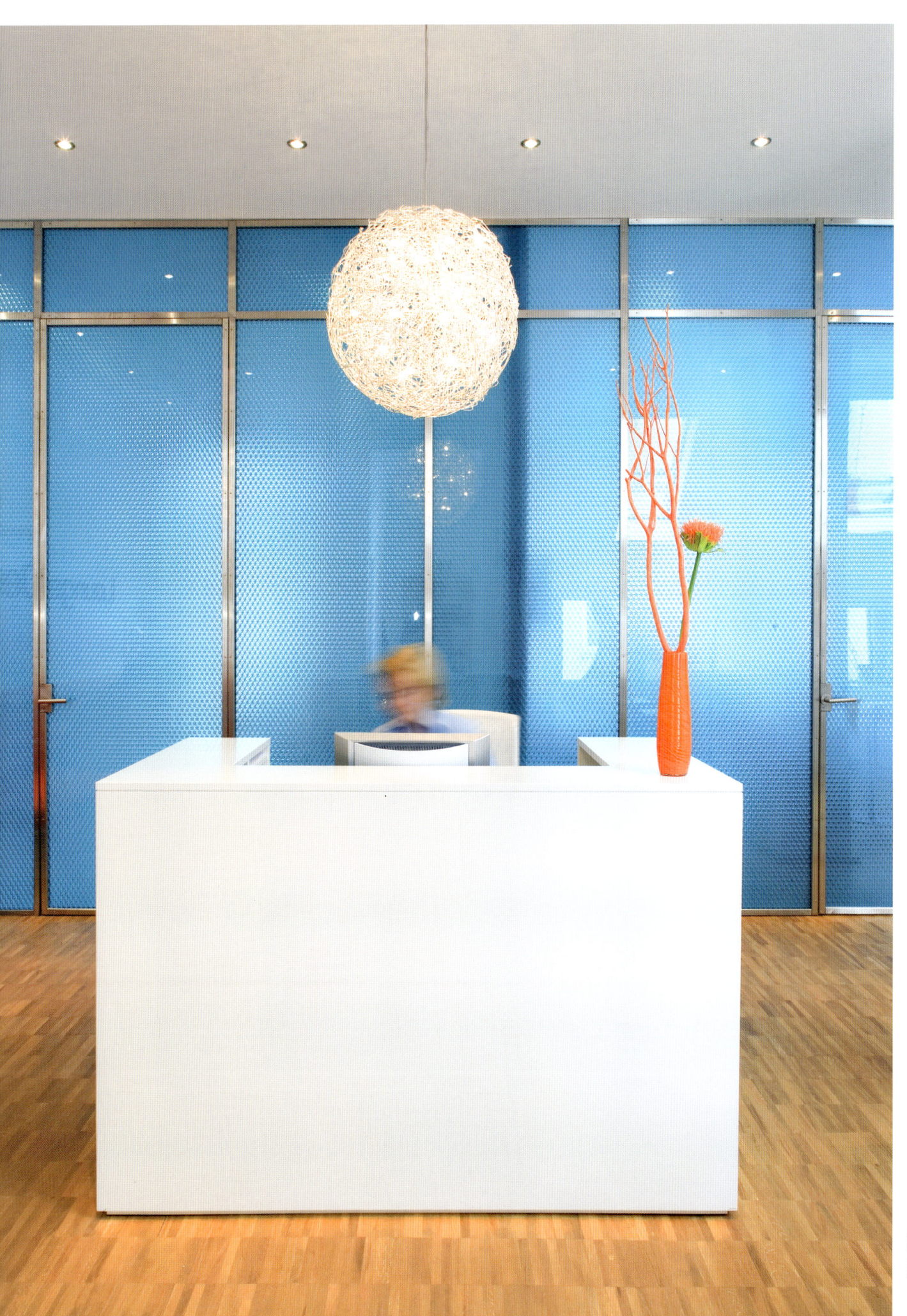

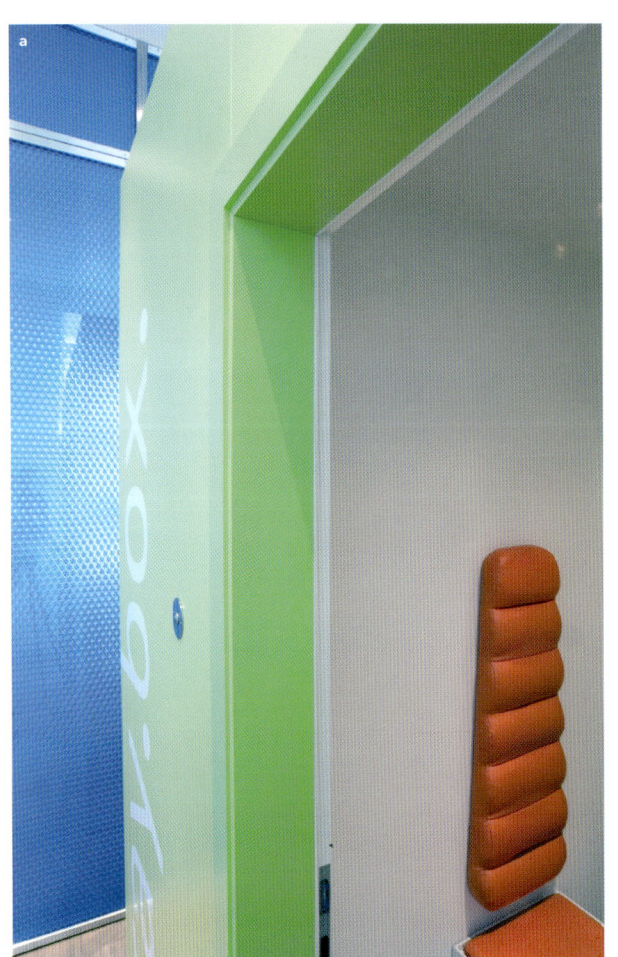
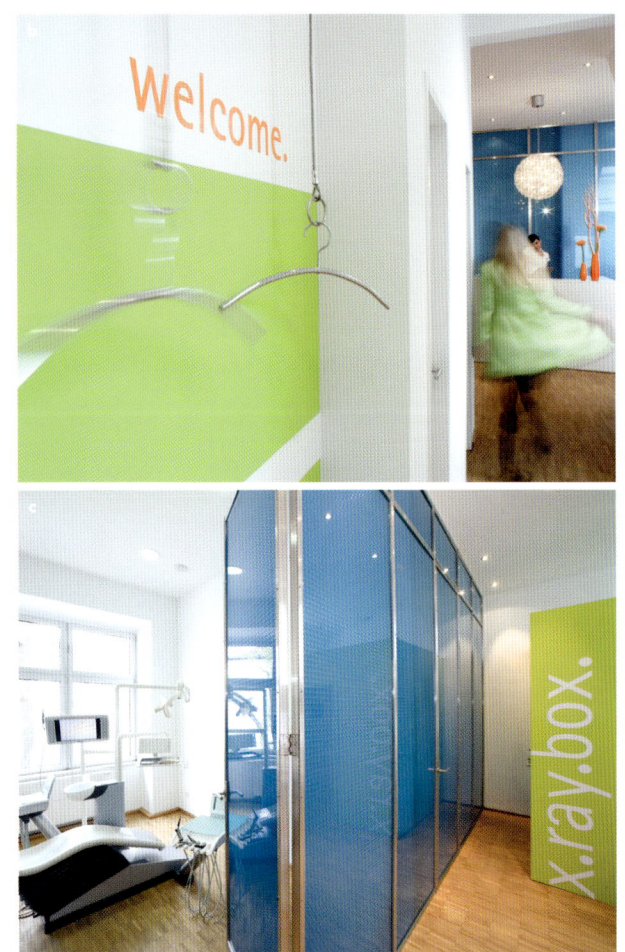

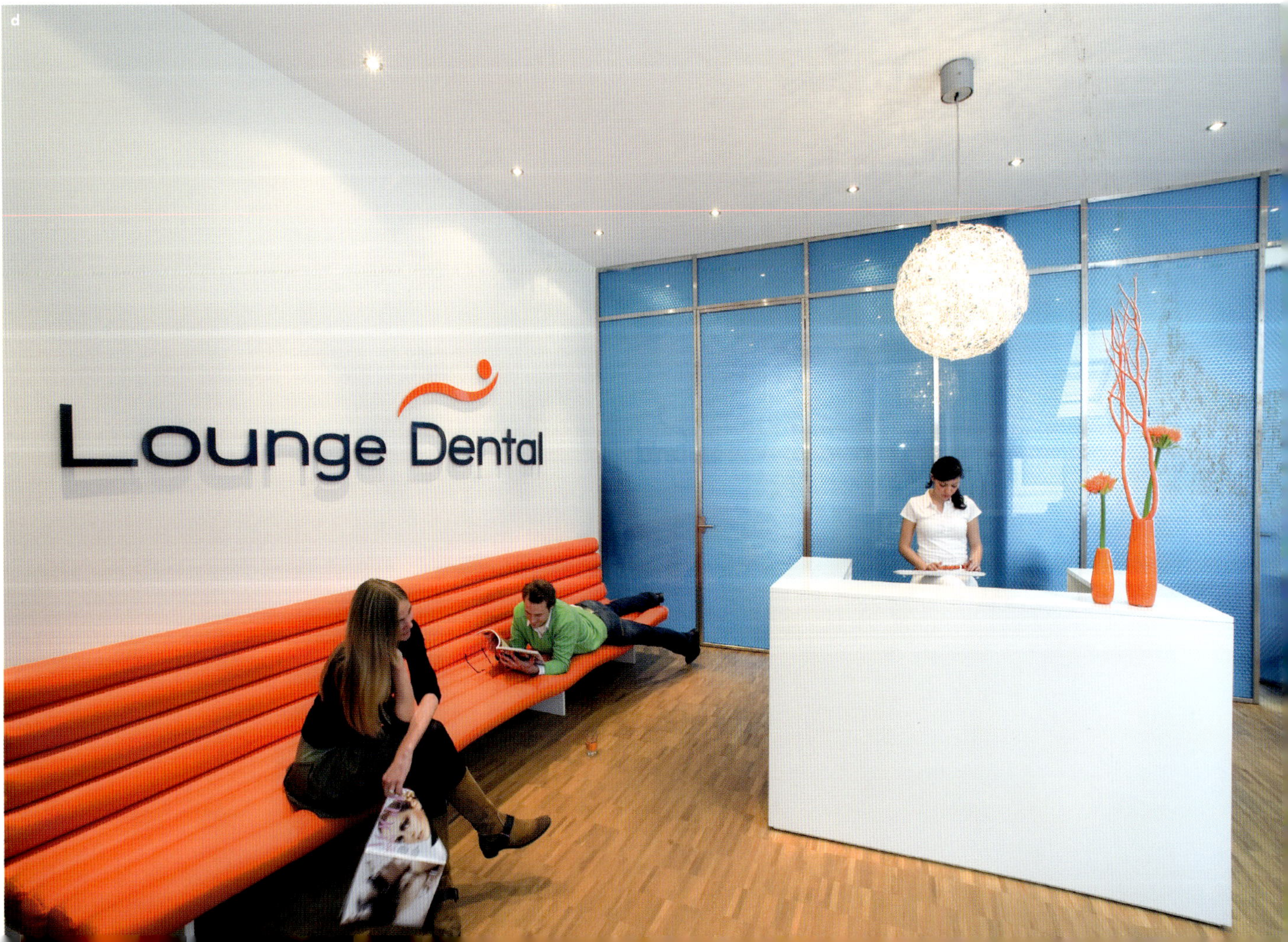

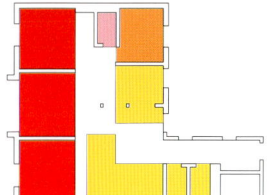

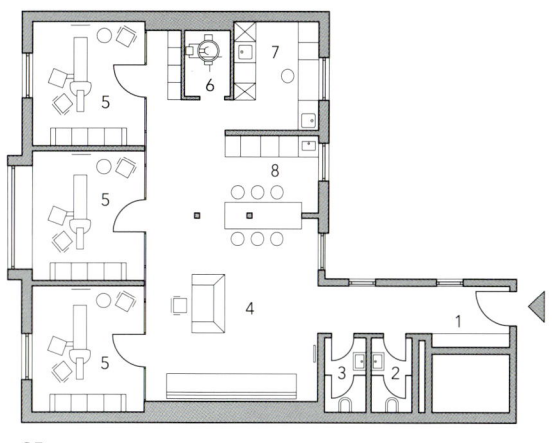

GF

Client | Operator   Riadh Ben Hamid
Planning time   05 2004 – 07 2004
Construction time   09 2004 – 11 2004
Usable floor space   71 sqm
Construction cost   130,000 EUR
Total cost   390,000 EUR

a The latest technology is used in the green X-ray box, where the patient sits on a softly upholstered "X-ray throne".

b A short entrance corridor with a coat-rack takes patients straight to the reception and waiting area.

c Behind the aquamarine blue clear PEP wall are the three treatment rooms.

d White walls, light oak parquet flooring and colourful accents such as the orange waiting bench create a refreshing and pleasant environment.

Diagrammatic plans, to scale 1:400
Floor plans, to scale 1:200

Floor plan layout

1 Coat-rack	**4** Reception	**7** Staff lounge
2 Toilet G	**5** Treatment room	**8** Waiting area
3 Toilet L	**6** Examination X-ray	

Optimal use has been made of the floor area in the single handed practice. From the entrance, patients make their way along a short corridor, on which the patient toilets are located, to a large room opening on to all the function groups. All the rooms that need daylight benefit from natural lighting. A small office and a storage room or a cleaning cupboard would be useful additions.

Usable floor spaces

Patient rooms	**yellow**	26 sqm	37 %
Examination	Treatment rooms	**red**	35 sqm	49 %
Specialist rooms	**pink**	2 sqm	3 %
Offices	Staff rooms	**orange**	8 sqm	11 %
Total		71 sqm	100 %

Performance data

Outpatients per year	1,100
Number and type of services per year	Cosmetic dentistry
	Paradontology
	Endodontics
	Implantology
	Prophylaxis
Clinic opening hours	5 days	50 hours
Waiting time	5 – 15 min.
Type and number of staff	1 doctor
	4 employees

A uFO has landed! Right in the middle of a modern dental practice! This elliptical structure separates the two sections of the practice, orthodontics and dentistry, and also houses the waiting area, which wraps patients in a cocoon; its light and welcoming atmosphere making them feel safe and at ease. The orthodontic treatment rooms have a totally different look; they are specifically designed to be visible from outside. The treatment chairs sit on a platform facing the display window so that curious passers-by can watch young patients having their braces fitted – but only to a limited extent, of course, they cannot see right into their mouths.

The dental rooms occupy the other side of the building of this ground-level practice. Small rooms and a minimalist style draw the eye straight to the dental chair. Instruments are not kept here, everything is wheeled into the rooms on trolleys. Sloping walls angle towards the chair and the treatment unit, and the corridor gradually narrows and lowers at the end, clearly indicating that it is for staff access only.

**ETSCHMANN
NOACK**

DENTAL PRACTICE
ANSBACH | G

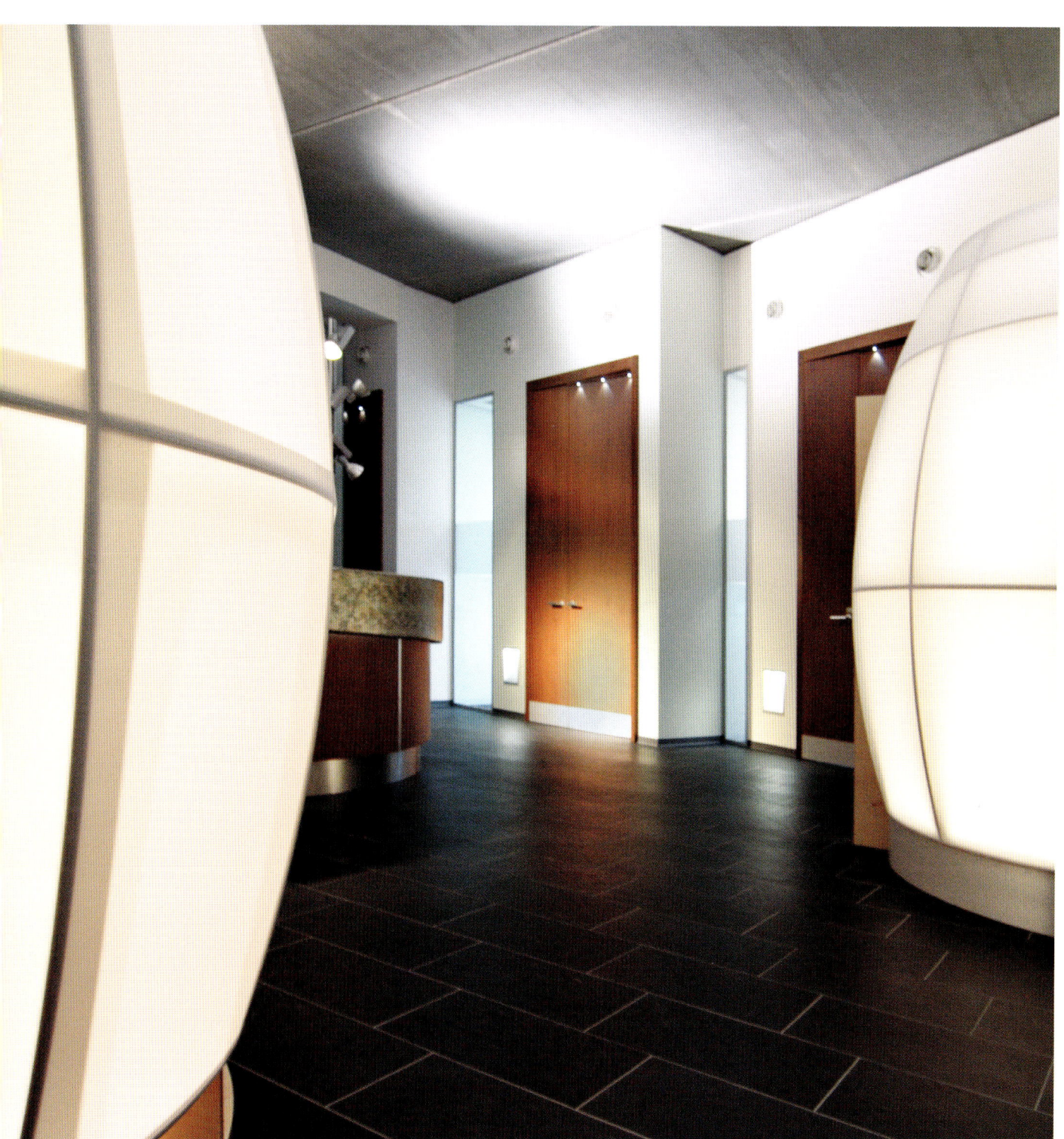

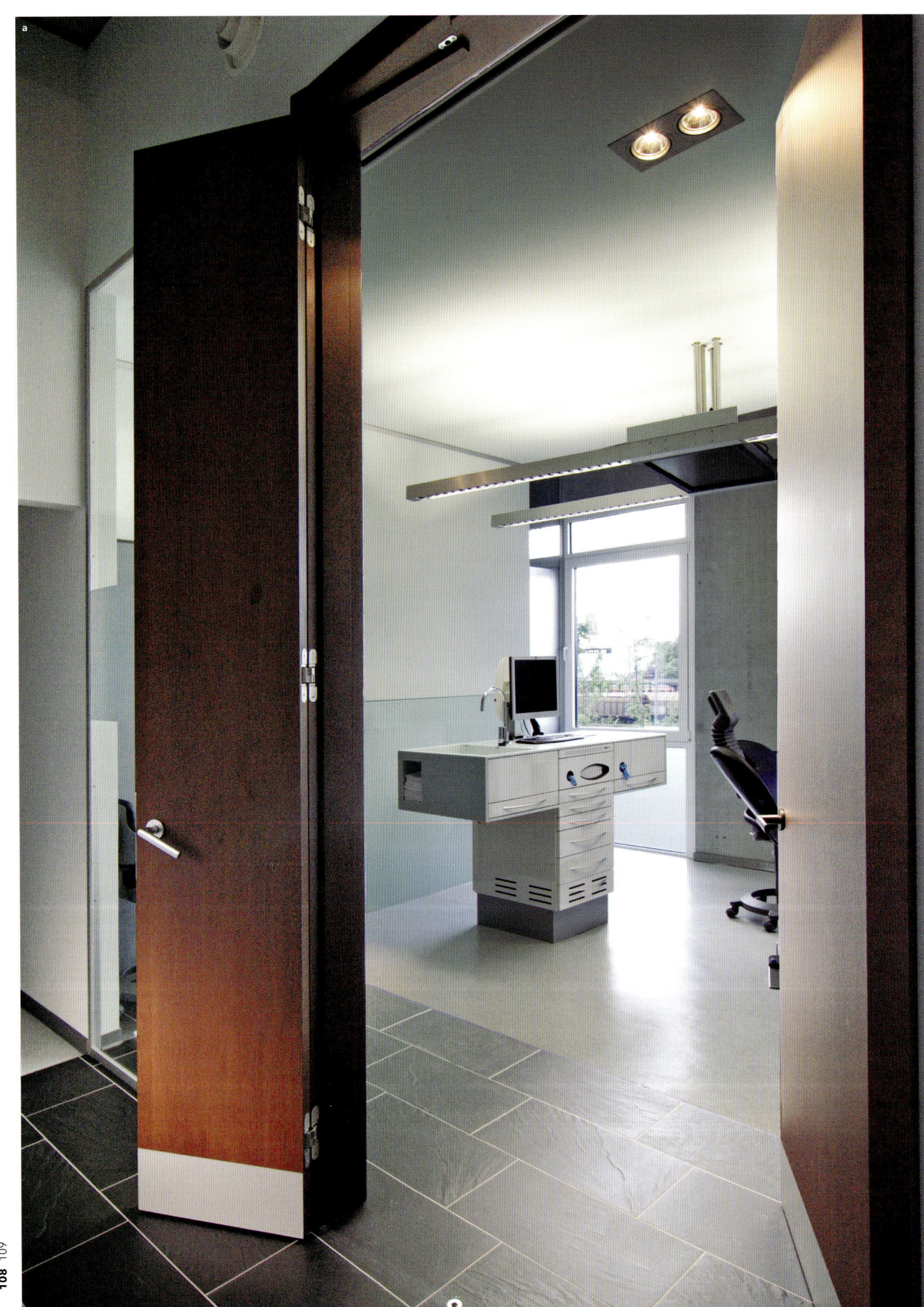

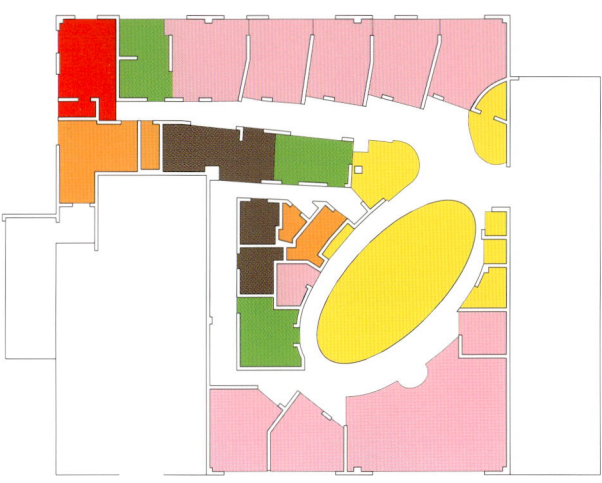

Diagrammatic plans, to scale 1:400
Floor plans, to scale 1:200

1	Reception		orthodontics	**13**	Staff toilet
2	Coat-rack	**8**	Treatment room	**14**	Office
3	Waiting area	**9**	Consultation room	**15**	Sterilisation room
4	Hygiene	**10**	Examination X-ray	**16**	Staff lounge
5	Patient toilet	**11**	Store room	**17**	Cast room
6	Pressroom	**12**	Staff changing	**18**	Laboratory
7	Treatment room		cubicle	**19**	Office

GF

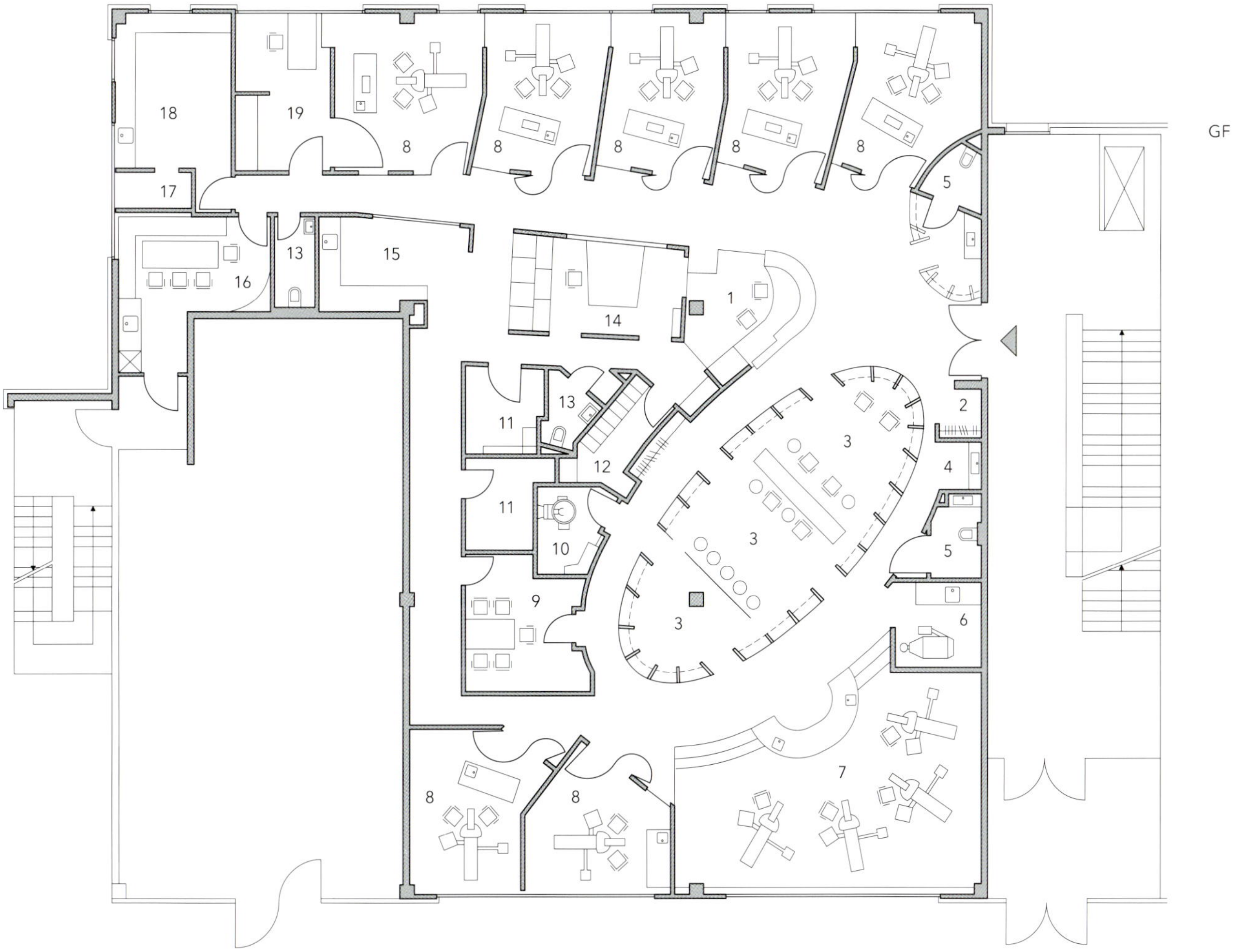

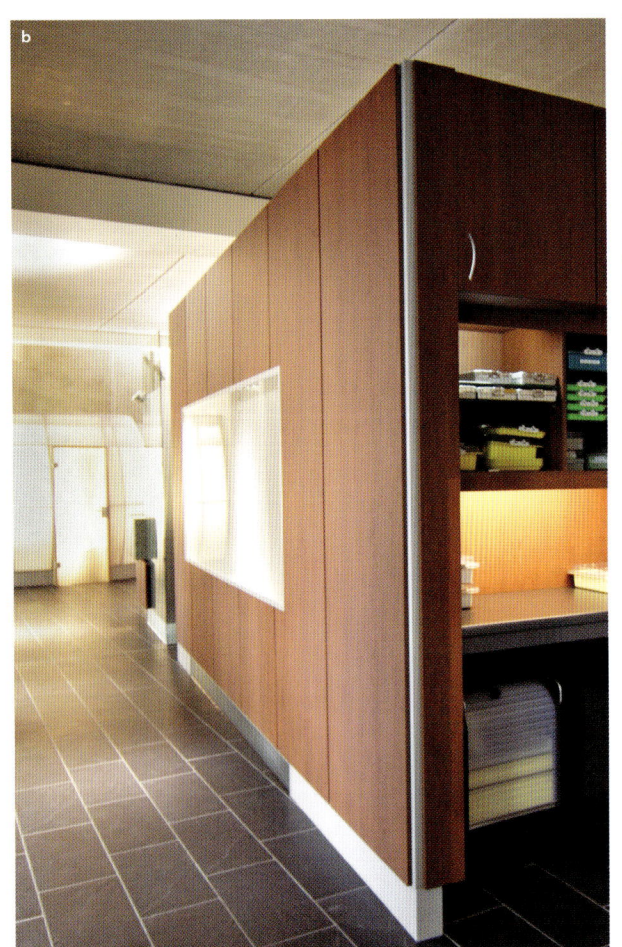

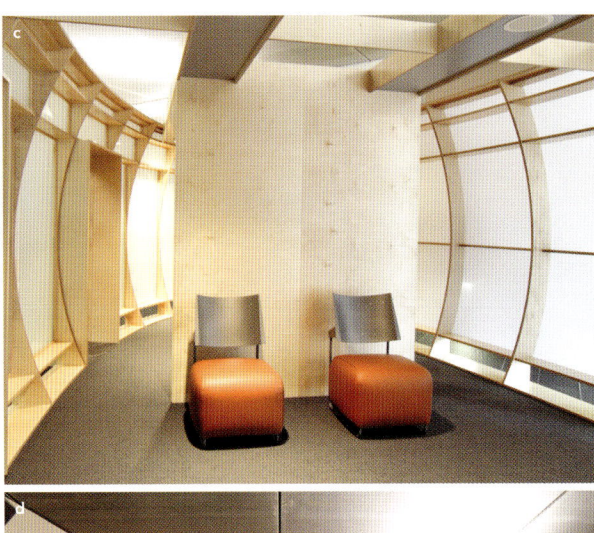

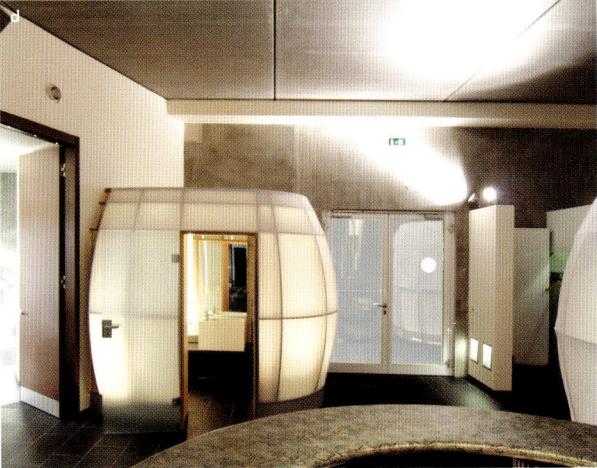

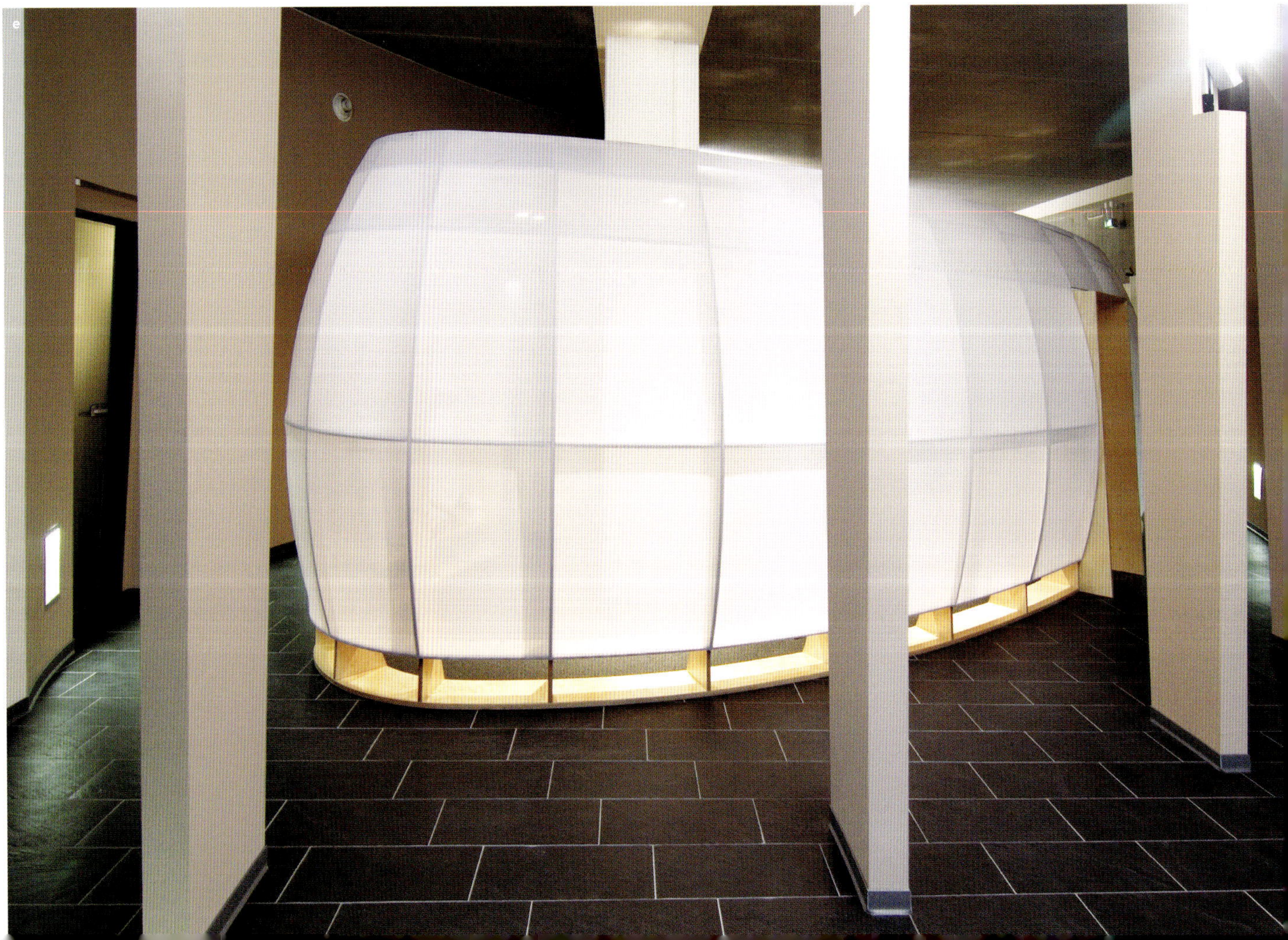

Client	Operator	Roland Madesta
	Dr. Volker Arendt
	Dr. Katrin Franzke
Planning time	10 2005 – 12 2005
Gross floor area	420 sqm
Usable floor space	370 sqm
Gross cubic capacity	1,175 cbm

a The treatment room's compact floor plan and a minimalist style draw the eye straight to the dental chair.

b The corridor from the treatment rooms narrows and lowers at the end, clearly indicating that it is for staff access only.

c The unusual waiting area enables patients to relax, screened from the busy reception area.

d The patient toilet is shaped like a "waiting UFO" and creates a room continuum.

e The elliptical waiting area is divided into three waiting areas: adults, young people and children each have their own separate space.

Floor plan layout

From the entrance patients of the multiple practice come directly into the cleverly structured waiting area, which is visible from reception. From there they enter three corridor sections housing the special rooms for examination and treatment. A large proportion of the practice rooms receives no direct natural light, including a consultation room and an office as well as the sterilisation room, a limitation which should perhaps be remedied.

Usable floor spaces

Patient rooms	**yellow**	78 sqm	21 %
Examination |			
Treatment rooms	**red**	18 sqm	5 %
Specialist rooms	**pink**	180 sqm	49 %
Administrative rooms	**green**	38 sqm	10 %
Offices | Staff rooms	**orange**	27 sqm	7 %
Supply | Waste disposal	**brown**	29 sqm	8 %
Total		370 sqm	100 %

High-grade Canadian grey elm and coated glass – the exquisite fittings reflect the dentist's area of expertise, namely the preparation of top quality ceramic inlays. The transparent light-flooded architecture of the building is replicated in the interior design, with a glass wall running parallel to the slightly curved outer façade. This separates the treatment rooms and offices from the through corridor, which therefore also has the benefit of natural light. The field of vision on the glass wall is coated with a translucent film that varies in texture, ensuring patient privacy during treatment. The natural light illuminates the mainly orange film and gives what is actually a narrow passage the illusion of spaciousness. Ceiling height sliding doors punctuate the almost twelve metre long glass wall. The practice rooms on the other side have wood laminate flooring to the corridor, creating a design counterpoint to the glass wall opposite. High quality is also the hallmark of the reception area, with its cosy sofas and a small but stylish counter.

This practice has a bespoke nameplate concept: pithy inscriptions such as "Aesthetics" and "Rivestident" [for the insertion of ceramic inlays] designate the individual rooms.

GFG

DENTAL PRACTICE
BREMEN | G

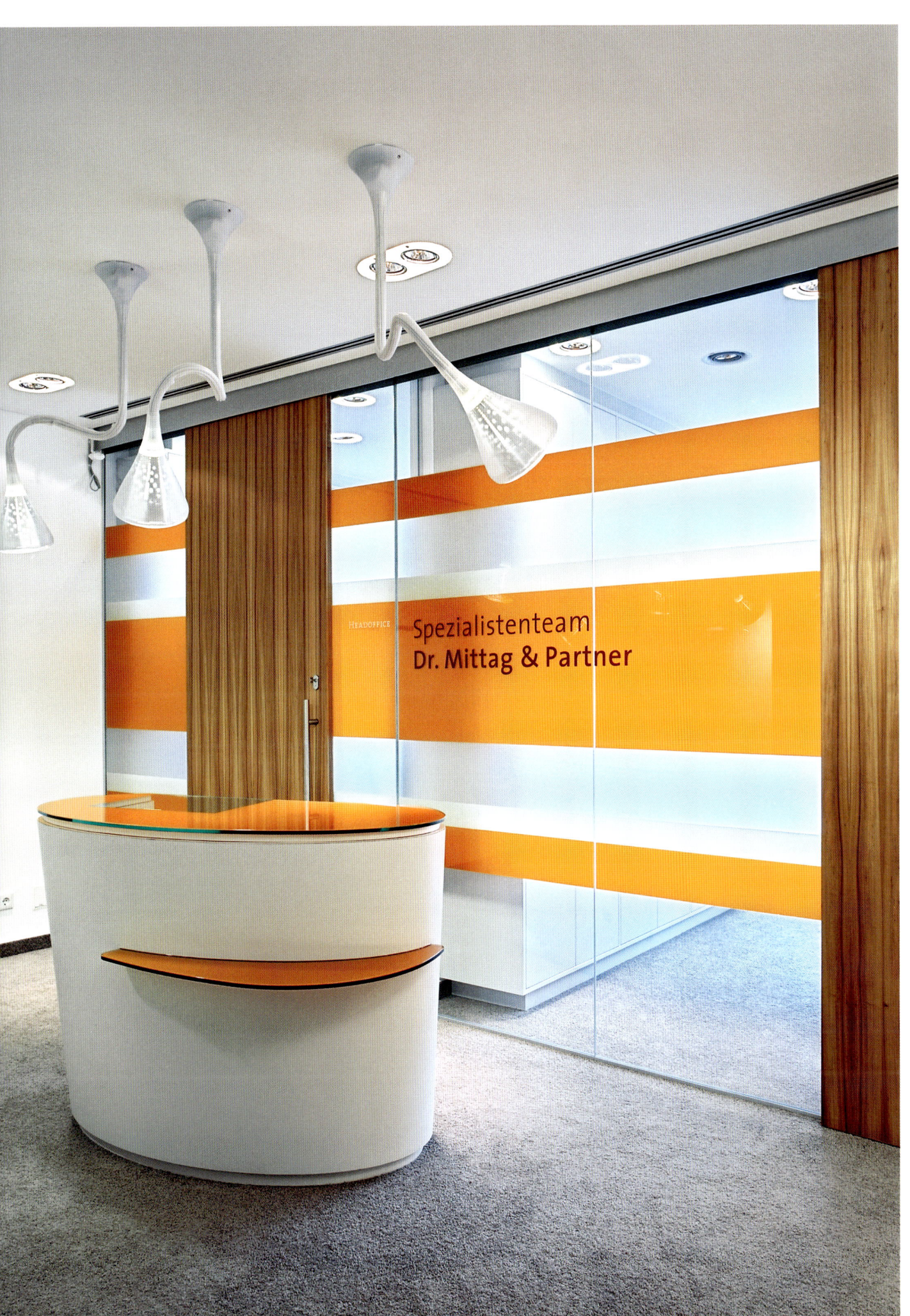

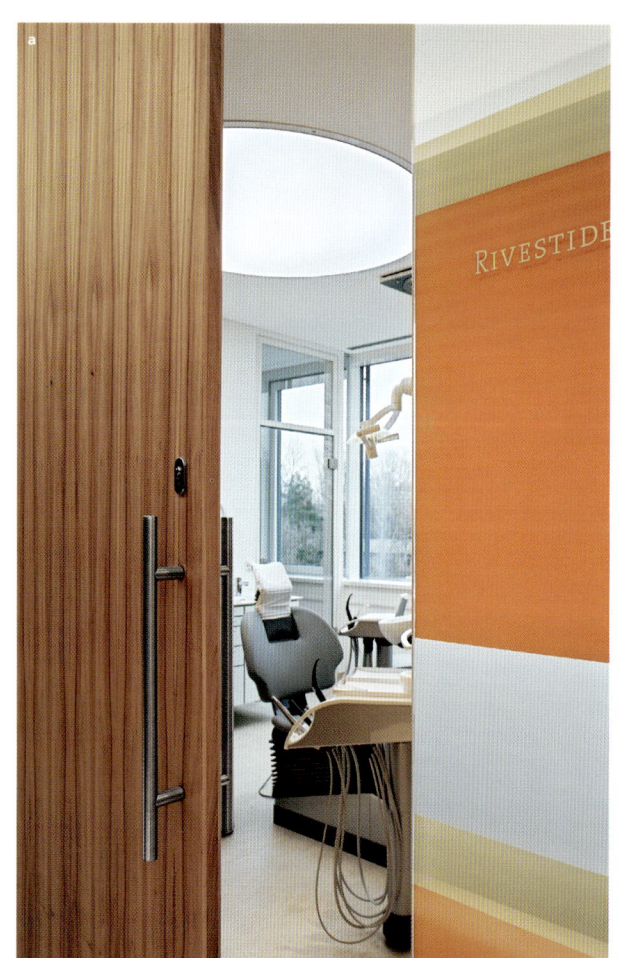
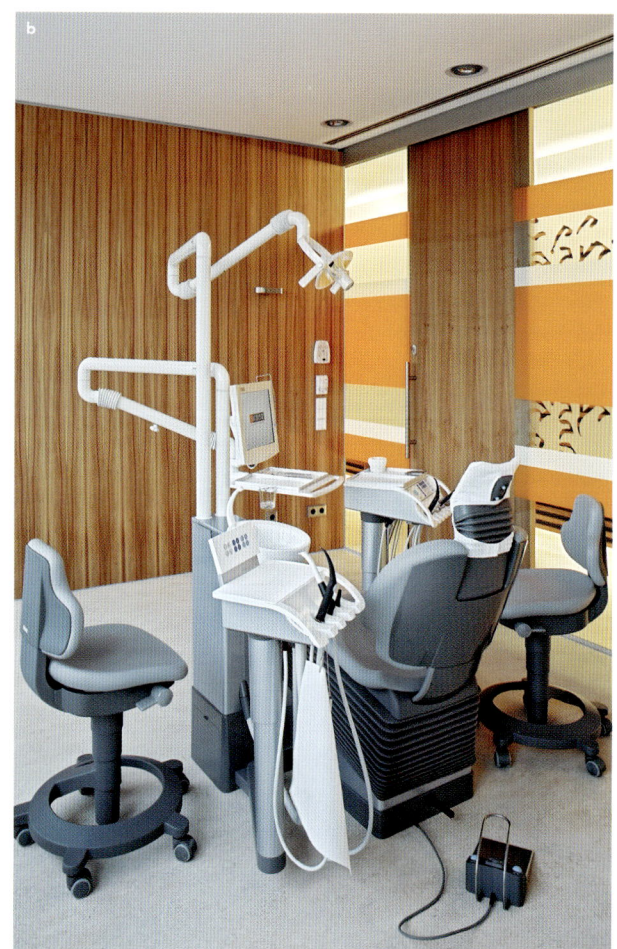

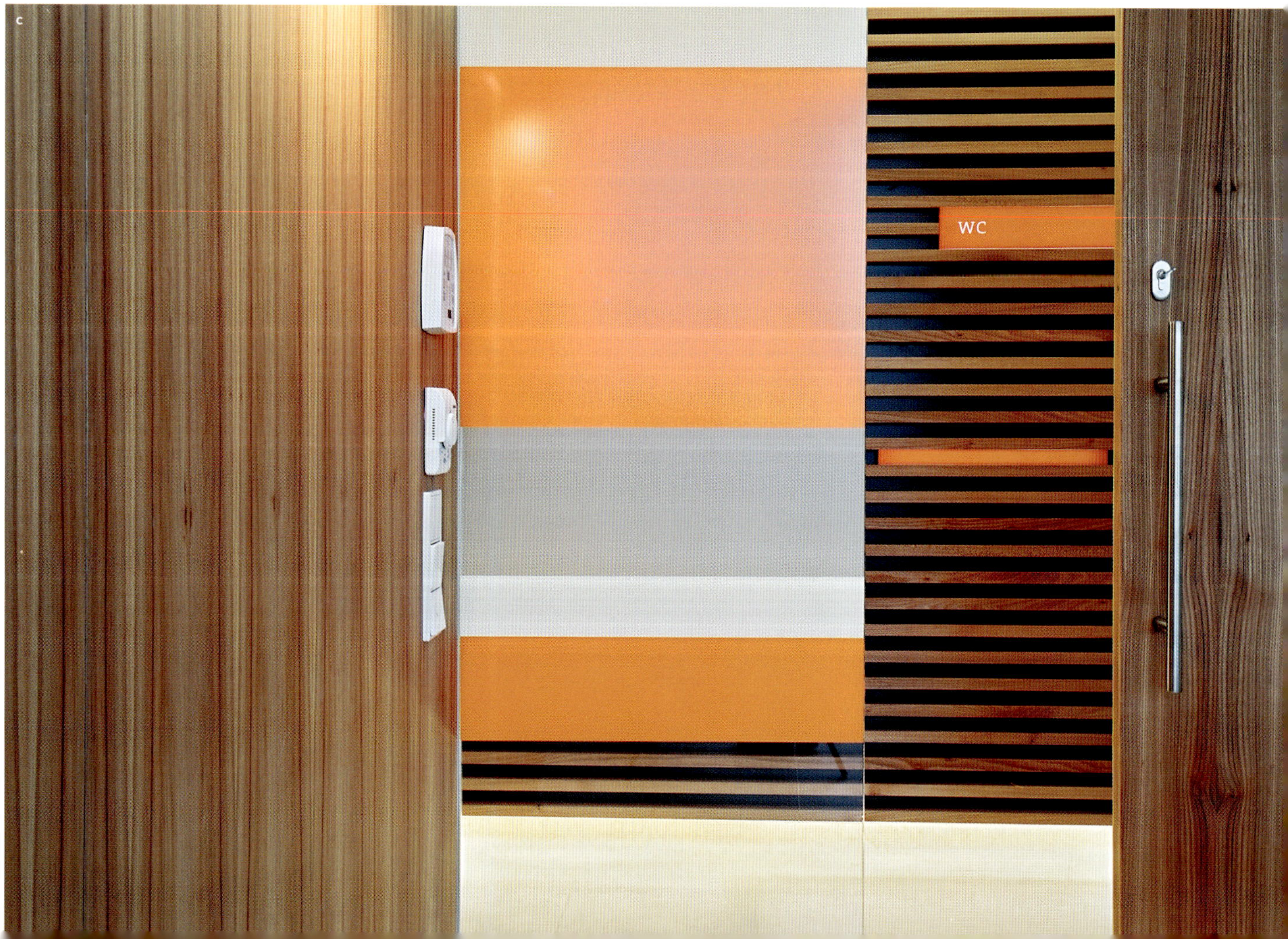

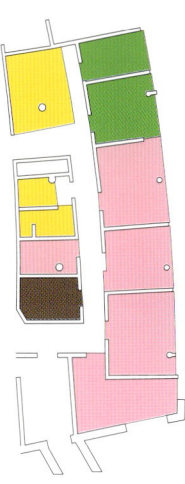

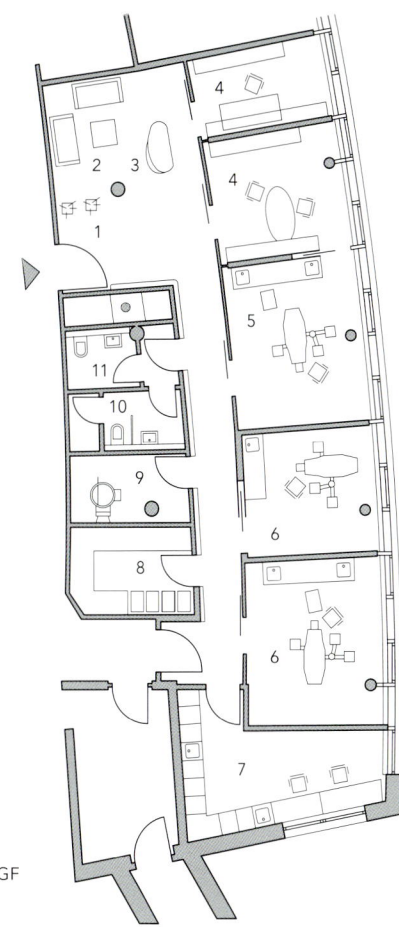

GF

Client   Dr. Inge Mittag
                          BCB Building Consult
                          Bremen GmbH
Operator   Dr. Inge Mittag
Planning time   05 2004 – 02 2005
Construction time   02 2005 – 03 2005
Gross floor area   170 sqm
Usable floor space   129 sqm
Gross cubic capacity 518 cbm

a The building's transparent, light-flooded
   exterior architecture mirrored by its interior
   design, with a glass wall running parallel to the
   slightly curved outer façade.
b The field of vision on the glass wall is coated
   in a translucent film that varies in texture,
   ensuring patient privacy during treatment.
c The luxurious fittings reflect the practice's area
   of expertise, the preparation of high quality
   ceramic inlays.

Diagrammatic plans, to scale 1:400
Floor plans, to scale 1:200

Floor plan layout

1 Coat-rack	**6** Treatment room	**9** Examination X-ray
2 Reception	prevention	**10** Toilet G
3 Waiting area	**7** Ceramic room	**11** Toilet L
4 Office	**8** Sterilisation room	
5 Treatment room	and store room	

From the main entrance in the first third of the slightly curved, long rectangular building that houses the partnership practice, patients proceed to the
treatment rooms, most of which are on the convex side. A second entrance
in the rear section of the floor plan is used for deliveries. While the rooms on
the convex side benefit from natural light, those on the concave side have
no windows.

Usable floor spaces

Patient rooms	**yellow**	24 sqm	19 %
Specialist rooms	**pink**	75 sqm	58 %
Administrative rooms	**green**	22 sqm	17 %
Supply | Waste disposal	**brown**	8 sqm	6 %
Total		129 sqm	100 %

Performance data

Outpatients per year	1,000
Number and type of services per year	Root canal treatment [200]
Services to other clinics	CT [50]
Clinic opening hours	5 days | 50 hours
Waiting time [with | without appointment]	10 min. | 45 min.
Type and number of staff	2 doctors
	4 full-time staff
	2 part-time staff
	1 dental technician
Clinic planning advice	Another office would be useful.

When designing this maxillofacial clinic, special attention was paid to the layout of the reception area – entering, registering and waiting forming the normal prelude to any practice visit. This area extends the full depth of the room along the whole window frontage and is defined by a twelve metre long light wall decorated with floral motifs and fitted with a state of the art dimmer system. The open structures of the loft-like reception area are picked up in the furnishings – the leather-lined reception desk "floating" on glass has a light filigree appearance. The room is defined by restrained but strong colours, dark leather and honey-coloured wood. Behind the illuminated motif wall are the treatment rooms, two of which have direct access to the recovery room. All fittings and cupboards are inset into the wall, leaving only the treatment chair free-standing. Everything is colour coordinated or in toning shades, preserving harmony of the rooms.

The practice's signature blend of strong lines, restrained, high-quality materials and an opulent, colourful wall structure mirrors the professional combination of precision and aesthetics, indirectly creating an atmosphere of calm and trust.

**GNOSA
ARCHITEKTEN**

CLINIC AT OPERNPLATZ
HANOVER | G

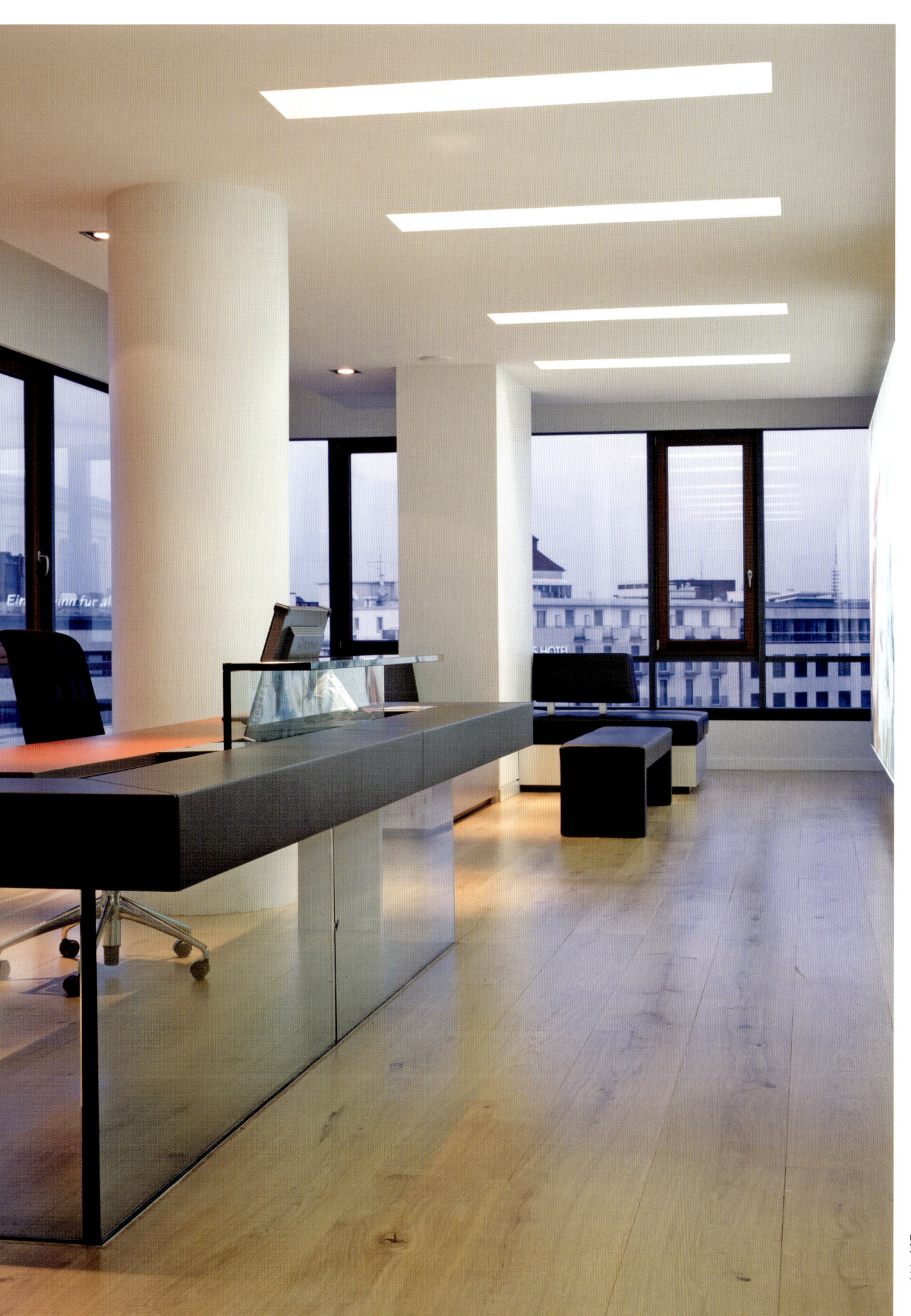

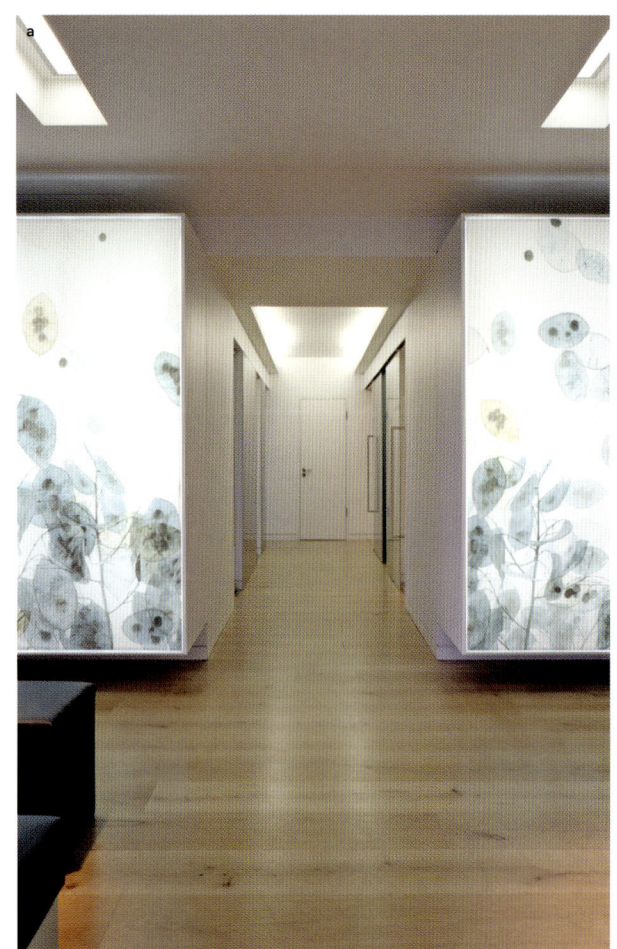

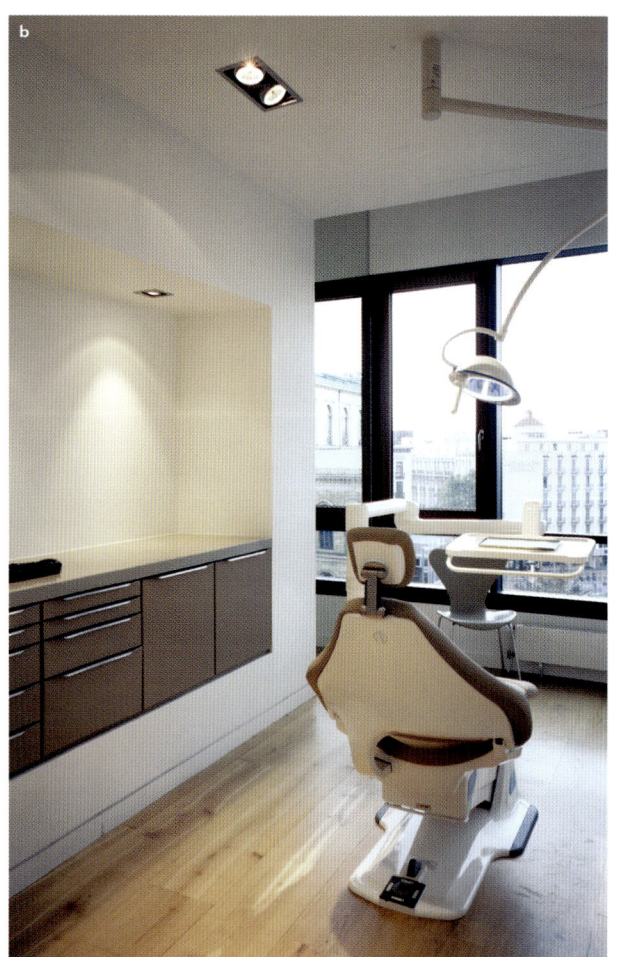

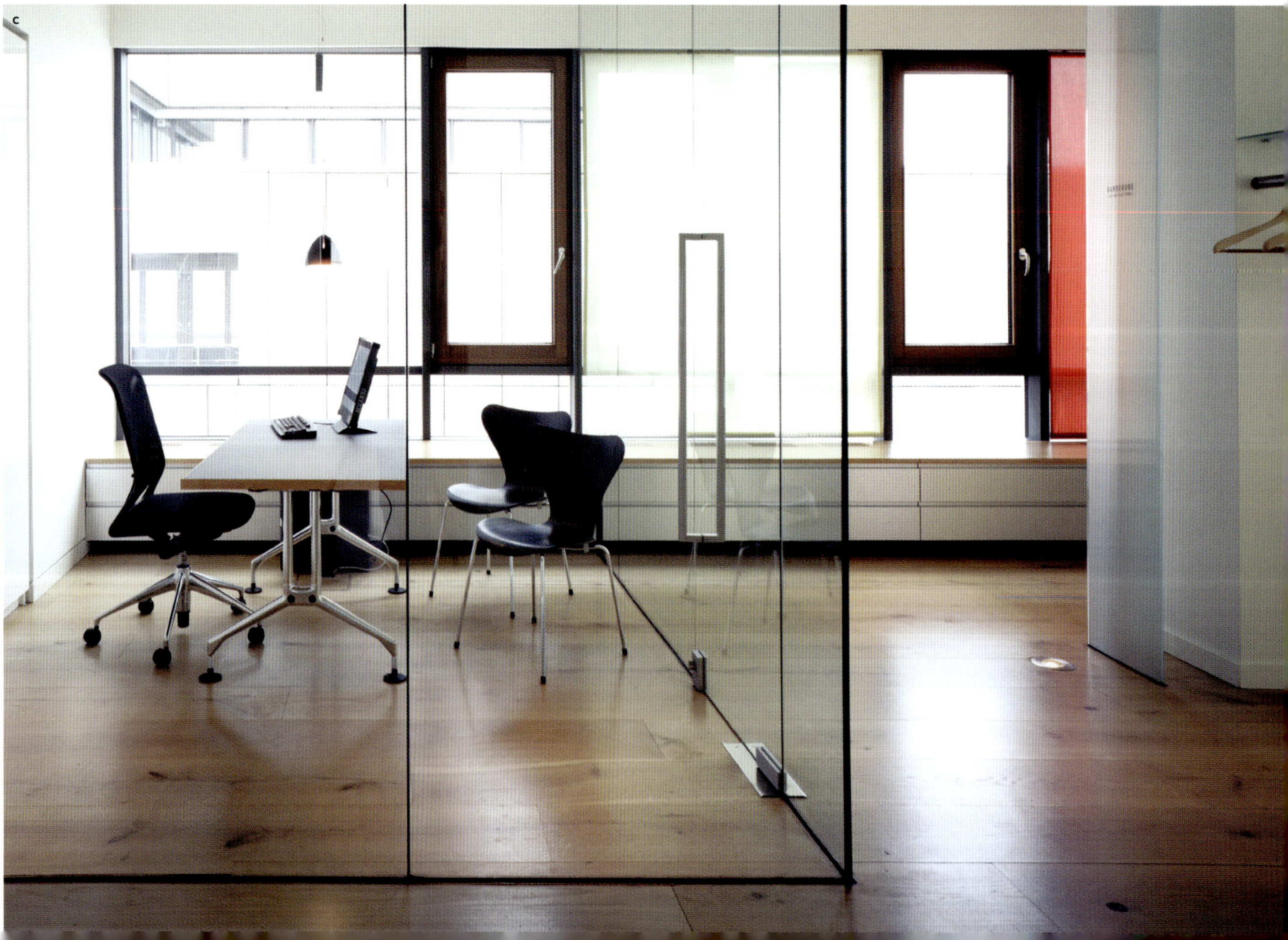

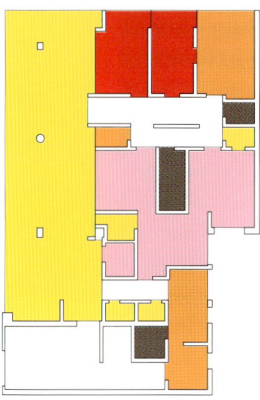

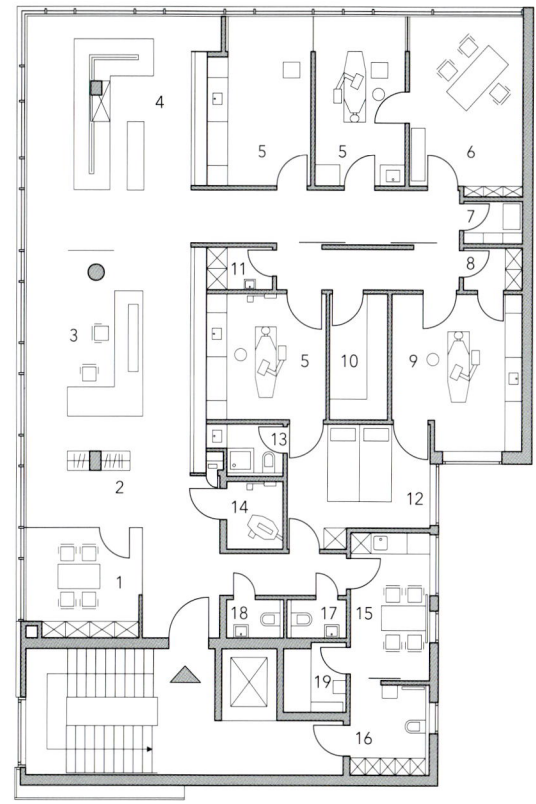

3. FL

Client | Operator   Clinic at Opernplatz
                            Dr. Stephan Vogt
Planning time   04 2003 – 11 2003
Construction time   06 2003 – 11 2003
Gross floor area   293 sqm
Usable floor space   220 sqm
Gross cubic capacity   923 cbm

a The spacious reception and waiting area is
   defined by a twelve metre long light wall
   decorated with floral motifs.
b All fittings and cupboards in the treatment
   rooms are inset into the walls, leaving only the
   treatment chair free-standing.
c The consultation room, separated from the
   coatrack by a glass wall, provides transparency.

Diagrammatic plans, to scale 1:400
Floor plans, to scale 1:200

Floor plan layout

1 Consultation room	cubicle	**14** Examination X-ray
2 Coat-rack	**9** Procedure room	**15** Staff lounge
3 Reception	**10** Sterilisation room	**16** Staff toilet and
4 Waiting area	**11** Staff changing	toilet for disabled
5 Treatment room	cubicle	**17** Toilet L
6 Doctor's office	**12** Recovery room	**18** Toilet G
7 Store room	**13** Patient toilet and	**19** Cleaning room
8 Patient changing	shower	

The treatment rooms in the split-level floor plan of this single-handed practice are accessed from a spacious foyer with reception, waiting area and
consultation room, through two connecting corridors. For some functional
groups this has resulted in short passageways, but it also means that some
rooms have no natural light. The recovery room is rather small.

Usable floor spaces

Patient rooms	**yellow**	103 sqm	47 %
Examination |			
Treatment rooms	**red**	27 sqm	12 %
Specialist rooms	**pink**	45 sqm	21 %
Offices | Staff rooms	**orange**	34 sqm	15 %
Supply | Waste disposal	**brown**	11 sqm	5 %
Total		220 sqm	100 %

Performance data

Outpatients per year	2,000
Inpatients per year	200
Clinic opening hours	5 days | 50 hours
Waiting time	10 – 15 min.
Number of staff	6 – 8

At the entrance to this Berlin dental practice specialising in the treatment of children, young children and their parents stare in amazement at the curling blue wave that "flows" through the whole building and serves as ceiling, wall, reception and lounge. A structural space has been created in which the rooms are interwoven by the movements of the wave. The split-level design draws people entering the building "beneath the wave" into an underwater world. Children, their dread of a visit to the dentist quite forgotten, dive into a mysterious universe, where shoals of fish swim along the walls and light points adorn the ceiling like rising bubbles. The architects spurned the conventional white colour scheme and sterile, hygienic atmosphere normally found in dental practices, opting instead for soft, flowing shapes. An atmosphere has been created in which children can forget the world around them – and in particular the fact that they have come to see the dentist. The underwater theme permeates every area of the practice and is emphasised by targeted use of light and materials. Echoing the wave that "rolls" through the rooms, a sea-blue colour concept was devised for the practice in collaboration with STRAUSS & HILLEGAART, embracing ceilings, walls and floors and even the furniture and dental equipment. A visit to this practice is a special experience – and not just for the children!

GRAFT

CHILDREN'S DENTAL PRACTICE
BERLIN | G

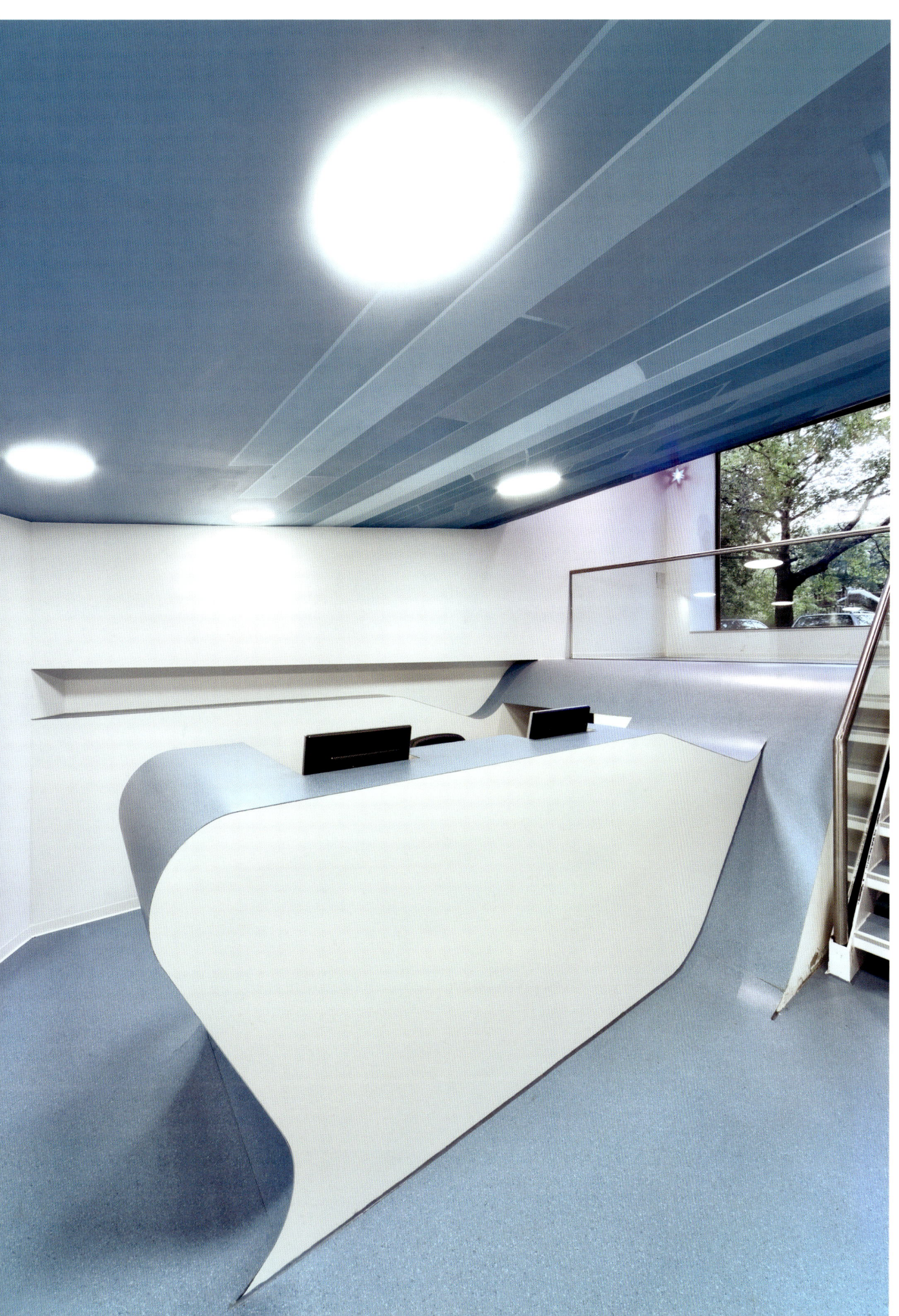

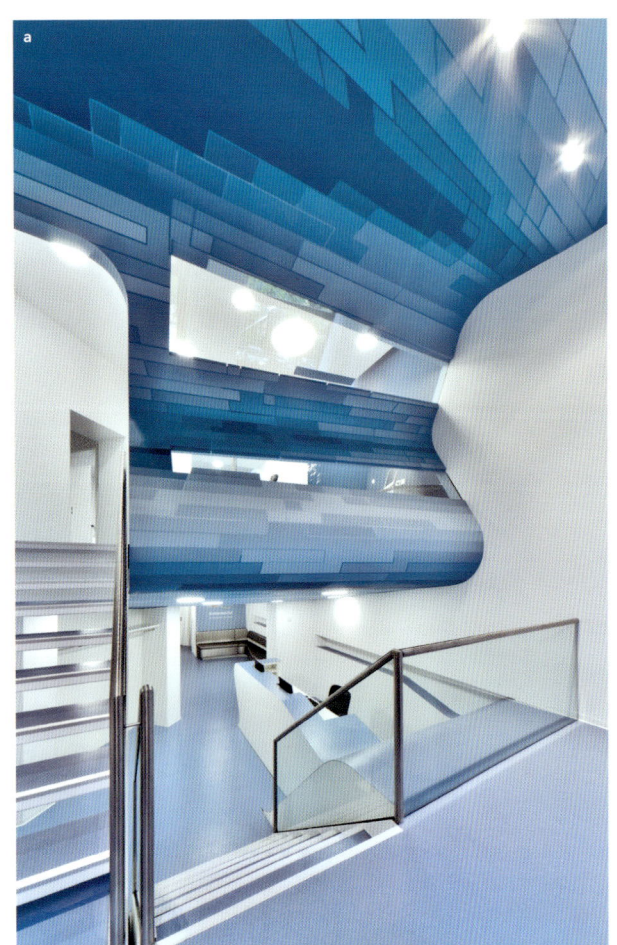

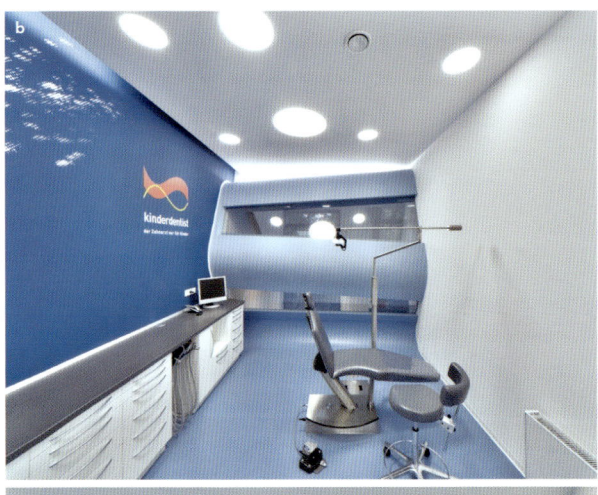

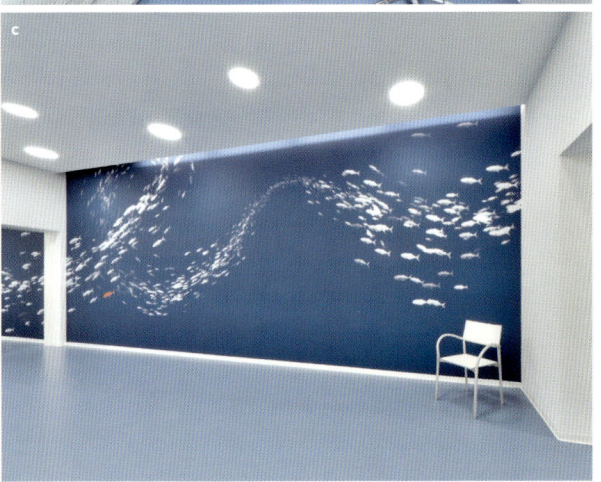

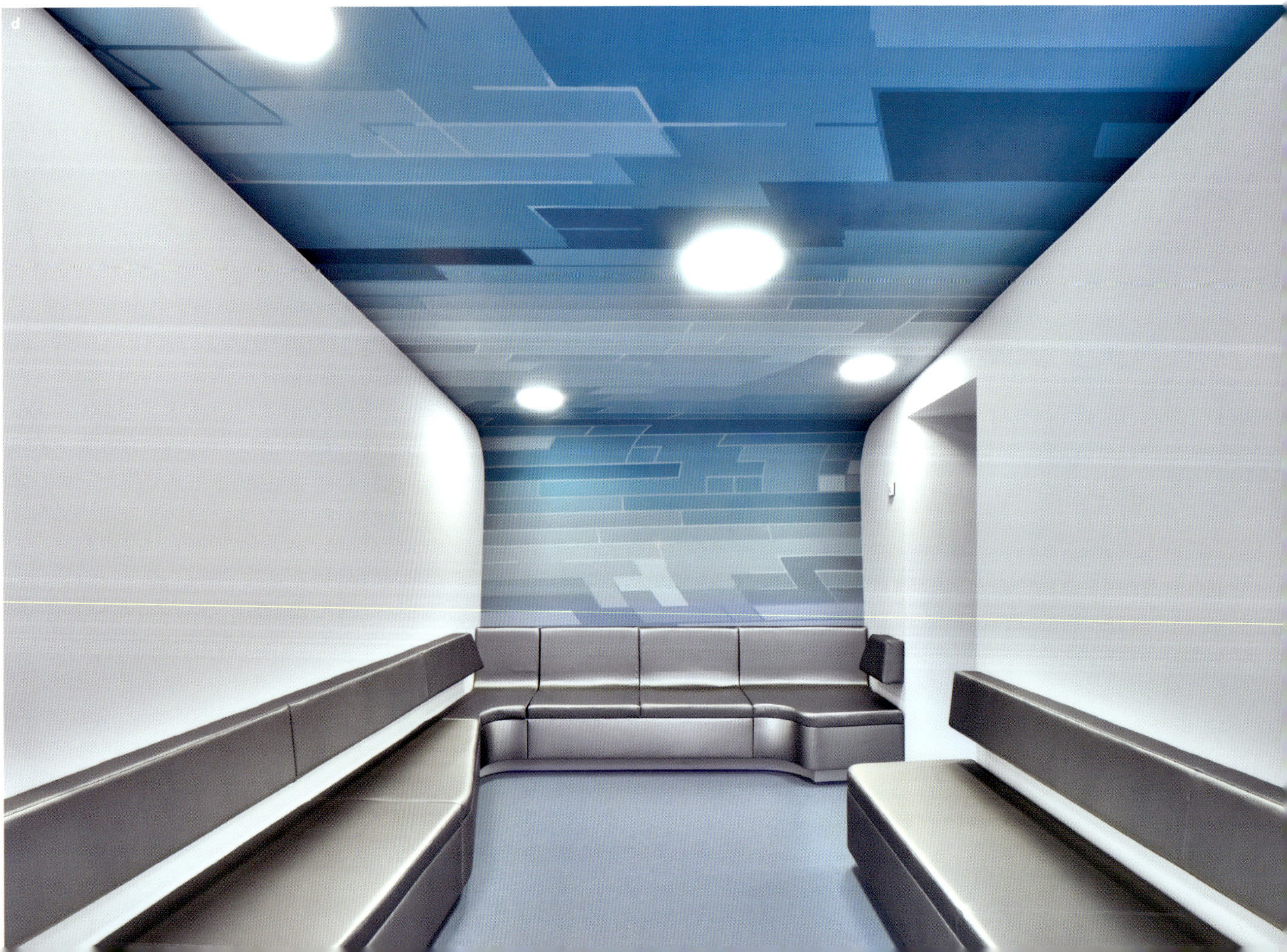

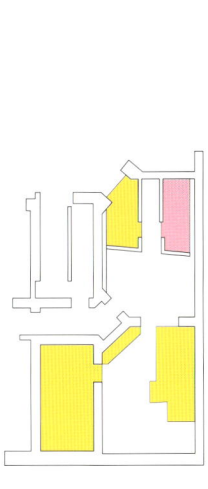
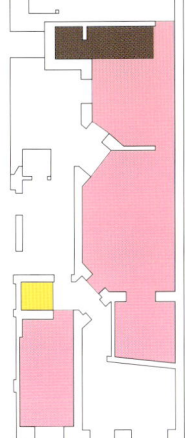

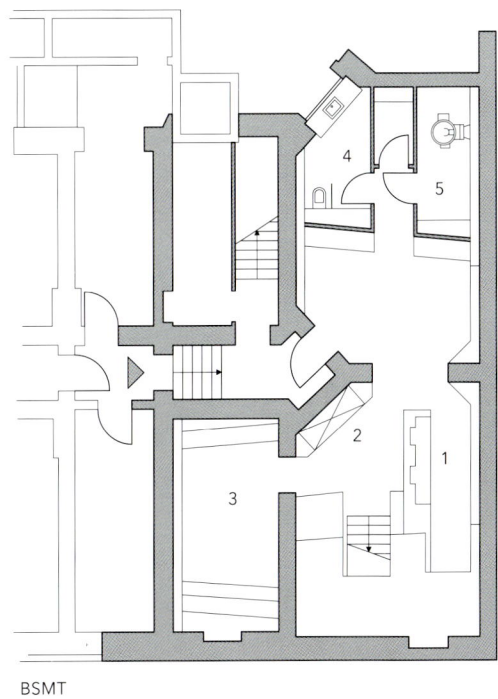

BSMT

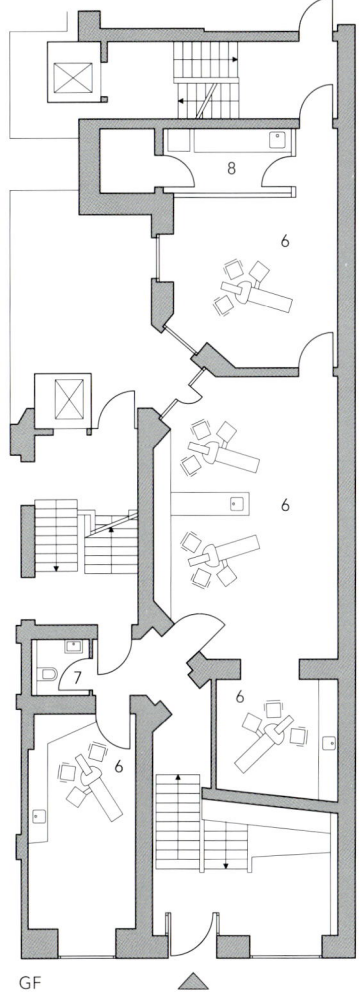

GF

Client | Operator   Dr. A. Mokabberi
Construction time   02 2007 – 08 2007
Gross floor area   177 sqm
Usable floor space   157 sqm

a A curling blue wave "flows through" the foyer, interweaving the two floors of the practice.

b The sea-blue colour concept devised for the practice embraces ceilings, walls and floors and even the furniture and dental equipment.

c Shoals of fish on the walls and light points dotting the ceiling like some rising bubbles create a mysterious world.

d The basement waiting area, which creates the illusion of diving into the ocean depths.

Diagrammatic plans, to scale 1:400
Floor plans, to scale 1:200

Floor plan layout

1	Reception	**4**	Patient toilet L		dentist
2	Coat-rack	**5**	Examination X-ray	**7**	Patient toilet G
3	Waiting area	**6**	Treatment room	**8**	Sterilisation room

Basement steps take patients into the spacious area housing reception, coat-rack and waiting area. The X-ray room is also located here, while all other treatment is provided at ground floor level. On the upper ground floor, natural light shines through doors into two of the four treatment rooms.

Usable floor spaces

Patient rooms	**yellow**	43 sqm	27 %
Specialist rooms	**pink**	104 sqm	66 %
Supply | Waste disposal	**brown**	10 sqm	7 %
Total		157 sqm	100 %

Few other environments have such negative connotations as a dental practice. Here the architects made a conscious decision to shun the normal practice setup, replacing it with a spectacular red and yellow interior themed on a landscape of sand-dune.

Patients visiting this practice are made to feel like beachgoers choosing a quiet spot in the sand, spreading their towels and settling down to enjoy the peace and quiet. The floor curves and waves billow on the ceiling. In the middle of this undulated landscape, flat built-in furniture – the unusual loungers and sofas are more than just seats – provide an idyllic beach setting, and a sundeck represents the sea. An open wood-burner suspended from the ceiling conjures up a campfire idyll in Charlottenburg practice. The dental treatment room is fitted out as spa area: a geometric, subtly lit "spring grotto" with a large basin reflects gentle water movements on the ceiling; glass washbasins float like islands in this artistic waterworld. As a counterpoint to the colourful and vibrant design of the public areas, the high-tech treatment rooms are more restrained. The two practice levels are connected by an open staircase at the end of the main corridor; a canyon-like passageway offers stunning views over the surrounding roofscape.

GRAFT

"KU64" DENTAL PRACTICE
BERLIN | G

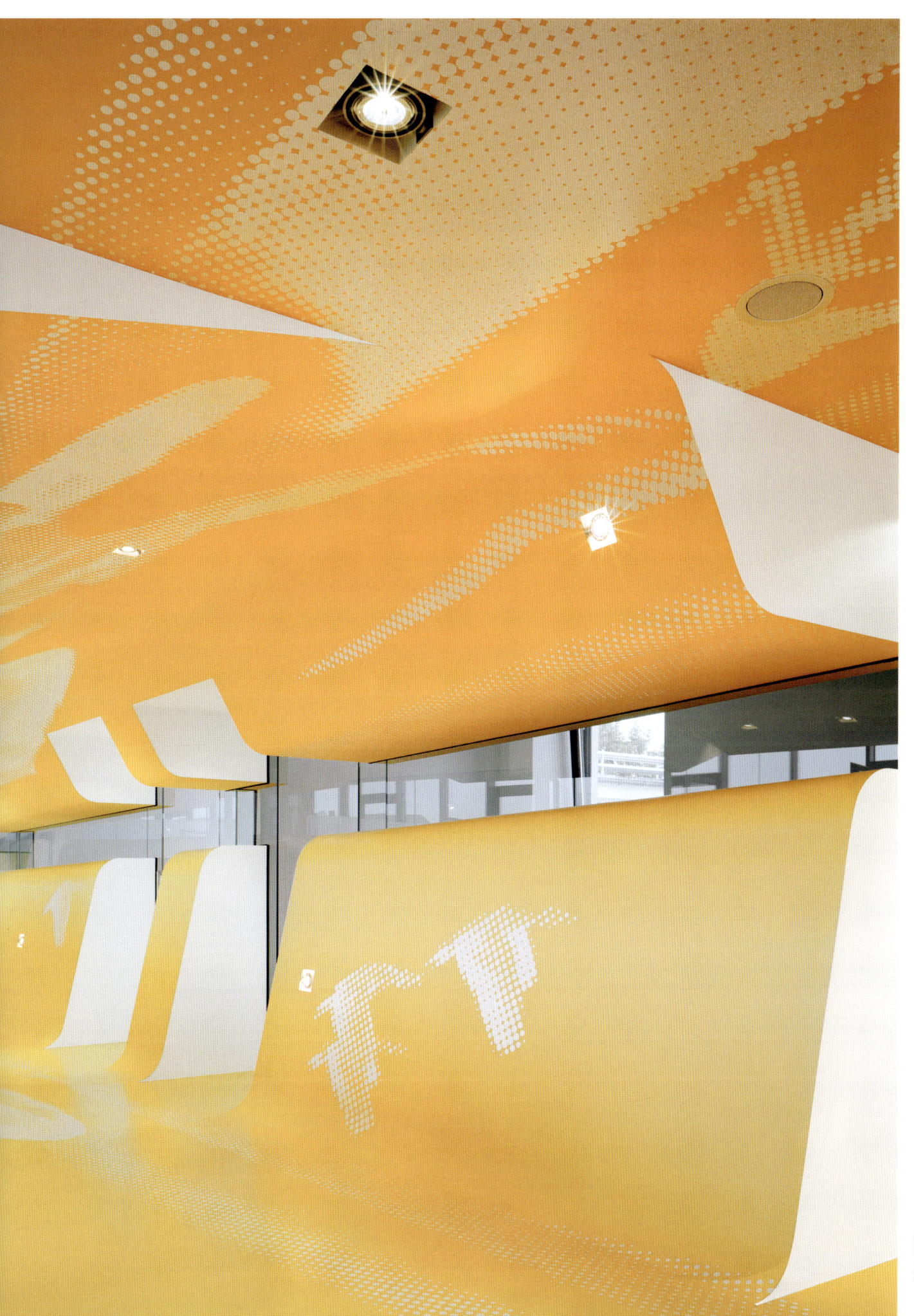

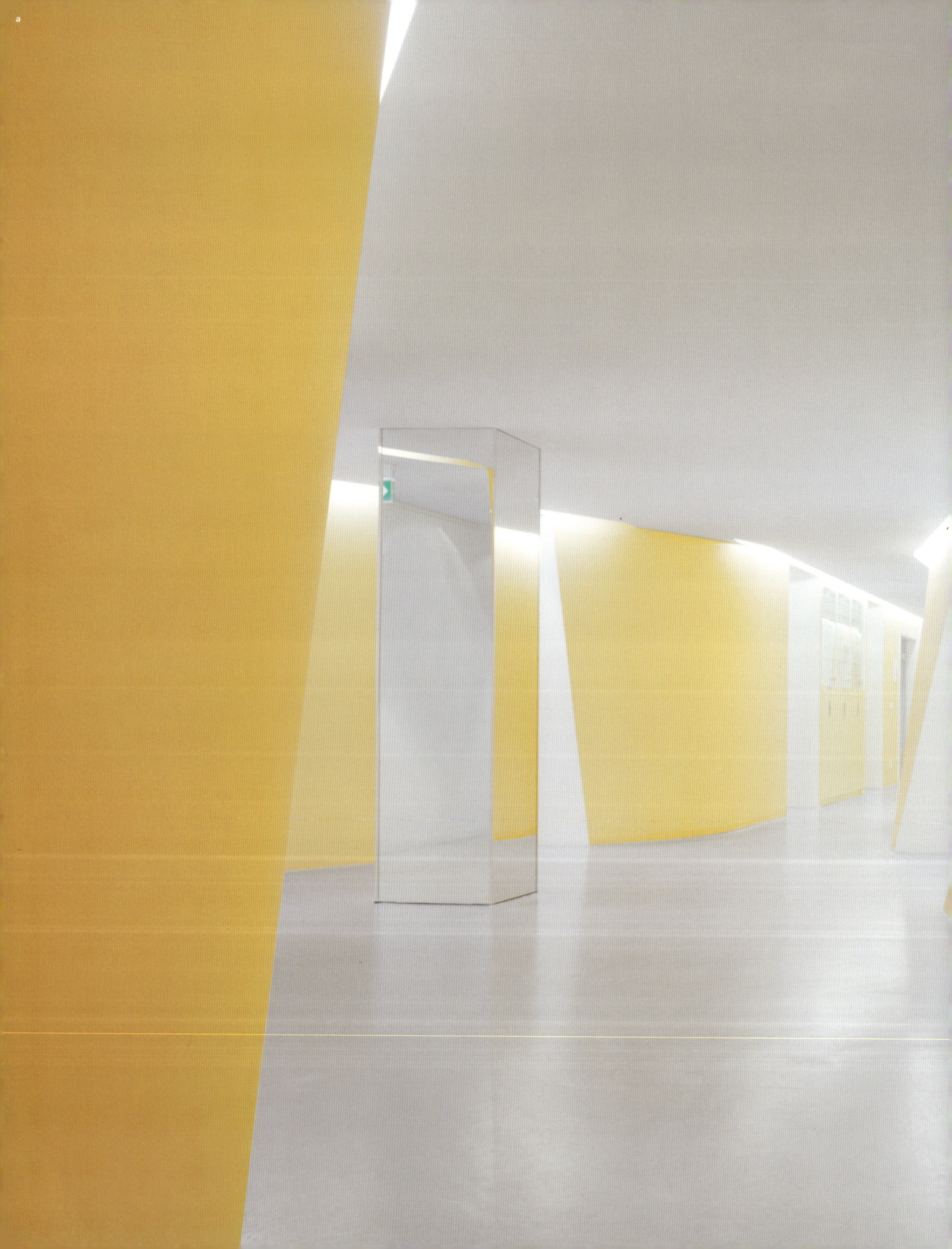

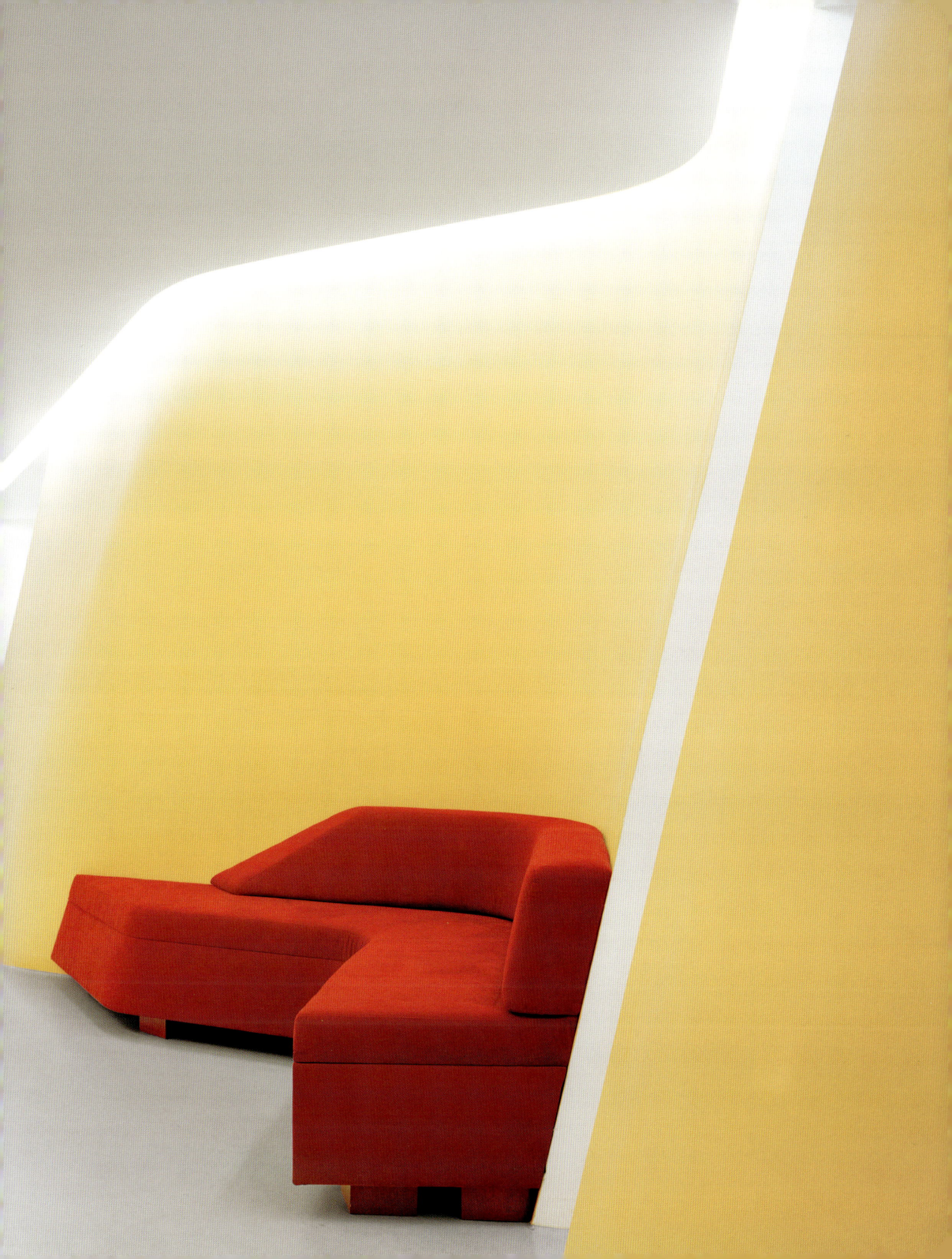

Diagrammatic plans, to scale 1:400
Floor plans, to scale 1:200

1 Installations room	**9** Sterilisation room	**17** Staff toilet G
2 Patient toilet L	**10** Prep room	**18** Staff shower G
3 Patient toilet G	**11** Office	**19** Staff changing
4 Patient toilet and	**12** Laboratory	cubicle G
shower	**13** Staff lounge	**20** Toilet for the
5 Quiet room	**14** Staff changing	disabled
6 Treatment room	cubicle L	**21** Waiting area
7 Consultation room	**15** Staff shower L	**22** Reception
8 Ceramic room	**16** Staff toilet L	

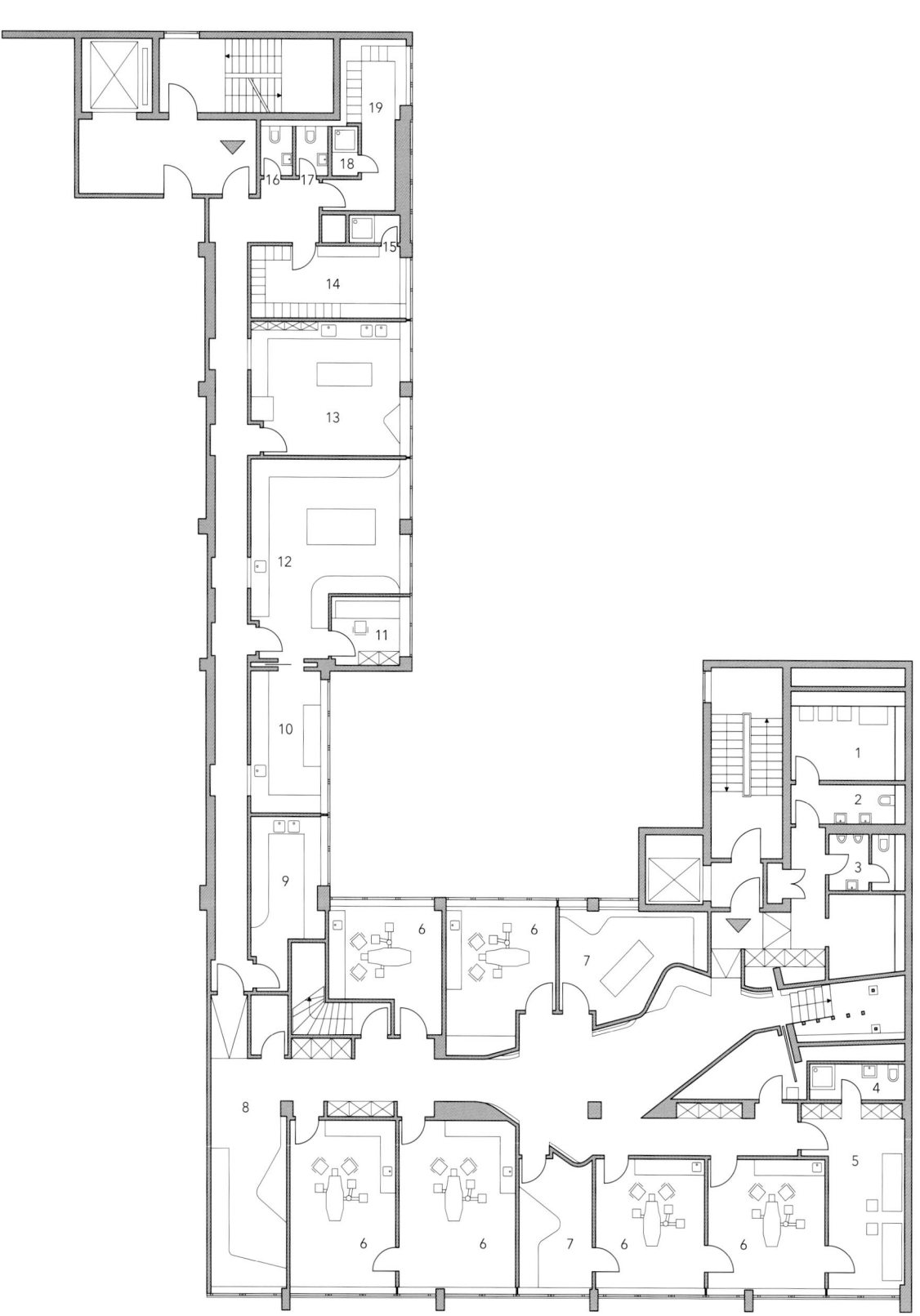

5. FL

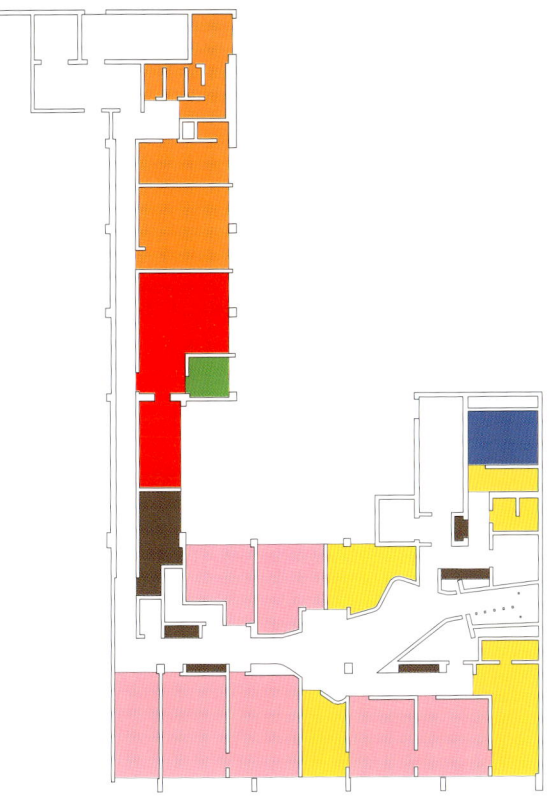

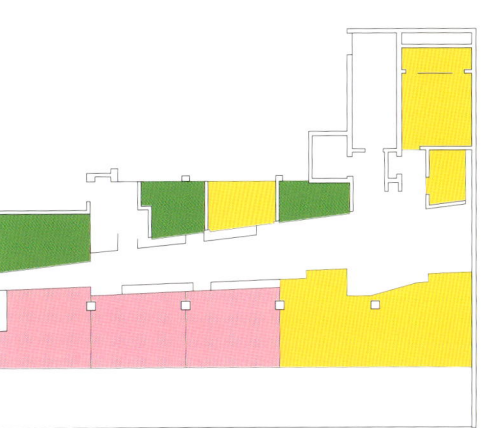

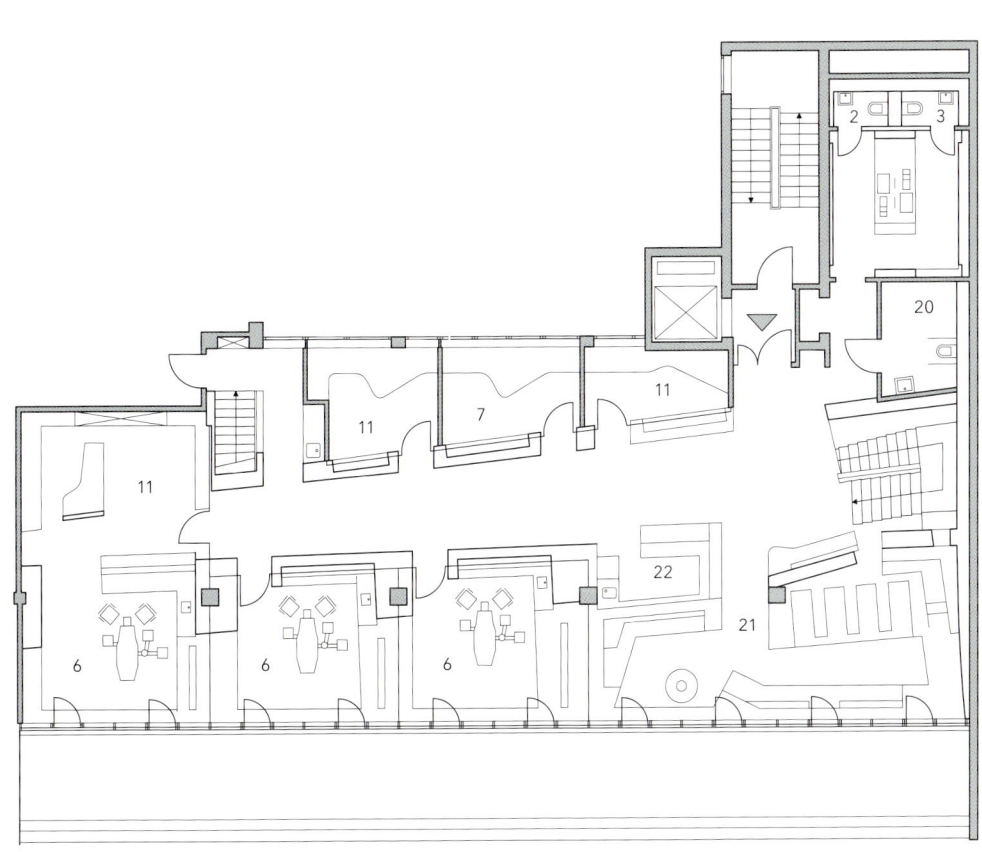

6. FL

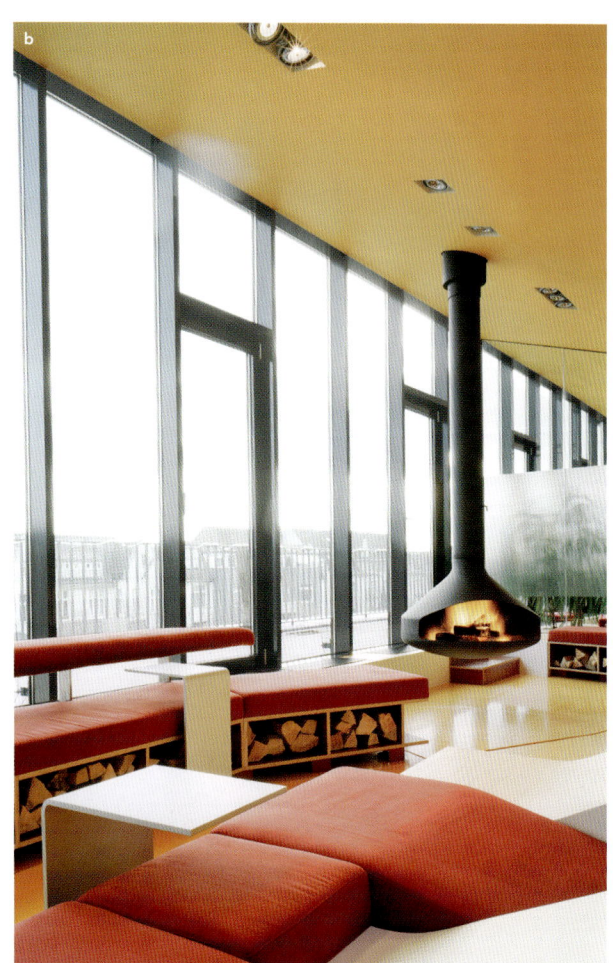

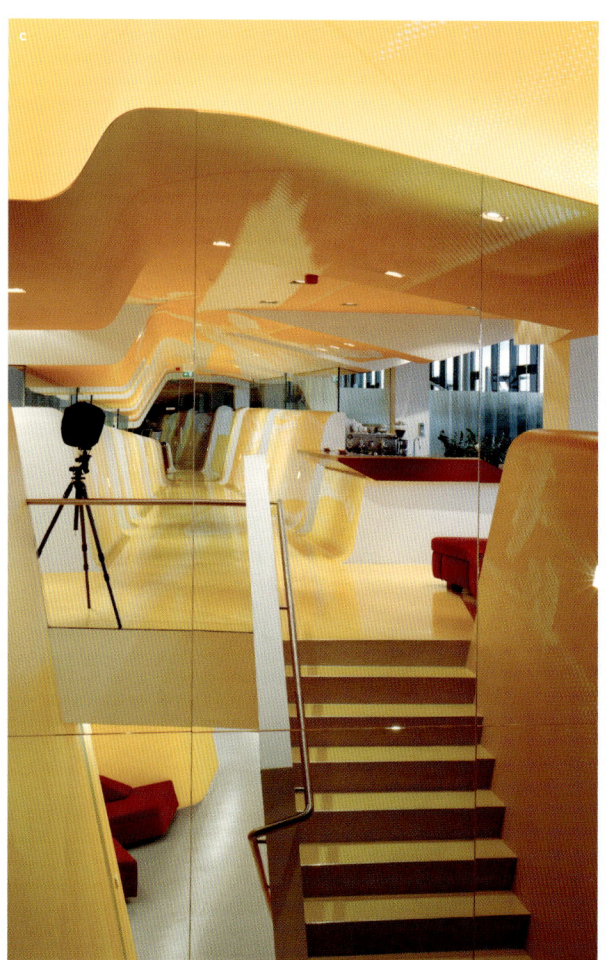

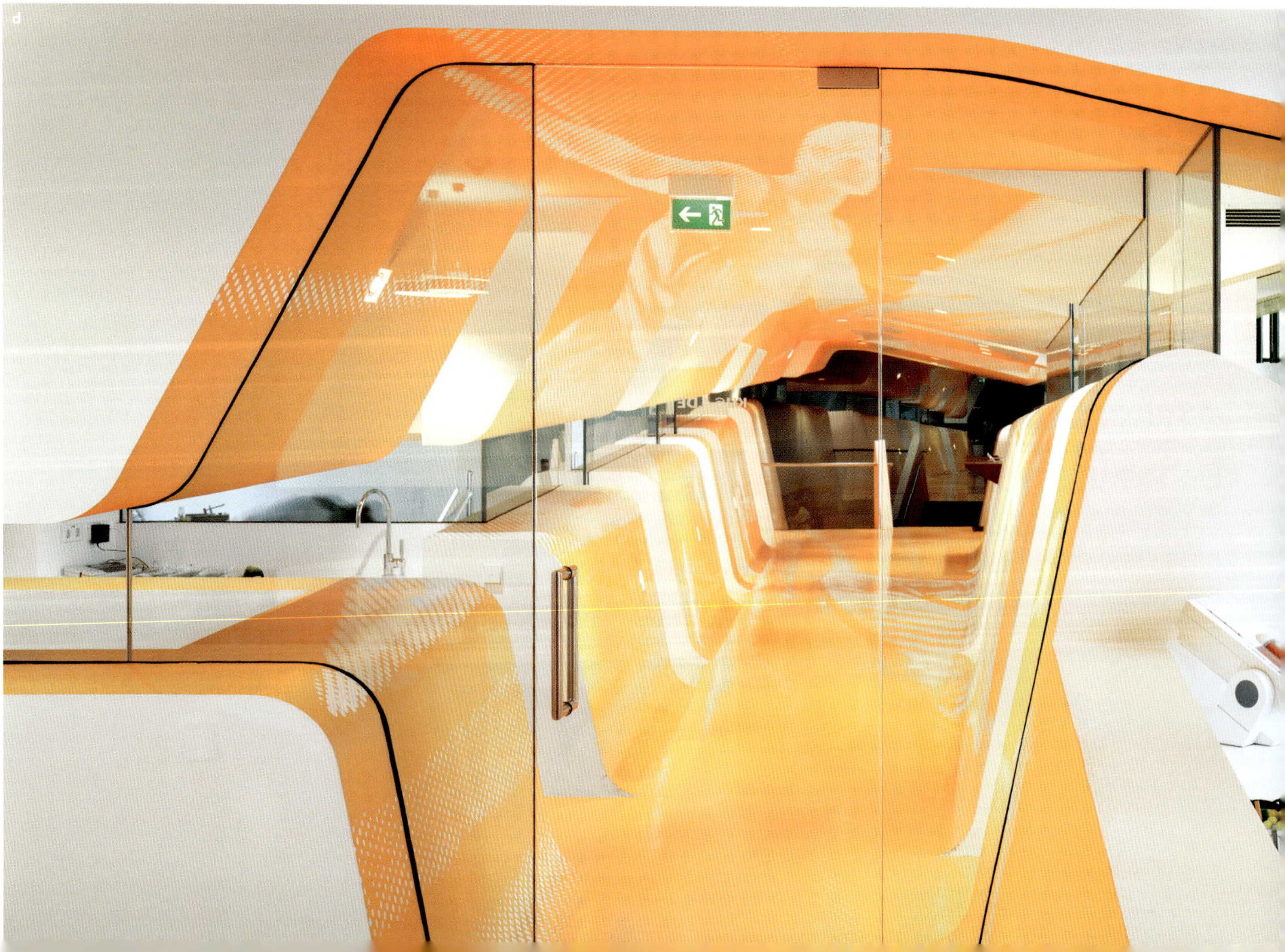

Client | Operator	Dr. Stefan Ziegler
Construction time	01 2005 – 07 2005
Gross floor area	940 sqm
Usable floor space	536 sqm
Gross cubic capacity	3,077 cbm
Total cost	519,680 EUR

a   The surprisingly colourful and vibrant
    corridor on the 5th floor.
b   An open wood-burner suspended from
    the ceiling conjures up a campfire idyll in
    the waiting area above the roofs of Berlin.
c   A staircase at the end of the corridor
    connects the practice's two levels.
d   The wall motifs, which appear normal or
    distorted always depending on the angle
    of view, were designed in collaboration
    with STRAUSS & HILLEGAART.

Floor plan layout

The main patient entrance into this large, two-level multi-doctor practice is
through the upper level which houses the reception and a spacious waiting
area. On the lower level are two secondary entrances. All the rooms apart
from a few side-rooms benefit from natural light.

Usable floor spaces

Patient rooms	**yellow**	160 sqm	30 %
Examination |			
Treatment rooms	**red**	43 sqm	8 %
Specialist rooms	**pink**	203 sqm	38 %
Administrative rooms	**green**	41 sqm	8 %
Offices | Staff rooms	**orange**	57 sqm	11 %
Supply | Waste disposal	**brown**	19 sqm	3 %
Plant rooms	**blue**	13 sqm	2 %
Total		536 sqm	100 %

The working area of every dentist is the mouth cavity. In this small practice at the edge of Munich's S-Bahn ring, the "Cavitas oris propria" is not only the theme of the treatment, but also of its interior design.

Dazzling white teeth shine out of an orange and red pulsing mouth cavity. Tooth caries is represented in the shape of customised pieces of furniture. The dentist and her assistants – clad in white – can be seen in the middle of an incomplete tooth image. Practice rooms are dominated by white against an orange and red background. Especially striking are the two architect-designed furniture pieces in the open-plan reception and waiting area: they represent two "teeth" in a huge mouth some 40 square metres. The filing system, almost one metre deep and accessible from both sides, incorporates 20 metres of file pullouts, a writing desk, broom and supply cupboards and adjoins the toilet and the laboratory. The reception desk forms another boundary, allowing the visitors to see over but not into the public area, and giving waiting patients as well as reception staff a measure of privacy. Treatment rooms, staff lounge and office line the long side of the practice.

GÜNTHER & SCHABERT

DENTAL PRACTICE
GILCHING | G

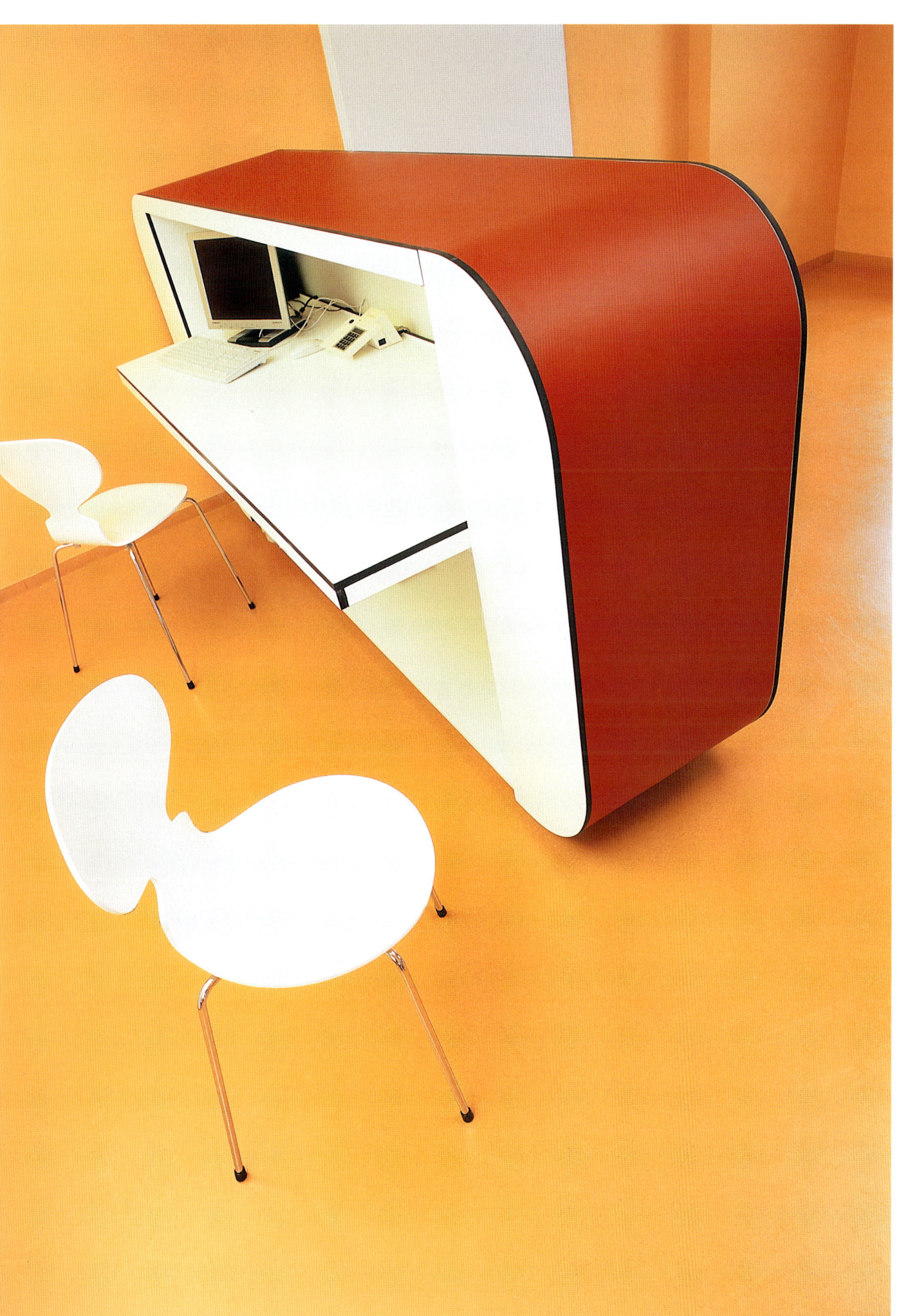

a

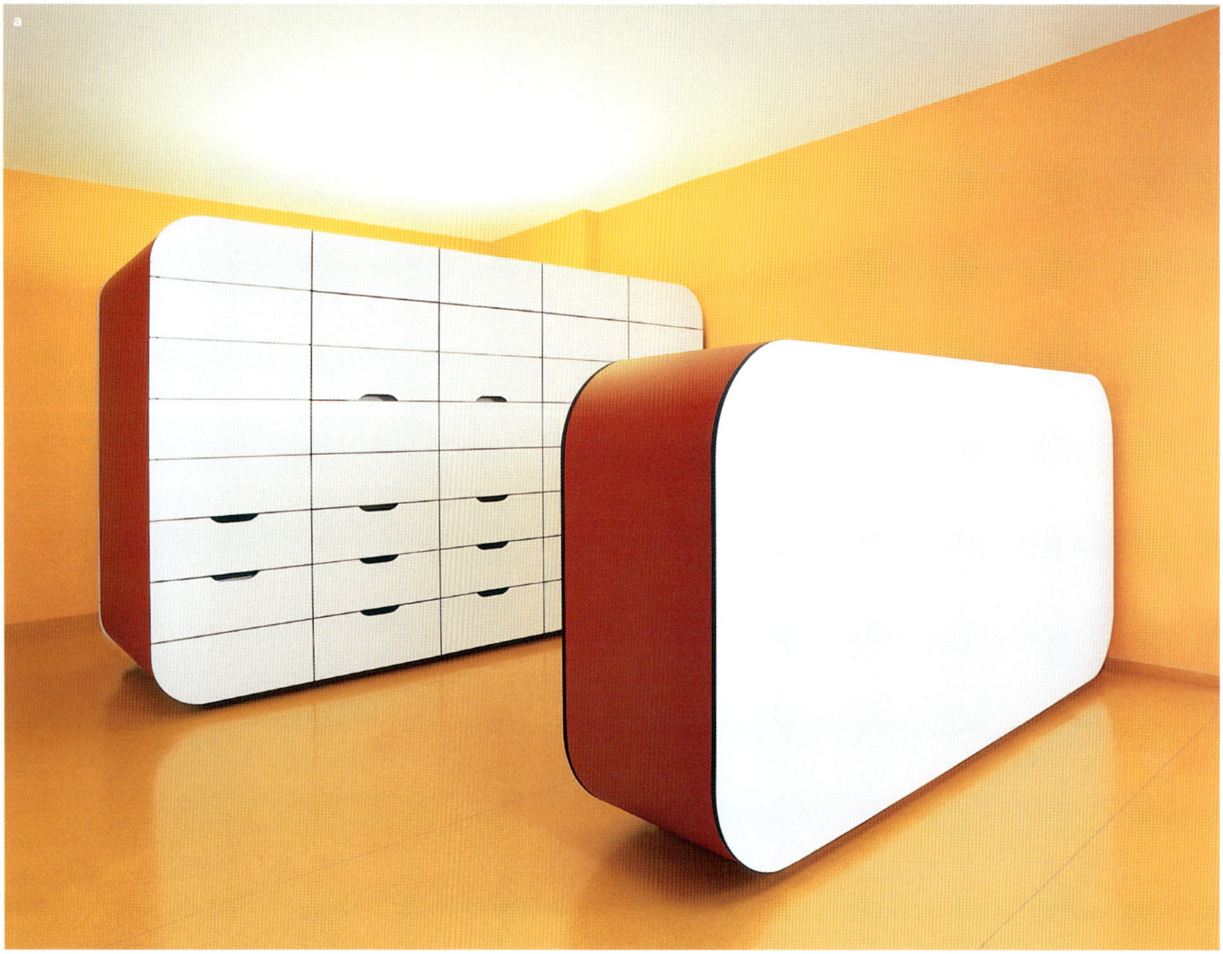

b

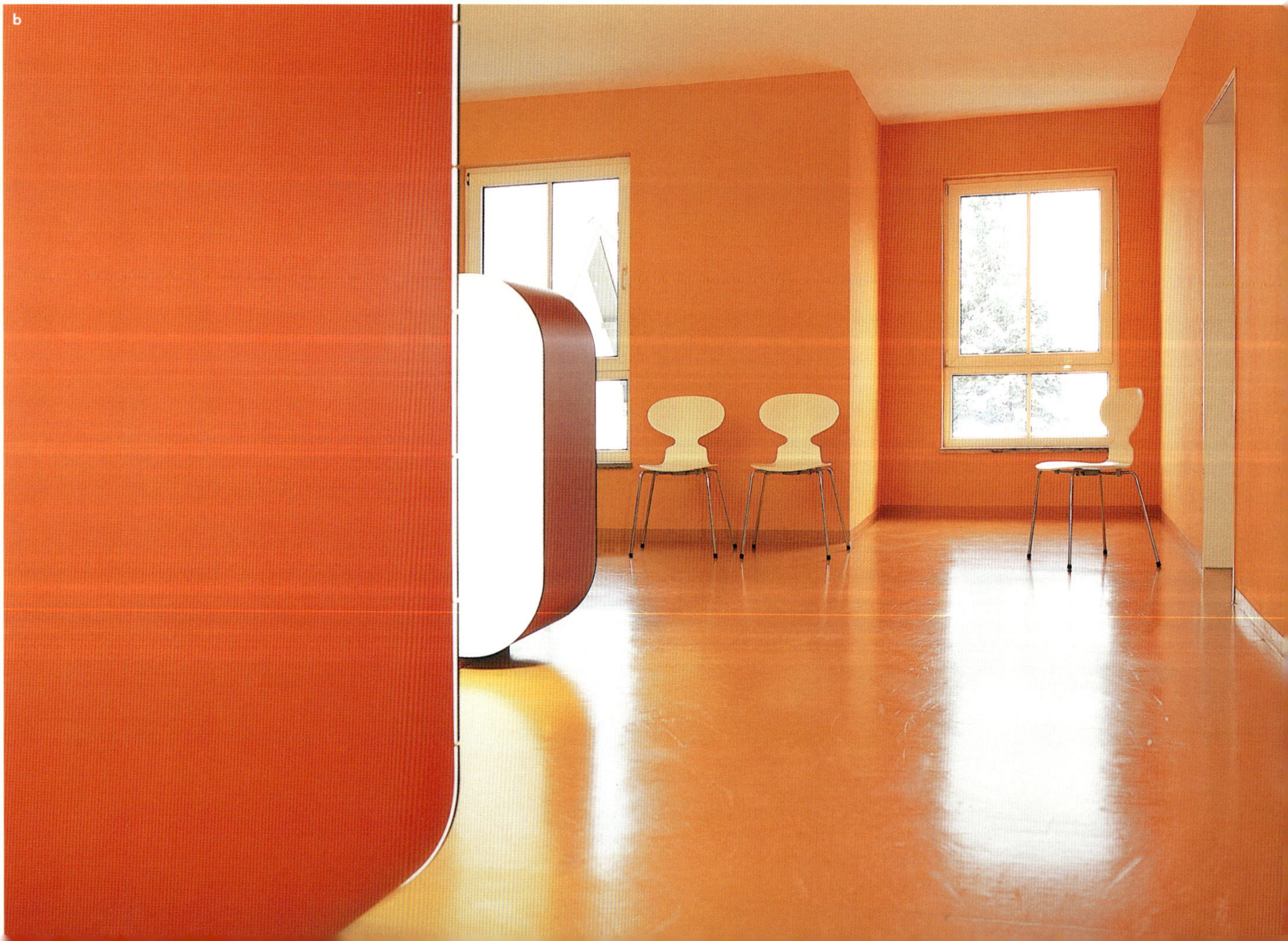

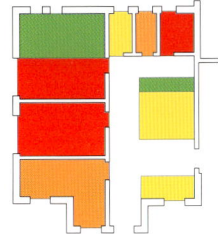

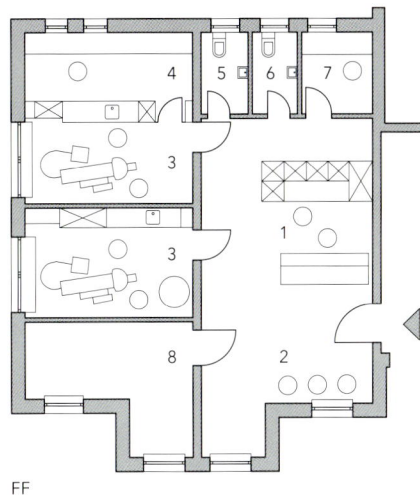

FF

Client	Operator	Dr. Kerstin Schlattner
Planning time	09 2002 – 10 2002
Construction time	10 2002 – 11 2002
Gross floor area	115 sqm
Usable floor space	80 sqm
Gross cubic capacity	295 cbm
Construction cost	65,000 EUR
Total cost	76,000 EUR

a The almost one metre deep filing cabinet, accessible from both sides, incorporates file pullouts and writing desk, broom cupboard and supply cupboard and also adjoins the toilet and laboratory.

b The two custom-made furniture pieces in the open-plan reception and waiting area of the practice are shaped like two "teeth" in a huge "mouth".

Diagrammatic plans, to scale 1:400
Floor plans, to scale 1:200

Floor plan layout

1	Filing room	**4**	Office	**7**	Laboratory
2	Waiting area	**5**	Patient toilet	**8**	Social room
3	Treatment room	**6**	Staff toilet		

The compact rectangular floor plan of the single-doctor practice makes good use of the public traffic areas needed to access the rooms [reception and waiting area]. The office, however, can only be accessed through one of the treatment rooms, and this could be problematic. All the practice's rooms, including side-rooms, benefit from natural light. The spaces needed for storage and cleaning purposes are cleverly integrated in the free-standing filing system in the foyer.

Usable floor spaces

Patient rooms	**yellow**	17 sqm	21 %
Examination |			
Treatment rooms	**red**	32 sqm	40 %
Administrative rooms	**green**	14 sqm	18 %
Offices | Staff rooms	**orange**	17 sqm	21 %
Total		80 sqm	100 %

Performance data

Outpatients per year	800
Services to other clinics	Orthodontics
	Implant surgery
Clinic opening hours	5 days | 44 hours
Waiting time	5 – 15 min.
Type and number of staff	1 doctor
	1 full-time staff
	1 trainee
	1 part-time staff

A spacious reception and waiting lounge welcomes visitors to the "Eye Do" eye clinic in Rotterdam's city centre. Custom-made upholstered furniture in silver-blue leather forms a curved semi-circle that invites patients to relax and admire the panoramic view of Rotterdam's breathtaking harbour skyline. The minimalist reception desk is backed by a large wall-mounted flat-screen monitor. In addition to three examination rooms, this former office floor houses the OP section with two operating rooms. The examination and operating rooms are fitted out in a more sober style than the rest of the clinic, and could almost be described as stark. Here the high-tech equipment stands alone in the middle of the otherwise simple space. The large recovery room resembles a trendy lounge rather than a clinic, with gold leather chairs and sofas, bright striped wallpaper and a long window frontage, affording wonderful views over the green area beyond.

A cafeteria and conference room are located on the upper floor, where a bold ornamental wall decoration and modern 1960s style tubular steel furniture have been adopted.

HELL UND FREUNDLICH

"EYE DO" EYE CLINIC
ROTTERDAM | NL

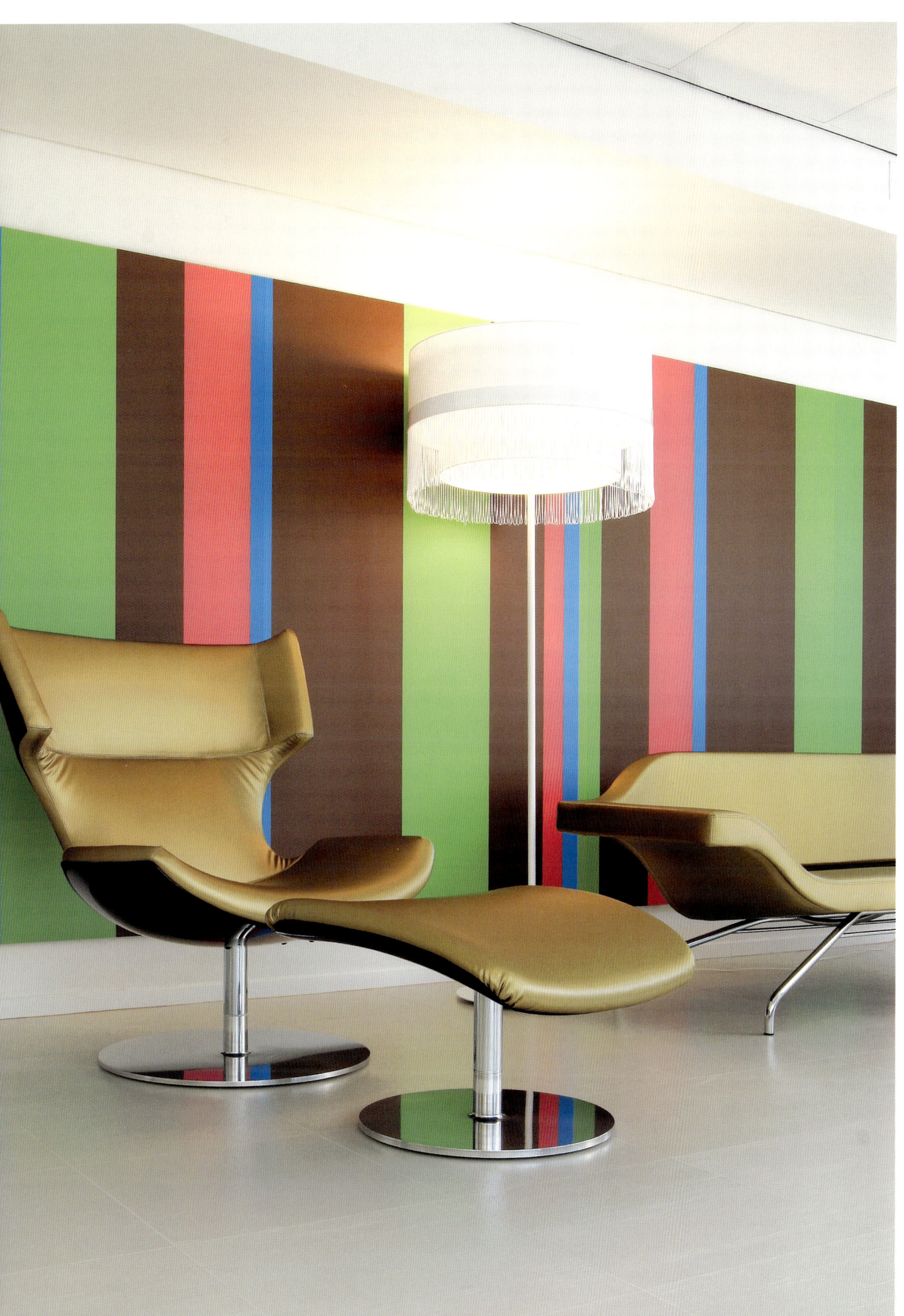

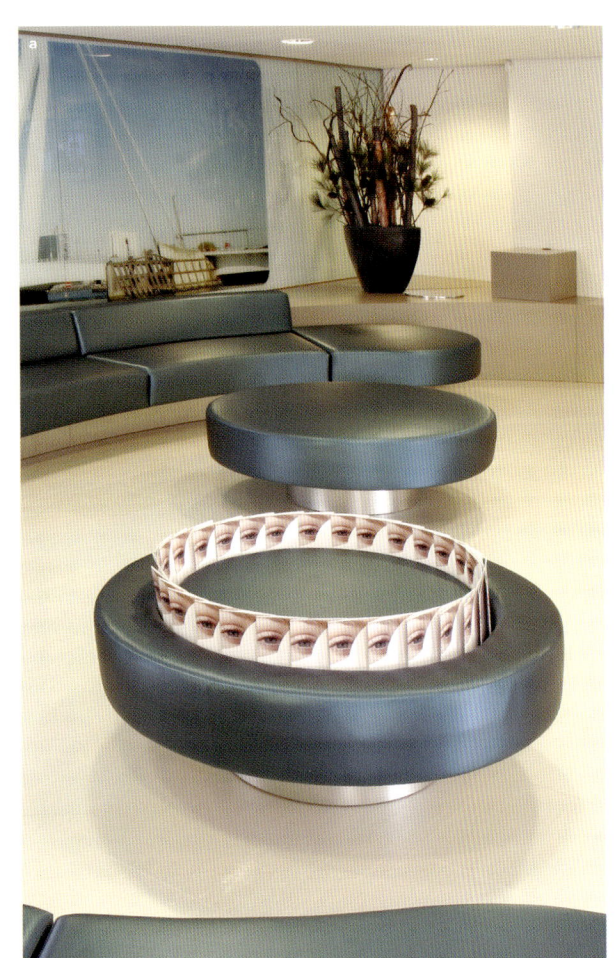

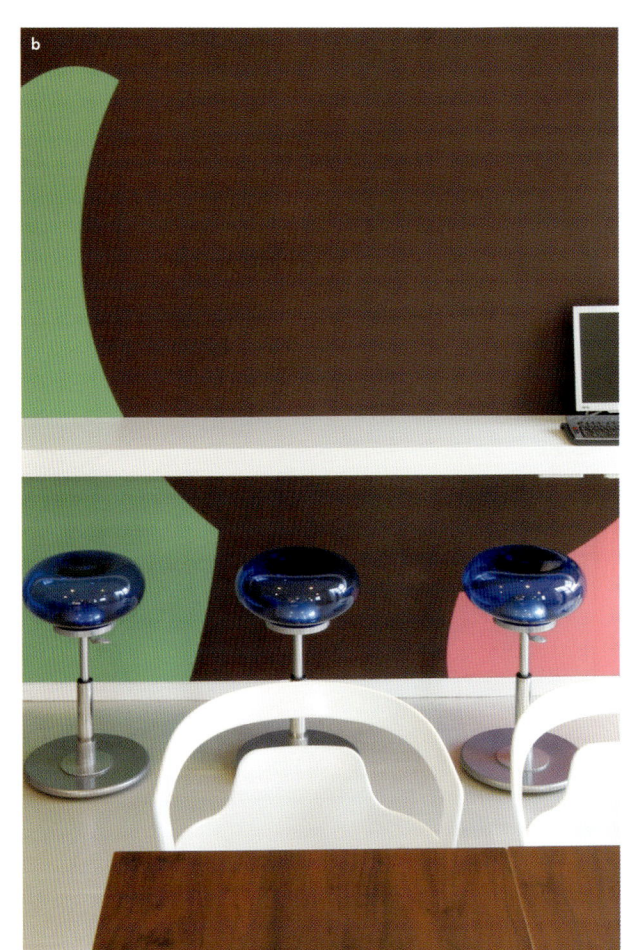

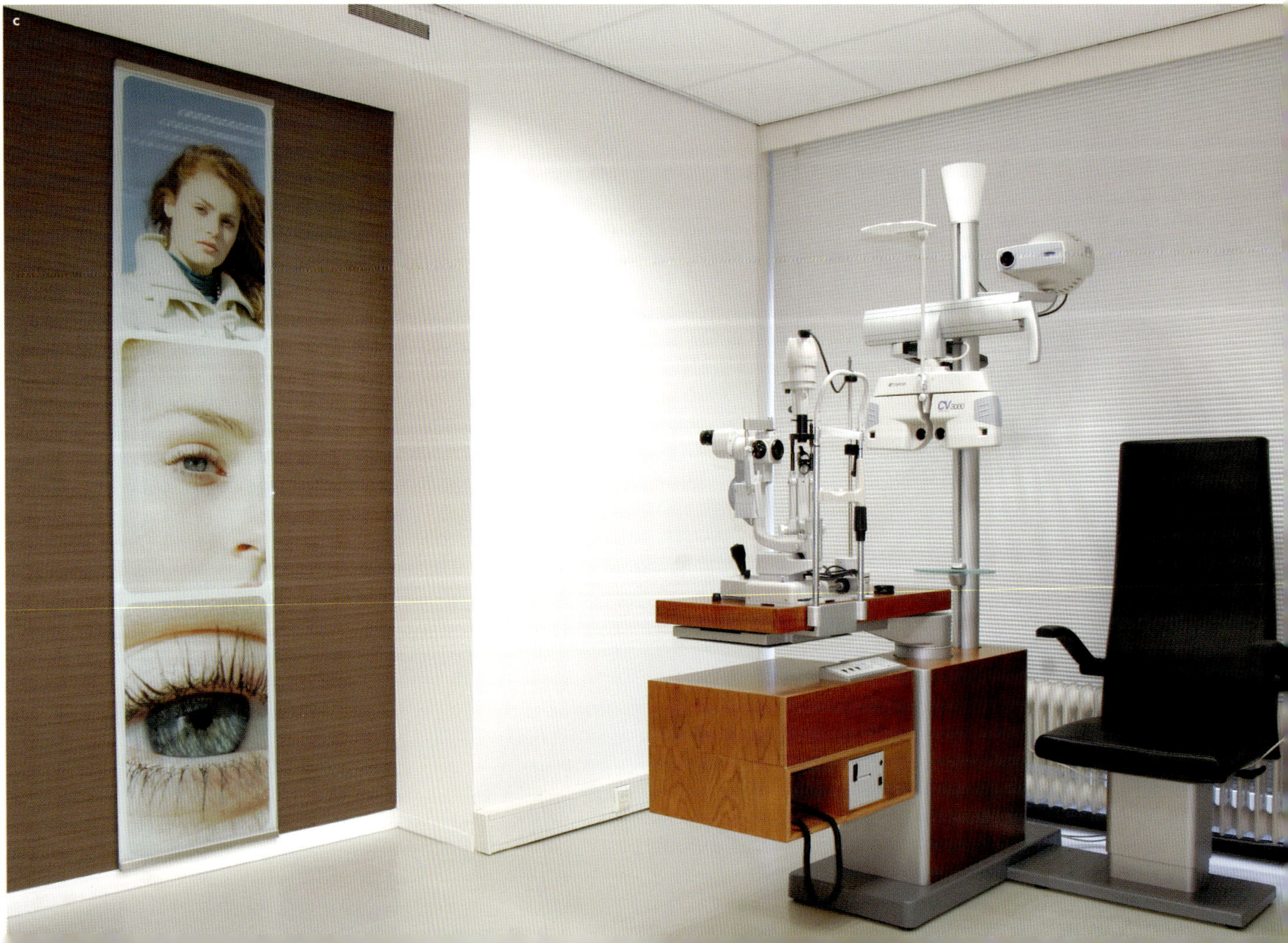

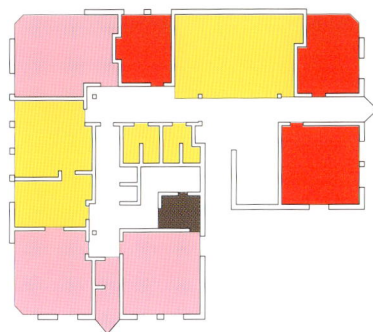

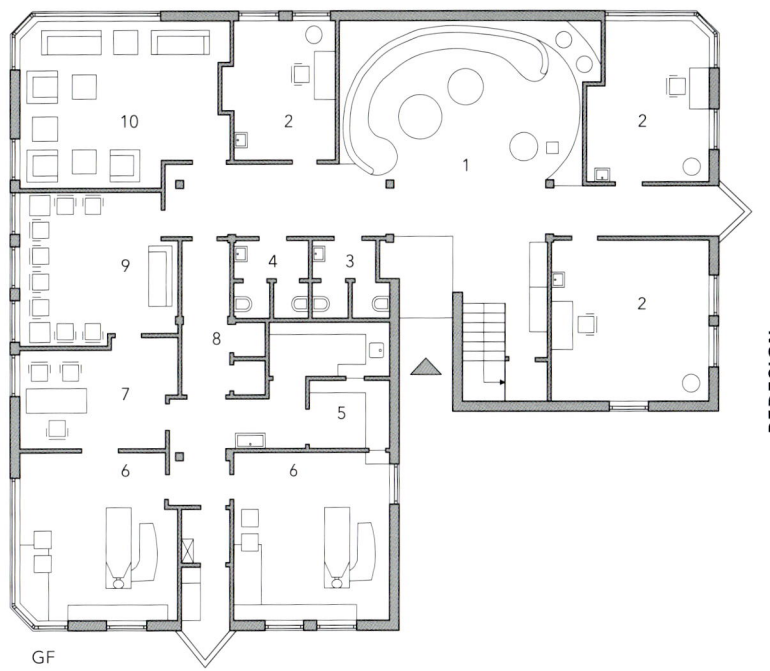

GF

Client	Operator	"Eye Do" Eye Clinic
Planning time	07 2005 – 10 2005
Construction time	11 2005 – 02 2006
Gross floor area	550 sqm [GF+FF]
Usable floor space	203 sqm [GF]
Gross cubic capacity	1,485 cbm [GF+FF]

a The recovery room resembles a lounge
rather than a clinic, with gold leather chairs
and sofas and bright striped wallpaper.
b The cafeteria on the upper floor boasts
eye-catching ornamental wall decoration in
strong colours.
c The examination rooms contain high-tech
equipment in an otherwise stark decor.

Diagrammatic plans, to scale 1:400
Floor plans, to scale 1:200

Floor plan layout

1	Waiting area	**5**	Sterilisation room	**9**	Waiting area
2	Examination	**6**	Operating theatre	**10**	Recovery room
3	Patient toilet G	**7**	Consultation room		
4	Patient toilet L	**8**	Patient sluice		

The angular structure of the eye clinic means that there is only one corridor
giving access to all the rooms. The entrance side of the corridor houses the
reception and waiting area and also the examination rooms, while the operating department is located in the connecting side and is accessible via a
rather narrow sluice. The upper level houses a cafeteria and conference
room that can be reached via a staircase located by the entrance [no lift].

Usable floor spaces

Patient rooms	**yellow**	71 sqm	35 %
Examination			
Treatment rooms	**red**	47 sqm	23 %
Specialist rooms	**pink**	80 sqm	39 %
Supply	Waste disposal	**brown**	5 sqm	3 %
Total		203 sqm	100 %

The large reception area forms the focal point of the practice. Patients enter a vast and welcoming environment, reminiscent of a spacious foyer in a hotel lobby, where the customary large reception desk has been replaced by a small standing desk. The accounts office is housed in a separate room behind. The foyer stands out like a beacon thanks to the orange stained cast plaster floor and the slightly darker orange luminous borders positioned between the walls and the light ceiling. All the treatment rooms, offices, consultation and waiting areas are accessed from here. Adjoining rooms are separated by ceiling height glass partition walls with frosted mid-sections, which provide natural light to the internal reception area.

At the rear of the practice are the OP area and the sterile, X-ray and staff rooms, dominated by rusty orange, white and warm brown tones. The walls are covered in gleaming PVC tiles, whose mother of pearl effect creates a real feeling of depth. The treatment rooms are fitted with high-grade synthetic cherrywood floors and radiate cosiness. In general, the focus on white furniture gives the practice rooms a clarity and freshness appreciated by both patients and staff.

HELL UND FREUNDLICH

PRACTICE FOR ORAL AND MAXILLOFACIAL SURGERY
OBERHAUSEN | G

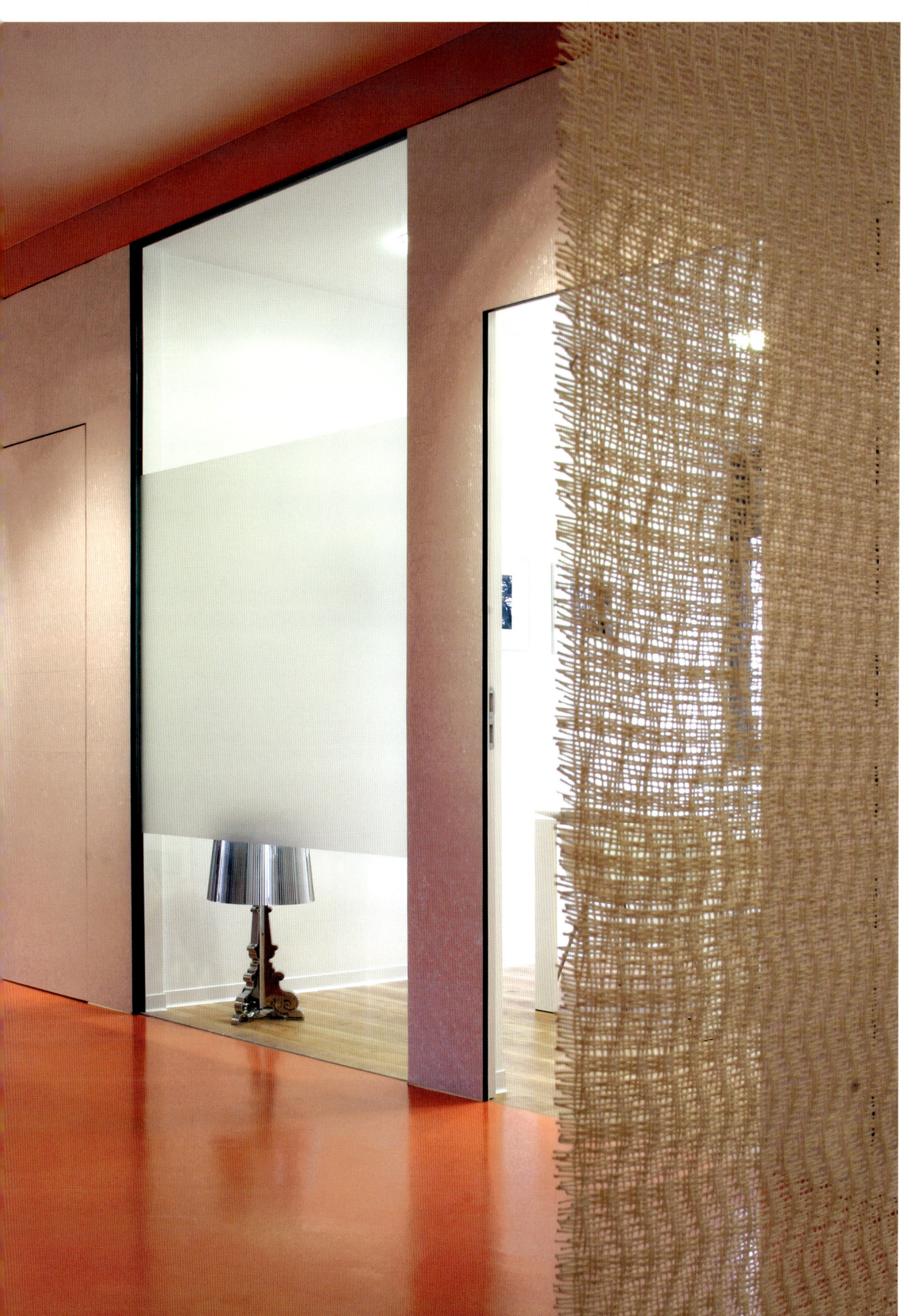

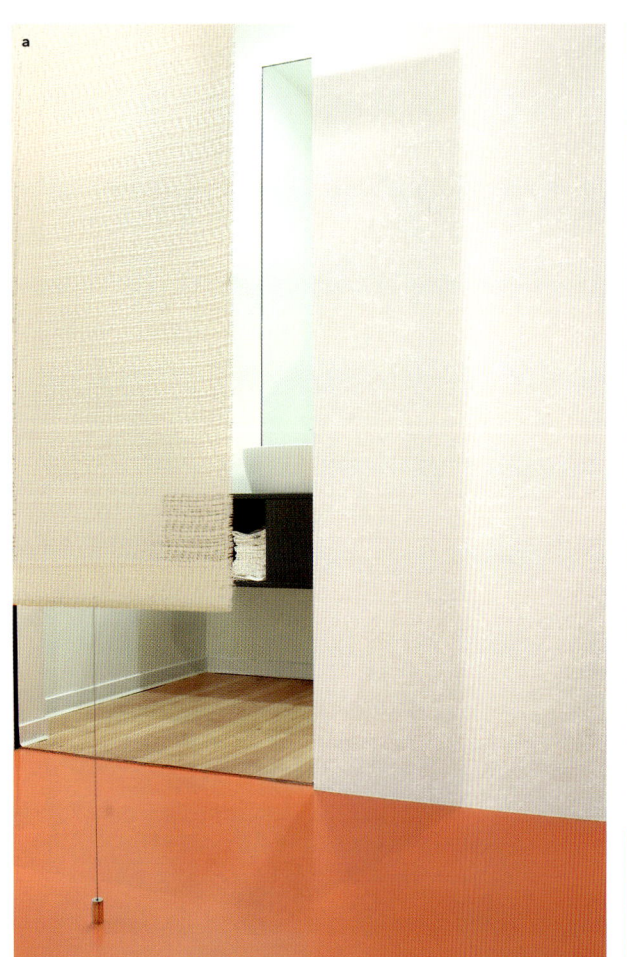

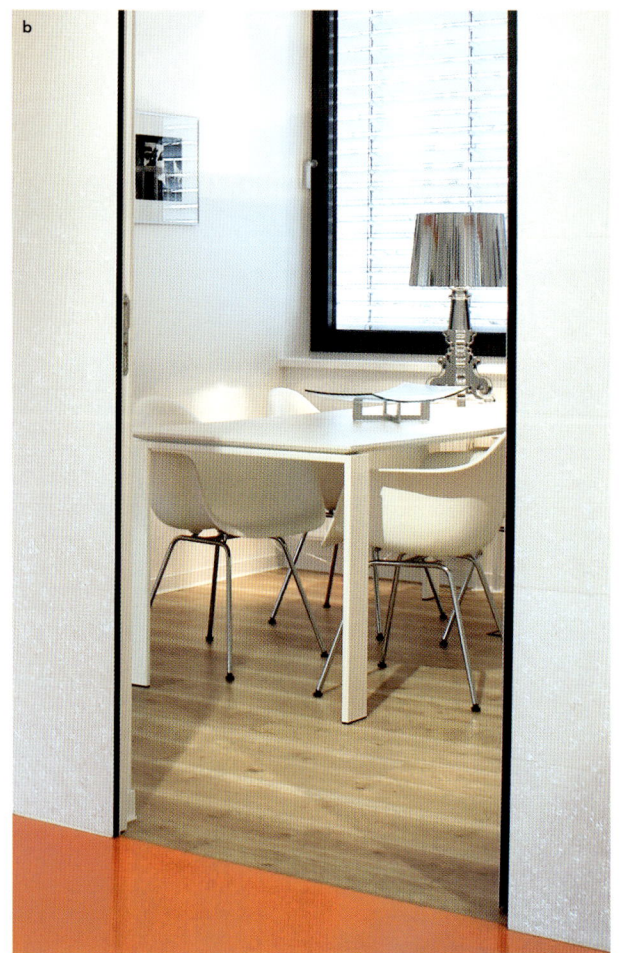

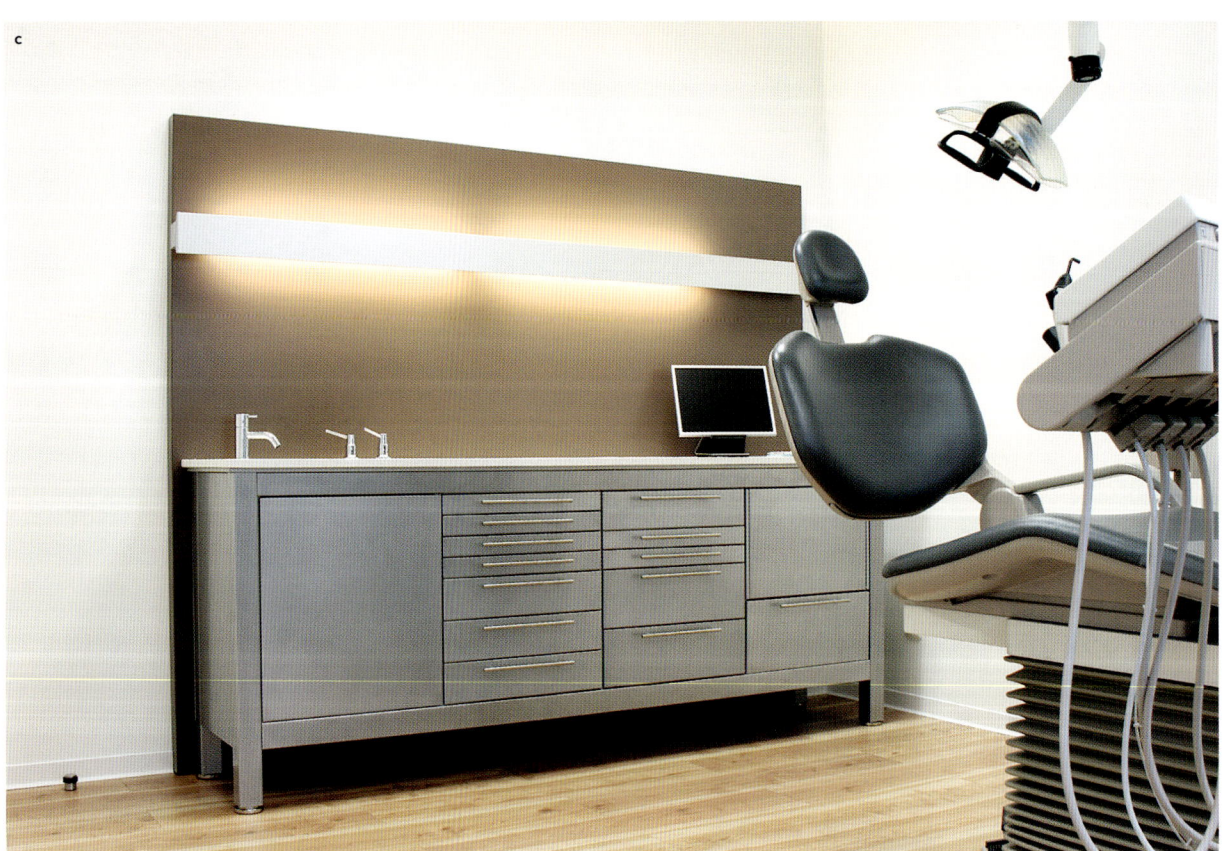

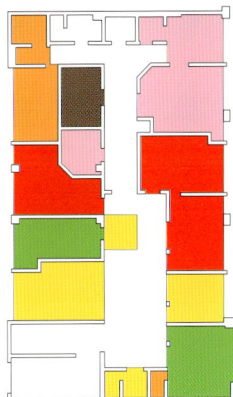

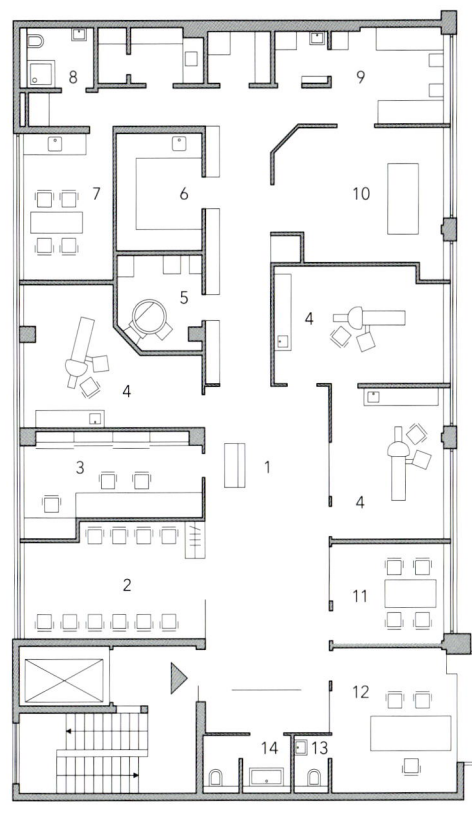

GF

Client	Operator	Dr. Dr. Thomas Betz
Planning time	04 2004 – 08 2004
Construction time	08 2004 – 10 2004
Gross floor area	250 sqm
Usable floor space	169 sqm
Gross cubic capacity	795 cbm

a Rusty orange, white and brown tones define
   the interior spaces of the practice.
b The focus on white furniture gives the practice
   a pleasing clarity and freshness.
c The treatment rooms are fitted with high-
   quality synthetic cherrywood floors, while
   gleaming PVC tiles decorate the walls.

Diagrammatic plans, to scale 1:400
Floor plans, to scale 1:200

Floor plan layout

1	Reception	**6**	Sterilisation room	**10**	Operating theatre
2	Waiting area	**7**	Staff lounge	**11**	Consultation room
3	Office	**8**	Staff toilet and	**12**	Office
4	Treatment room		shower	**13**	Staff toilet
5	Examination X-ray	**9**	Recovery room	**14**	Patient toilet

The rectangular floor plan of the single-doctor practice is accessed from
one corner. A initially wide but gradually narrowing central corridor leads
to the waiting area and the other practice rooms, opening up to a further
cross-corridor, at the rear of the practice, used by recovering patients. All
the rooms needing natural light have windows. No storage or cleaning
areas are provided.

Usable floor spaces

Patient rooms	**yellow**	34 sqm	20 %
Examination			
Treatment rooms	**red**	45 sqm	27 %
Specialist rooms	**pink**	35 sqm	21 %
Administrative rooms	**green**	29 sqm	17 %
Offices	Staff rooms	**orange**	18 sqm	11 %
Supply	Waste disposal	**brown**	8 sqm	4 %
Total		169 sqm	100 %

Unsurprisingly, eyes are the focus of the newly built three-storey eye centre in Cologne. At reception a rolling display at eye level sets the tone for visitors. Its figures and letters are reminiscent of the charts used for testing eyesight. Curved walls divide the ground floor into several sections, which in addition to reception, house the offices and examination and treatment rooms. Light colours and a cosy atmosphere create a pleasant environment for patients. The coat-rack fashioned from young birch saplings is particularly striking, as are the trendy furniture and the bold wallpaper in the examination rooms. The two sight test cubicles encircled by helical double cord screening resemble transparent changing cubicles. In the examination rooms the "eye" motif comes to the fore once again: large pairs of eyes watch the seated patient. On a backlit wall a group of verbs all connected with eyes is prominently displayed: "… twinkle, peek, weep, wink …"

HELL UND FREUNDLICH

EYE CENTRE
COLOGNE | G

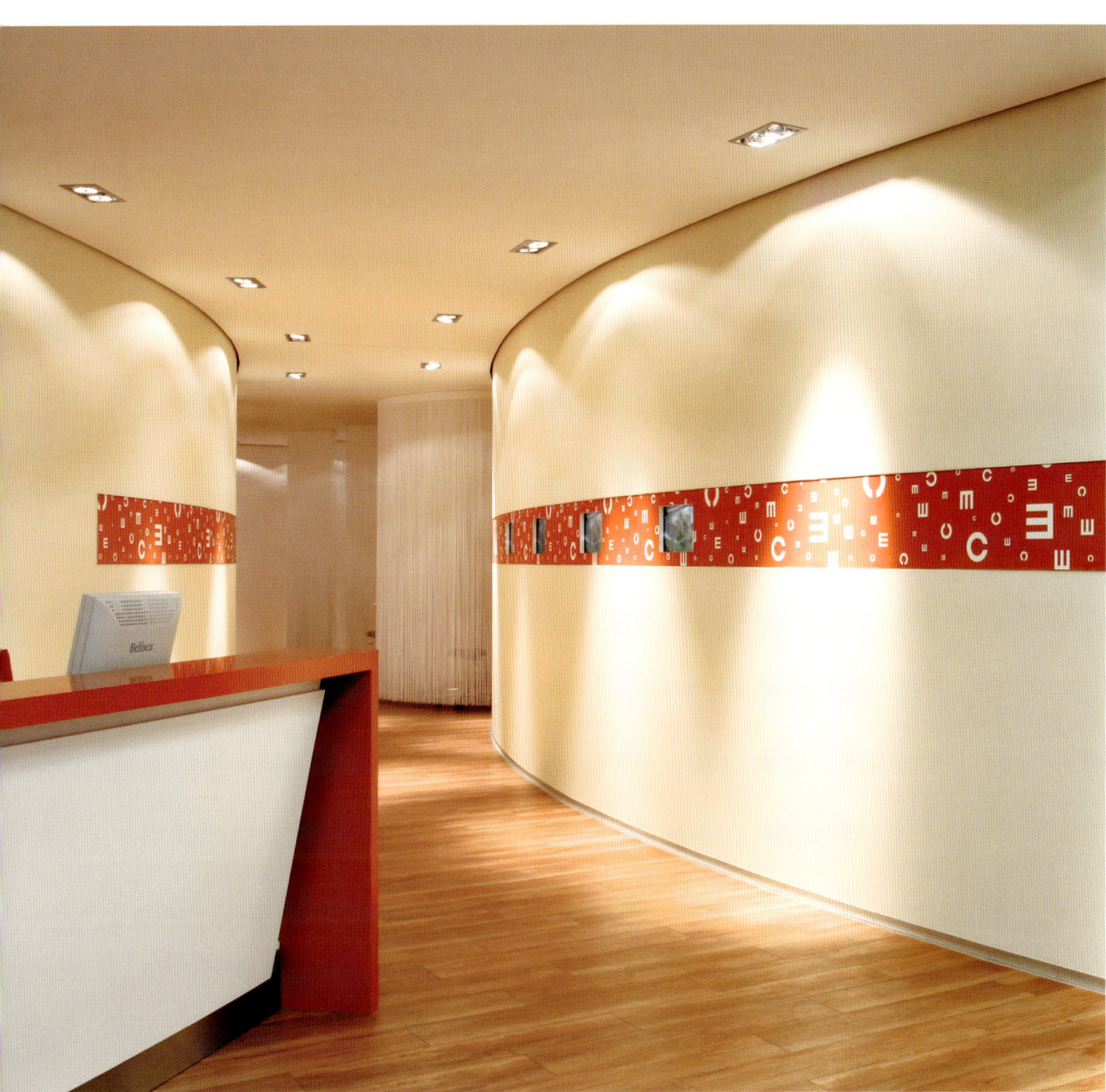

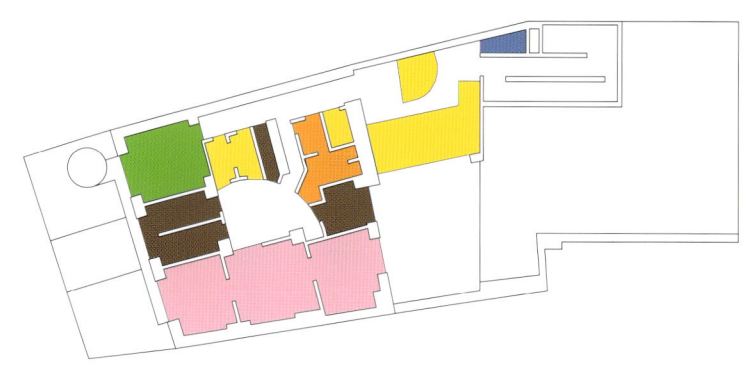

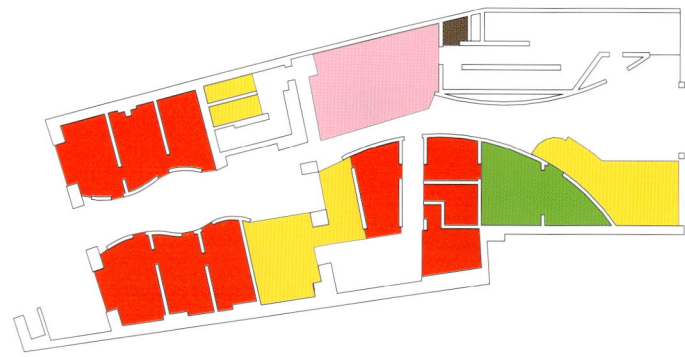

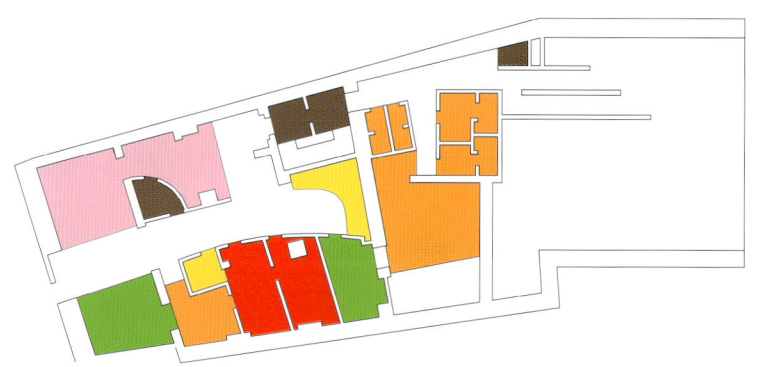

Diagrammatic plans, to scale 1:400
Floor plans, to scale 1:200

1 Reception	shower	**20** Staff changing
2 Office	**12** Staff sluice	cubicle L
3 Treatment room	**13** Operating theatre	**21** Staff changing
4 Examination	**14** Prep room	cubicle G
5 Waiting area	**15** Sterilisation room	**22** Staff lounge
6 Patient toilet L	unsterile	**23** Quiet room
7 Patient toilet G	**16** Sterilisation room	**24** Examination and
8 Examination eye test	sterile	treatment room
9 Store room	**17** Patient sluice	optician
10 Server room	**18** Waste disposal room	**25** Staff toilet L
11 Patient toilet and	**19** Supply room	**26** Staff toilet G

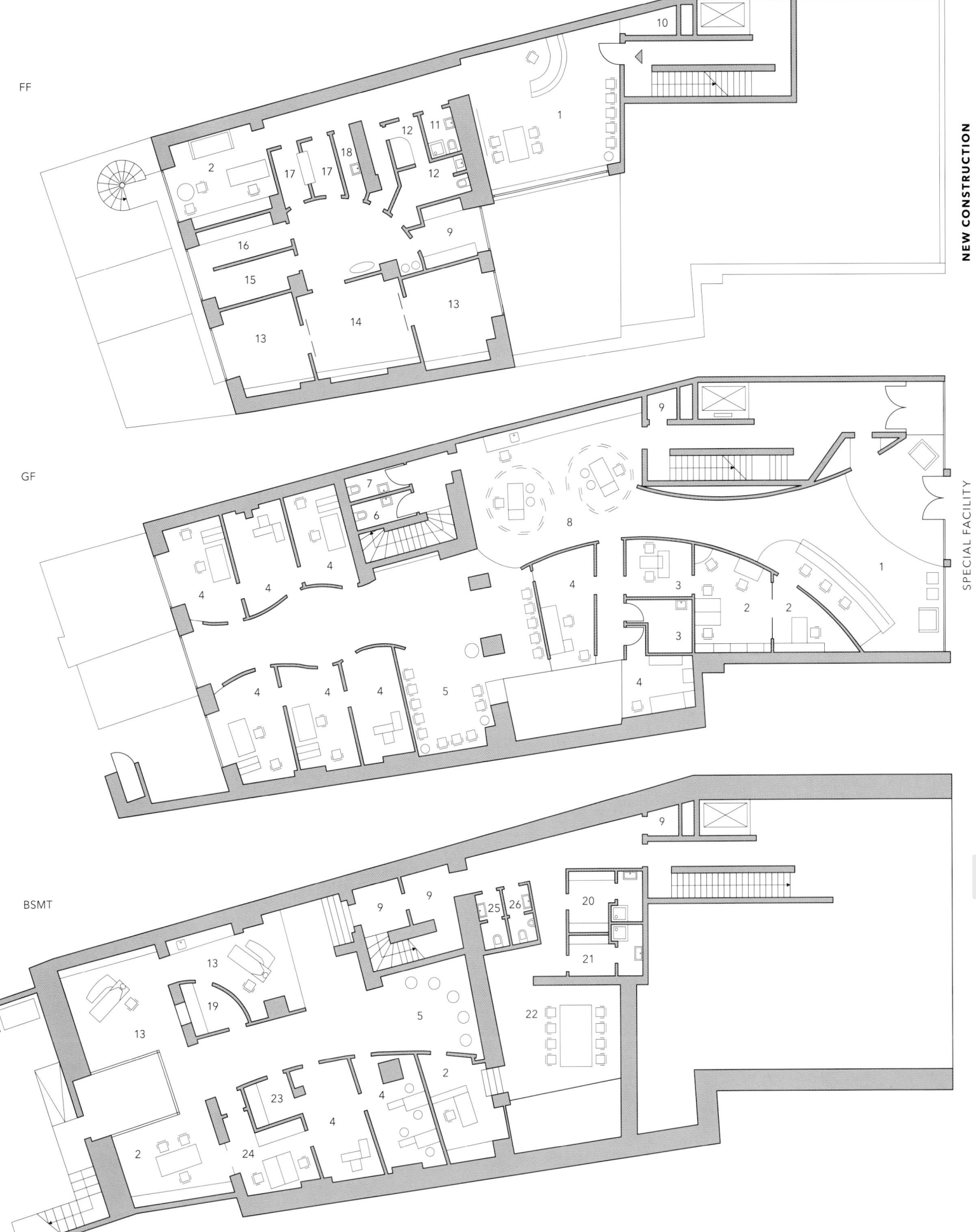

FF

GF

BSMT

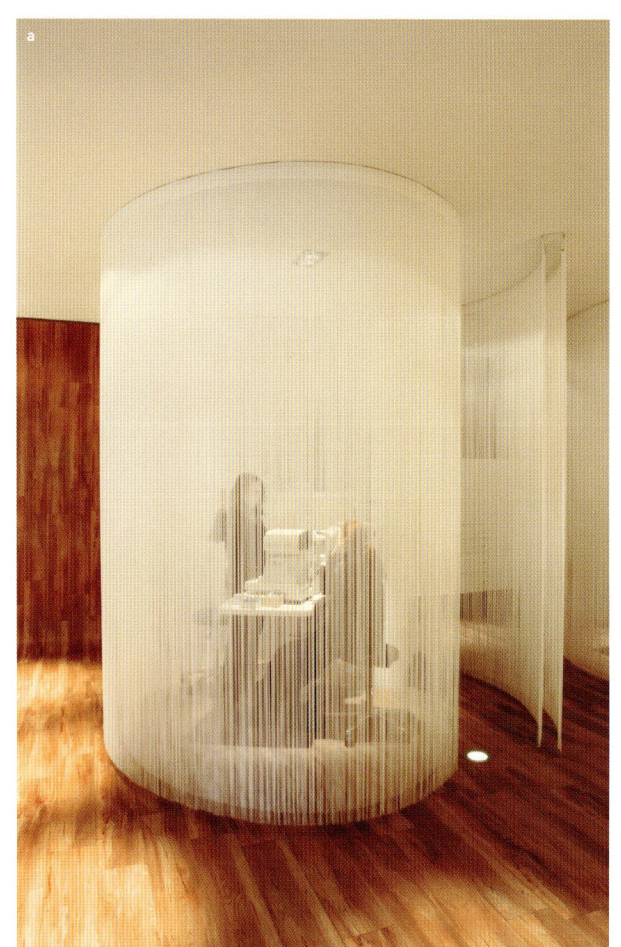

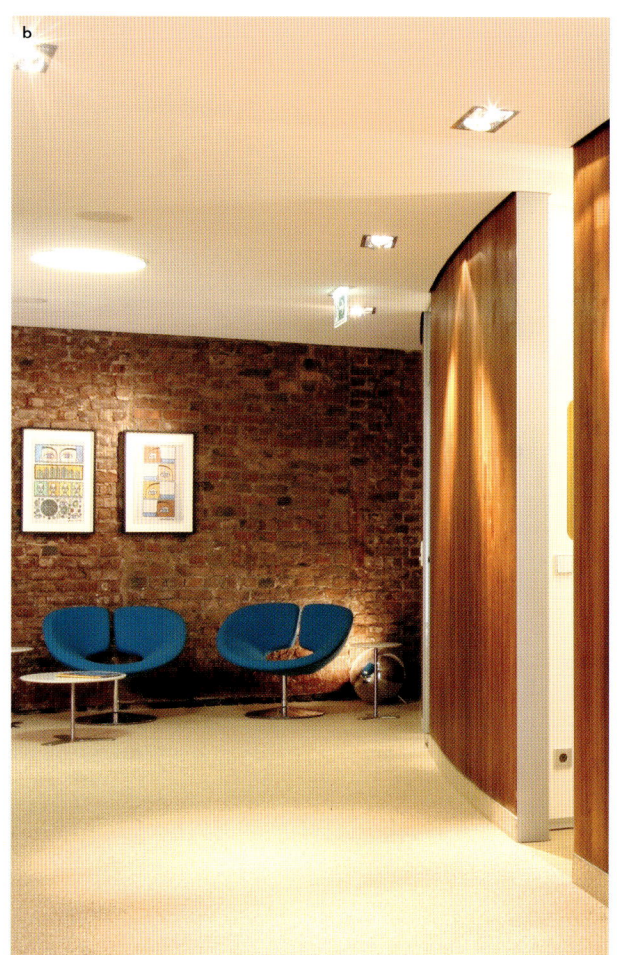

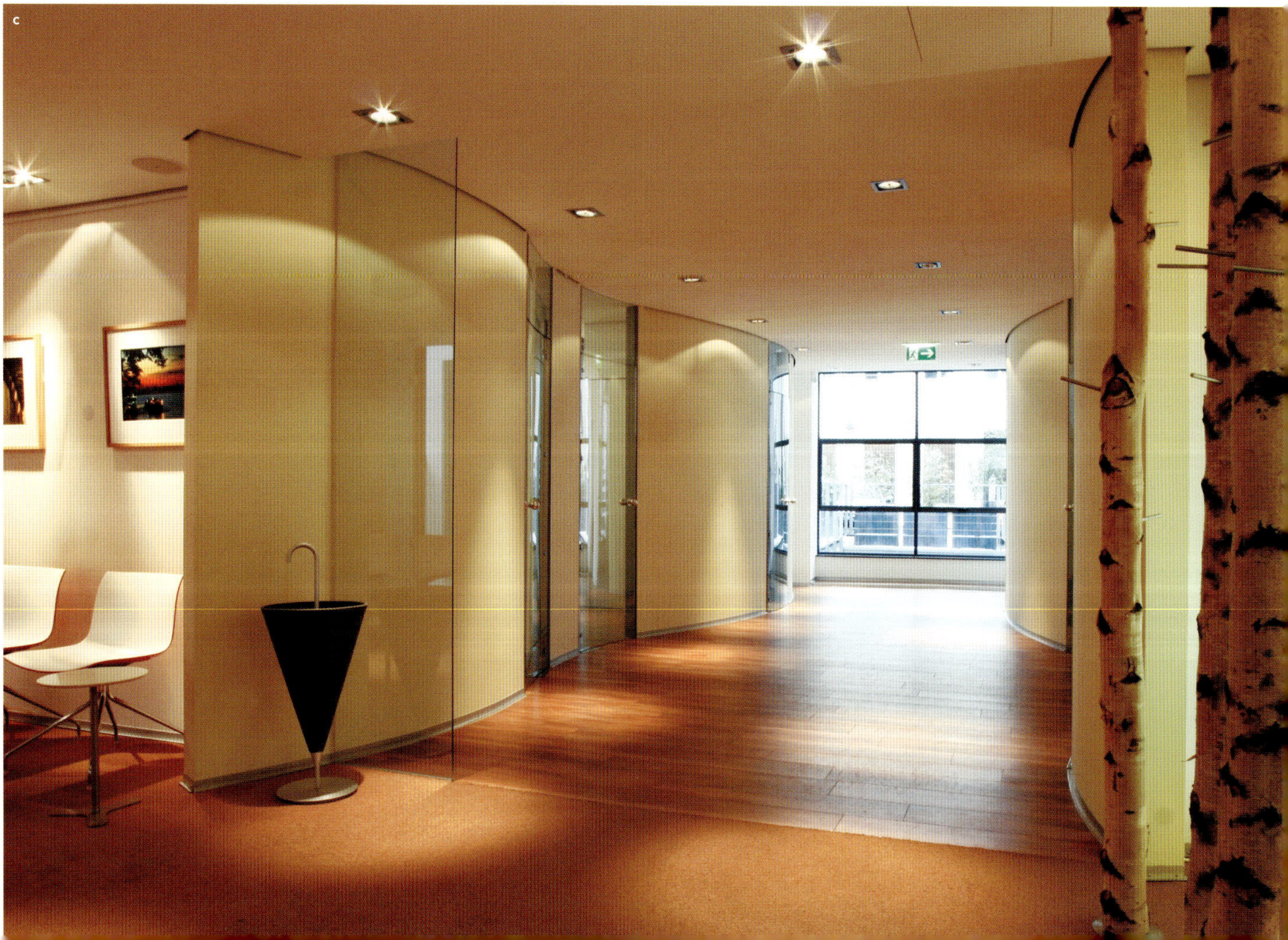

Client	Operator	Eye Centre
Planning time	04 2003 – 10 2003
Construction time	10 2003 – 02 2004
Gross floor area	900 sqm
Usable floor space	563 sqm
Gross cubic capacity	2,838 cbm

a Although transparent, the eye test booth encircled by helical double cord screening protects patient privacy.

b The basement walls are made of brickwork and lightweight elements in real wood.

c Curved walls divide the ground floor into several sections.

Floor plan layout

The eye centre extends over three levels. Access to the basement level is via a central staircase, while a staircase and lift located near reception take patients up to the 1st floor. Two light-wells provide the basement with natural light.

Usable floor spaces

Patient rooms	**yellow**	110 sqm	19 %
Examination | Treatment rooms	**red**	139 sqm	25 %
Specialist rooms	**pink**	125 sqm	22 %
Administrative rooms	**green**	72 sqm	13 %
Offices | Staff rooms	**orange**	71 sqm	13 %
Supply | Waste disposal	**brown**	43 sqm	7,5 %
Plant rooms	**blue**	3 sqm	0,5 %
Total		563 sqm	100 %

Mobility keeps you healthy. This motto seems to have provided inspiration also for the dynamic architecture of the building which, in keeping with the adjoining AWD Arena [the former Lower Saxony stadium], is replicated inside the practice, dominated by a fluid room continuum.

A central corridor – which is also the backbone of the practice – takes patients to the white boomerang-shaped reception desk, behind which a panoramic window affords a breathtaking view of the surrounding green area. The same spatial concept is reflected in the floating ceiling panel above the reception desk. After registering, patients are invited to take a seat and maybe enjoy an espresso from the coffee bar in the open-plan waiting area, where integrated benches and a coat-rack are set into the curved wall panels. The fresh white and light blue tones of the walls combined with the warm shade of the parquet floor give the practice a soothing atmosphere. In a simple nod to the corporate design, the sky-blue accenting over the rear walls in the waiting area graduates into full colour in the computed tomography functional unit. The innovative treatments used in the practice find a visual counterpoint in the interior design.

ROLAND HOLZ

SPINAL COLUMN CENTRE
HANOVER | G

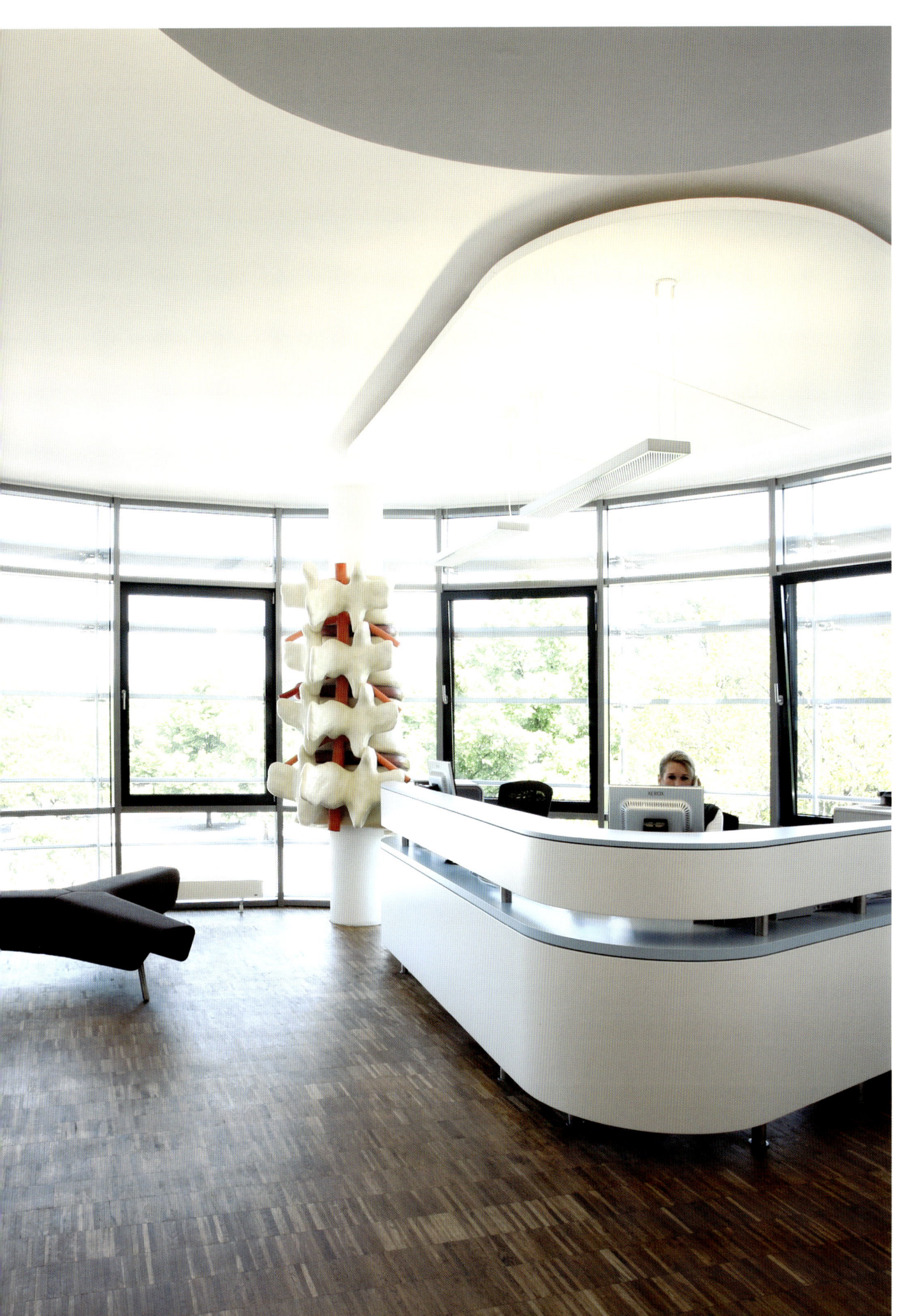

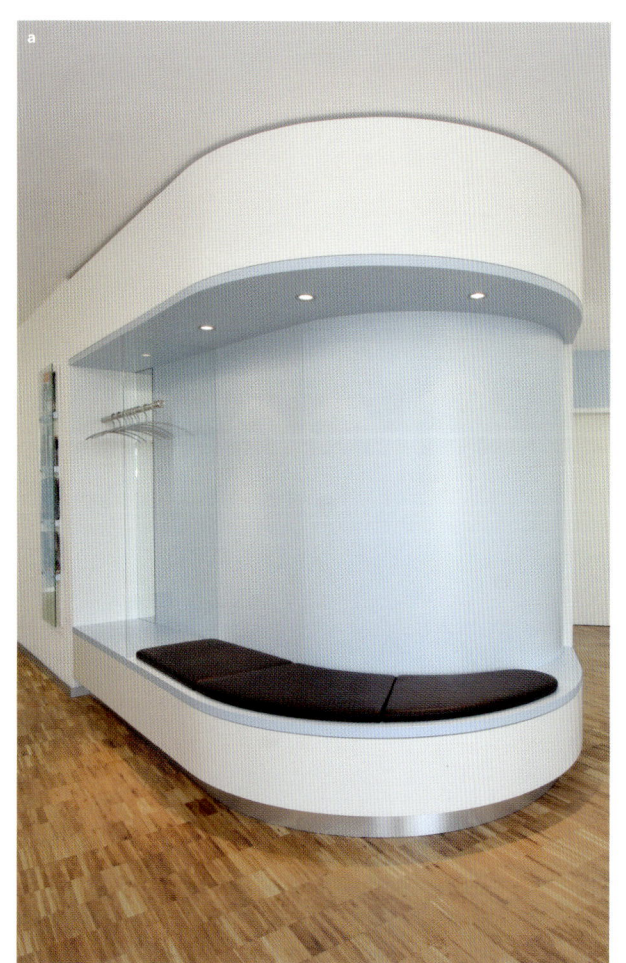

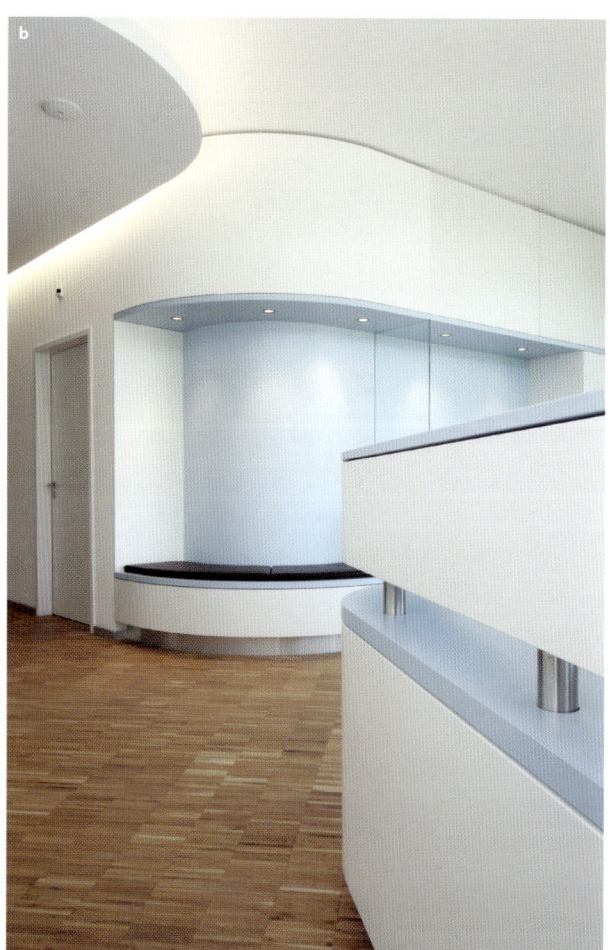

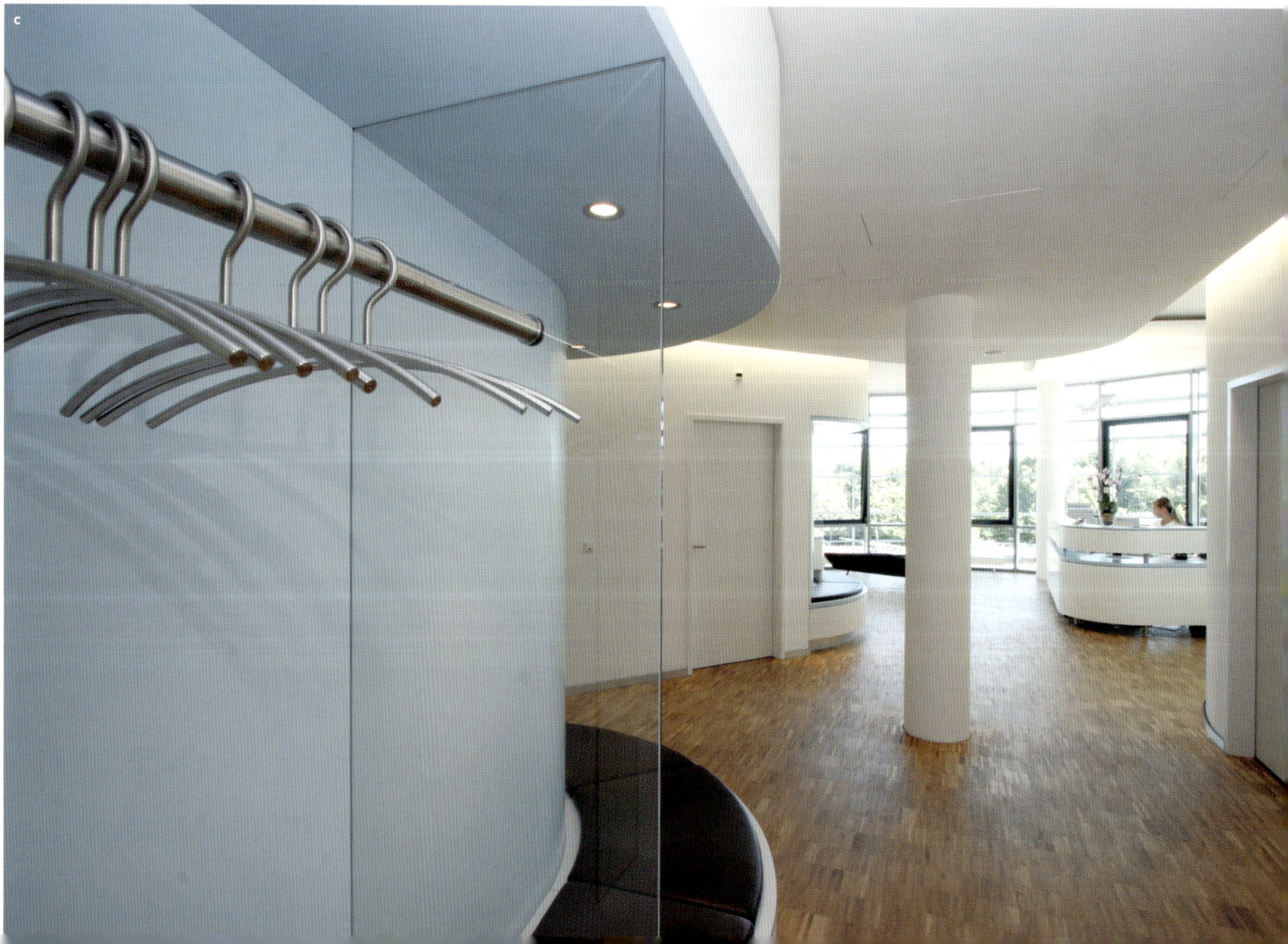

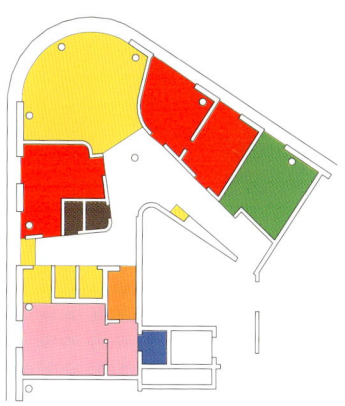

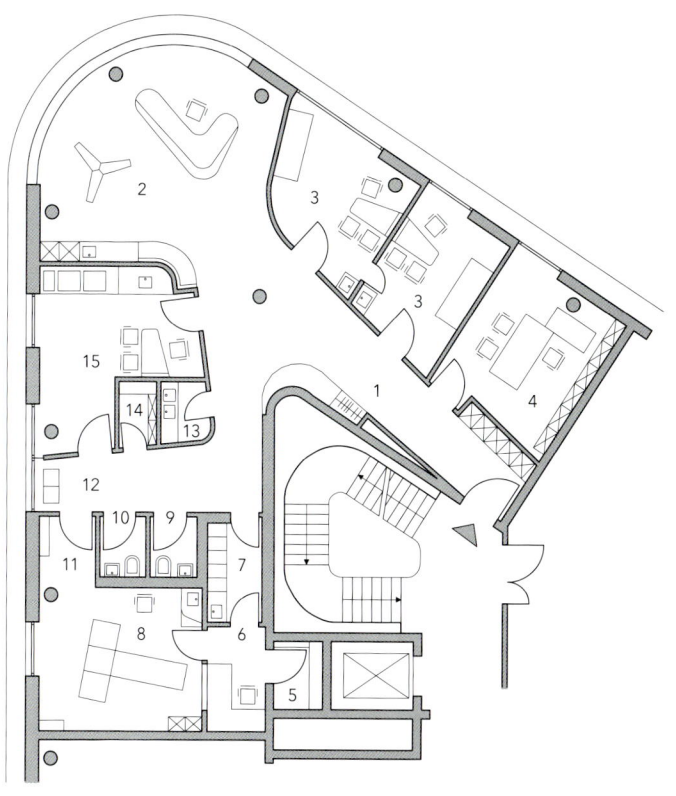

GF

Client	Baum Consortium
Operator	Prof. Dr. Axel Piepgras
Planning time	2005
Construction time	2006
Gross floor area	210 sqm
Usable floor space	148 sqm
Gross cubic capacity	672 cbm
Construction cost	135,000 EUR
Total cost	285,000 EUR

a Integrated benches and a coat-rack are set
   into the curved wall panels.
b Fresh white and light blue tones give the
   practice a soothing atmosphere.
c The eye-catching white boomerang-shaped
   reception desk is positioned in front of the
   large panoramic window.

Diagrammatic plans, to scale 1:400
Floor plans, to scale 1:200

Floor plan layout

1	Coat-rack	6	Control room	11	Patient changing cubicle
2	Waiting area	7	Staff changing cubicle	12	Waiting area CT
3	Treatment room	8	Examination CT	13	Cleaning room
4	Office and consultation room	9	Patient toilet G	14	Store room
5	Installations room	10	Patient toilet L	15	Quiet room

The floor plan of the multiple practice with its V-shaped main corridor has
been designed so that patients only have a short distance to walk between
the spacious, centrally located reception and waiting area and the other
rooms in the practice. Windows provide natural light where needed the most.
Despite the economical layout, administrative, storage and cleaning areas
have been included.

Usable floor spaces

Patient rooms	yellow	47 sqm	32 %
Examination | Treatment rooms	red	46 sqm	31 %
Specialist rooms	pink	25 sqm	17 %
Administrative rooms	green	5 sqm	3 %
Offices | Staff rooms	orange	18 sqm	12 %
Supply | Waste disposal	brown	4 sqm	3 %
Plant rooms	blue	3 sqm	2 %
Total		148 sqm	100 %

Performance data

Outpatients per year	7,500
Inpatients per year	500
Clinic opening hours	5 days | 40 hours
Waiting time [with | without appointment]	0 – 15 min. | 30 – 60 min.
Number of staff	3 – 4

A pleasantly relaxed atmosphere greets visitors to the practice for women's health care in Braunschweig's renovated health centre. From the reception area with its modern steel design and attached wooden seating, patients reach the large waiting area via a rather narrow corridor. The fittings in this "lounge room" extend almost to ceiling, while seating alcoves, wooden benches lined in brown leather and striped wall panelling in warm red tones invite relaxation. The panelling provides ample storage space while concealing the high-tech units required for ventilation and air conditioning. The windowless room, from which all the examination, treatment and consultation rooms are accessible, is bathed in indirect light from plentiful cove lighting fixtures.

The colour and material concept was deliberately chosen to create a relaxing and calming environment. The windows in the practice rooms, some to ceiling height, are shielded from bright sunlight by an external awning, while adjustable internal blinds protect patient privacy in the examination rooms. In the ultrasound rooms, where the latest technology monitors the growth of new life, simple functional furniture underpins the ergonomics of the medical treatment. The same wood motive present in the waiting area is repeated on the bespoke examination beds, giving the patient a sense of security and continuity.

ROLAND HOLZ

WOMEN'S HEALTH CARE PRACTICE
BRAUNSCHWEIG | G

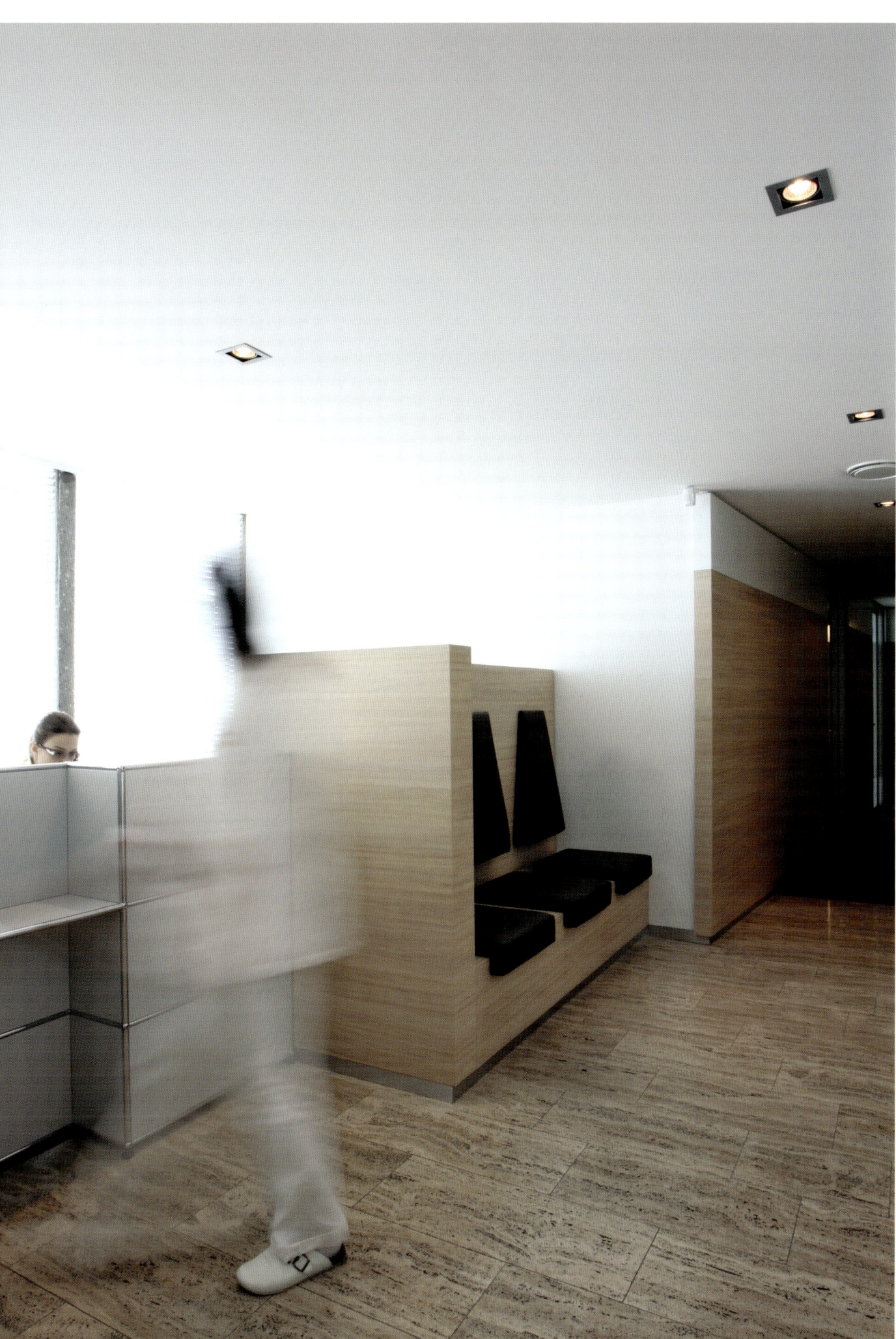

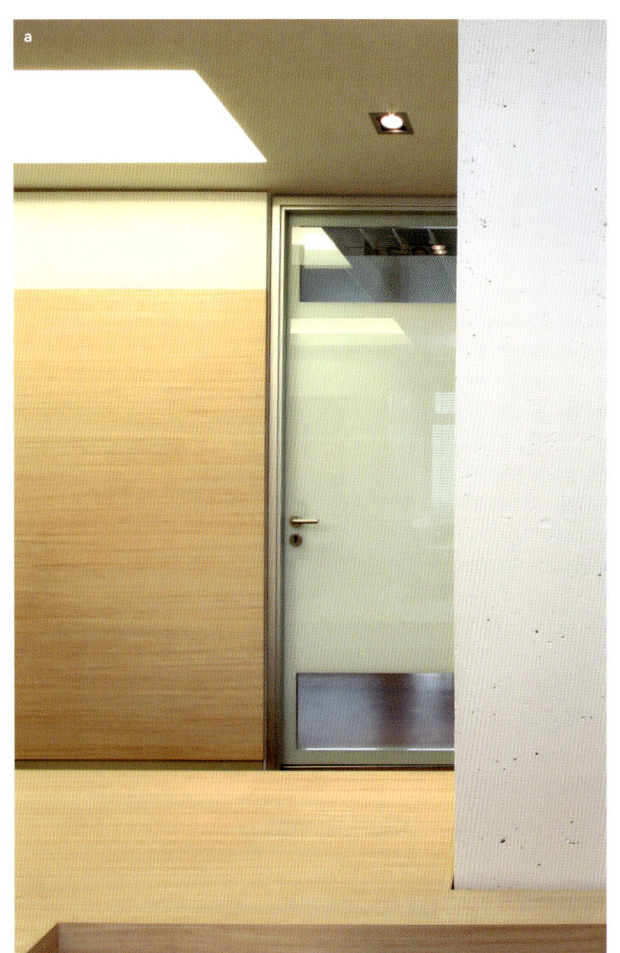

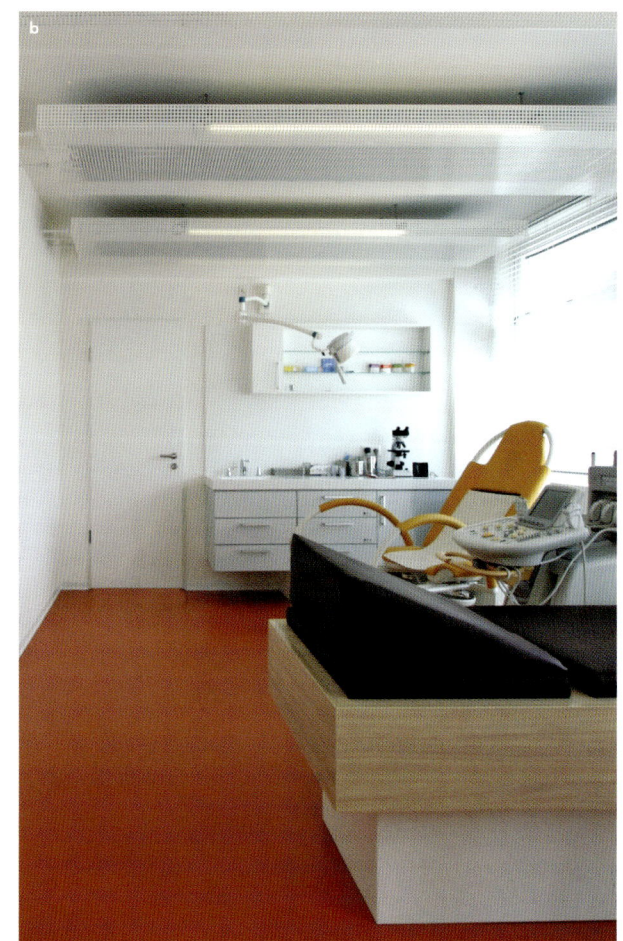

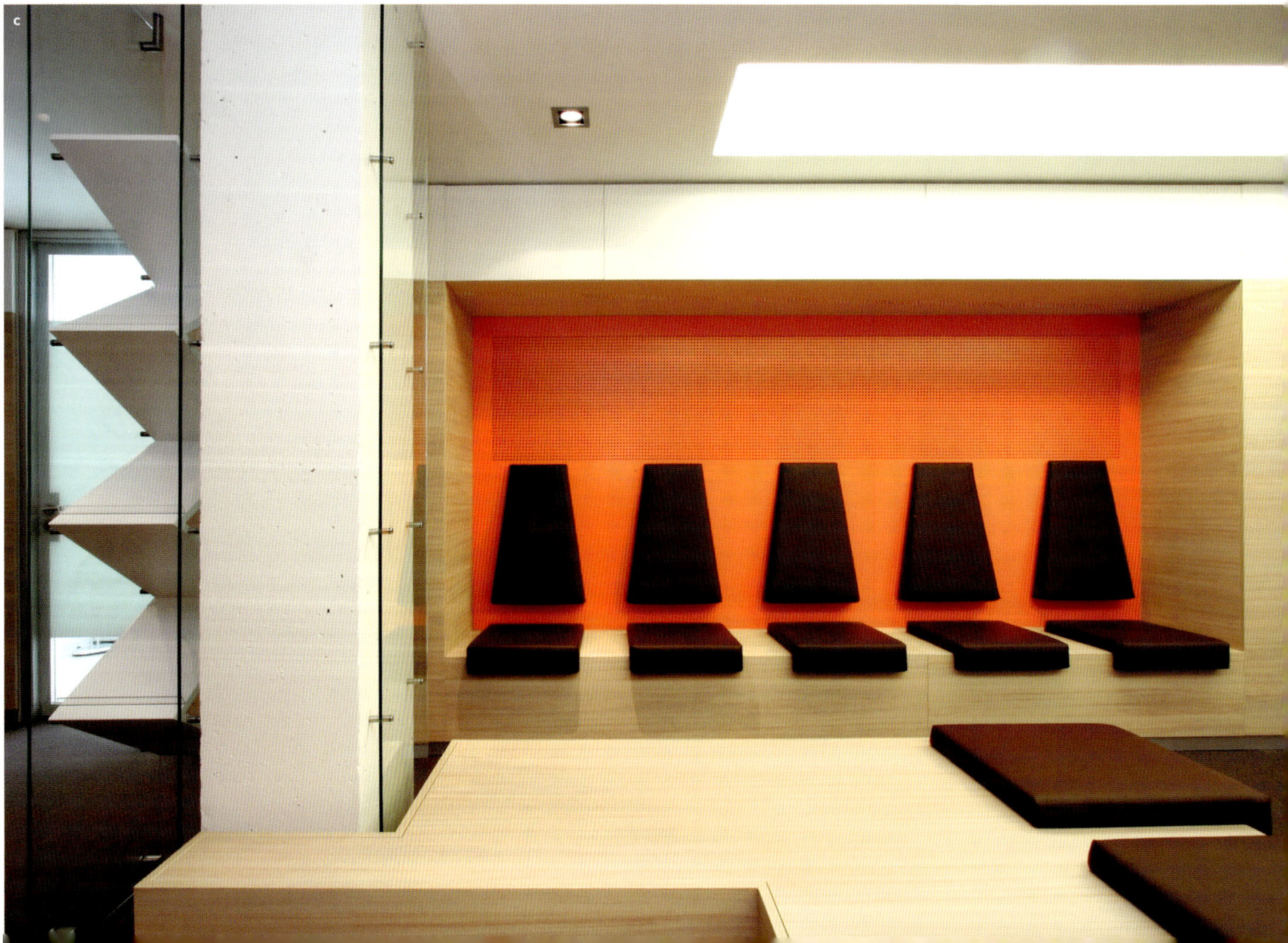

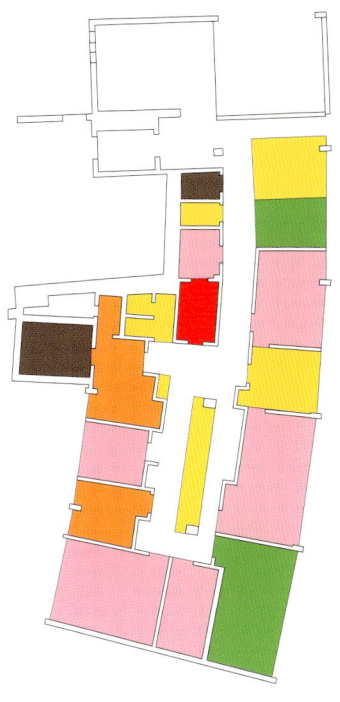

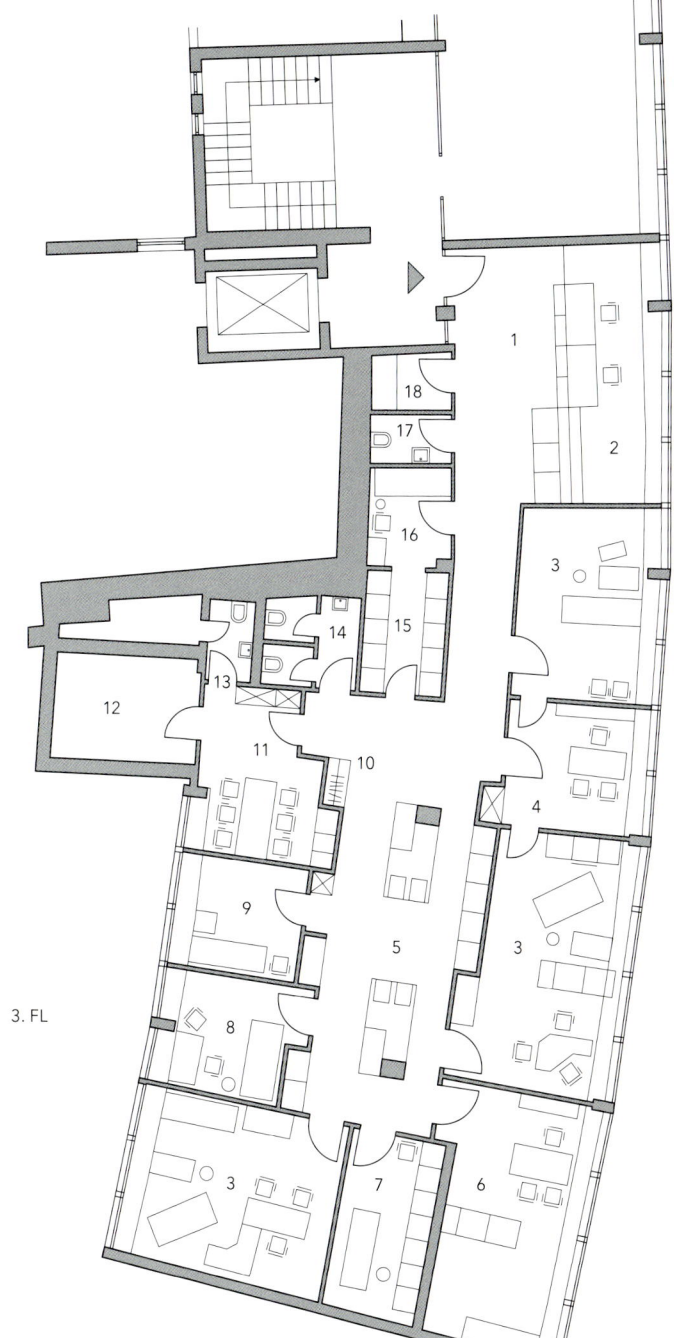

Diagrammatic plans, to scale 1:400
Floor plans, to scale 1:200

3. FL

1 Reception
2 Office
3 Examination and
treatment room
gynaecology
4 Consultation room
5 Waiting area
6 Office
7 Procedure room
8 Office
9 Examination
10 Coat-rack

11 Staff lounge and
small kitchen
12 Store room and
filing room
13 Staff toilet
14 Patient toilet L
15 Laboratory
16 Examination
blood pressure
17 Patient toilet G
18 Cleaning room

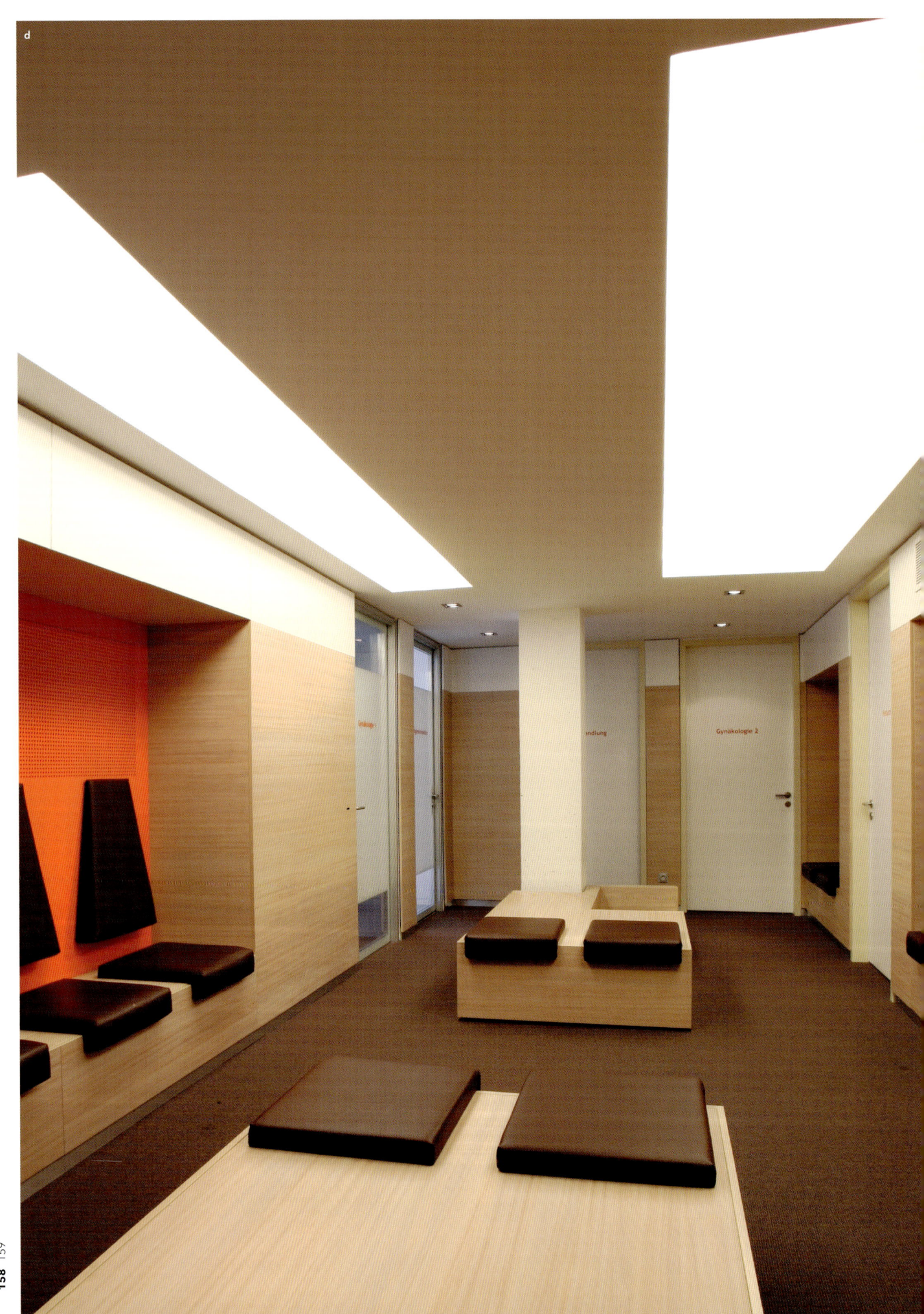

Gynäkologie 2

Client	Perschmann GmbH
	& Co. KG
	Dr. Christian Schütte
Operator	Dr. Christian Schütte
Planning time	2004
Construction time	2004–2005
Usable floor space	266 sqm
Gross cubic capacity	756 cbm
Construction cost	165,000 EUR
Total cost	215,000 EUR

a Choice of colours and materials was intended to provide a calming environment.

b The bespoke examination beds repeat the wood motif of the waiting area.

c The waiting area has fittings almost to ceiling height: seating alcoves, wooden benches and red striped wall panelling all invite relaxation.

d Plentiful cove lighting bathes the windowless waiting area in indirect light.

Floor plan layout

The entrance and reception of the practice are located at one end of the slightly curved rectangular floor plan. Through a rather narrow corridor the patients are then lead to the waiting area. Situated in the widened, windowless main corridor, it does not benefit from natural light. From there it is only a short distance to most of the rooms in the practice. The store room is accessed directly through the staff lounge.

Usable floor spaces

Patient rooms	**yellow**	51 sqm	19 %
Examination | Treatment rooms	**red**	8 sqm	3 %
Specialist rooms	**pink**	117 sqm	44 %
Administrative rooms	**green**	41 sqm	16 %
Offices | Staff rooms	**orange**	33 sqm	12 %
Supply | Waste disposal	**brown**	16 sqm	6 %
Total		266 sqm	100 %

Performance data

Outpatients per year	10,000
Number and type of services per year	Antenatal diagnostics Therapy [IGel 10 %]
Clinic opening hours	5 days | 45 hours
Waiting time	10–15 min.
Number of staff	5

After climbing the long entrance staircase with its back-lit handrail and ball lights set at different heights, visitors to the Freising Airport Clinic reach a reception area that is impressive in its minimalist design and affords a wide view of the surrounding neighbourhood through frameless fixed glazing. The centrally located oak veneer wooden box, which houses the reception area and other functional rooms, forms the heart of the practice. The rounded corners of the corridor walls seem to emphasise the angularity of the platform-mounted wood-frame structure, while the surrounding light gap further accentuates the already imposing cube. The waiting area opposite, with its low ceiling, indirect lighting and felt covered rear walls, creates a cosy space for patients, that can relax during their wait by watching the programmes of their choice on the TV set into the wall. A smooth levelled grey-black concrete floor provides a strong counterpoint to the matt white walls. Both wooden box and walls indicate directions and emergency exits; these are slightly offset to avoid the impression of long monotonous passages. The light points of the recessed spots in the public area do not follow any pattern, but are randomly placed.

The orange corporate identity colour is a repeating element throughout the practice rooms – handrail, taps and desk – adding an opulent bright touch to the deliberately simple colour scheme.

HOLZRAUSCH

MKG-SURGERY AIRPORT CLINIC
FREISING | G

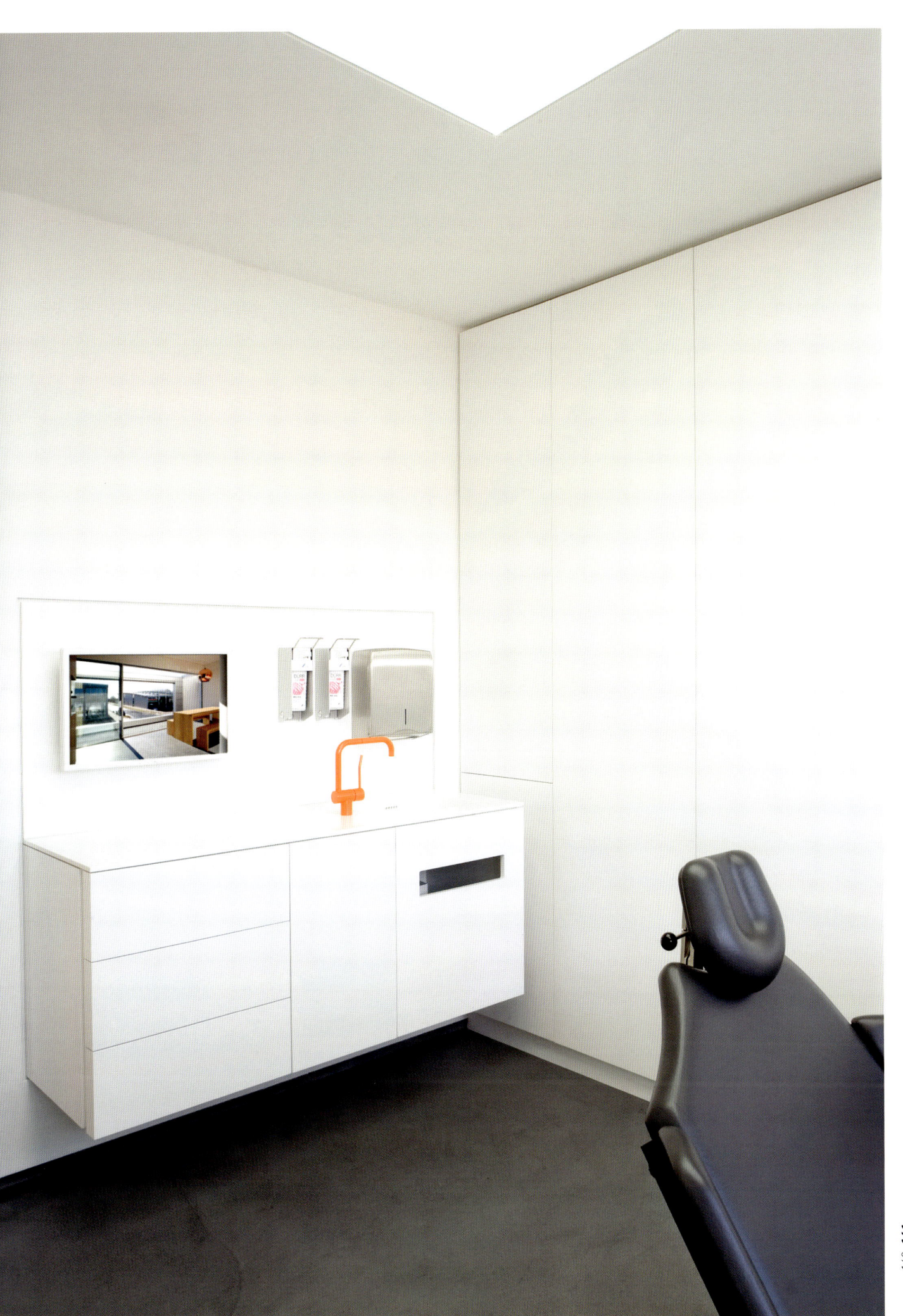

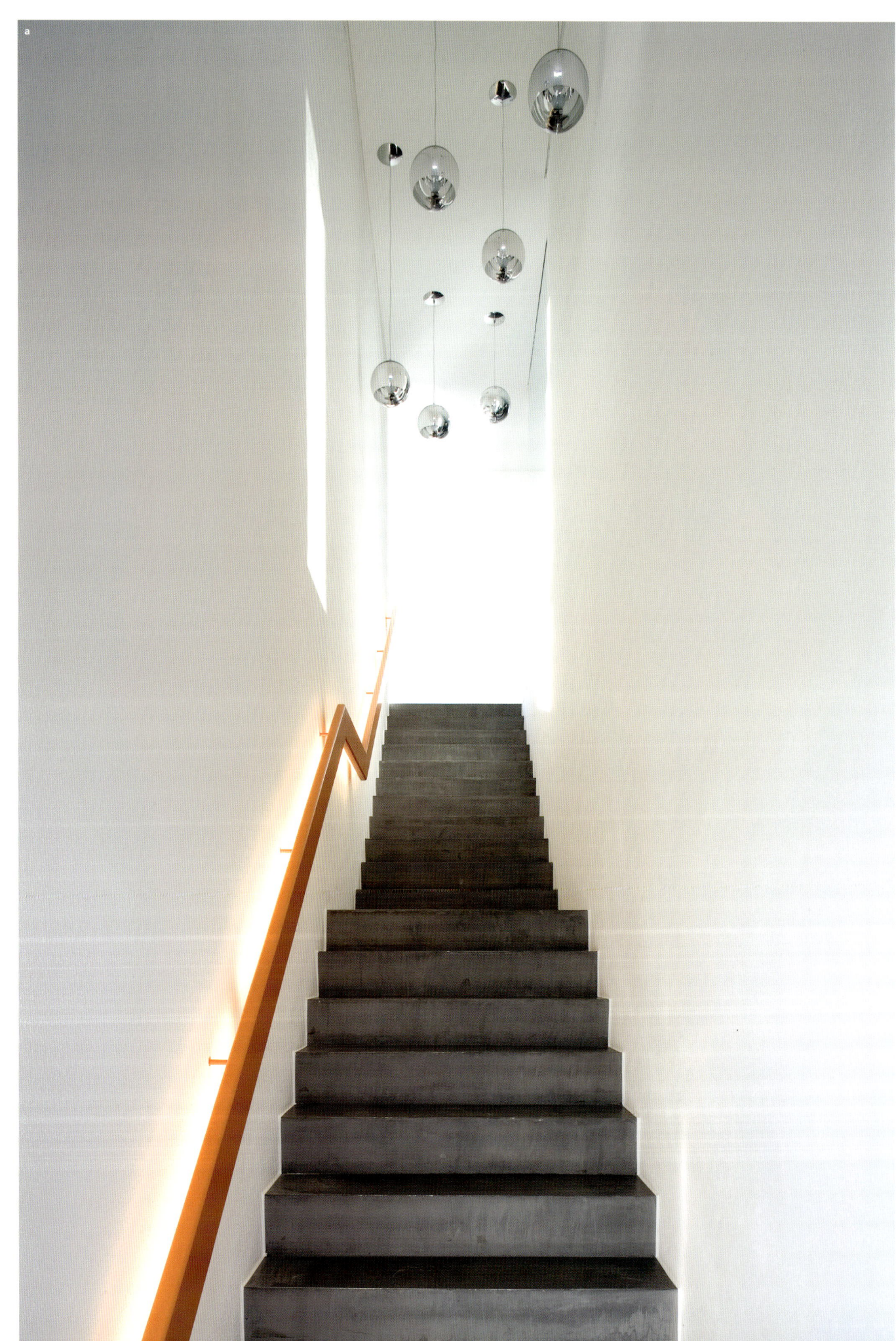

b

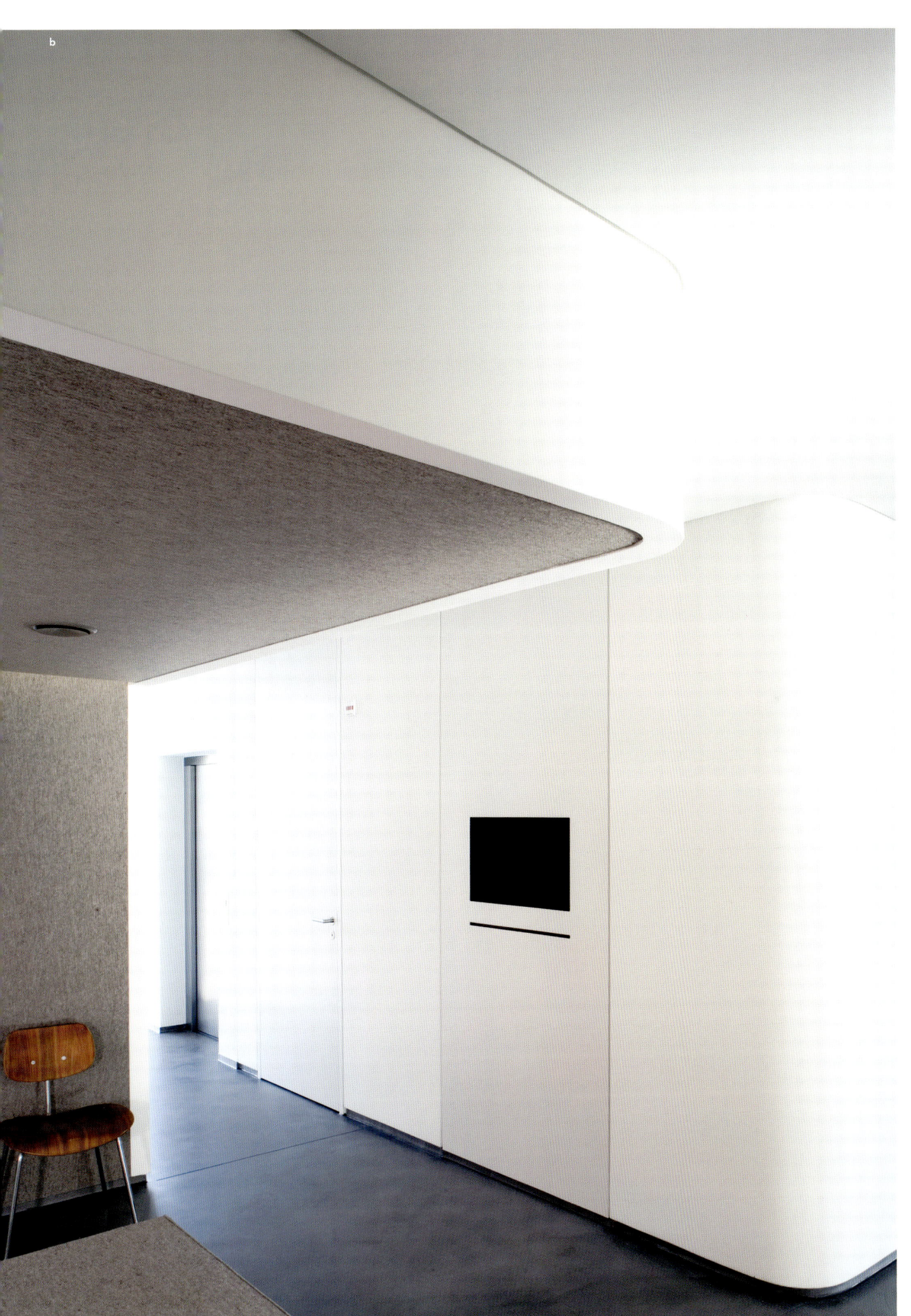

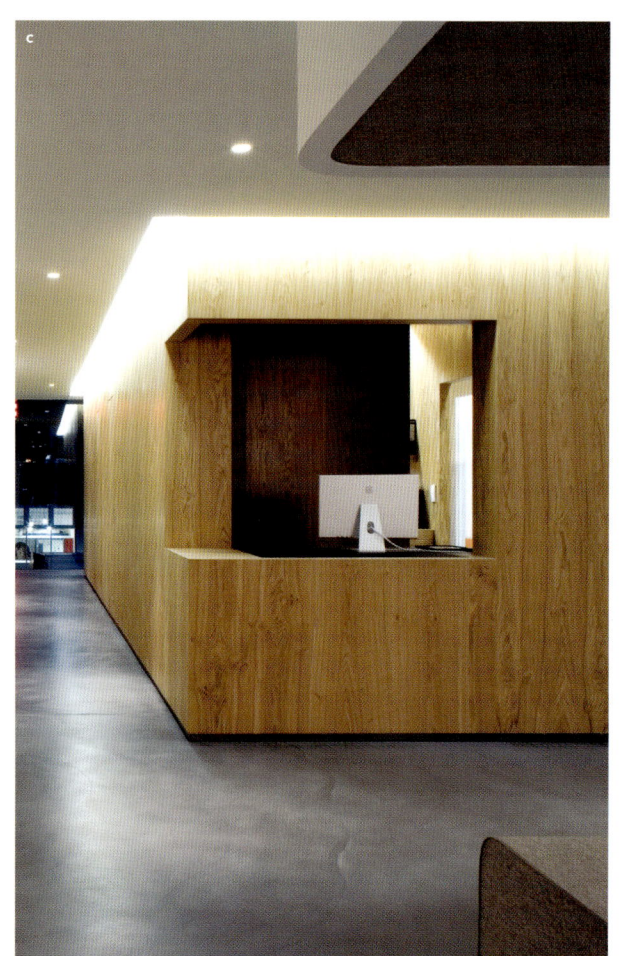

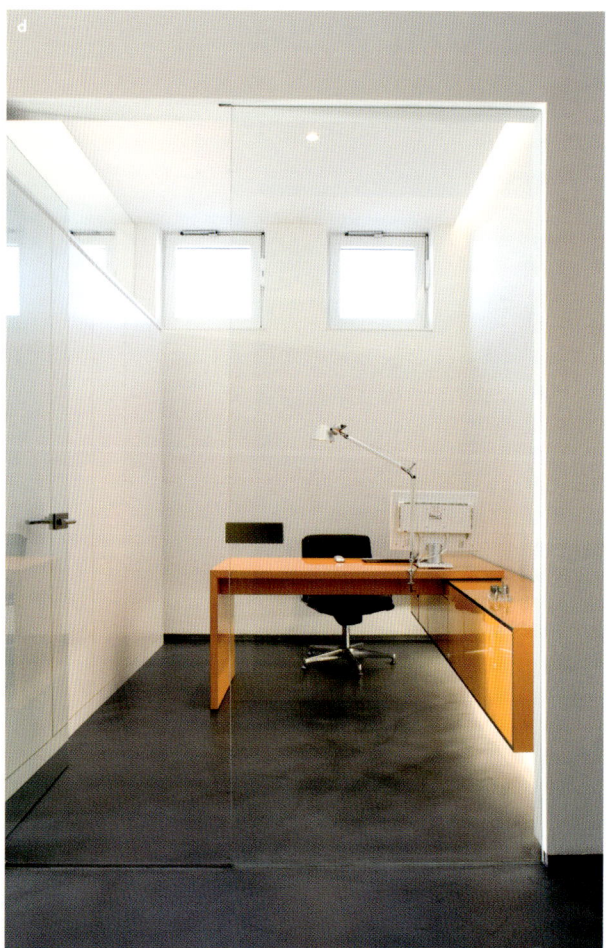

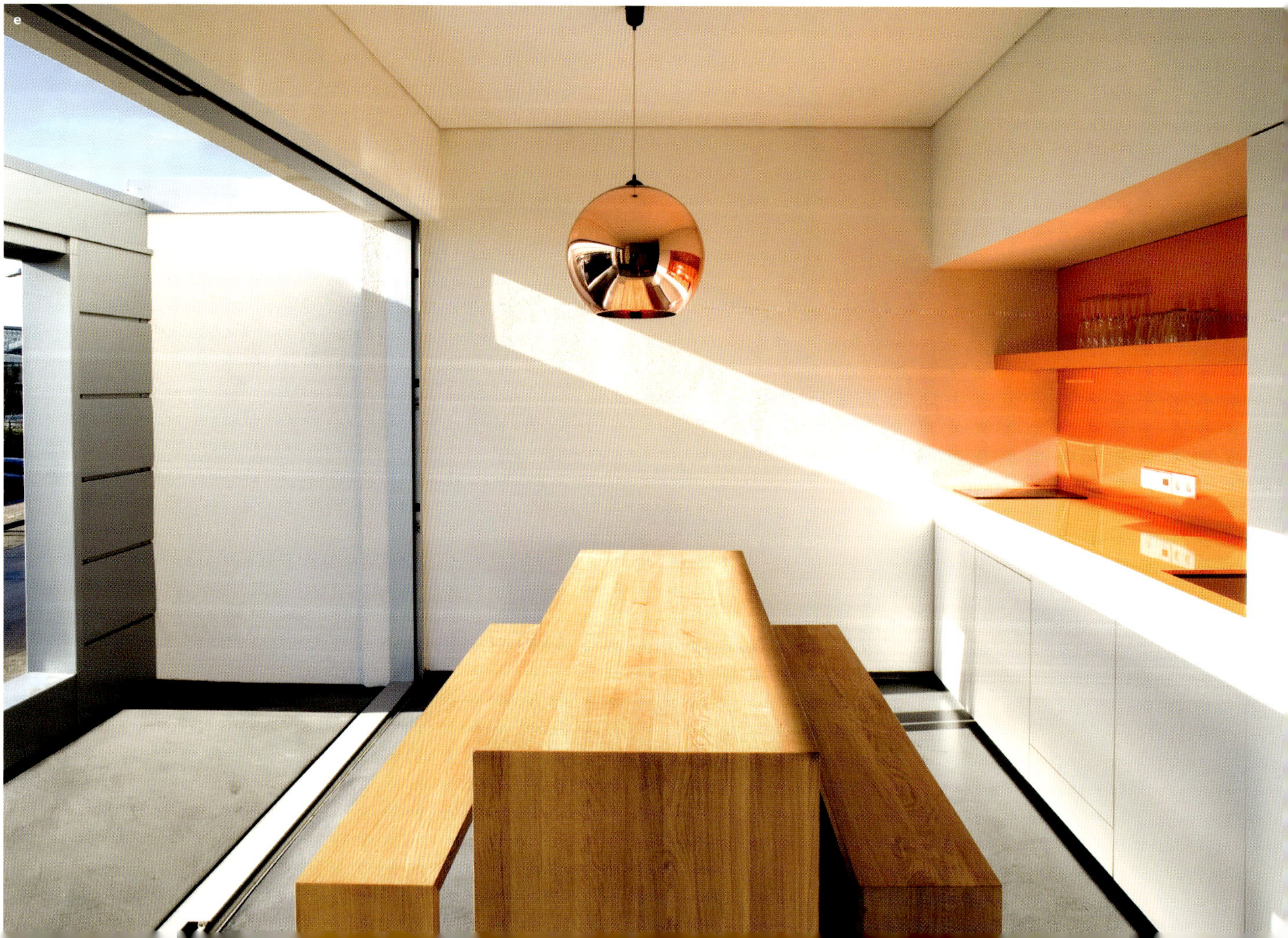

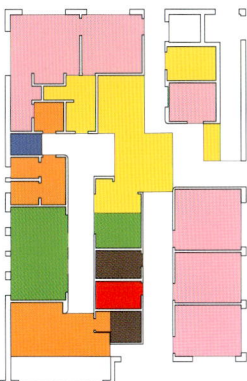

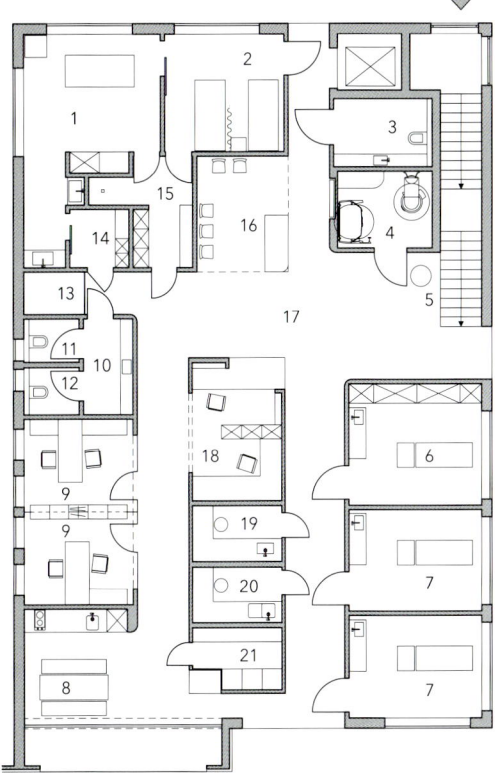

FF

Client | Operator Dr. Andreas Jauch
Gross floor area 250 sqm
Usable floor space 157 sqm

a Visitors to the Airport Clinic are greeted by
   a long staircase with illuminated handrail.
b A cosy corner for patients: the television set
   into the wall informs and entertains them as
   they wait.
c Entrance area with the high-quality wood
   reception desk.
d Simple, classical functionality in the treatment room.
e Large Sky-Frame sliding doors open out-
   wards from the staff lounge and provide
   plenty of natural light.

Diagrammatic plans, to scale 1:400
Floor plans, to scale 1:200

Floor plan layout

1	Operating theatre		small kitchen	**16**	Waiting area
2	Recovery room	**9**	Office	**17**	Reception
3	Patient toilet	**10**	Toilet anteroom	**18**	Office
4	Examination X-ray	**11**	Staff toilet L	**19**	Sterilisation room
5	Coat-rack	**12**	Staff toilet G	**20**	Laboratory
6	Treatment room	**13**	Installations room	**21**	Staff changing
	prevention	**14**	Staff sluice		cubicle and store
7	Treatment room	**15**	Patient changing		room
8	Staff lounge and		cubicle		

Patients ascend a staircase or use a lift in one corner of the rectangular floor plan
to reach the upper floor with its central reception and waiting area, from which
they can then access all the rooms in the multiple practice via two corridors. The
operating area is favourably located in a corner section and most of the rooms
benefit from natural light.

Usable floor spaces

Patient rooms	**yellow**	24 sqm	15 %
Examination			
Treatment rooms	**red**	39 sqm	25 %
Specialist rooms	**pink**	37 sqm	24 %
Administrative rooms	**green**	25 sqm	16 %
Offices	Staff rooms	**orange**	24 sqm	15 %
Supply	Waste disposal	**brown**	6 sqm	4 %
Plant rooms	**blue**	2 sqm	1 %
Total		157 sqm	100 %

Performance data

Outpatients per year	1,000
Number and type of services per year	Implantology [200]
	Cosmetic surgery [100]
	Orthodontics [200]
	Dentistry [300]
Services to other clinics	Tumour surgery
Clinic opening hours	5 days	50 hours
Waiting time [with	without appointment]	5 min.	15 min.
Type and number of staff	1–3 doctors
	4 specialists

The unusual design of the central aisle catches the eye as soon as you enter the new Zurich West School Dental Clinic housed in a 1930s building. Glass elements alternate at regular intervals with cupboards supported on glass feet. The L-shaped wooden fittings are secured to the supporting wall opposite to form an arcade. The glass partition wall thus held in place acts as a decorative feature, while providing ample natural light to the centre of the building. The wooden elements above the central aisle are transformed into a gleaming canopy, concealing the open installation area above and creating a pleasing proportional relationship by dint of the lowered ceiling height. The four treatment rooms and the sterilisation and X-ray rooms are located to the left of the entrance, with the patient rooms – excluding the laboratory and prophylaxis room – to the right. Patient and staff passageways have been separated by relocating the administrative and staff rooms to the upper floor.

American cherrywood veneer, indirect lighting and lime-green tones create a warm and soothing atmosphere in the practice.

HÖNIG ARCHITEKTEN

ZURICH WEST SCHOOL DENTAL CLINIC
ZURICH | CH

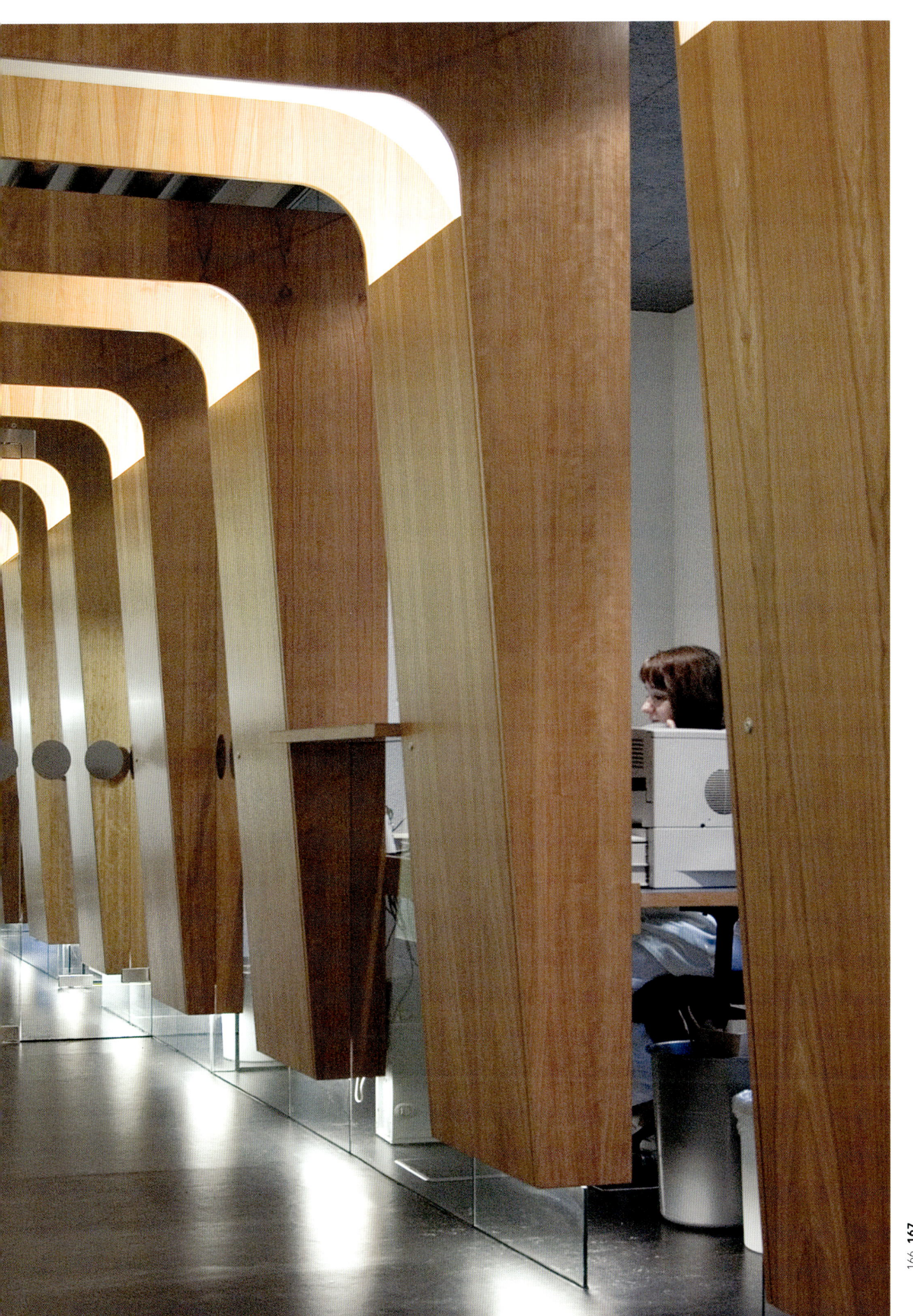

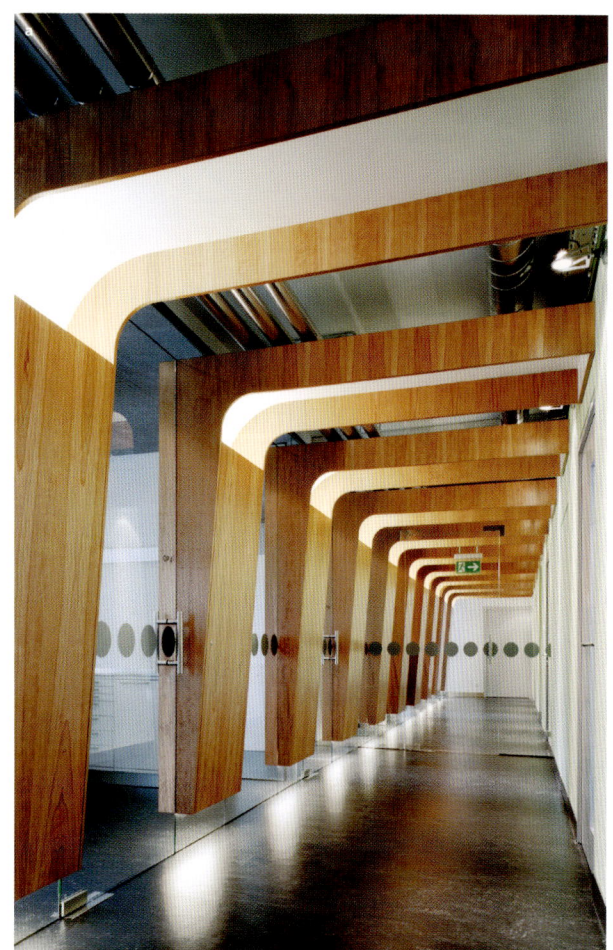

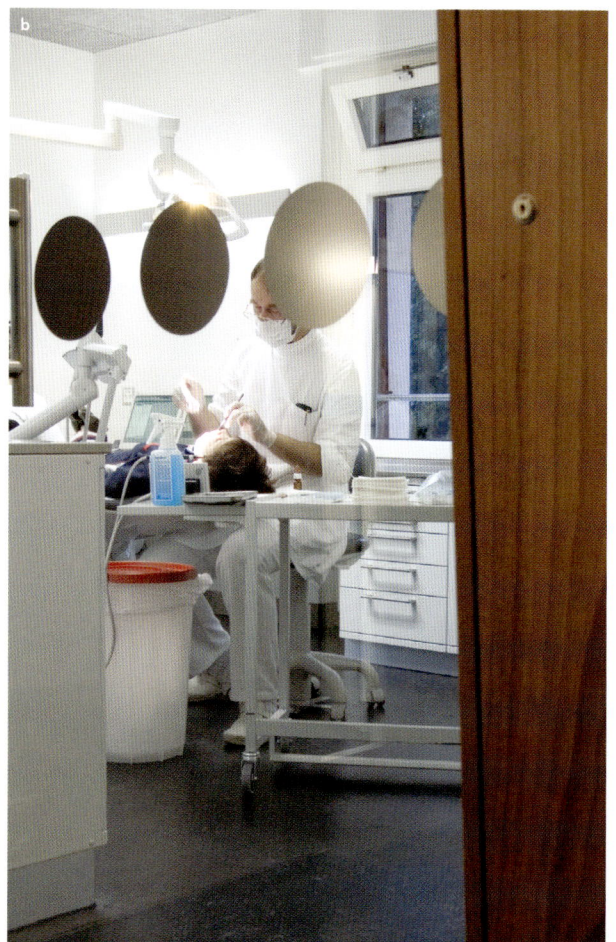

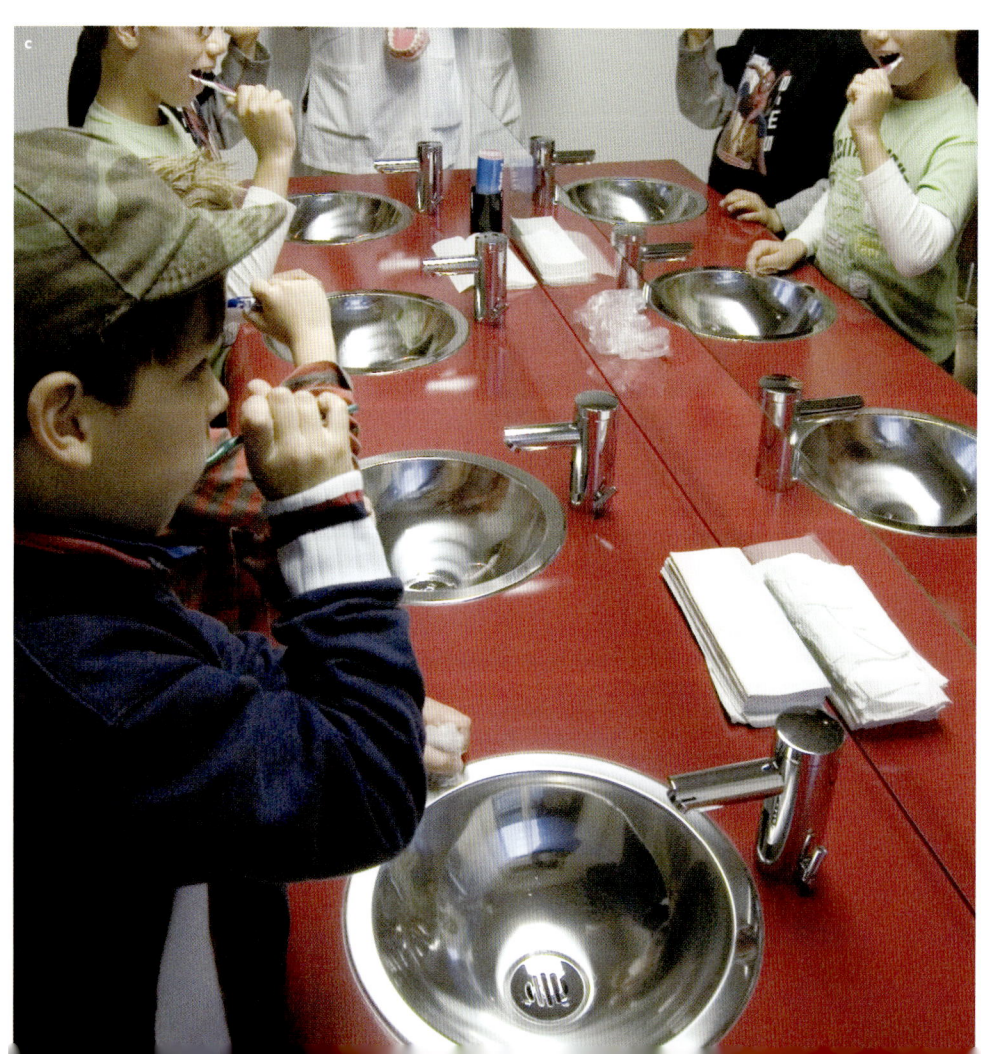

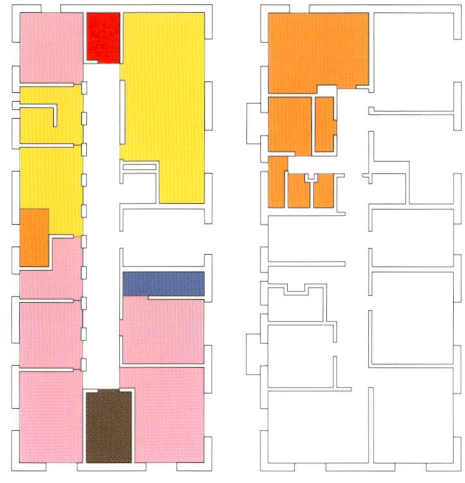

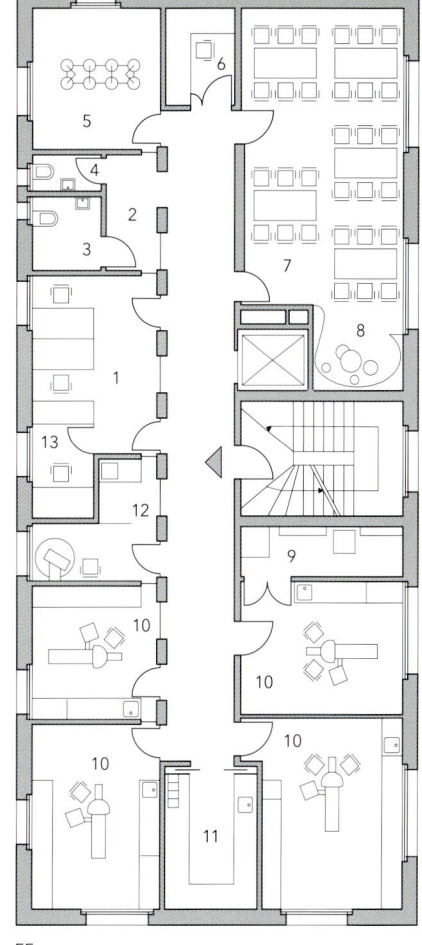

FF

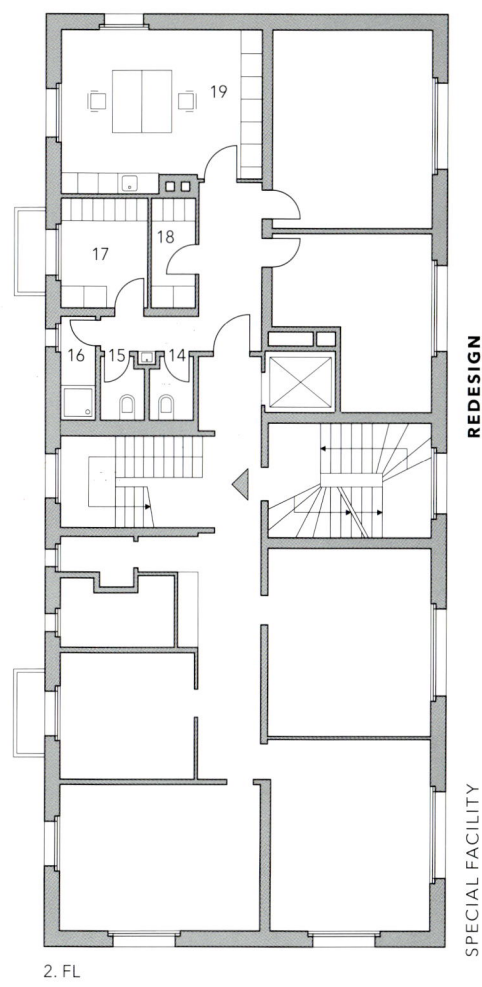

2. FL

**Client	Operator**	Zurich
Planning time	06 2005 – 09 2006
Construction time	01 2006 – 09 2006
Usable floor space	246 sqm
Gross cubic capacity	1,000 cbm
Construction cost	1,183,000 CHF
Total cost	1,703,000 CHF

a Wooden elements over the central aisle are transformed into a gleaming canopy, lowering the original ceiling height and making room for installations above.

b Childish curiosity satisfied: The doors to the four treatment rooms along the access passageway are transparent.

c Everything at child height: communal teeth-cleaning in the large prophylaxis room.

Diagrammatic plans, to scale 1:400
Floor plans, to scale 1:200

Floor plan layout

1	Reception and administrative office	**7**	Waiting area	**14**	Staff toilet L
2	Anteroom	**8**	Kid's corner	**15**	Staff toilet G
3	Patient toilet [L and disabled]	**9**	Installations room	**16**	Staff shower
4	Patient toilet G	**10**	Treatment room	**17**	Staff changing cubicle L
5	Prevention	**11**	Sterilisation room	**18**	Staff changing cubicle G
6	Laboratory	**12**	Orthopantomography	**19**	Staff lounge
		13	Office		

Thanks to the specialist clinic's rectangular floor plan with its straight corridor and central access and clear room layout, patients have no difficulty finding their bearings. A useful addition could be provided by downlights at both ends of the corridor. The practice design was further improved by the relocation of administrative and staff rooms to the floor above. Nearly all the rooms benefit from natural light.

Usable floor spaces

Patient rooms	**yellow**	73 sqm	30 %
Examination	Treatment rooms	**red**	6 sqm	3 %
Specialist rooms	**pink**	98 sqm	40 %
Offices	Staff rooms	**orange**	51 sqm	20 %
Supply	Waste disposal	**brown**	11 sqm	4 %
Plant rooms	**blue**	7 sqm	3 %
Total		246 sqm	100 %

Performance data

Outpatients per year	6,000
Services to other clinics	Orthodontics
Clinic opening hours	5 days	40 hours
Waiting time	0 – 15 min.
Type and number of staff	3 dentists
	4 dental assistants
	1 trainee

Cantonal legislation requires every schoolchild in Switzerland to be examined by the school dentist at least once a year and special school dental clinics have been set up for this purpose in the larger cities. Zurich has a total of six clinics caring for children's dental health; two of them stand out for their modern and welcoming design.

At the access to the staircase of this dental clinic, an extended "threshold" has been installed to make it easier for children to enter the clinic rooms. Dark reds, low ceilings and built-in wooden furniture create a warm and cosy atmosphere. The ramp leading to the waiting area and the passageway past the brightly lit treatment rooms gently prepare children for a new, unfamiliar environment. The waiting area gives on to the large bright and open treatment area, where the treatment stations are insulated cubicles dotted round the room. Separated from the surrounding rooms by glass partition walls, these cubicles protect the children from inquisitive eyes, while at the same time providing transparency and openness – avoiding any feeling of "vulnerability". Separate corridors for doctor and patient allow work to proceed cleanly and calmly in the four treatment units stationed one behind the other.

HÖNIG ARCHITEKTEN

ZURICH CITY SCHOOL DENTAL CLINIC
ZURICH | CH

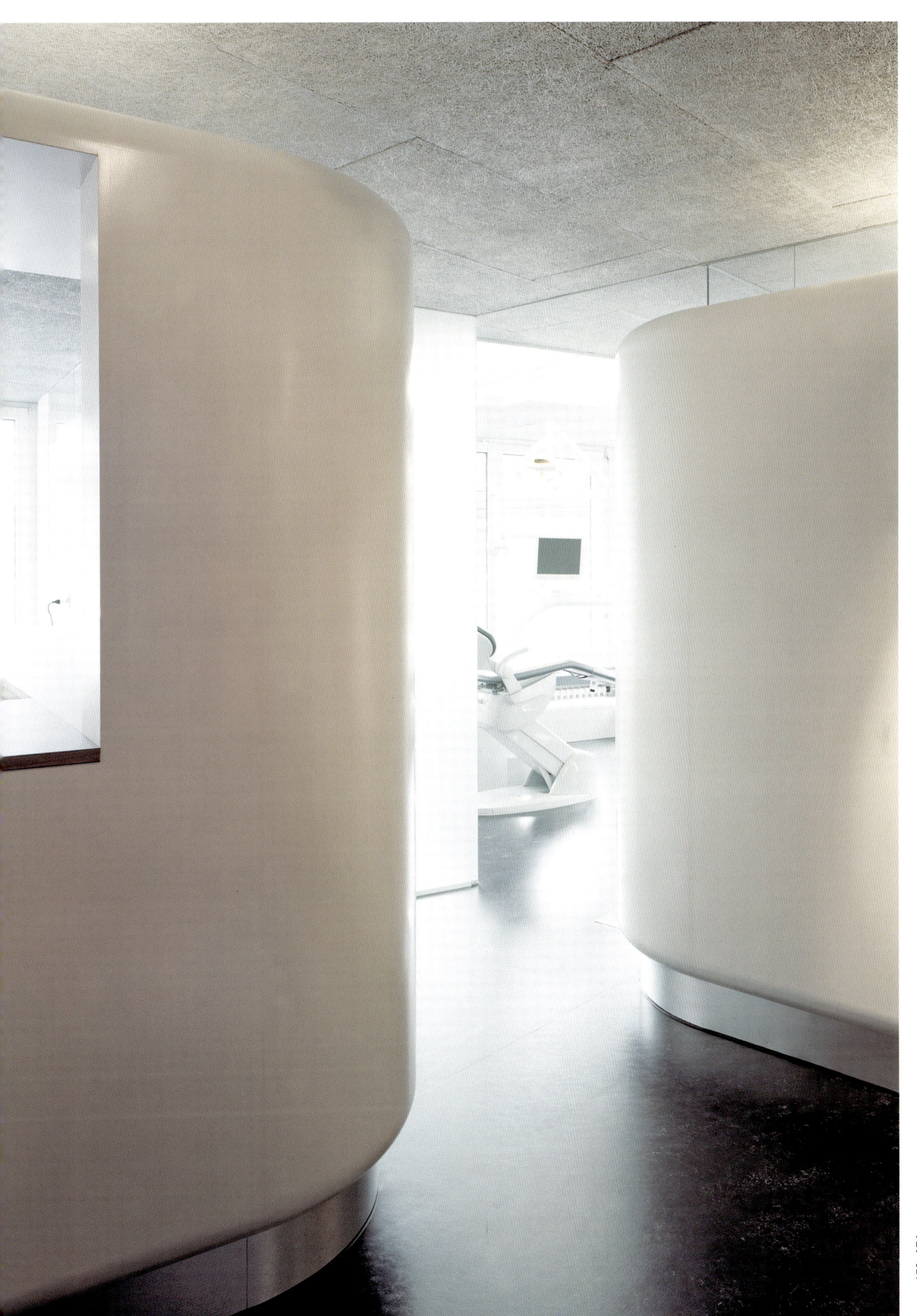

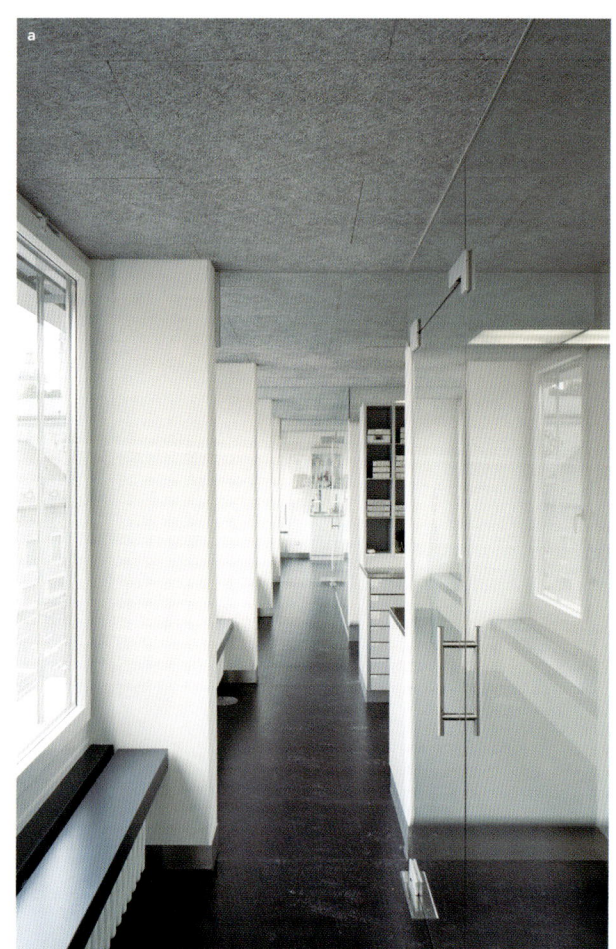
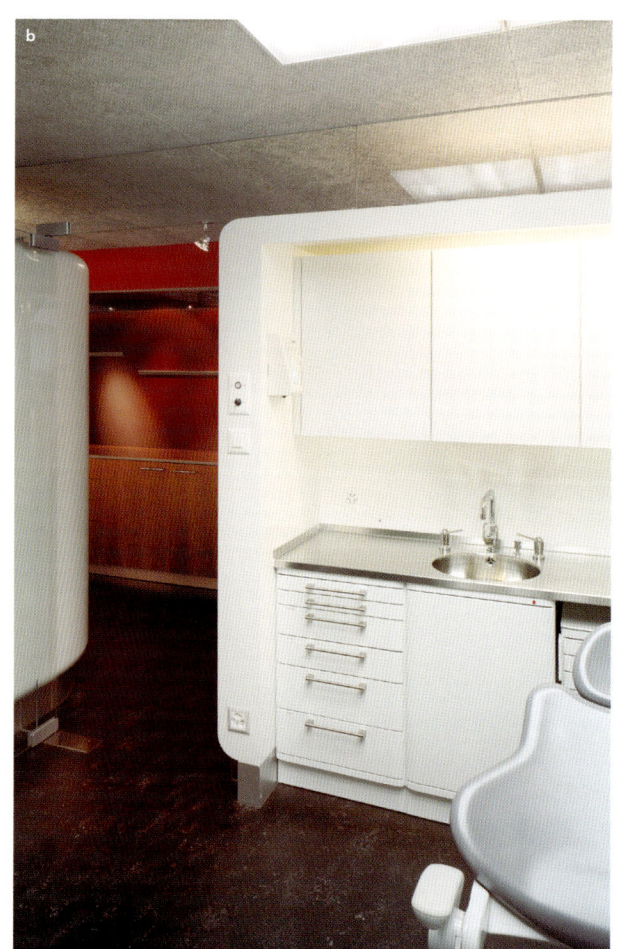

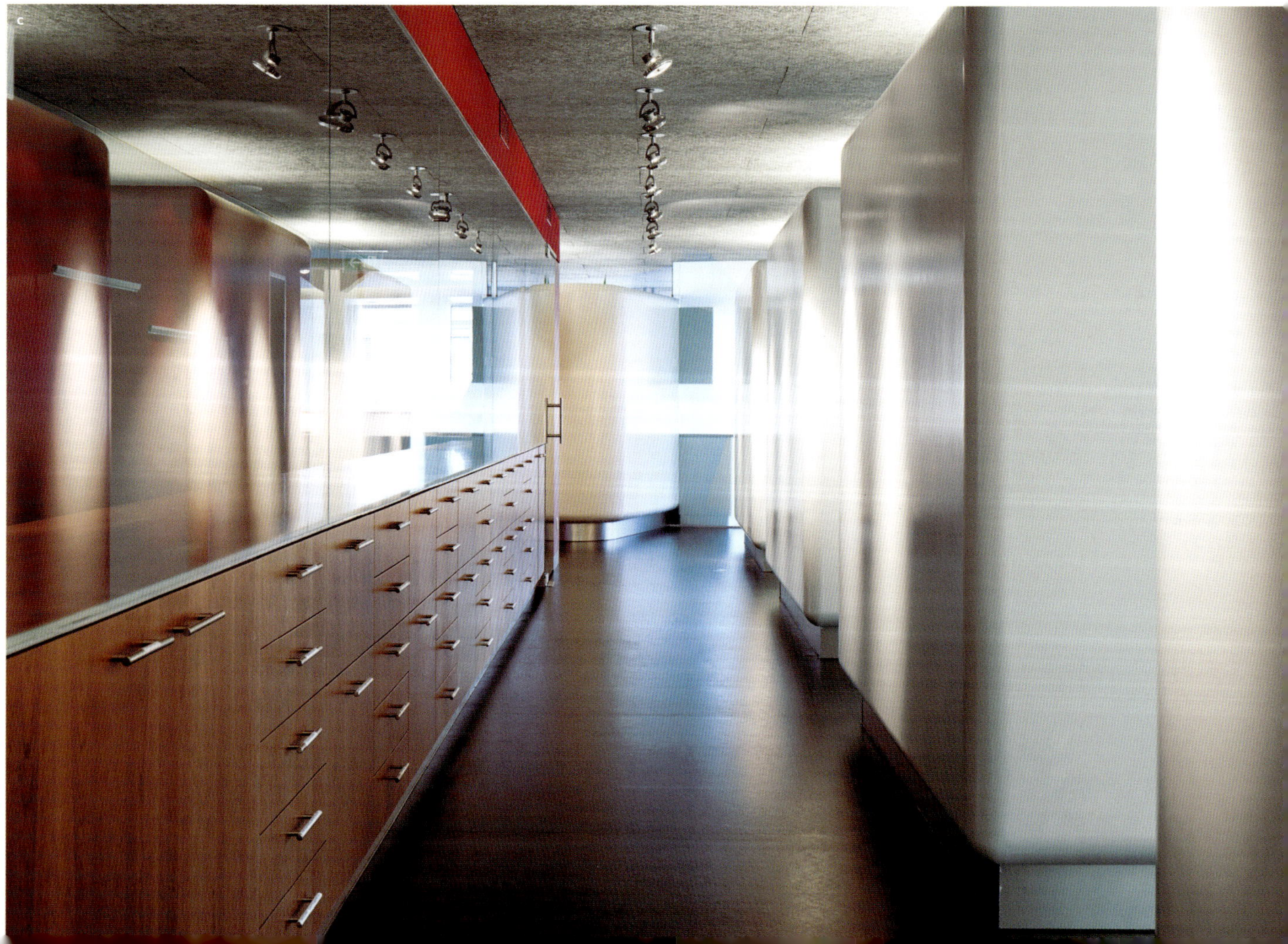

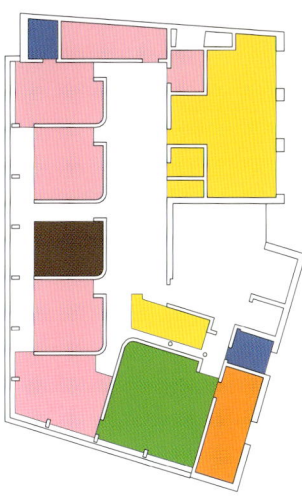

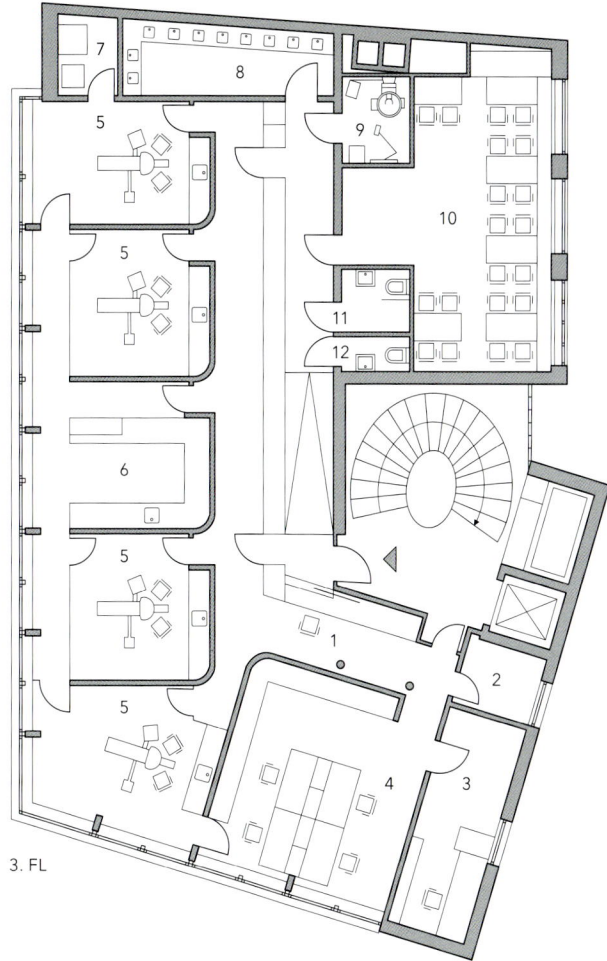

3. FL

Client | Operator Zurich
Planning time 11 2003 – 02 2005
Construction time 08 2004 – 02 2005
Usable floor space 221 sqm
Gross cubic capacity 806 cbm
Construction cost 1,363,000 CHF
Total cost 1,660,000 CHF

a A dedicated staff corridor enables work to proceed cleanly and calmly in the four treatment units stationed one behind the other.
b Dark red walls, low ceilings and built-in wooden furniture create a warm and cosy atmosphere.
c Three of the four treatment stations are freestanding insulated booths; drawers built into the corridor wall provide the necessary storage space.

Diagrammatic plans, to scale 1:400
Floor plans, to scale 1:200

Floor plan layout

1 Reception	**5** Treatment room	**9** Examination X-ray
2 Installations room	**6** Sterilisation room	**10** Waiting area
3 Manager's office	**7** Installations room	**11** Patient toilet L
4 Office	**8** Prevention	**12** Patient toilet G

On arrival at the special clinic, patients proceed past reception to this large waiting area. A more accentuated visual connection between the two rooms could however be beneficial. After a possible diversion via the prophylaxis room, patients reach the four treatment rooms on the main corridor, which are interconnected by an internal staff corridor. Staff rooms and supply and waste disposal rooms are located on the floor above.

Usable floor spaces

Patient rooms	**yellow**	55 sqm	25 %
Specialist rooms	**pink**	88 sqm	40 %
Administrative rooms	**green**	33 sqm	15 %
Offices	Staff rooms	**orange**	15 sqm	7 %
Supply	Waste disposal	**brown**	13 sqm	6 %
Plant rooms	**blue**	17 sqm	7 %
Total		221 sqm	100 %

Performance data

Outpatients per year	6,000
Services to other clinics	Orthodontics
Clinic opening hours	5 days	40 hours
Waiting time	0 – 15 min.
Type and number of staff	3 dentists
	4 dental assistants
	1 trainee

A UFO in the lily pond? The architectural design for the oral and maxillofacial surgery is indeed extremely striking. A blue illuminated room divider, housing a small auditorium and kitchen, appears to float above the shallow pool in the entrance area. The curved body of the training room, open to the top, is made of glass-fibre reinforced, translucent plastic. Advanced technology allows surgical operations in the adjacent treatment rooms to be observed live. The entrance to the practice is styled as a wooden footbridge: bamboo parquet leads from the stairs to the reception desk and accentuates the Asian feel of the waterscape. The surrounding floors are fitted with black porcelain stoneware tiles, the functional area with linoleum. The individual treatment rooms are divided by cuboid boxes lined with reddish doussie parquet and provide fire integrity.

The sophisticated interior design, complementing the high aesthetic demands of the surgical practice, provides an exciting contrast to the building's basic technical structure – pillars and ceilings have been left in their natural state and painted in coordinating colours.

**HÖNIG
ARCHITEKTEN**

**PRACTICE FOR ORAL AND
MAXILLOFACIAL SURGERY**
ST. GALLEN | CH

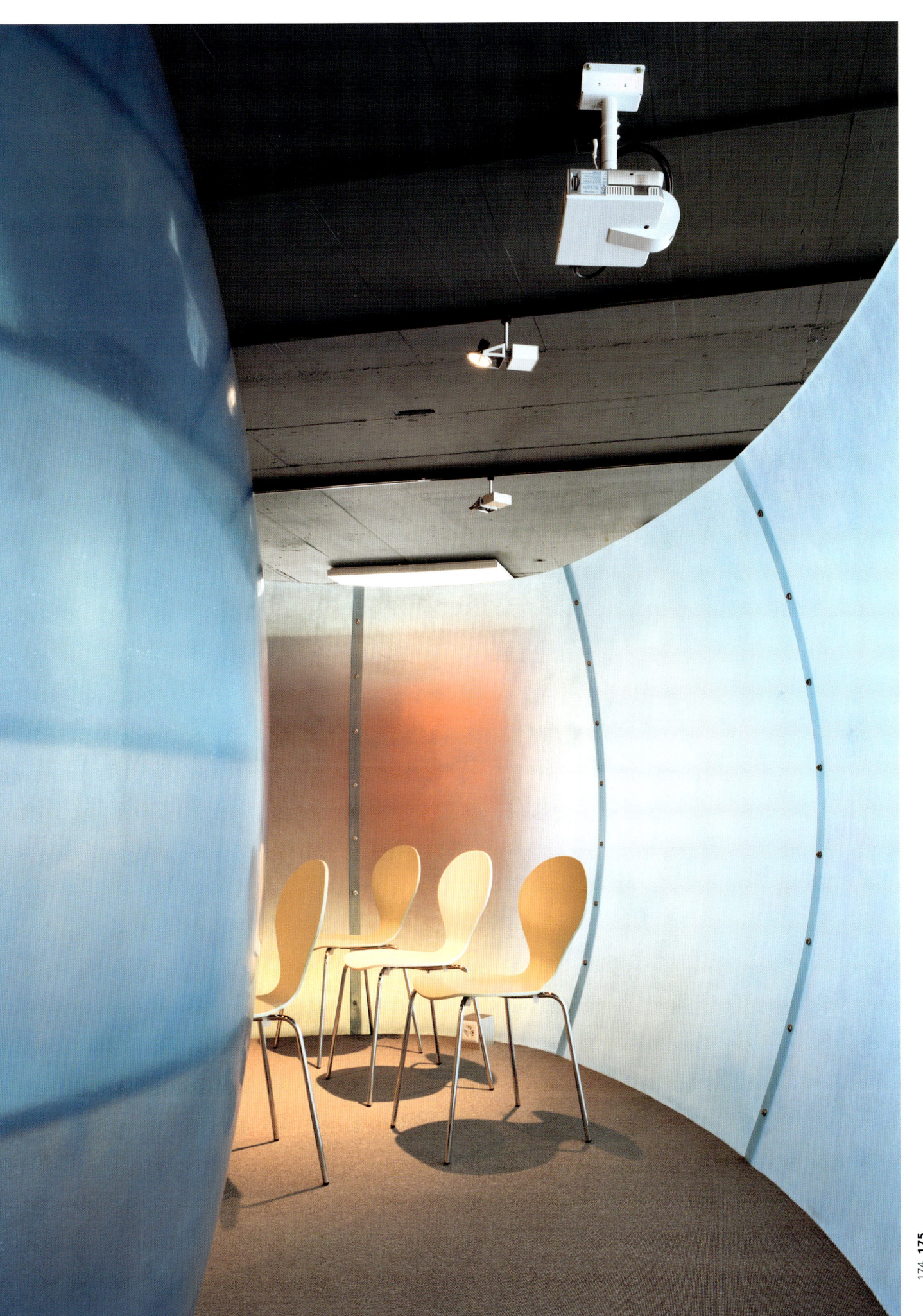

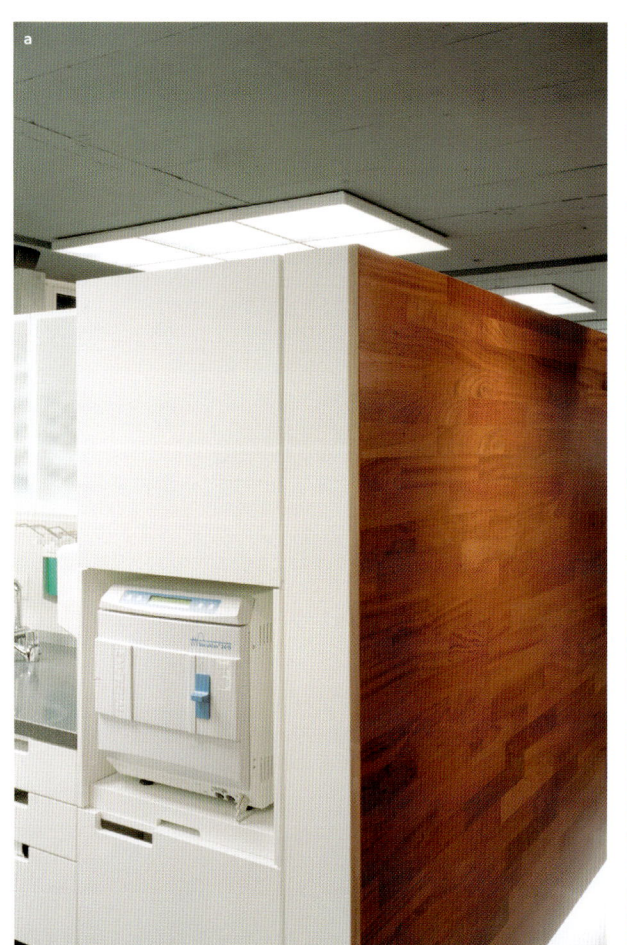

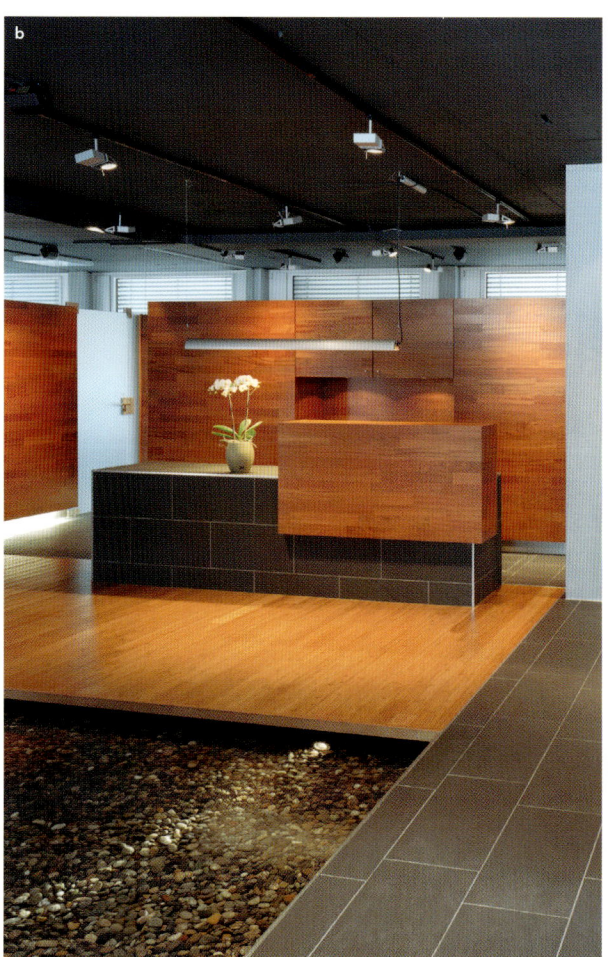

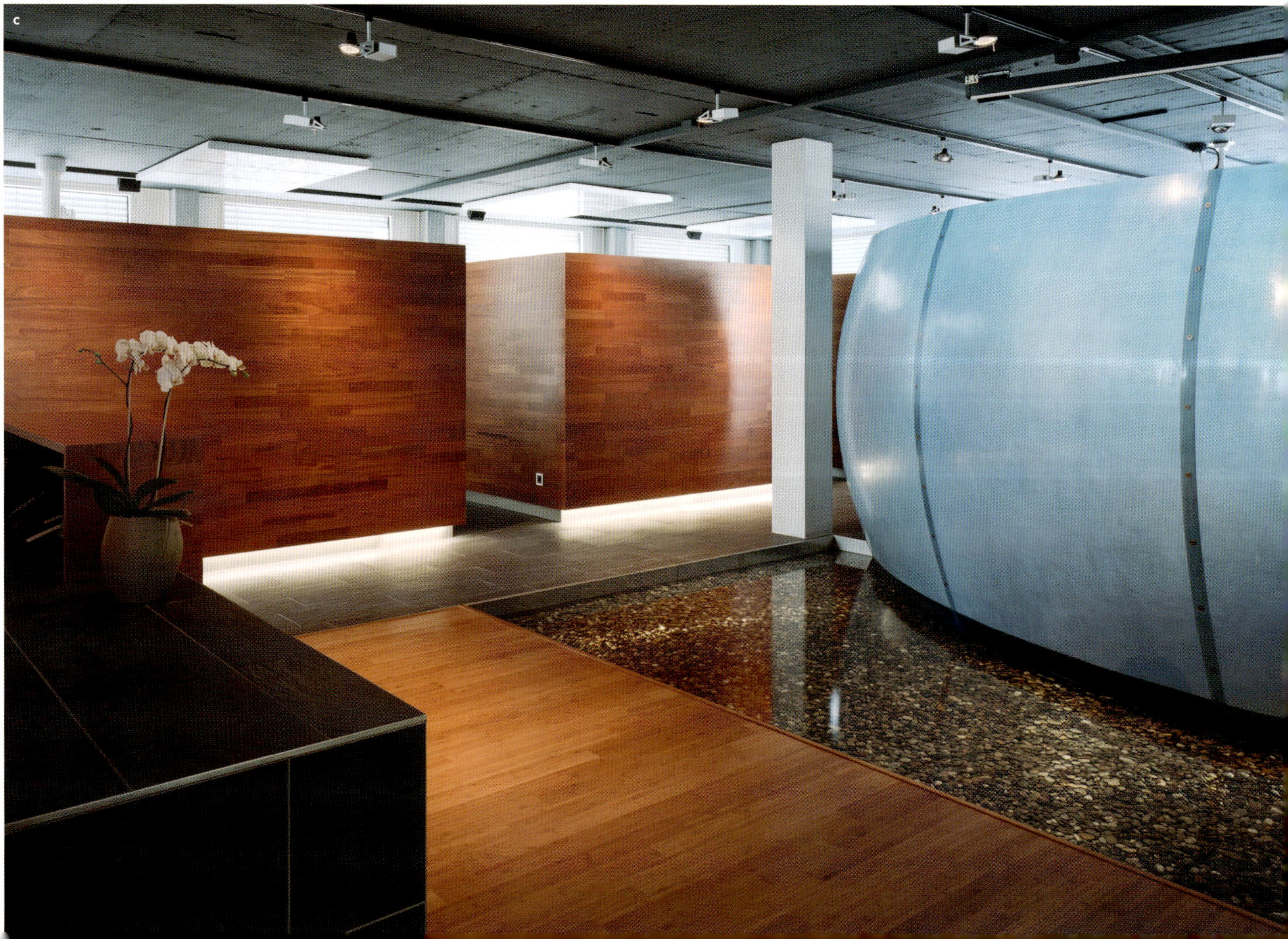

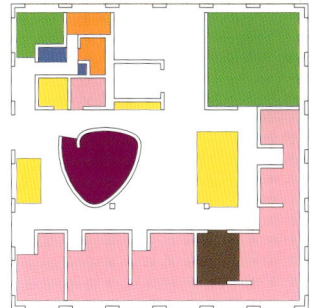

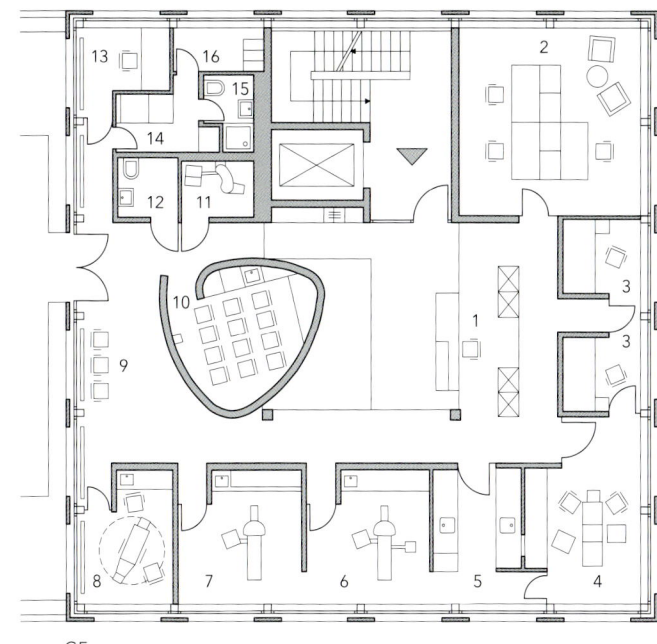

GF

Client	Dr. Dr. Ronald Bucher
Operator	Dr. Dr. Ronald Bucher
	Dr. Tanja Lemm
Planning time	10 2003 – 02 2004
Construction time	11 2003 – 02 2004
Usable floor space	147 sqm
Gross cubic capacity	630 cbm
Construction cost	500,000 CHF

a The treatment rooms are divided by cuboid boxes lined with reddish doussie parquet; these provide fire integrity.

b The entrance area is defined by dark materials.

c The curved body of the training room, open to the top, is made of glass-fibre reinforced, translucent plastic.

Diagrammatic plans, to scale 1:400
Floor plans, to scale 1:200

Floor plan layout

1	Reception	**7**	Treatment room	**12**	Patient toilet
2	Office and	**8**	Treatment room	**13**	Office
	consultation room		laser	**14**	Installations room
3	Recovery room	**9**	Waiting area	**15**	Staff toilet and
4	Treatment room	**10**	Seminar and		shower
	surgery		refreshment room	**16**	Staff changing
5	Sterilisation room	**11**	Orthopantomog-		cubicle
6	Treatment room		raphy		

The square floor plan of the partnership practice with its U-shaped rooms set around an internal area has been clearly sub-divided. From the reception area however, there is no direct line of sight to the waiting seats at the window. All the treatment rooms are interconnected by an internal corridor, including the two recovery rooms, which appear quite small. Nearly all the rooms benefit from natural light.

Usable floor spaces

Patient rooms	**yellow**	18 sqm	12 %
Specialist rooms	**pink**	67 sqm	46 %
Administrative rooms	**green**	34 sqm	23 %
Offices | Staff rooms	**orange**	6 sqm	4 %
Supply | Waste disposal	**brown**	7 sqm	5 %
Training rooms	**violet**	13 sqm	9 %
Plant rooms	**blue**	2 sqm	1 %
Total		147 sqm	100 %

Performance data

Outpatients per year	3,000
Clinic opening hours	5 days | 45 hours
Waiting time [with | without appointment]	5 min. | 30 min.
Type and number of staff	2 doctors
	2 trainees
	3 full-time staff
	1 part-time staff

Dental-associative free-form fusions meet practical ascetic strength here: The architectural concept used in the conversion of the small Wuppertal dental practice is immediately apparent in the curved steps whose central location and unusual shape produce a striking effect. Three of the four steps rise to meet the reception desk, each following a different bold curve. A projection above one of the steps acts as a convenient bag shelf, where the customers can rest their bags or their papers while they are talking to the receptionist. The uniformly dark stone floor throughout the practice also covers the four steps and the bag shelf, creating an interesting contrast with the matt white Corian surfaces of the built-in furniture and the surrounding white walls. No embellishments were added during the conversion process, leaving the simple elegance of the very small practice to form a stark study in black and white.

As the practice has an exclusively private clientele and patients are seen as soon as they arrive for their appointment, there is no need for a waiting area. In addition to the reception area, there are two treatment rooms off to the side, a laboratory, a sterilisation room and a toilet. At the end of the short corridor is a large well-lit consultation room.

INSTANTCONCEPT OBJEKT DESIGN

PRIVATE DENTAL PRACTICE
WUPPERTAL | G

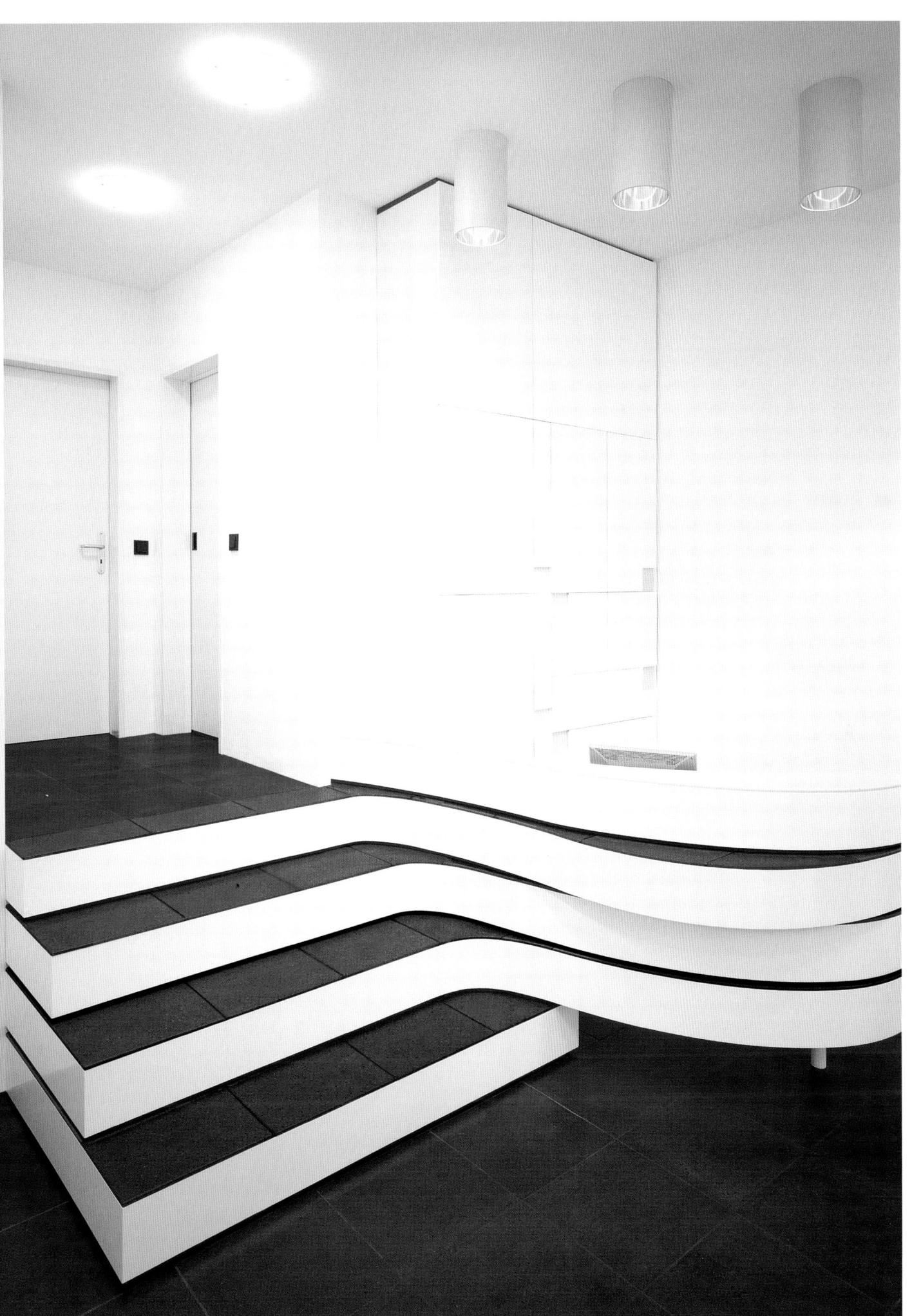

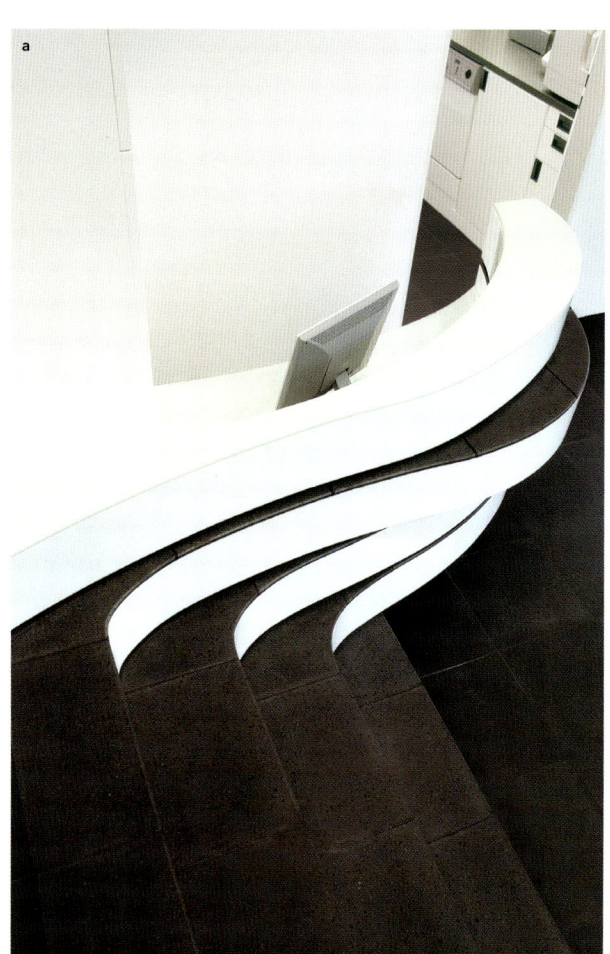

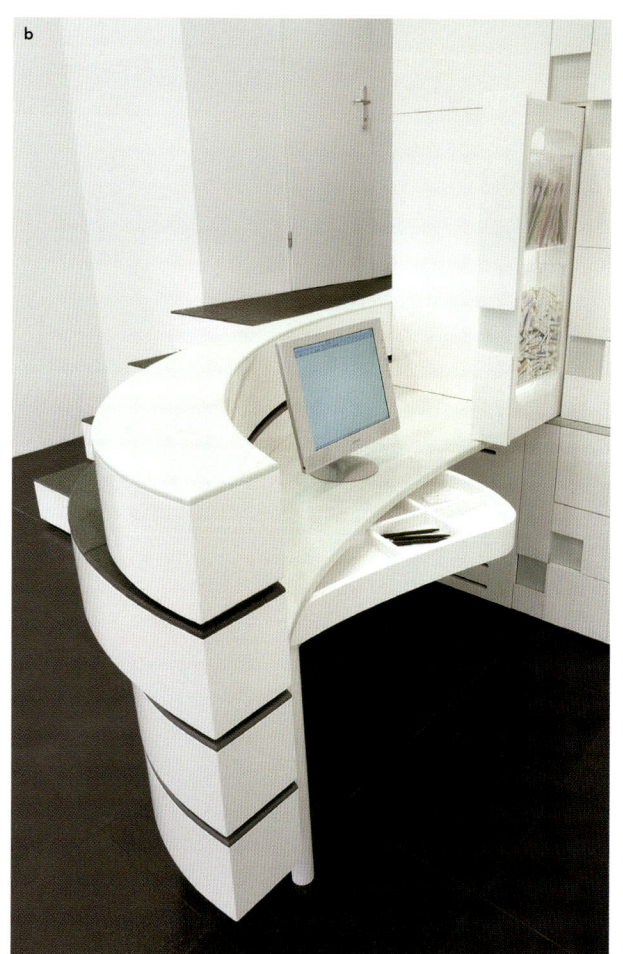

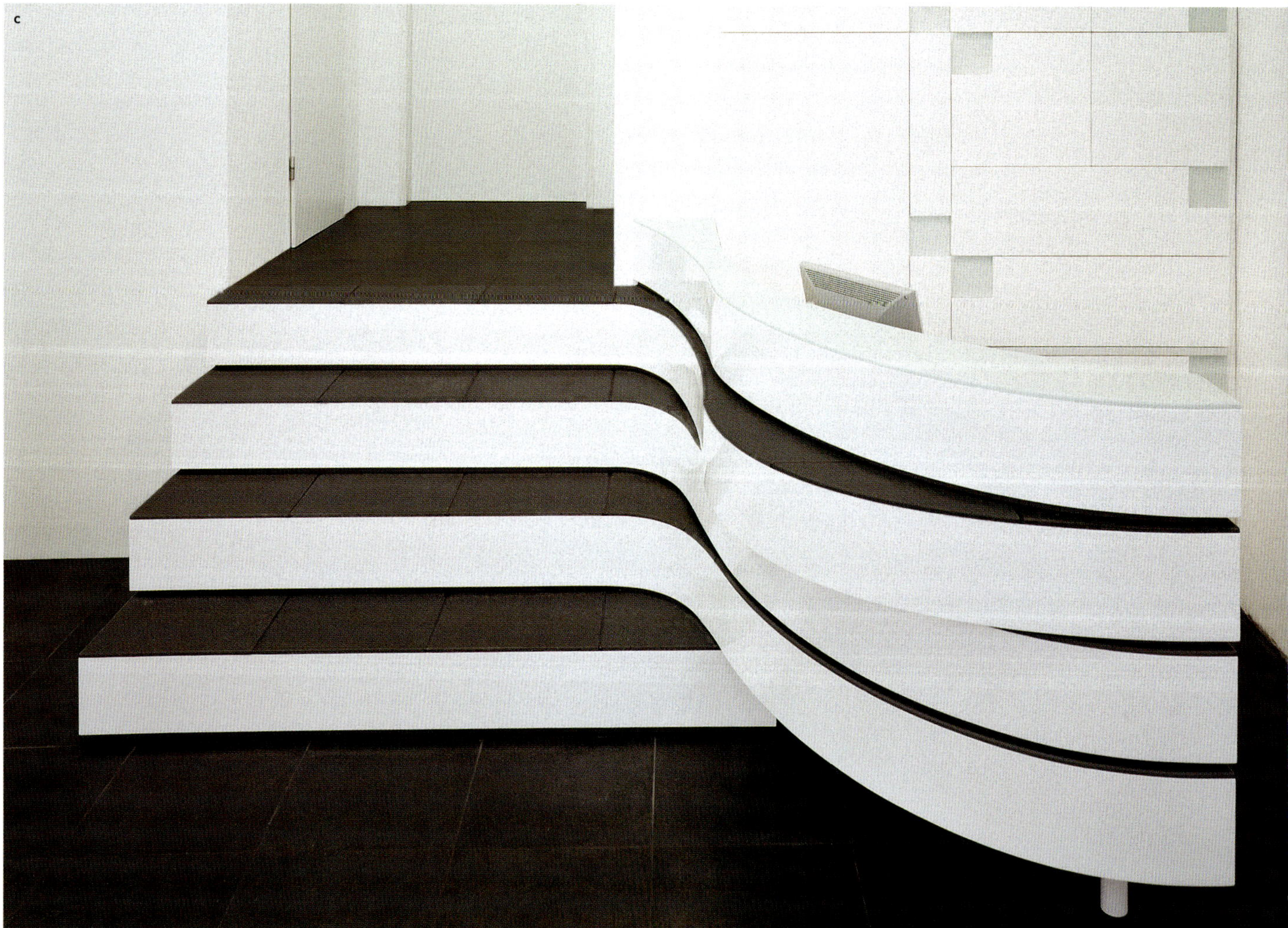

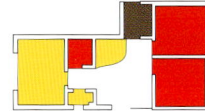

GF

Client | Operator Arnd Kauert
Planning time 2002
Construction time 01 2002 – 06 2002
Usable floor space 36 sqm
Construction cost 172,270 EUR
Total cost 198,980 EUR

a Three of the four steps forming the
curved stairway swing away in different
curves to meet the reception desk.
b The central position and unusual shape
of the reception desk make it particularly
eye-catching.
c A dark stone floor is laid throughout the
practice, creating a strong contrast with
the matt white surfaces of the built-in
furniture and with the walls.

Diagrammatic plans, to scale 1:400
Floor plans, to scale 1:200

Floor plan layout

1 Reception	**3** Consultation room	**5** Sterilisation room
2 Patient toilet	**4** Laboratory	**6** Treatment room

All the rooms required for a private solo medical practice – reception,
two treatment rooms, sterilisation room, laboratory, toilet and a large
consultation room – are functionally fitted out.

Usable floor spaces

Patient rooms	**yellow**	14 sqm	39 %
Examination | Treatment rooms	**red**	19 sqm	53 %
Supply	Waste disposal	**brown**	3 sqm	8 %
Total		36 sqm	100 %

Performance data

Outpatients per year	1,000
Services to other clinics	X-ray diagnostics Tissue diagnosis [around 20]
Clinic opening hours	5 days	40 hours
Waiting time	none
Type and number of staff	1 doctor 1 full-time staff
Clinic planning advice	One extra room would be useful [X-ray].

"And always clean thoroughly!" These four words inset into the mirror in the patient bathroom encapsulate the mission of the redesign of the dental practice that has occupied these rooms since the 1970s.

The concept focuses on two main ideas, light and colour. The reception and waiting area have been moved in a bid to improve patient processing and to make the premises as a whole appear brighter and more spacious. Reception is now adjacent to the entrance and screened from the waiting area by a long plexiglass wall embellished with oak slats. A sisal floor covering reduces noise and creates a cosy atmosphere. The multi-functional reception desk combines a variety of materials: Light beige, high-gloss laminate and wine-red linoleum make for an interesting combination. The straight reception desk stands at a 90 degree angle to the waiting area; in a lit alcove carved out of the counter, fruit and drinks are set ready for the waiting patients. The wine-red coat-rack projects from the wall. The colour theme is repeated in the treatment rooms, where wine-red metal furniture is paired with beige Corian work surfaces.

INSTITUT_ FEINER_DINGE

OTTO-SUHR-ALLEE DENTISTS
BERLIN | G

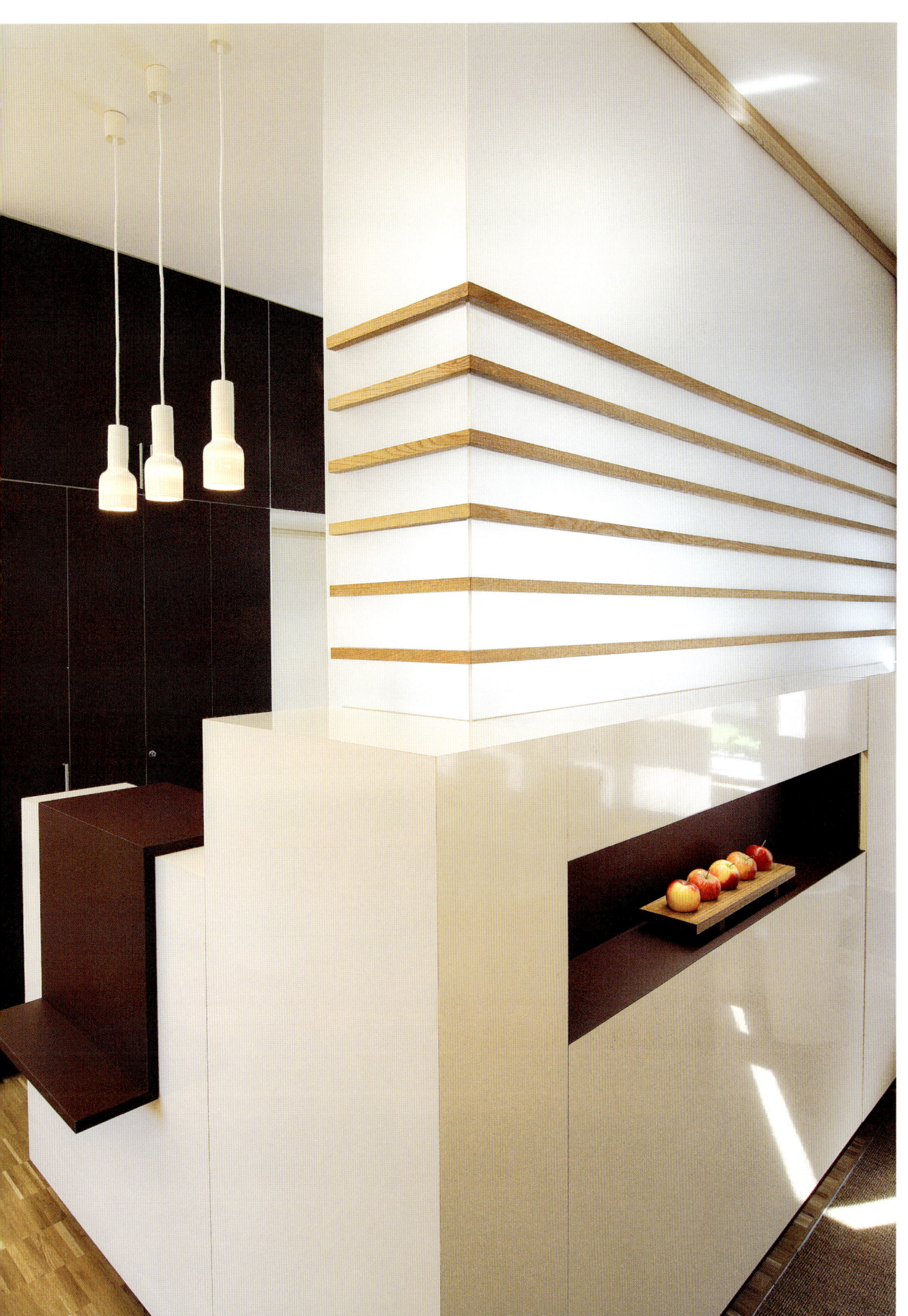

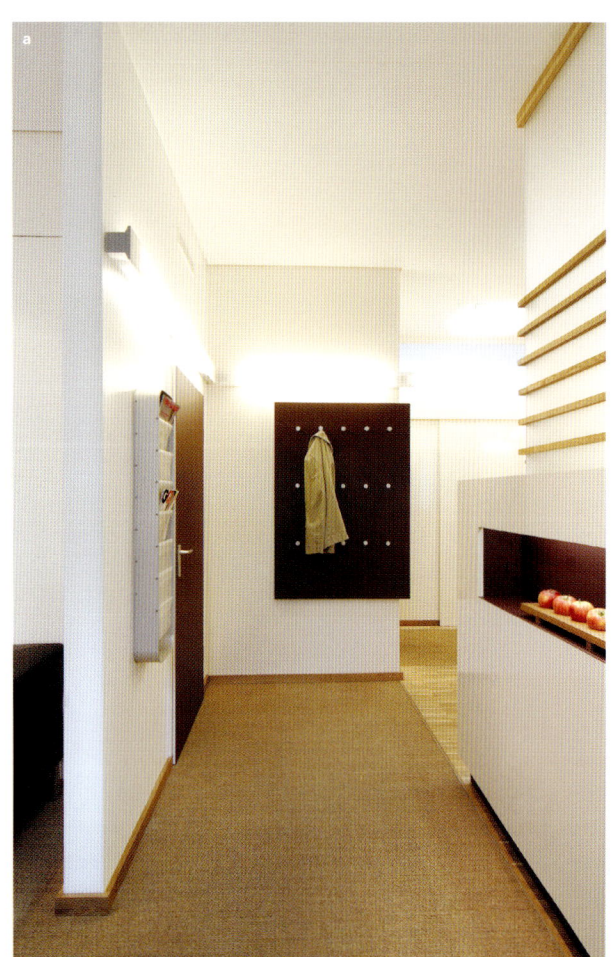
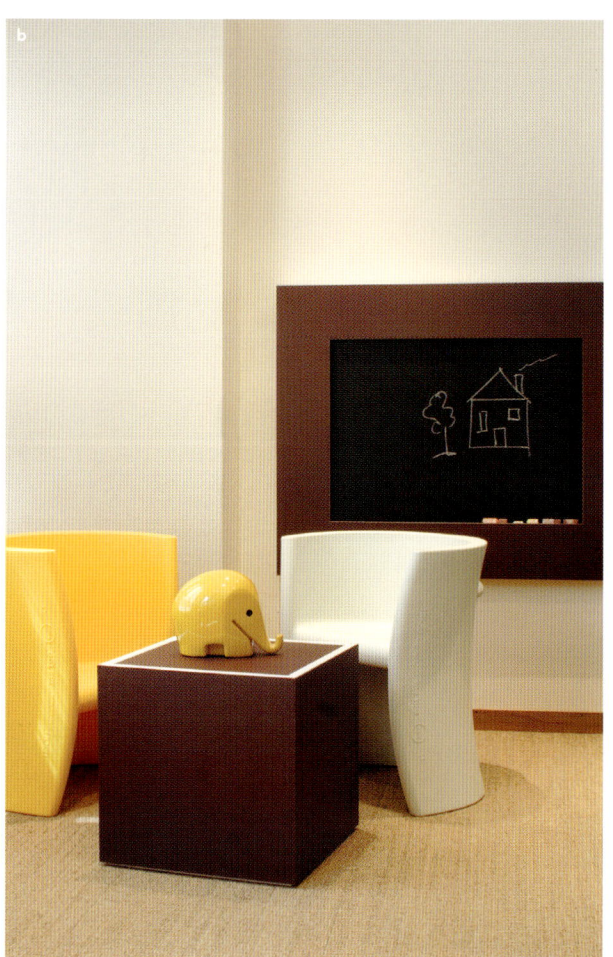

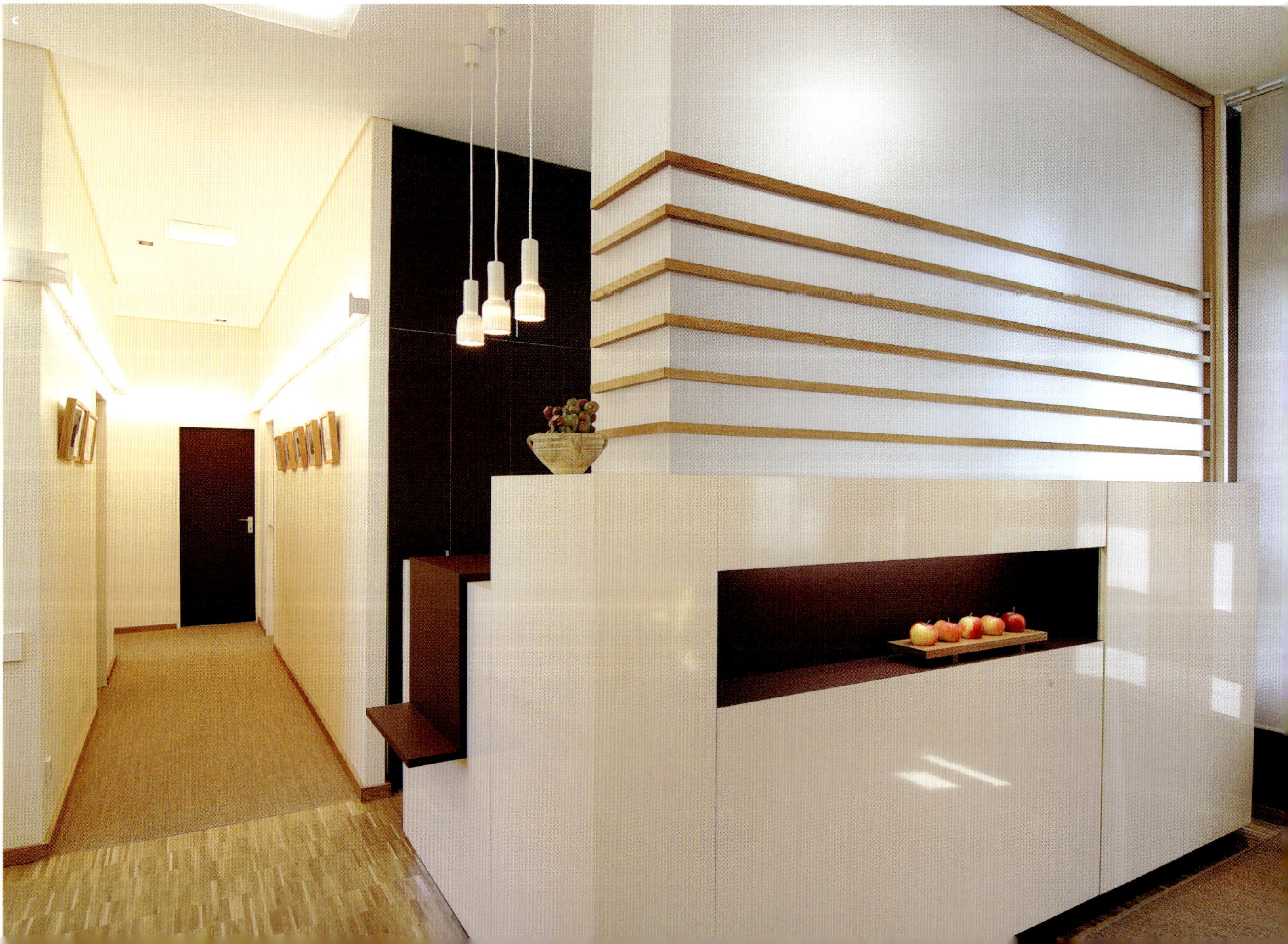

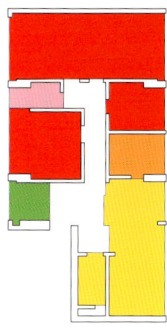

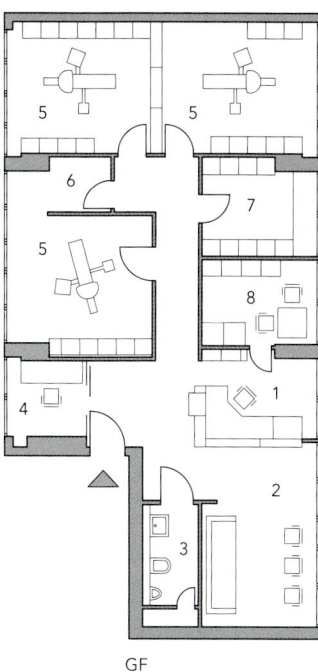

GF

Client	Dr. Markus Schramm
	Dr. Barbara Willigerodt
Operator	Dr. Markus Schramm
Planning time	01 2006 – 03 2006
Construction time	04 2006
Gross floor area	127 sqm
Usable floor space	107 sqm
Gross cubic capacity	381 cbm
Construction cost	65,000 EUR

a In a lit alcove carved out of the reception desk, fruit and drinks are set ready for waiting patients.
b The sisal floor covering in the waiting area reduces noise and creates a cosy atmosphere.
c Reception is screened from the waiting area by a plexiglass wall embellished with oak slats.

Diagrammatic plans, to scale 1:400
Floor plans, to scale 1:200

Floor plan layout

1	Reception	**4**	Office	**7**	Laboratory
2	Waiting area	**5**	Treatment room	**8**	Staff lounge
3	Patient toilet	**6**	Examination X-ray		

Reception faces the entrance and incorporates a speaker system for addressing patients in the waiting area. Patients walk down a short corridor to the practice rooms, which all benefit from natural light, except for the toilet. The room layout, which is ideal in terms of patient processing, cannot be faulted, the only slight drawback being the lack of space for storage and cleaning.

Usable floor spaces

Patient rooms	**yellow**	31 sqm	29 %
Examination | Treatment rooms	**red**	59 sqm	55 %
Specialist rooms	**pink**	4 sqm	4 %
Administrative rooms	**green**	5 sqm	5 %
Offices | Staff rooms	**orange**	8 sqm	7 %
Total		107 sqm	100 %

Performance data

Clinic opening hours	5 days | 40 hours
Number of staff	6

Dark red, light grey, ivory – these three distinctive colours define the interior of the dental practice in Berlin's new centre. They combine with the beech parquet flooring and brass-coloured sliding element to create a calm and restrained atmosphere in the converted loft space of an office complex. The previously open-plan floor has been divided up to form a clear, functional series of rooms. The entrance leads straight to the reception desk which is located in close proximity of waiting room, office and a small consultation room. Facing the main corridor, the glossy reception desk is framed by two light boxes made of white acrylic glass. Its white, high-gloss laminated counter appears to be floating weightlessly above the floor, thanks to two fluorescent tubes integrated in the base panel. The emphasis on airy lightness is also evident in the ceiling area – a skylight strip to the ceiling is set into the walls separating the treatment rooms from the corridor, giving the practice an open feel and maintaining the visual character of the loft.

An additional dedicated access for the staff has been incorporated into the internal layout, connecting all the treatment rooms and the laboratory. This solution prevents the reception and waiting area from becoming congested and too busy.

**INSTITUT_
FEINER_DINGE**

**DENTISTS IN
KRONPRINZENKARREE**
BERLIN | G

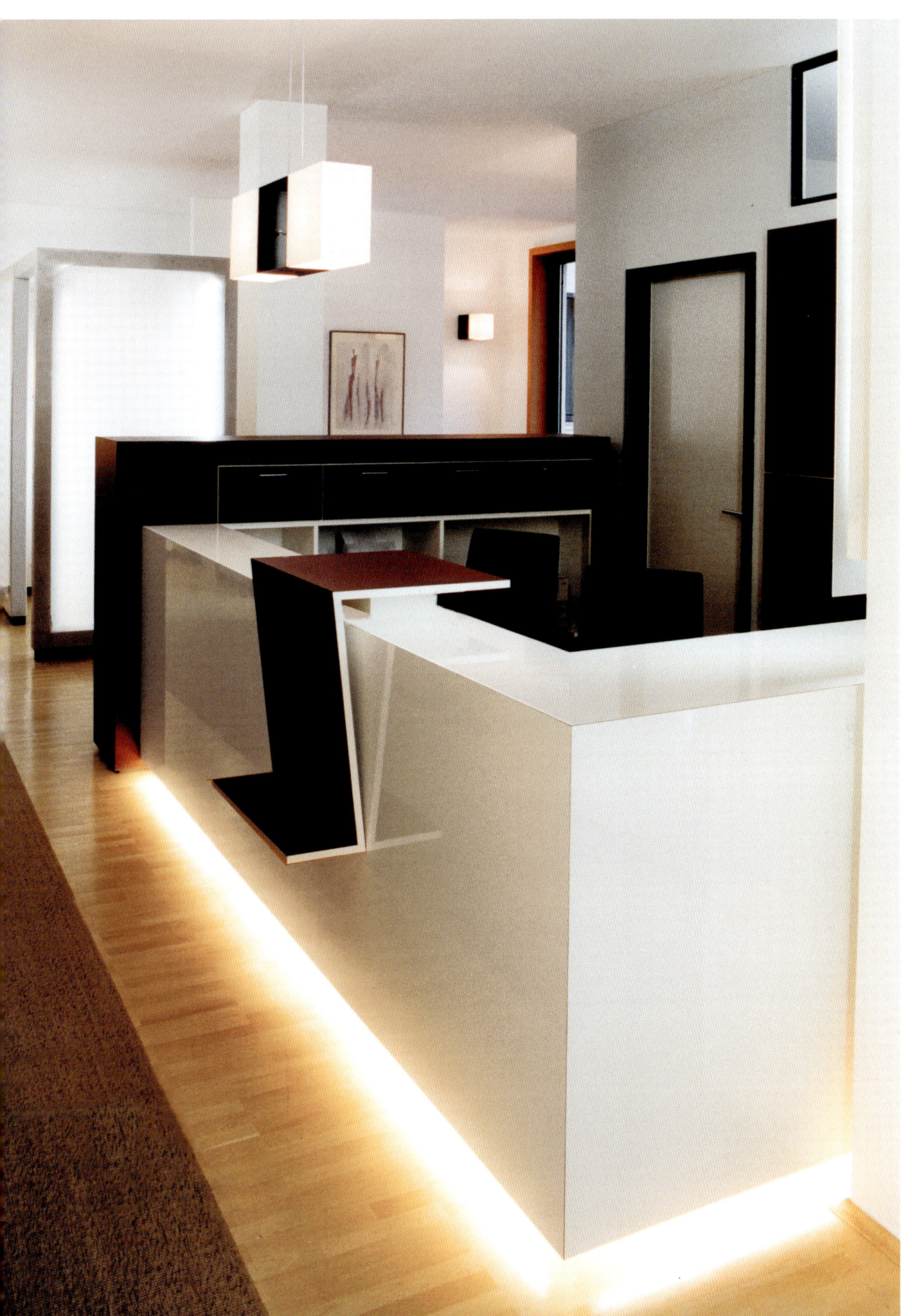

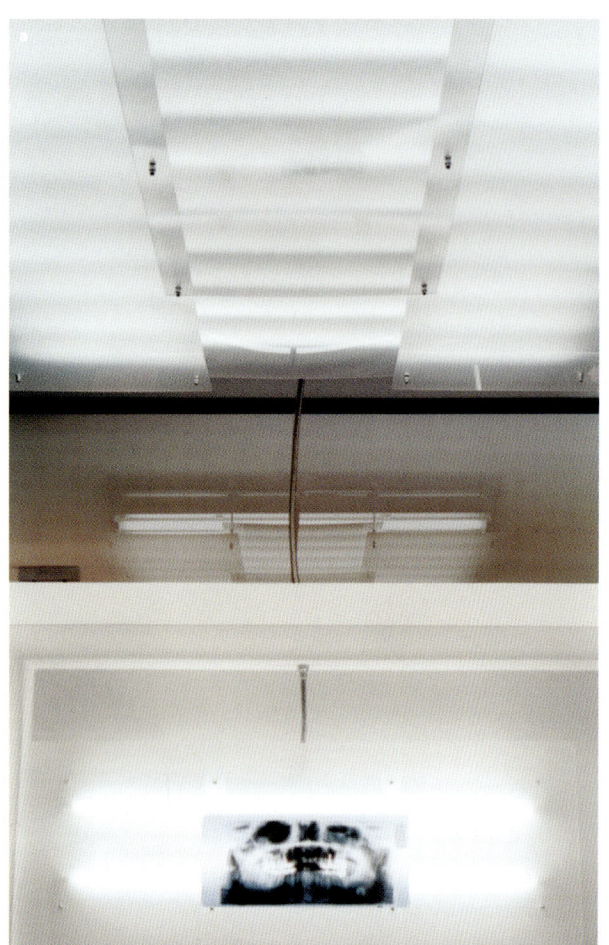

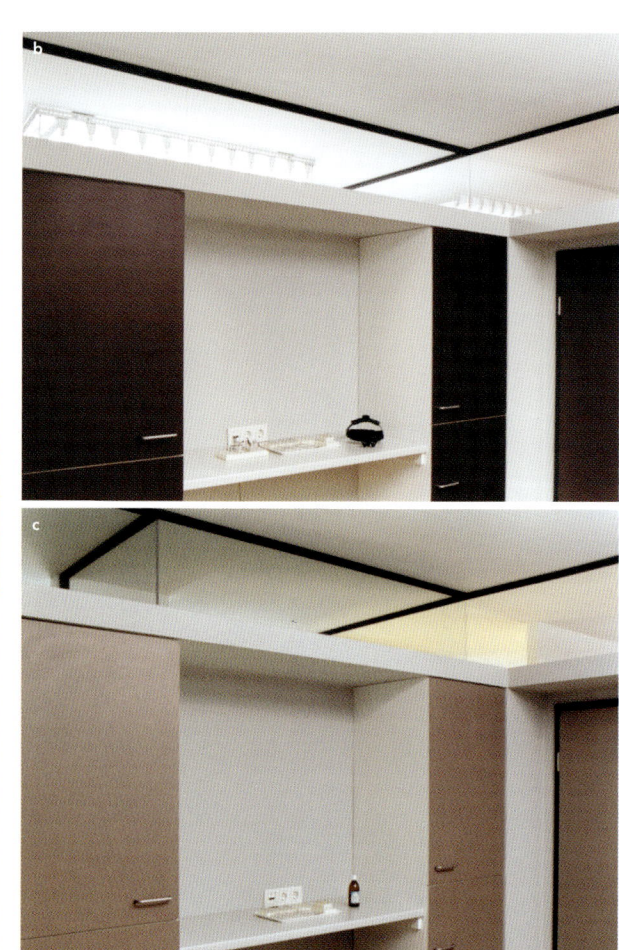

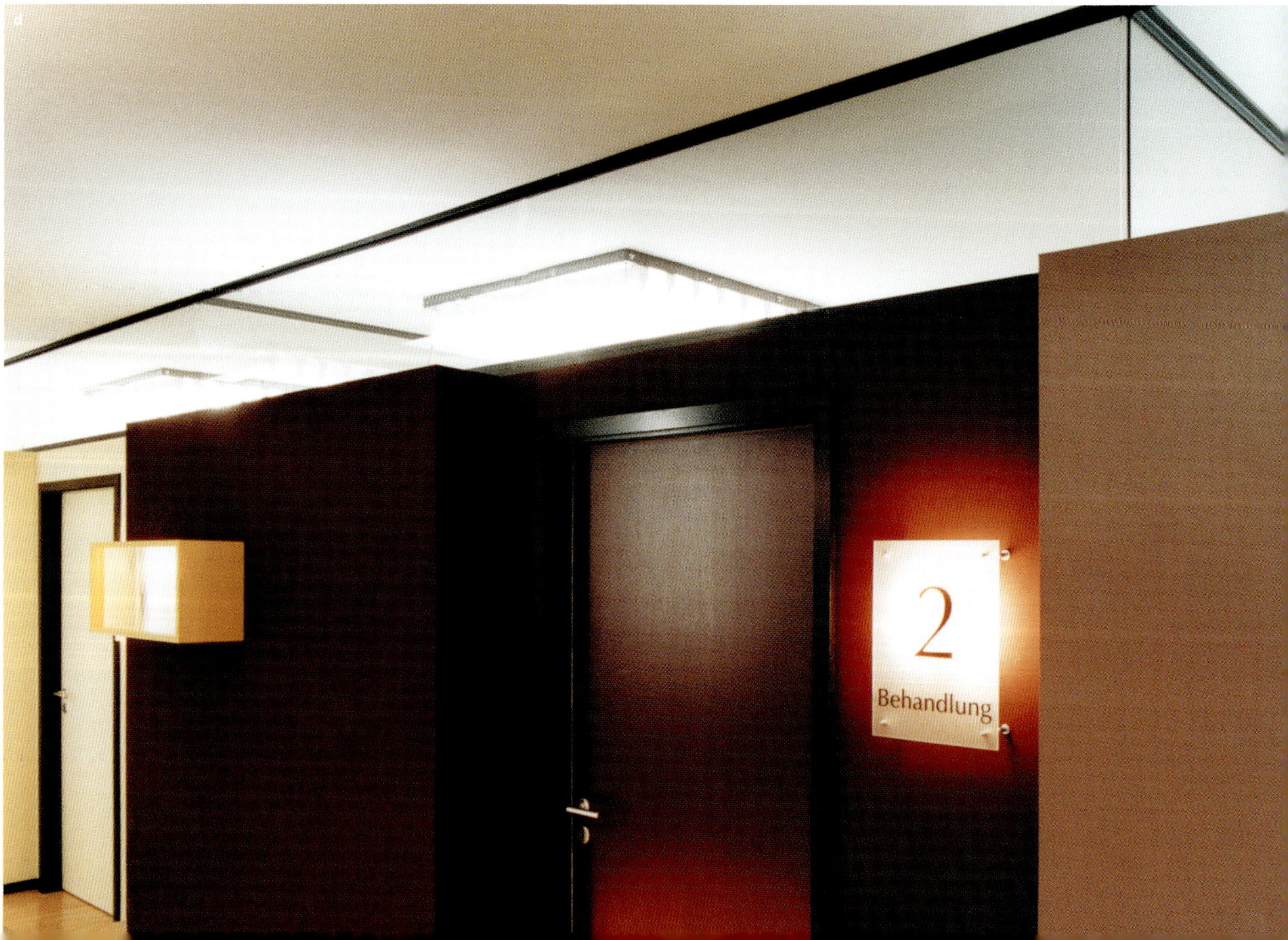

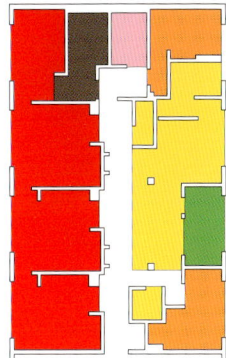

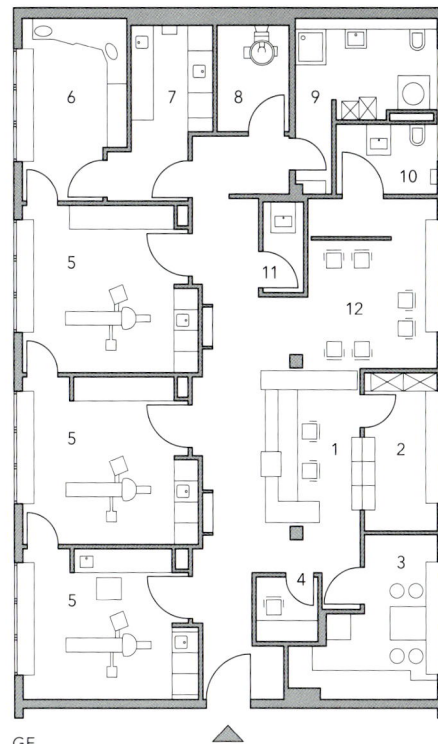

GF

Client	Dr. Matthias Bethig
Operator	Dr. Matthias Bethig
	Philipp Wedemeyer
Planning time	05 2004 – 07 2004
Construction time	08 2004 – 10 2004
Gross floor area	207 sqm
Usable floor space	187 sqm
Gross cubic capacity	536 cbm
Construction cost	150,000 EUR

a   Two white acrylic glass light boxes frame the
    glossy reception desk.
b   A skylight strip to the ceiling is set into the
    walls dividing the treatment rooms from the
    corridor.
c   The open ceiling design maintains the visual
    character of the loft.
d   Three distinctive colours define the straight
    lines of the interior design: dark red, light
    grey and ivory.

Diagrammatic plans, to scale 1:400
Floor plans, to scale 1:200

Floor plan layout

1	Reception	**6**	Laboratory	and shower
2	Office	**7**	Sterilisation room	**10** Patient toilet
3	Staff lounge	**8**	Examination X-ray	**11** Hygiene
4	Consultation room	**9**	Staff changing	**12** Waiting area
5	Treatment room		cubicle, toilet	

The gable end access to the compact rectangular floor plan of the partnership practice is rather unusual. From here, however, patients have a clear
view of the sectioned corridor and most of the rooms. Reception and
waiting area are located with the staff rooms on one side of the corridor,
with treatment rooms and laboratory on the other. All the rooms that need
natural light have windows.

Usable floor spaces

Patient rooms	**yellow**	48 sqm	26 %
Examination |			
Treatment rooms	**red**	84 sqm	45 %
Specialist rooms	**pink**	6 sqm	3 %
Administrative rooms	**green**	10 sqm	5 %
Offices | Staff rooms	**orange**	28 sqm	15 %
Supply | Waste disposal	**brown**	11 sqm	6 %
Total		187 sqm	100 %

Performance data

Outpatients per year	2,000
Clinic opening hours	5 days | 50 hours
Waiting time [with | without appointment]	up to 30 min.
	30 min. and longer
Type and number of staff	2 dentists
	6 assistants

Warm colours ranging from soft beige to strong terracotta define the holistic concept of this practice for naturopathy and general medicine.

The practice has dispensed with the customary waiting area. The focal point for patients entering the practice is the bespoke luminescent cube, a solitary light sculpture which illuminates the practice rooms. Natural light filters softly through translucent panel curtains.

Light installations with motifs of smooth expanses of water and representations of the heavens underpin the soothing atmosphere of the whole practice. Black accents in the form of leather armchairs and sofas contrast with the warm colour spectrum. The representation of a leaf contour symbolises naturopathy's status as a superior element, while the outline of the human body represents mankind as the focus of medicine. Both motifs are repeated in the wall decoration: instead of pictures, a leaf and a person in miniature are painted directly on to the walls. They are carefully placed to be visible from one room to another.

100% INTERIOR

**PRACTICE FOR NATUROPATHY
AND GENERAL MEDICINE**
COLOGNE | G

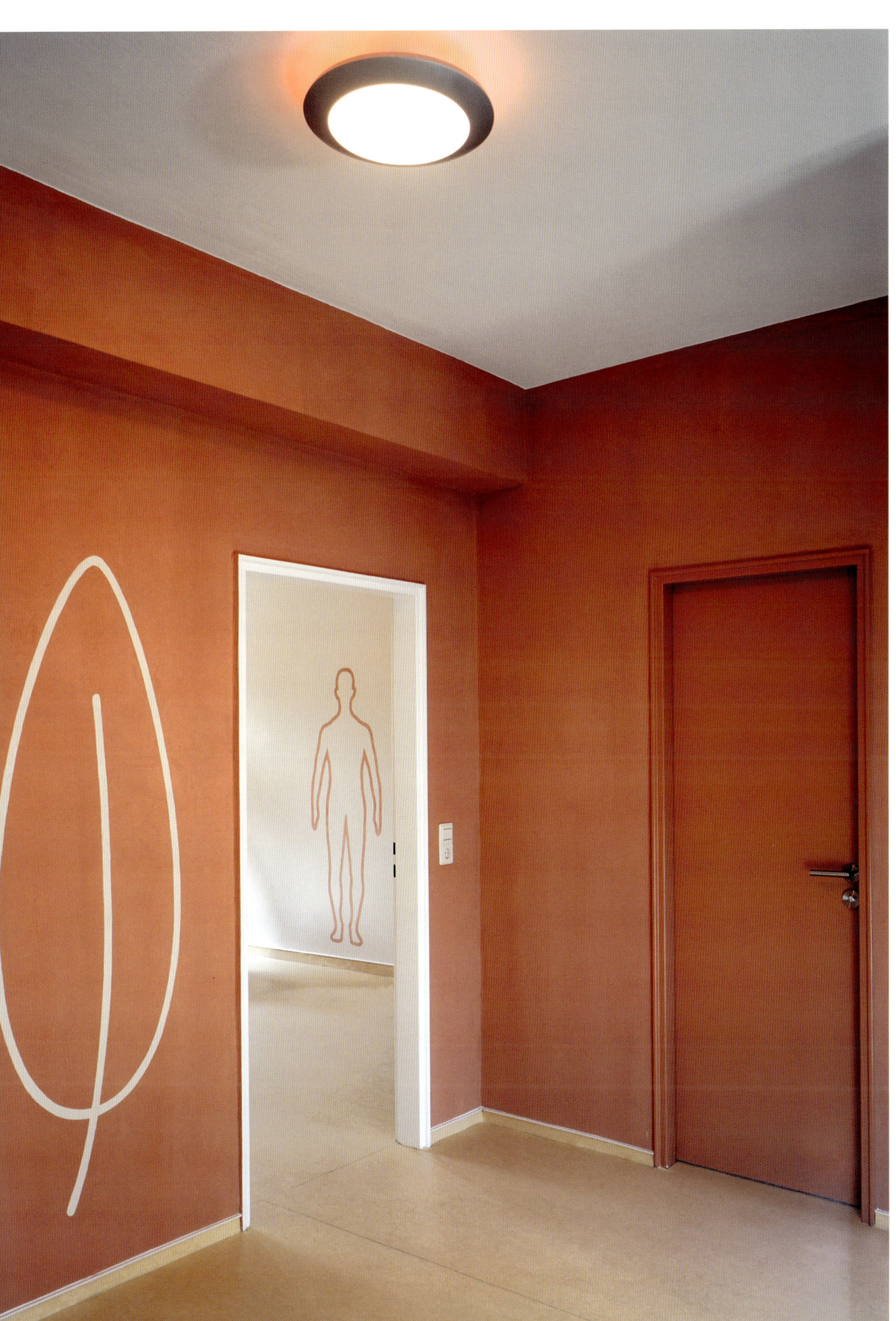

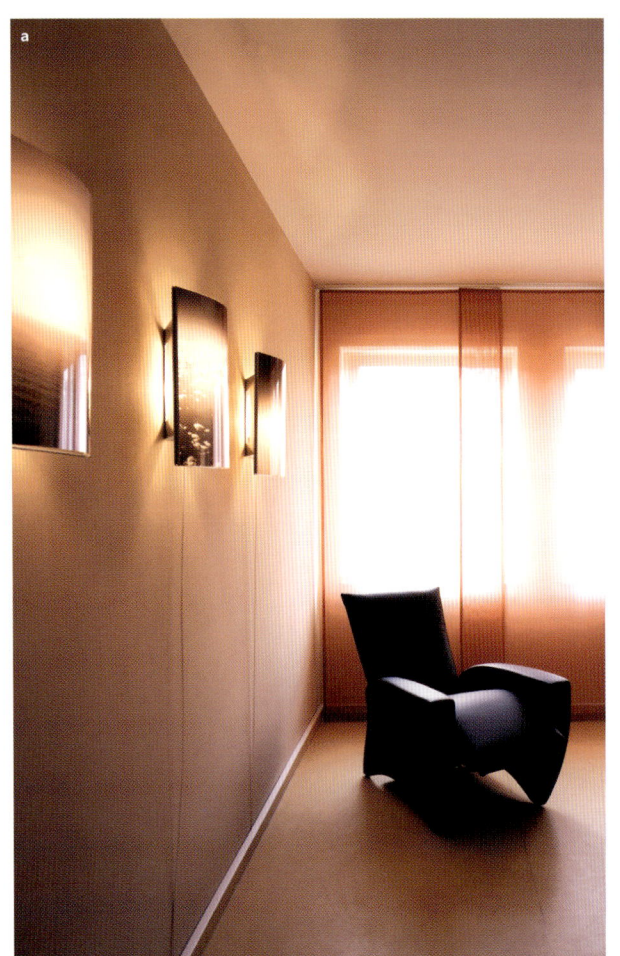

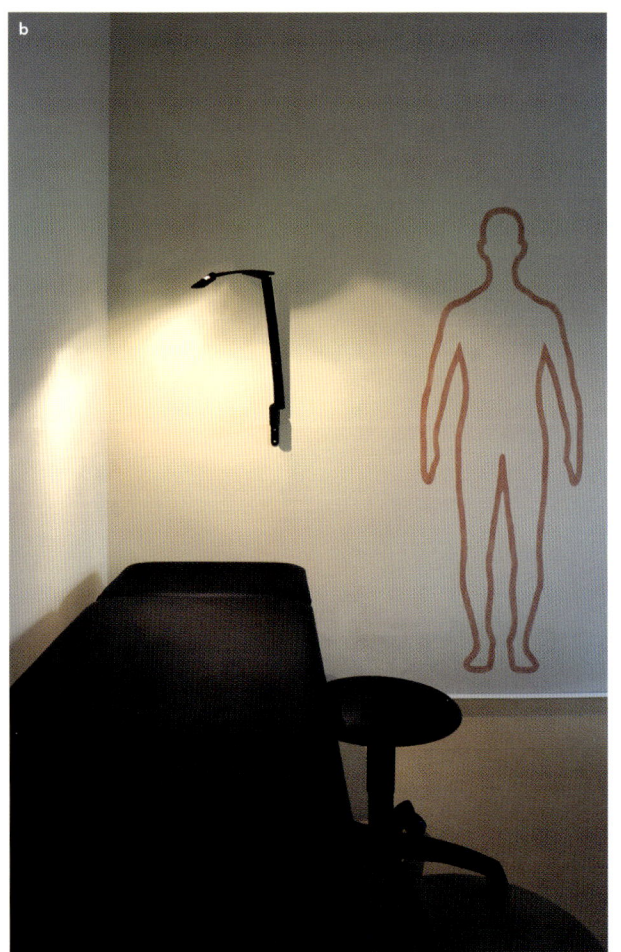

a

b

c

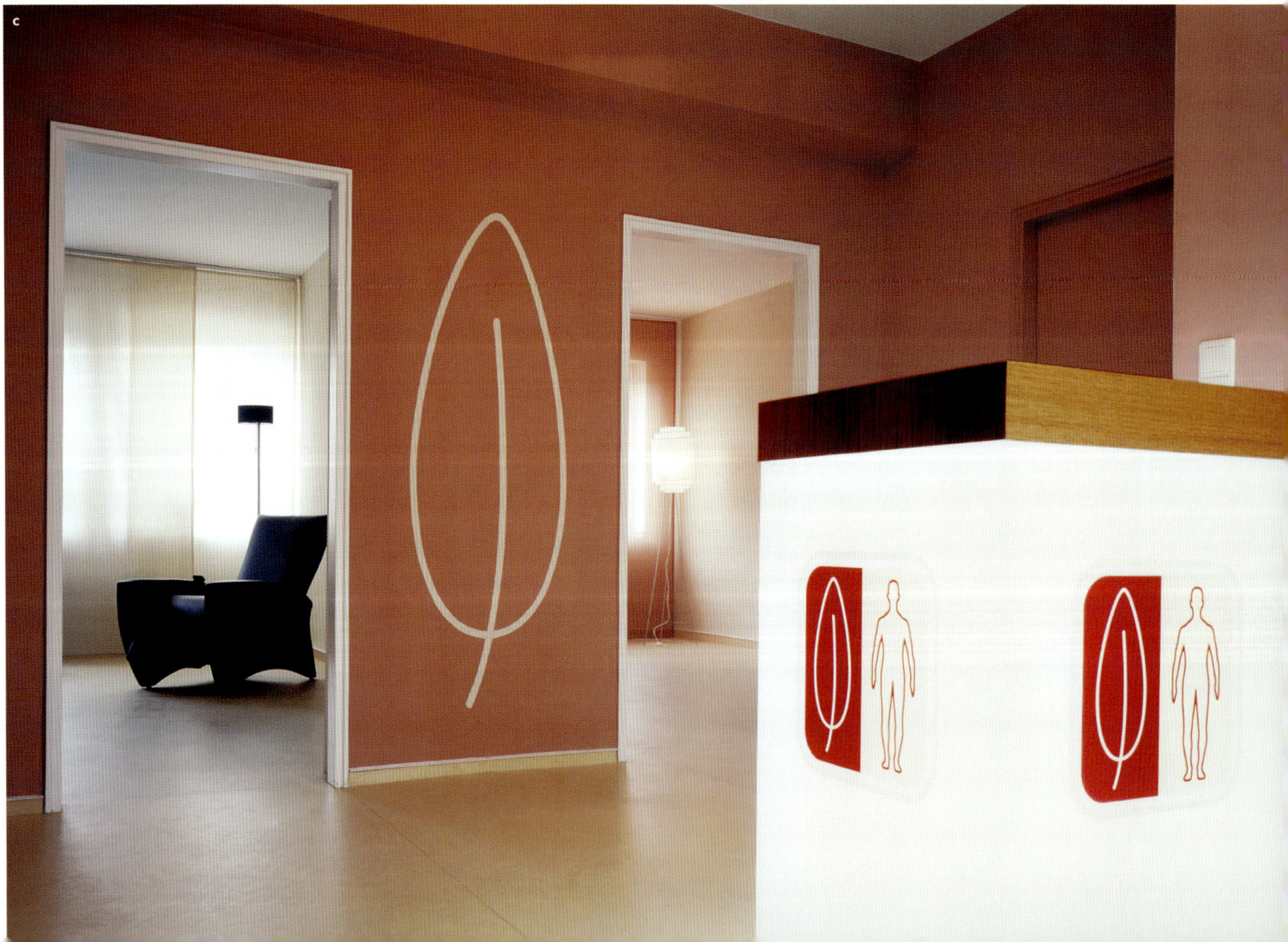

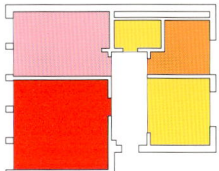

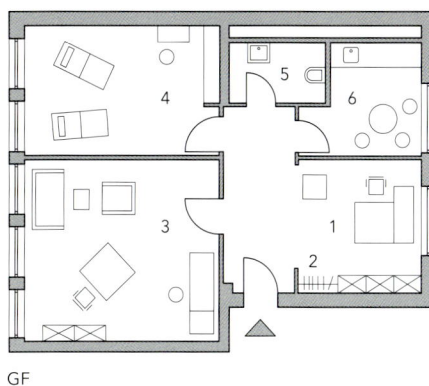

GF

**Client	Operator**	Dr. Michael Radecki
Planning time	2004
Construction time	2004
Usable floor space	79 sqm

a Black accents in the form of leather armchairs and sofas contrast with the otherwise warm colour spectrum.

b Instead of pictures, the outline of the human body is repeated as a decorative pattern, representing the holistic medicine practised here, which is entirely patient-focused.

c A solitary light sculpture in the form of a bespoke luminescent cube illuminates the entrance area.

Diagrammatic plans, to scale 1:400
Floor plans, to scale 1:200

Floor plan layout

1	Reception	**3**	Treatment room	**5**	Patient toilet
2	Coat-rack	**4**	Infusionsraum	**6**	Staff lounge

The small single-doctor practice is approached by a short, off-centre entrance corridor, giving on to five rooms in total. All rooms needing natural light have windows. Next to the joint patient and staff toilet is a staff lounge. There are no designated areas for administrative, storage and cleaning purposes.

Usable floor spaces

Patient rooms	**yellow**	19 sqm	24 %
Examination			
Treatment rooms	**red**	29 sqm	37 %
Specialist rooms	**pink**	21 sqm	27 %
Offices	Staff rooms	**orange**	10 sqm	12 %
Total		79 sqm	100 %

Performance data

Clinic opening hours	5 days
Waiting time	none
Number of staff	2

Following its move, the group radiology practice in the basement of the Schorndorf Health Centre now occupies an area of around 600 square metres. At the centre of this new practice is the spacious waiting area, decorated in light colours. Ceiling height, upholstered side walls keep waiting patients safe and cosy in keeping with the brief to the designers to make the patient experience as pleasant as possible.

A referral for radiological examination often has serious medical implications. Many of the patients arriving for their appointment are aware of this and feel particularly vulnerable. They need to be given a sense of security and a simple layout makes it easier for them to find their way around. In contrast, the technical installations are almost invisible. On entering, patients make their way along the tapering corridor to the central waiting area. Black and white backlit walls with cloud motifs – the unusual colour scheme references an X-ray image – frame the two reception desks in the waiting area. The various functional units for nuclear medicine, MRI and CT, X-ray, mammography and ultrasound and the doctor's offices are grouped around the central waiting area and reached via the U-shaped access hallway. As a deliberate counterpoint to the calming colours in the waiting area, a distinctive orange has been chosen here to assist with orientation and create a suitable backdrop to this busy area.

IPPOLITO FLEITZ GROUP

RADIOLOGY
SCHORNDORF | G

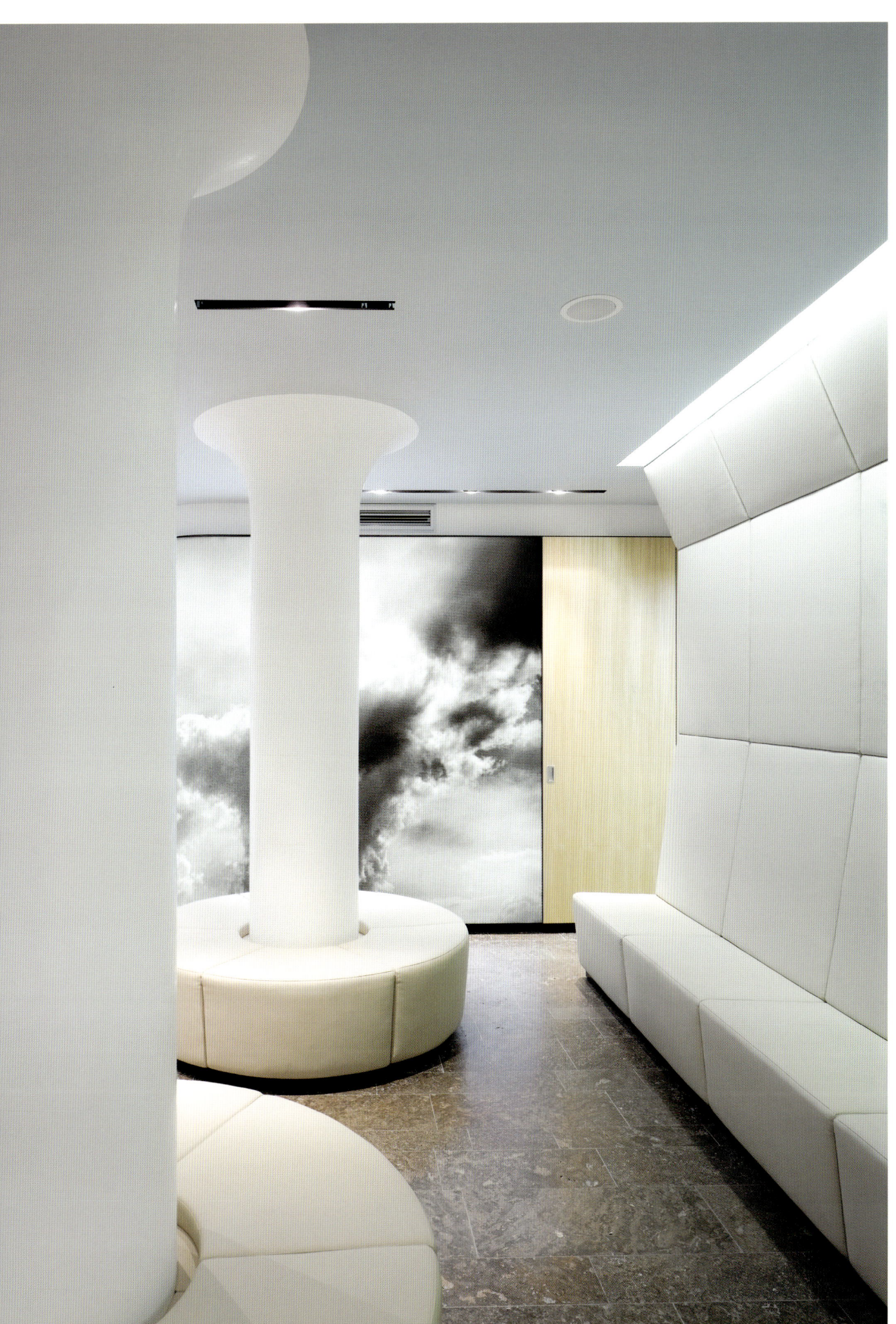

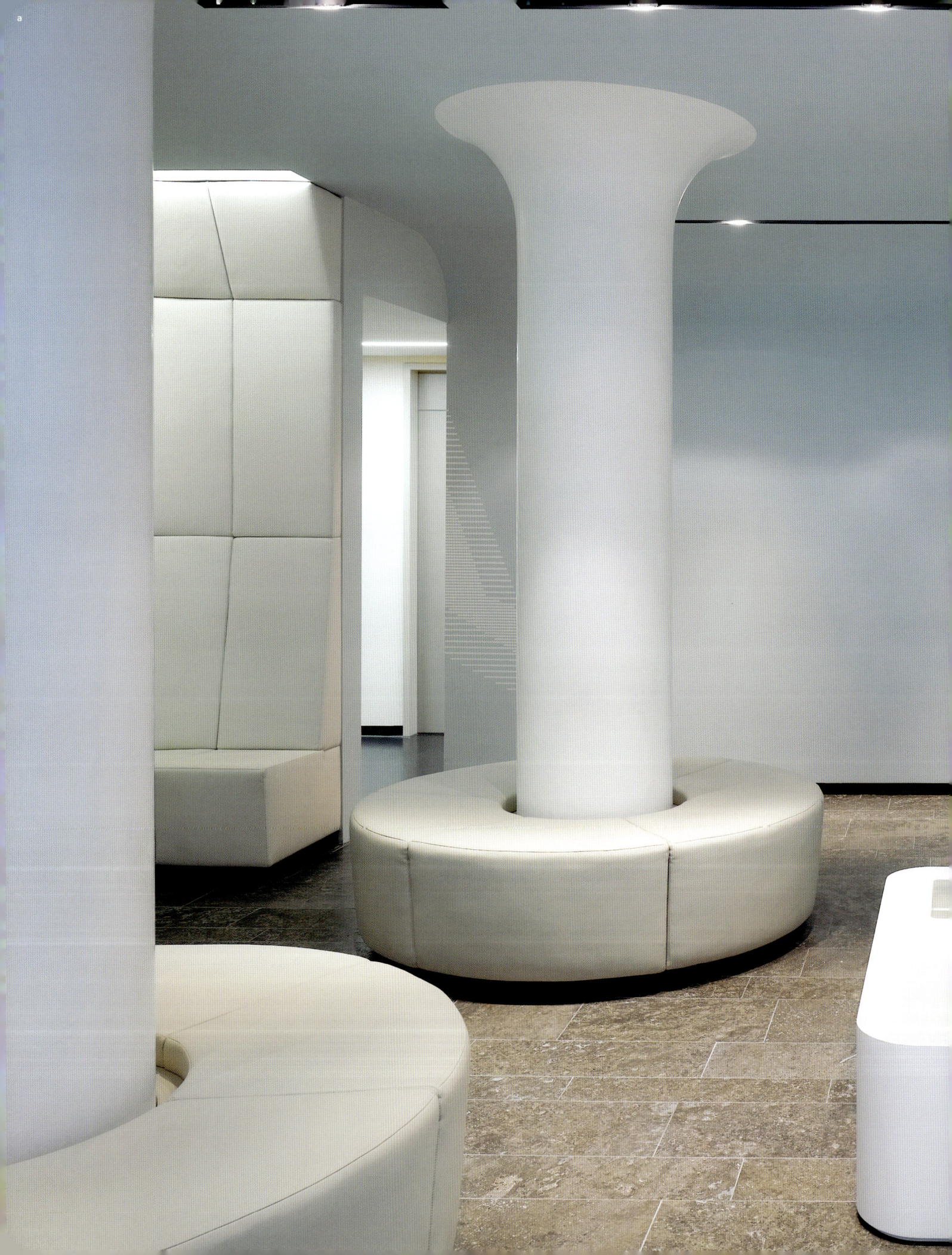

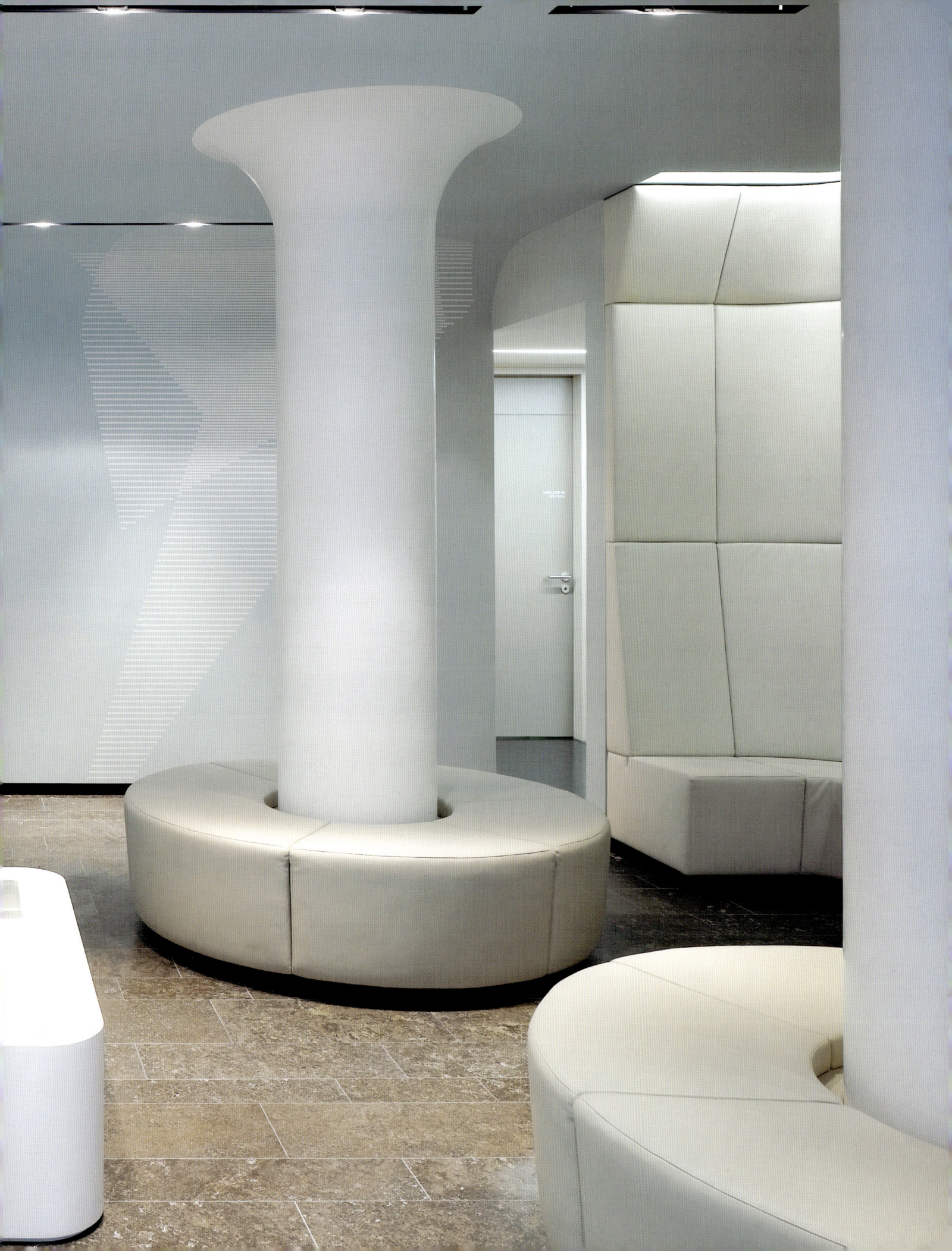

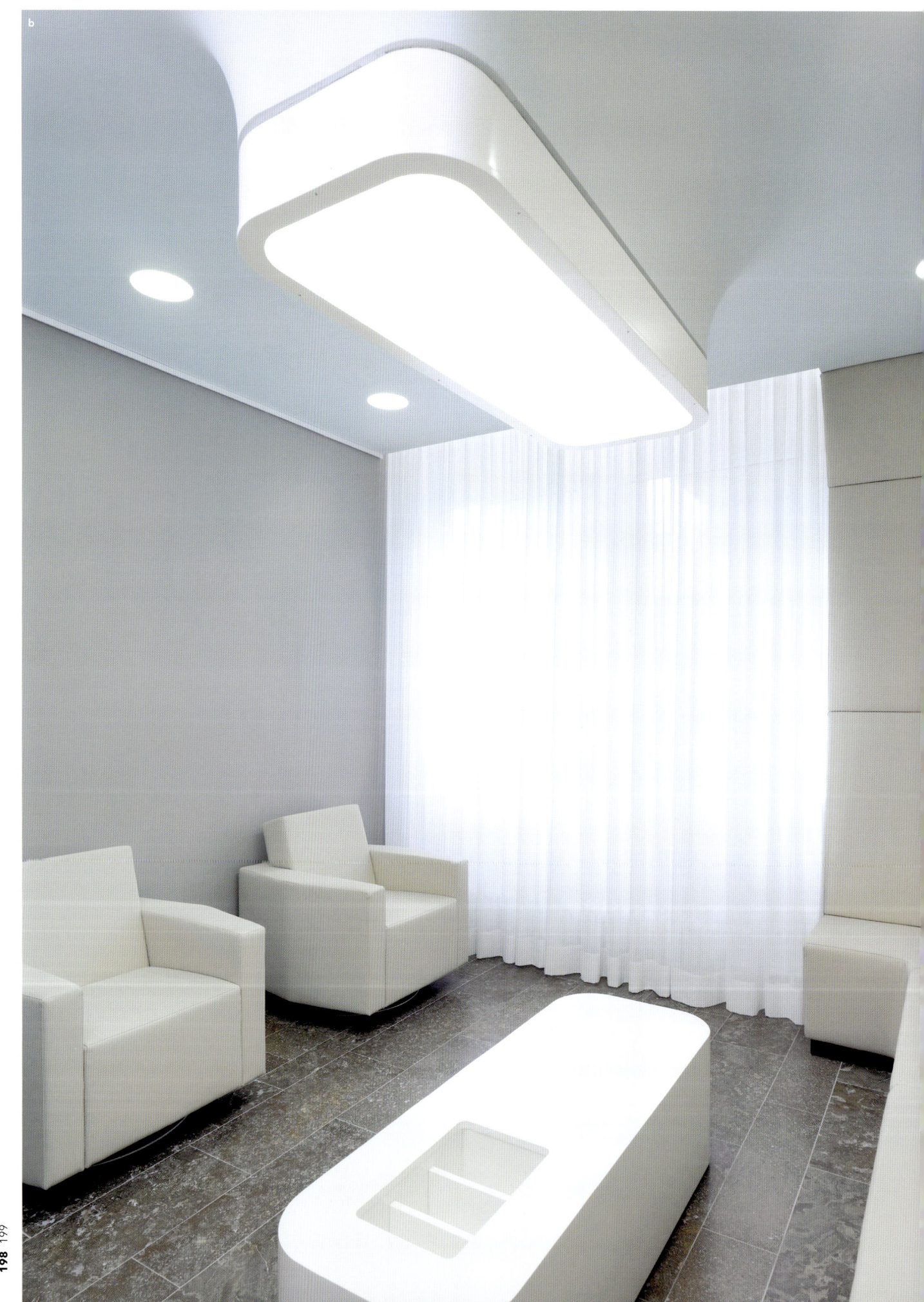

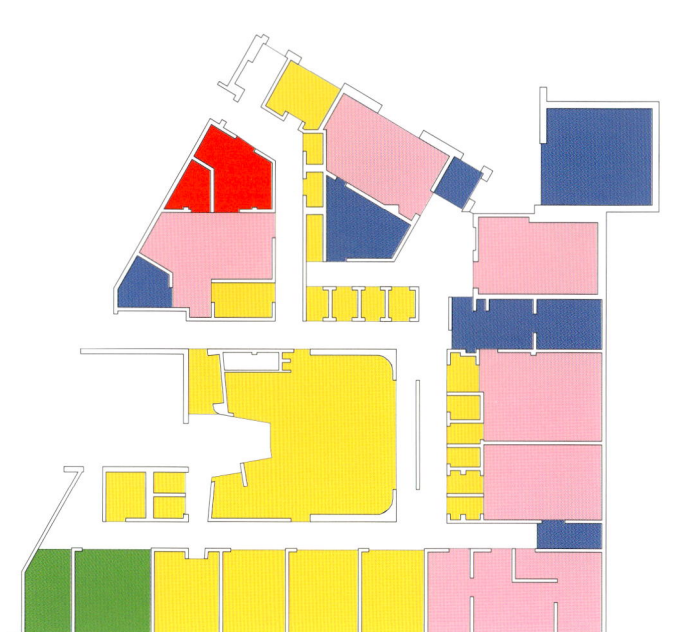

1	Coat-rack
2	Reception
3	Waiting area
4	Nuclear medicine switch room
5	Doctor's consultation room
6	Nuclear medicine treatment room
7	Laboratory
8	Treatment room spray booth
9	Sluice
10	Patient toilet
11	Staff toilet
12	Examination magnetic resonance tomography [MRI]
13	Installations room MRI
14	Patient changing cubicle
15	MRI switch room
16	Treatment room
17	CT switch room
18	Changing cubicle for the disabled
19	Examination CT
20	Examination X-ray
21	X-ray switch room
22	Examination ultrasound
23	Examination mammography
24	Private patients' waiting area
25	Office
26	Telephonist's office
27	Toilet for the disabled
28	Patient toilet L
29	Patient toilet G

Diagrammatic plans, to scale 1:400
Floor plans, to scale 1:200

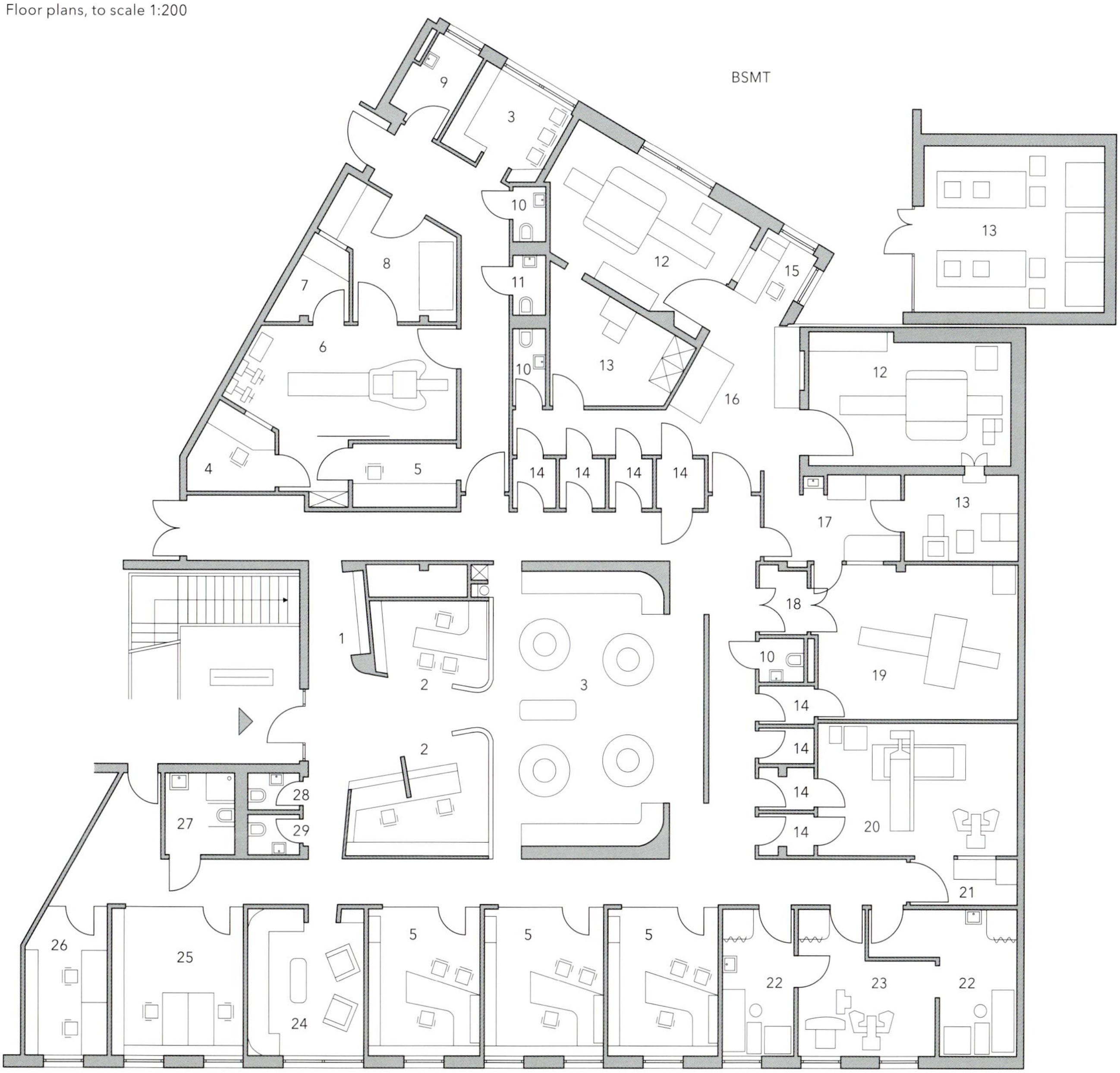

BSMT

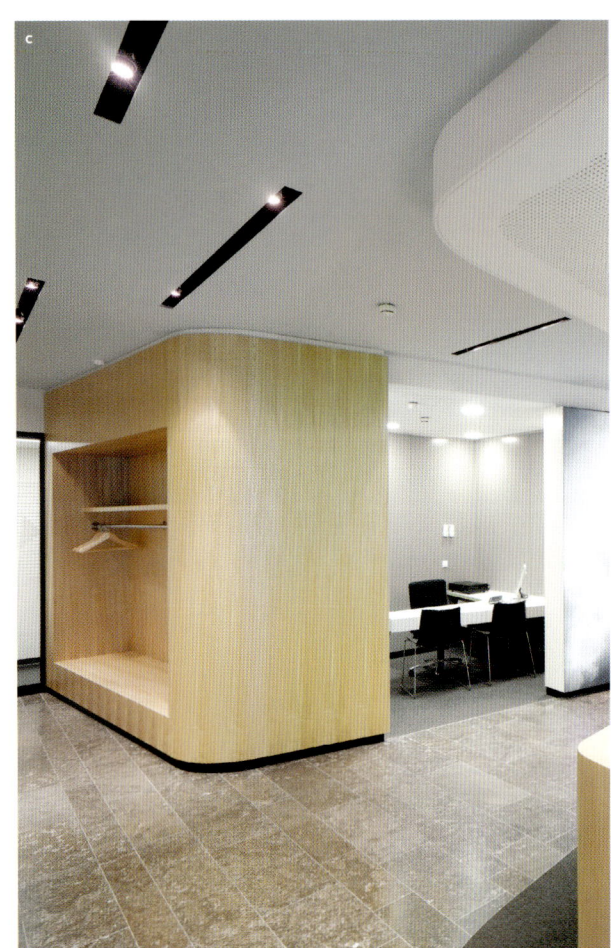

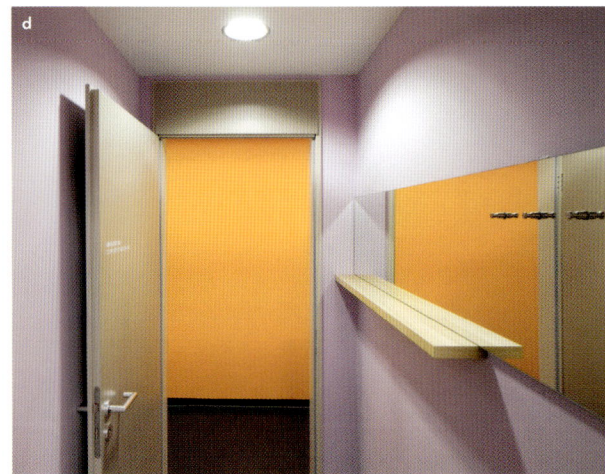

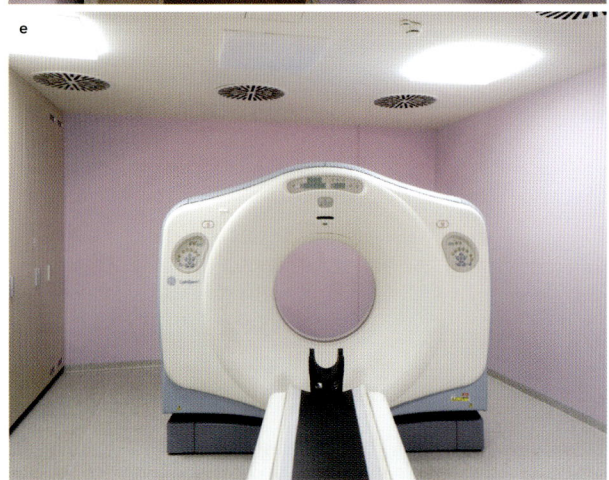

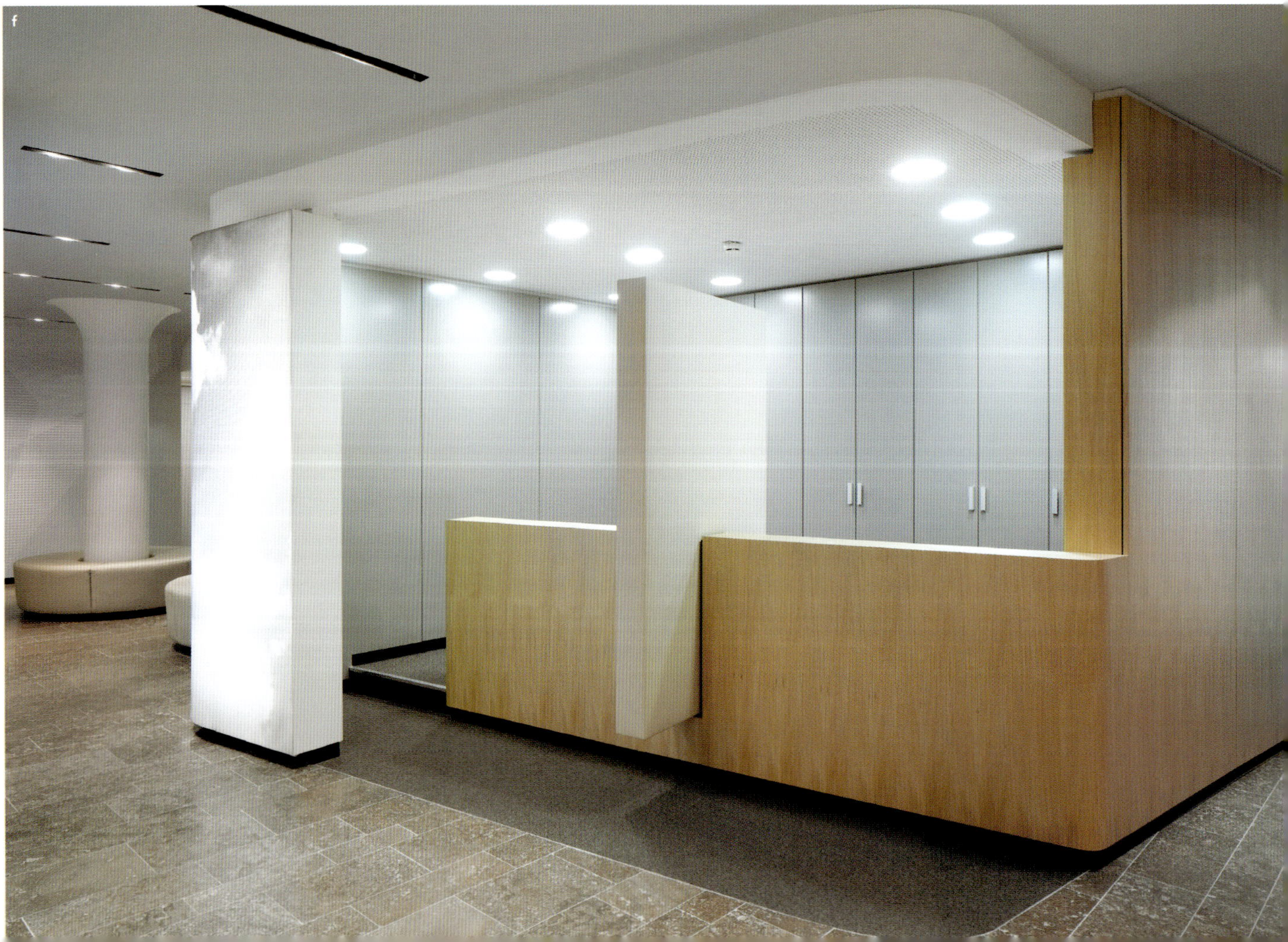

**Client	Operator**	Dr. Gebhard Wittlinger
	Dr. Christoph Hahn
	Dr. Wolfgang Stern
Planning time	06 2006
Construction time	04 2007
Gross floor area	800 sqm
Usable floor space	577 sqm
Gross cubic capacity	2,400 cbm

a   The waiting area is decorated in light colours with ceiling height upholstered side walls.

b   The waiting area for private patients.

c   Coat-rack and reception office in the centrally located entrance area.

d   As a deliberate counterpoint to the calming colours in the waiting area, the U-shaped access hallway is painted bright orange.

e   View into the examination room CT, where the latest technology takes centre stage.

f   Patients go past the reception desk straight to the central waiting area.

Usable floor spaces

Patient rooms	**yellow**	225 sqm	39 %
Examination			
Treatment rooms	**red**	20 sqm	3 %
Specialist rooms	**pink**	206 sqm	36 %
Administrative rooms	**green**	34 sqm	6 %
Plant rooms	**blue**	92 sqm	16 %
Total		577 sqm	100 %

Performance data

Outpatients per year	25,000
Number and type of services per year	Diagnostic radiology
Clinic opening hours	5 days	50 hours
Waiting time [with	without appointment]	15 min.	30 min.
Number of staff	25

At reception a slightly distorted circle with a floral motif symbolises the quest for a personal sense of beauty rather than homogenised perfection. It is also the logo of the Frankfurt clinic, which combines aesthetics and function in its respectful and individual treatment of patients. The practice boasts an organically shaped central island, with a corridor running past it. All the rooms are accessible from here. The two waiting areas are favourably situated one-third and two-thirds of the way along the series of rooms, which represent a visual voyage of discovery. The differentiation of the rooms is accentuated by varying wall surfaces: the central island with its soft floral motif is smoothly varnished, while a matt blue-grey dispersion paint coats the walls to the treatment rooms. An open-pore shell limestone laid in a random pattern was chosen for the floor in the public area, while the treatment rooms are laid with cosy, oiled ash block flooring.

The deliberate contrast between cold and warm, spaciousness and narrowness, playfulness and surgical precision is the theme throughout the practice.

IPPOLITO FLEITZ GROUP

KAISERPLATZ PRACTICE CLINIC
FRANKFURT ON THE MAIN | G

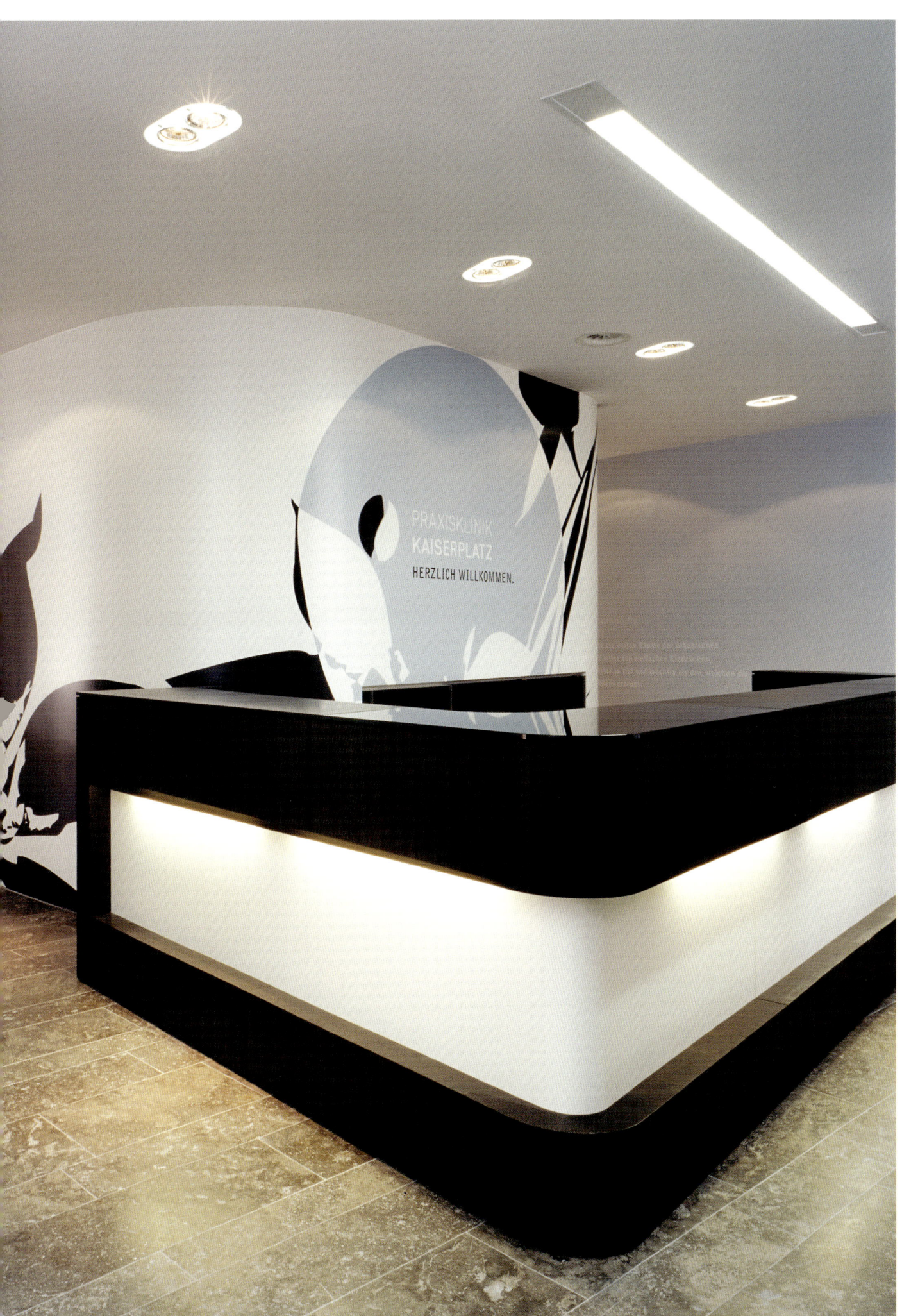

PRAXISKLINIK
KAISERPLATZ
HERZLICH WILLKOMMEN.

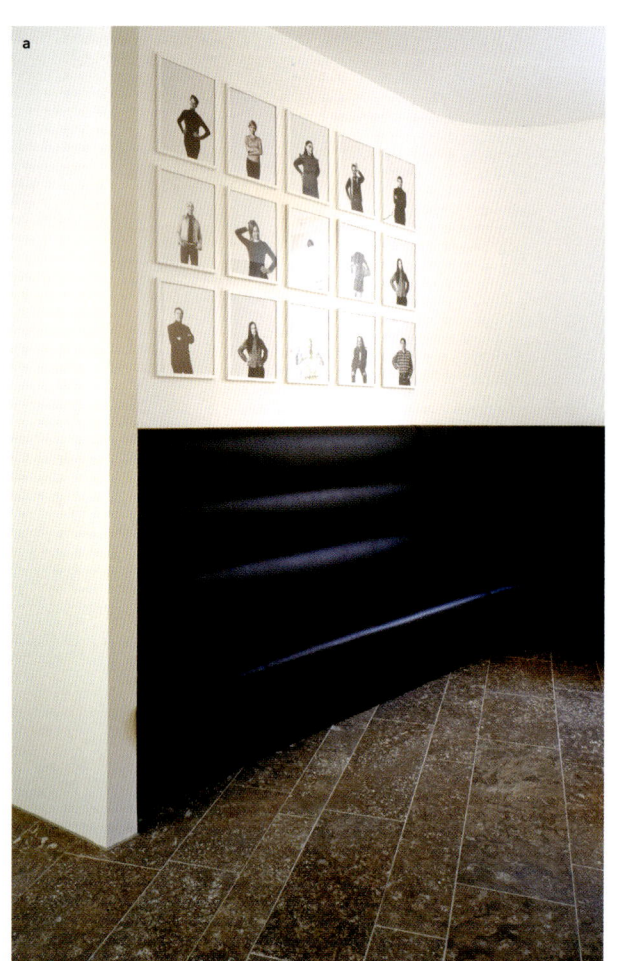

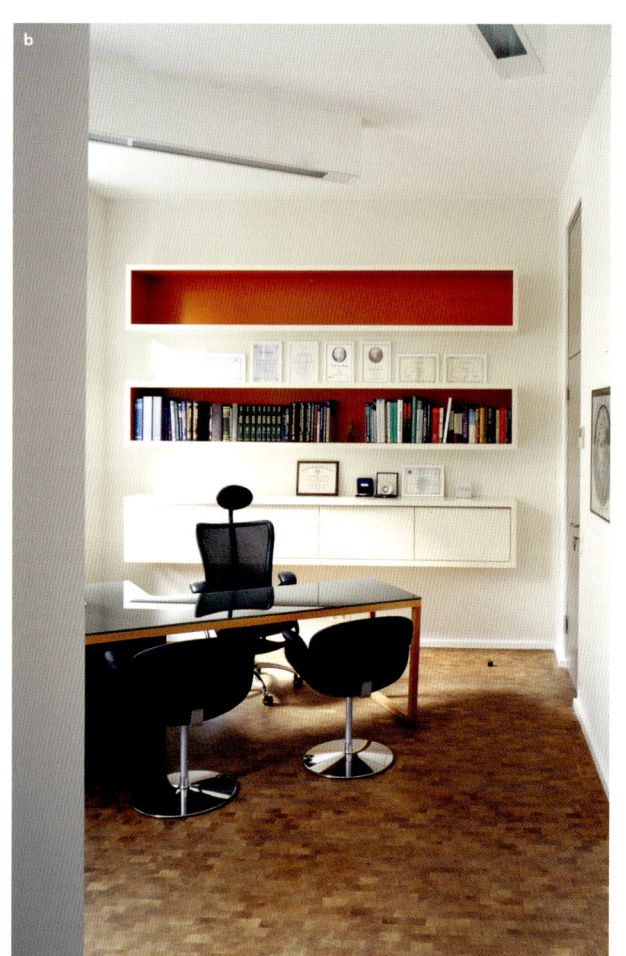

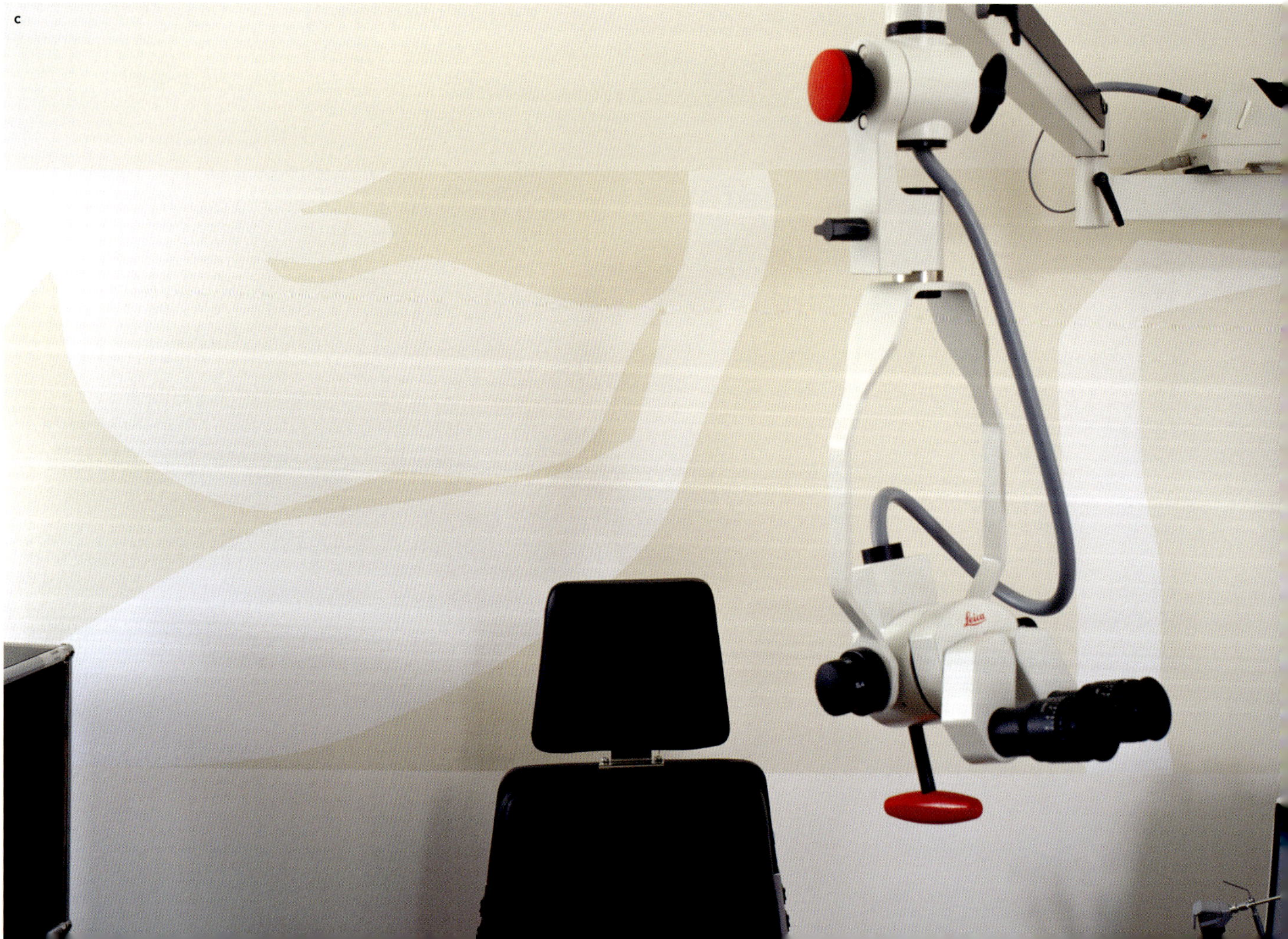

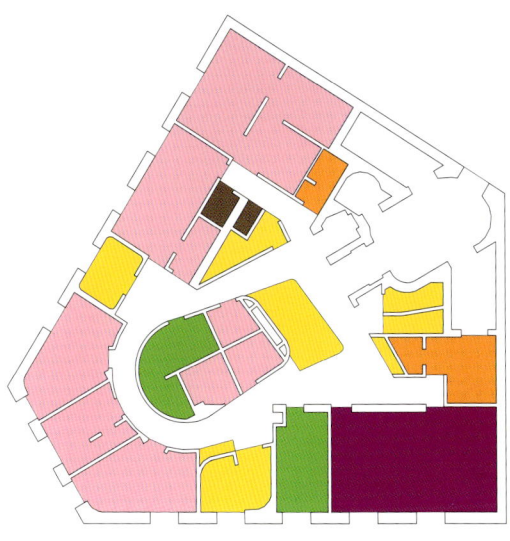

Diagrammatic plans, to scale 1:400
Floor plans, to scale 1:200

1 Reception
2 Coat-rack
3 Patient toilet G
4 Patient toilet L
5 Staff lounge
6 Seminar room
7 Office
8 Waiting area
9 Examination ENT

10 Examination
audiology
11 Filing room
12 Examination
ultrasound
13 Infusion
14 Bandage room
15 Examination and
treatment room

16 Patient changing
cubicle
17 Workroom
unsterile
18 Workroom sterile
19 Operating theatre
20 Recovery room
21 Staff toilet
and shower

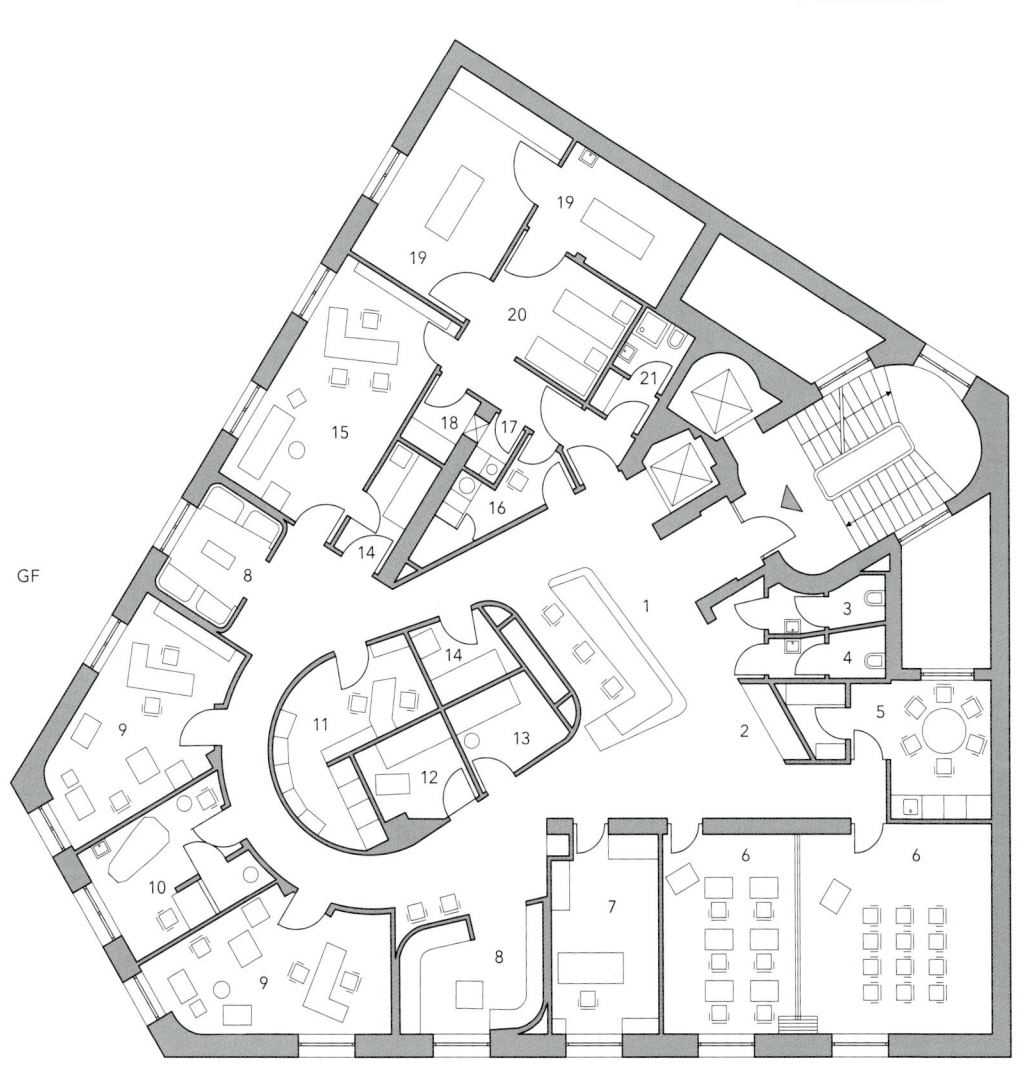

GF

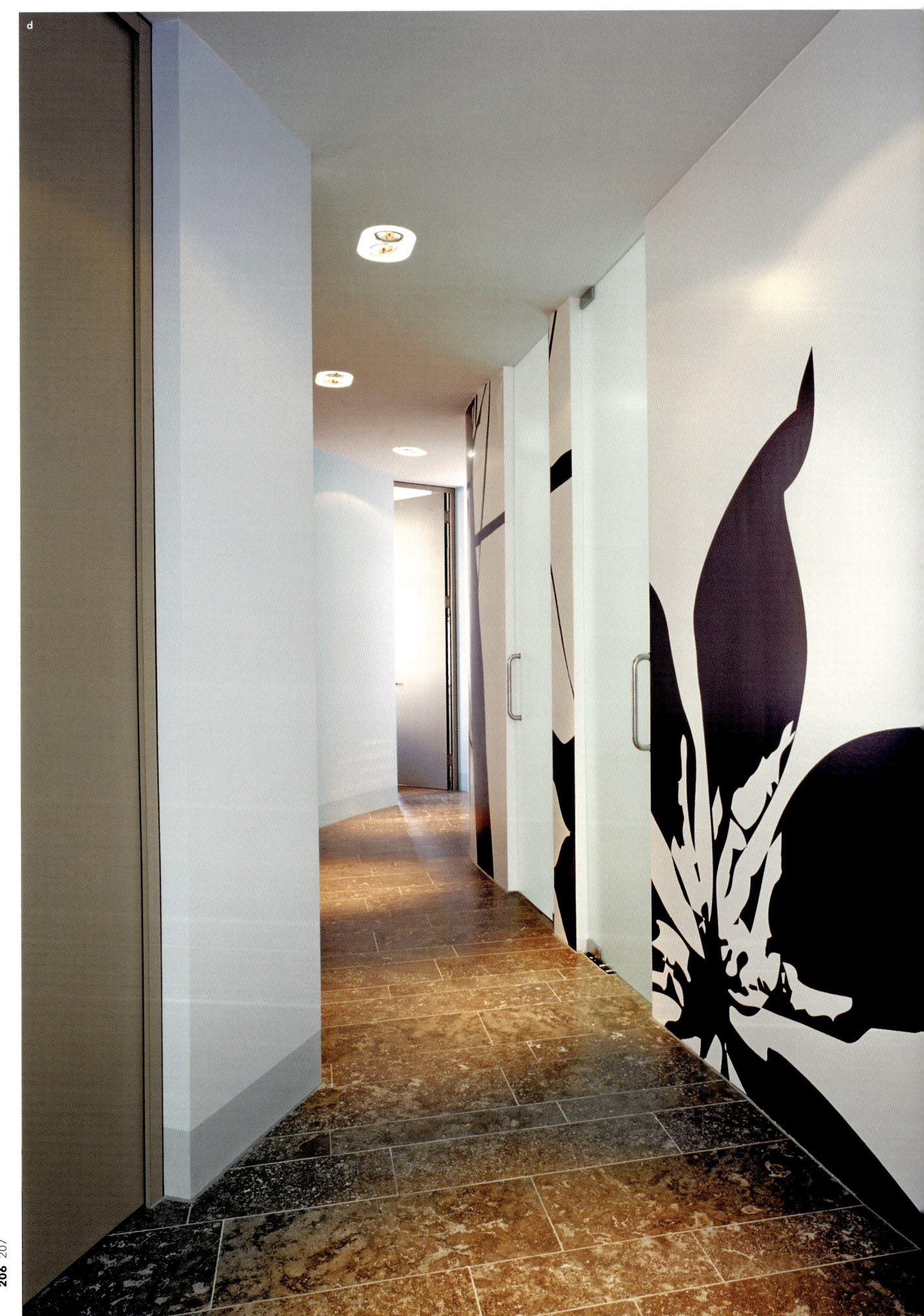

Client	Operator	Prof. Dr. Dennis
	von Heimburg
	Dr. Wibke von Heimburg
	Dr. Jens Feyh
Construction time	07 2003
Usable floor space	334 sqm
Gross cubic capacity	1,200 cbm

a An open-pored shell limestone laid in a random pattern was chosen for the floor in public areas.
b The treatment rooms are laid with cosy ash block flooring.
c Abstract flower shapes adorn the walls in the treatment rooms.
d The central island with its floral motif is coated in a smooth lacquer, while the walls to the treatment rooms are painted with a matt, blue-grey dispersion paint.

Floor plan layout

The majority of the rooms in the rhomboid multiple practice benefit from natural light; only in the operating wing and in the organically shaped central island are a few internal examination and treatment rooms. Patients proceed straight from the entrance to the reception and from there to two favourably situated waiting areas, which benefit from natural light but are not visible from the reception. The functional hallways would be shorter without the central island.

Usable floor spaces

Patient rooms	**yellow**	53 sqm	16 %
Specialist rooms	**pink**	164 sqm	49 %
Administrative rooms	**green**	33 sqm	10 %
Offices	Staff rooms	**orange**	22 sqm	7 %
Supply	Waste disposal	**brown**	5 sqm	2 %
Training rooms	**violet**	57 sqm	16 %
Total		334 sqm	100 %

Performance data

Outpatients per year	4,000 [40 %]
Number and type of services per year	Operations [1,000	15 % IGel]
	Wrinkle treatments [300	100 % IGel]
	ENT diagnostics [2,000	10 % IGel]
Services to other clinics	Imaging procedures [600]
Clinic opening hours	5 days	57,5 hours
Waiting time [with	without appointment]	15 min.	25 min.
Type and number of staff	4 doctors
	5 full-time staff
	1 trainee
	1 half-day staff

The clinic building, built in 1979, has attained a new, more patient-friendly look thanks to the extensive redesign work. The foyer | reception area has become the focal point, with a stand-alone elliptical pale wooden desk. A circular light in the ceiling above the reception desk emphasises its solitary position in the room. The backlit glass wall opposite is decorated with a yellow | orange floral motif and points the way to the three adjacent treatment rooms.

First room we come to is the spacious waiting area, designed in bright, friendly colours, which exudes a cosy atmosphere: here the foyer's orange floral motif is taken up in the form of a backlit glass wall. Behind this translucent wall are the treatment rooms, which have been extricated from their old wooden door leaves and are now boasting sliding glass doors, with the result of appearing much more open and light. Warm shades of the new, block-shaped wooden elements, such as the desk and cabinets, contrast with the predominant grey | white tones of the wall and ceiling. Only the colour-accentuated toilet block, which has been relocated in the foyer, catches the eye when entering. Black | white | grey patterned linoleum is laid throughout the practice.

JURETZKA ARCHITEKTEN

DENTAL CLINIC
ESCHENBACH | G

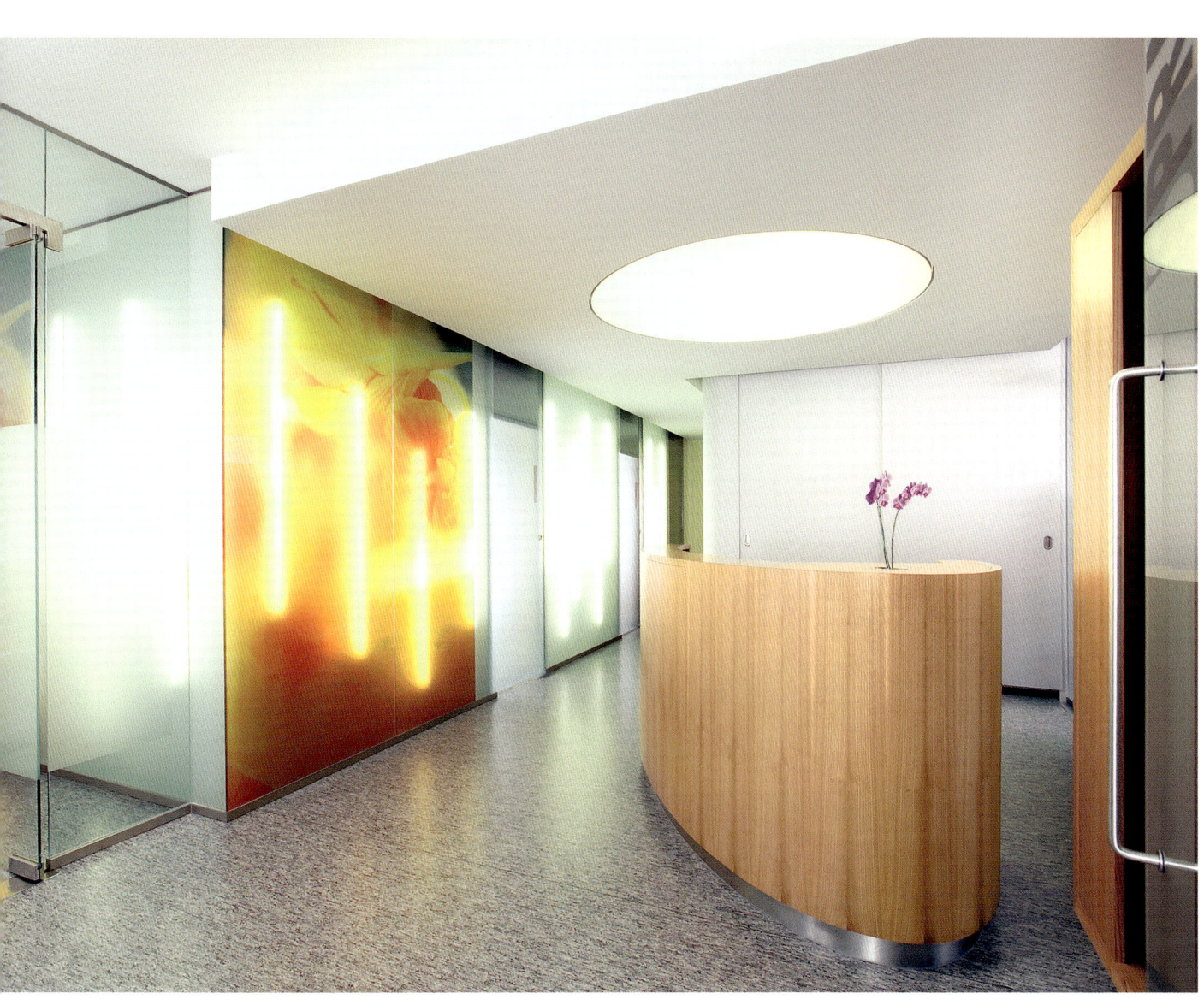

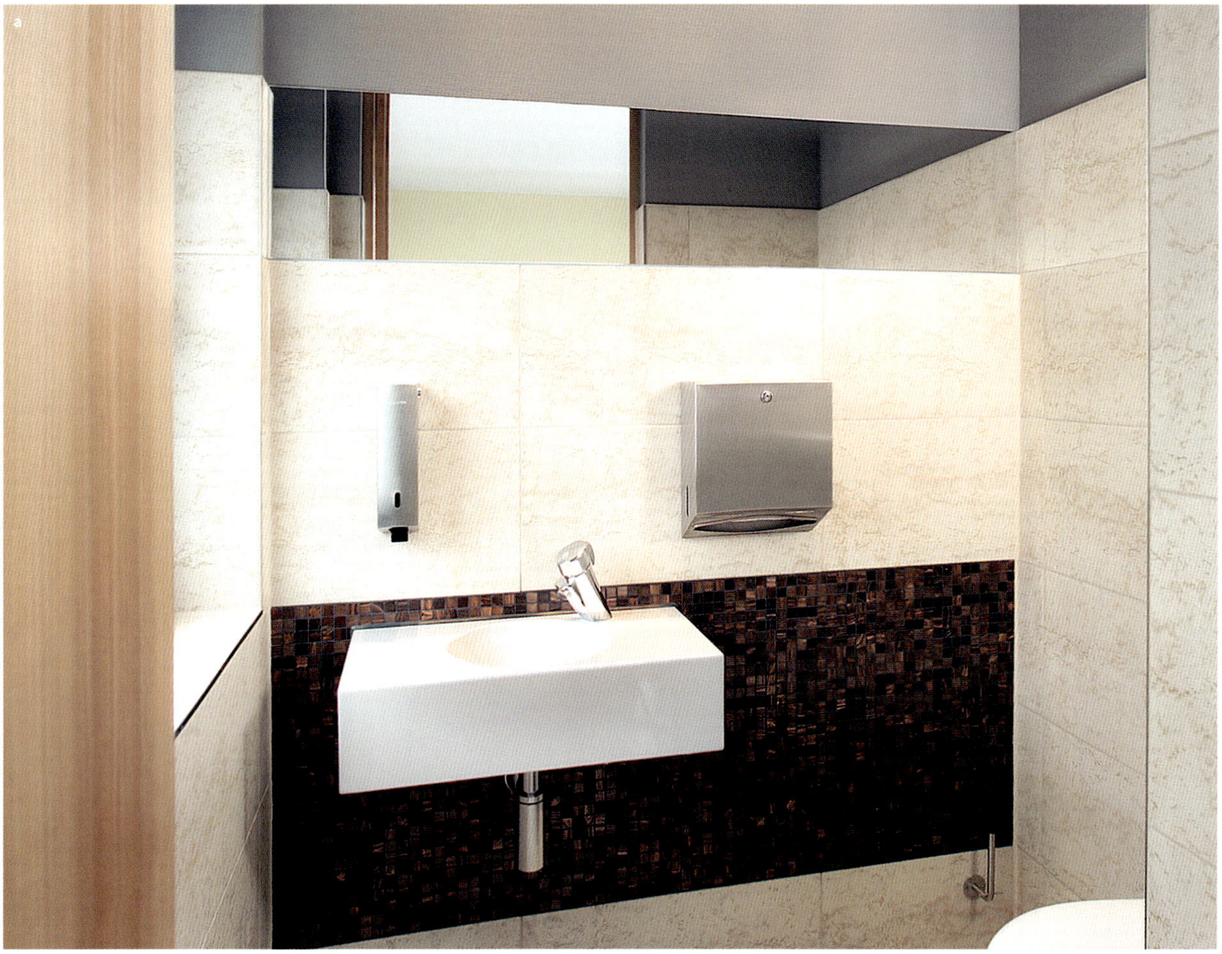

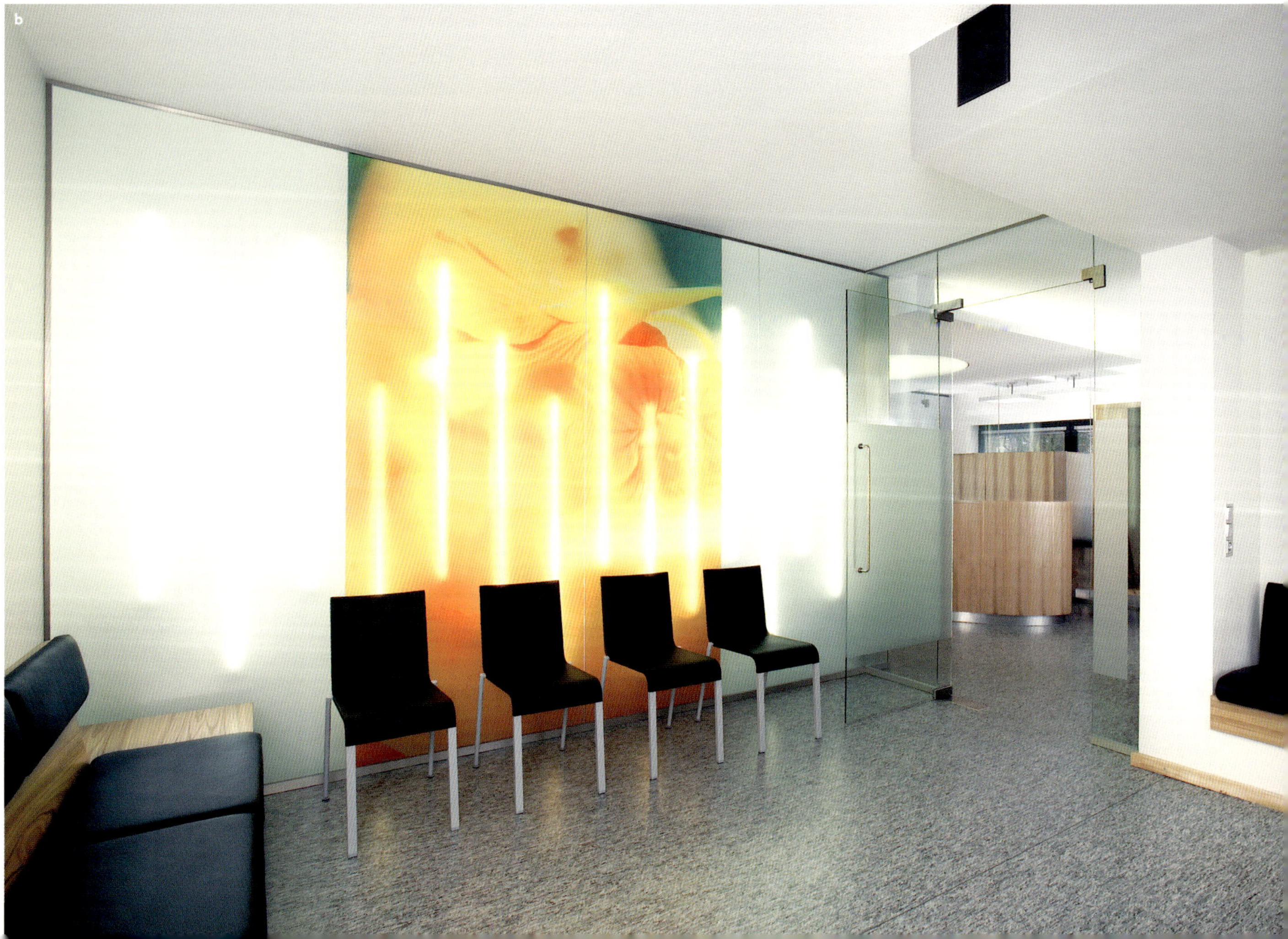

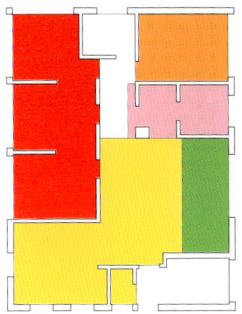

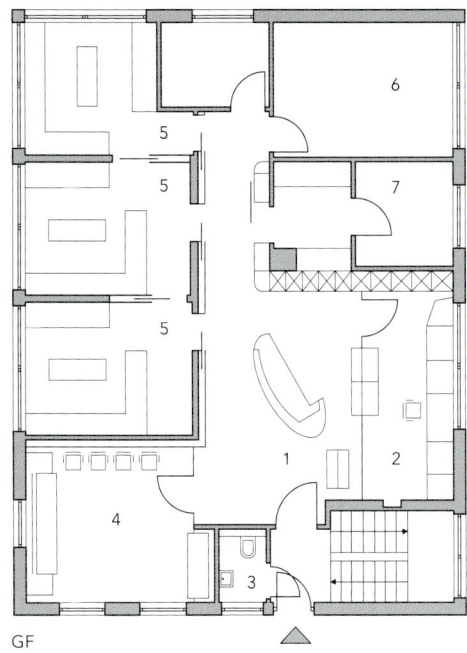

GF

Client	Operator	Dr. Wolfgang Gebel
Planning time	03 2003 – 07 2003
Construction time	08 2003 – 09 2003
Usable floor space	168 sqm
Gross cubic capacity	500 cbm
Construction cost	130,000 EUR
Total cost	165,000 EUR

a Simple elegance and high-quality materials are also found in the patients' toilet.
b The spacious waiting area, designed in bright colours with a backlit glass wall, exudes a cosy atmosphere.

Diagrammatic plans, to scale 1:400
Floor plans, to scale 1:200

Floor plan layout

1 Reception	**4** Waiting area	**7** Examination
2 Office	**5** Treatment room	X-ray
3 Patient toilet	**6** Lounge	

The floor plan for the single-doctor practice, with a large add-on corridor for reception and office and a short connecting corridor, could hardly be better planned. The internal connection between treatment rooms is proving convenient. All practice rooms receive natural light. There are no areas for supplies and cleaning. The staff lounge can be used if additional space is needed.

Usable floor spaces

Patient rooms	**yellow**	61 sqm	36 %
Examination |			
Treatment rooms	**red**	54 sqm	32 %
Specialist rooms	**pink**	16 sqm	10 %
Administrative rooms	**green**	17 sqm	10 %
Offices | Staff rooms	**orange**	20 sqm	12 %
Total		168 sqm	100 %

Performance data

Clinic opening hours	5 days
Number of staff	9 – 10

With the move to the new premises, the orthopaedic practice has not only become bigger, but it has also extended the range of medical services on offer, with pain and exercise therapy added.

The centre-point of the practice, which is accessible to the disabled, is the reception; from there, clients can reach all the rooms via a U-shaped corridor. The semi-circular, stand-alone reception desk is in keeping with the therapy room behind it. The examination and treatment rooms and the procedure room are all located on one side of the corridor. So-called room boxes [built-on room in the form of a box], which can be used as changing areas or for storing supplies, form small seating alcoves towards the open reception area. On the other side of the corridor are situated a waiting area and the therapy area, which can be divided into individual cubicles with curtains and sliding glass partition walls. If needed, this area can also be joined with the waiting area to form a large room. Natural light streams into the practice through green-shimmering translucent glass doors and walls. The atmosphere of the orthopaedic practice is defined by a bright maple veneer, red floor covering, lime-green fabrics and an extensive use of glass.

**ANDREAS
KANZIAN**

ORTHOPAEDICS CENTRE
GRAZ | A

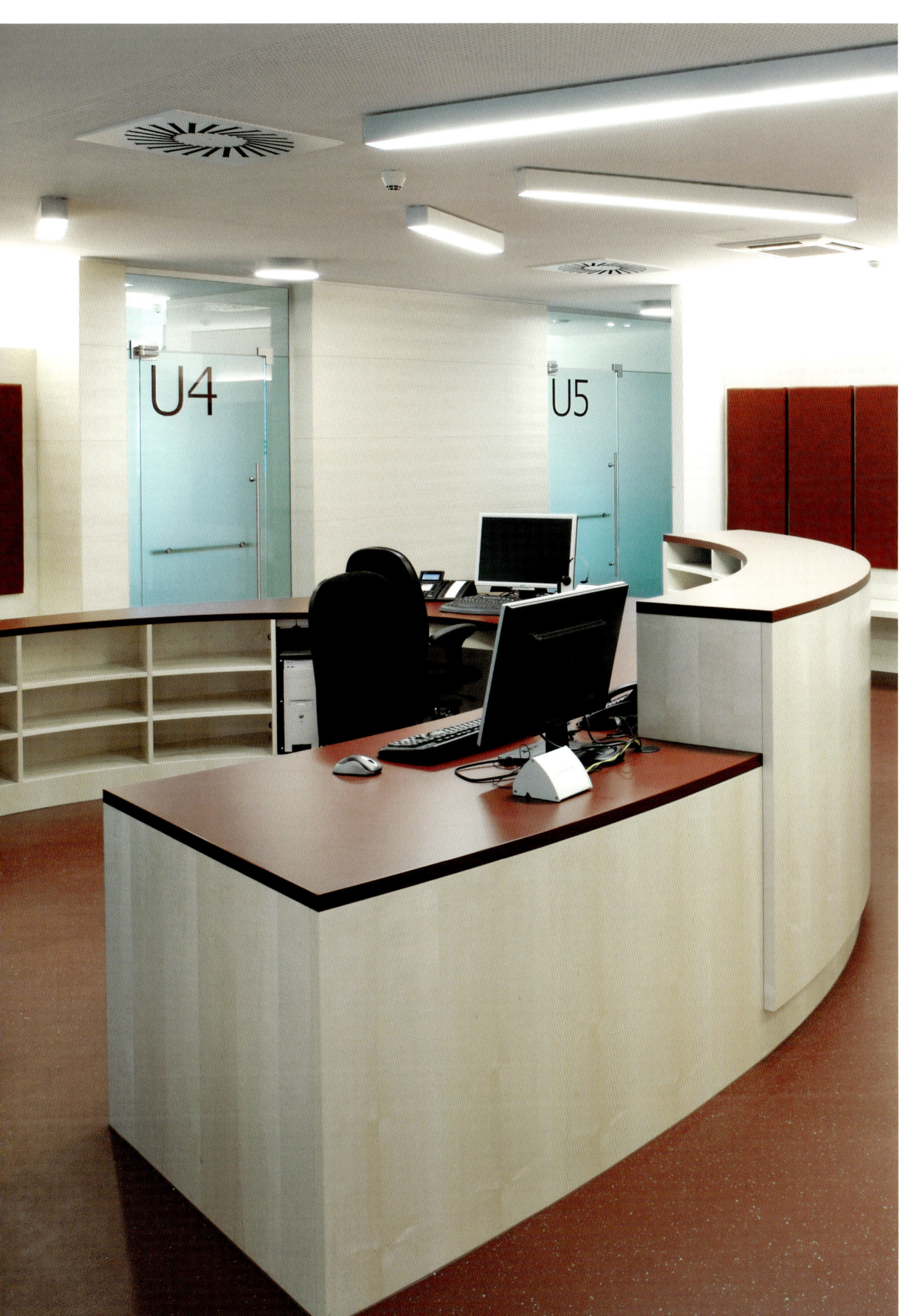

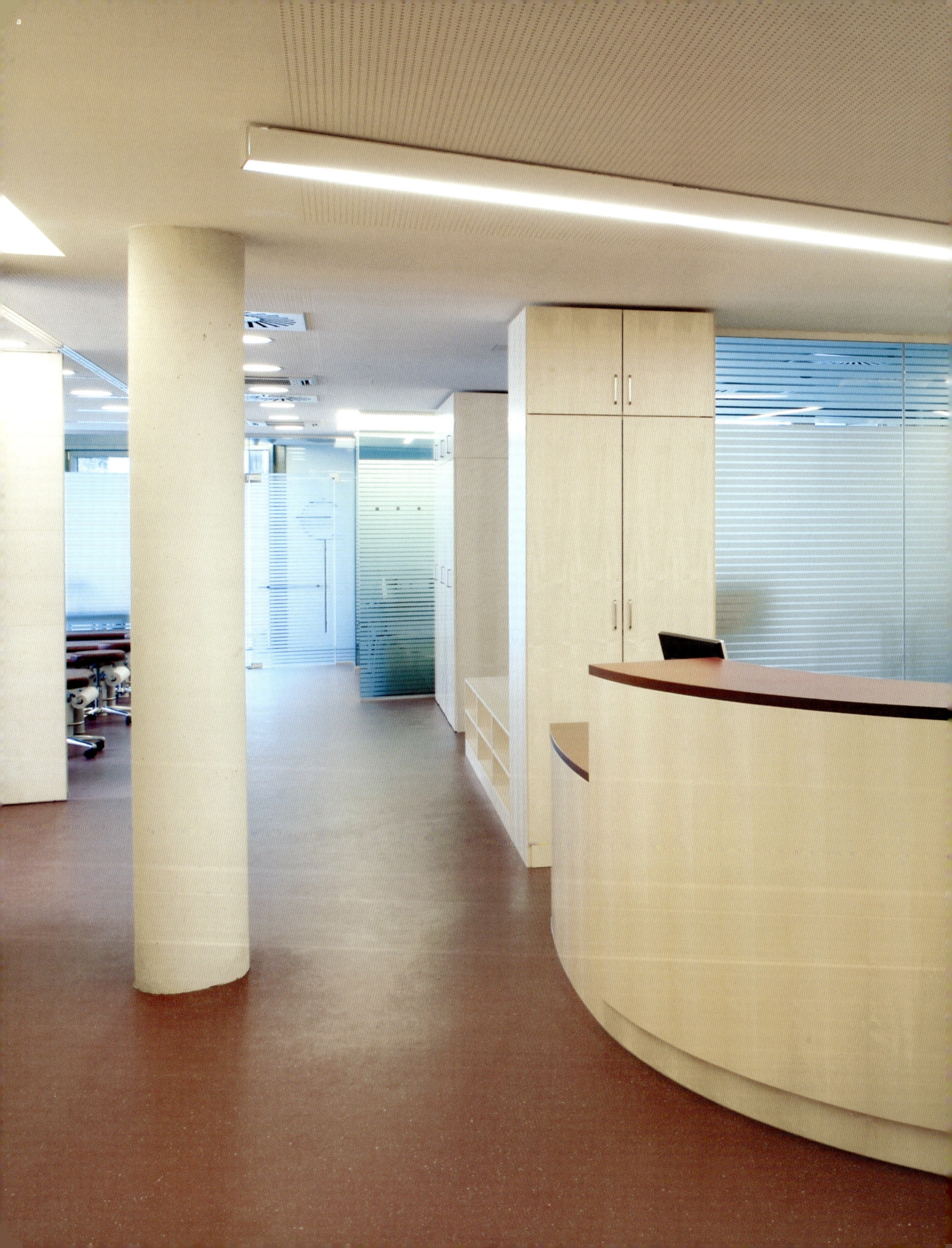

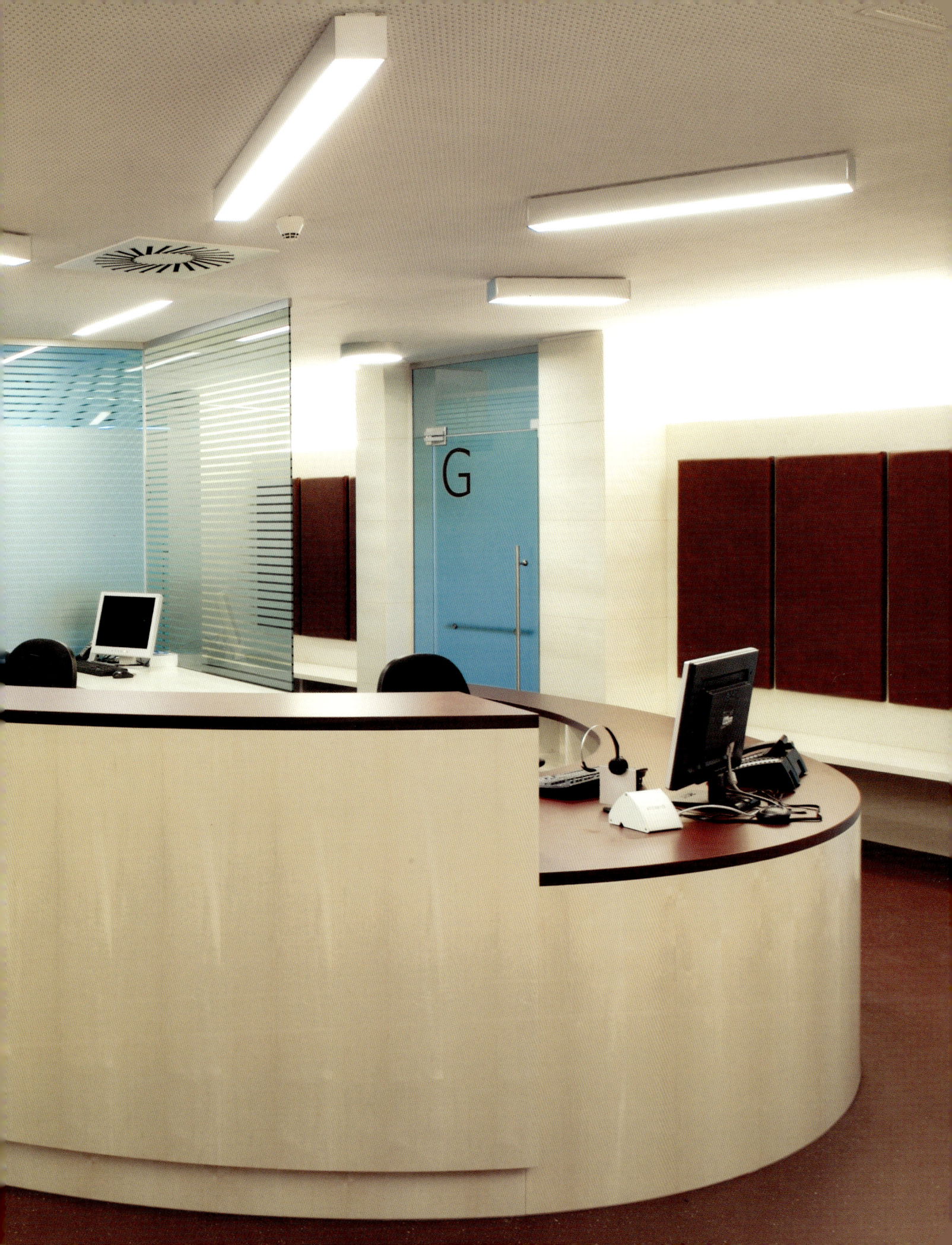

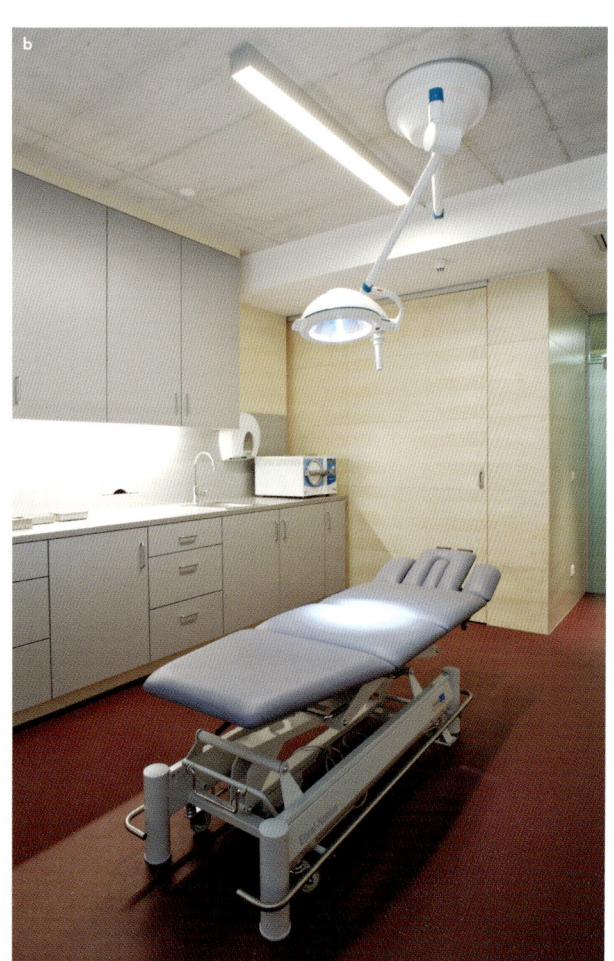

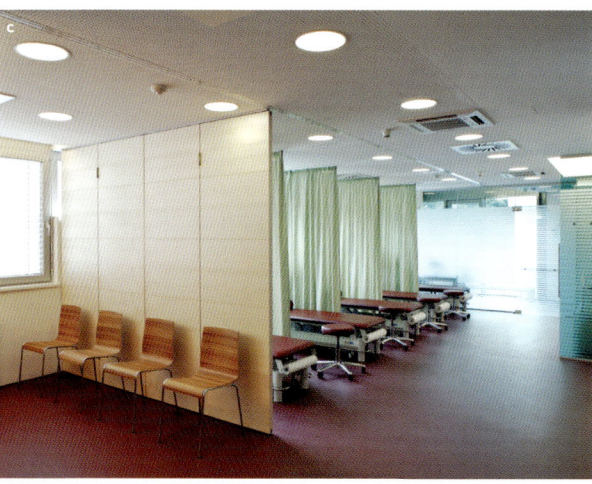

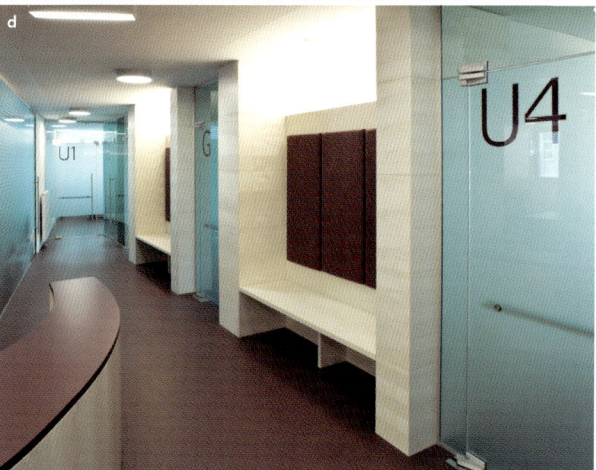

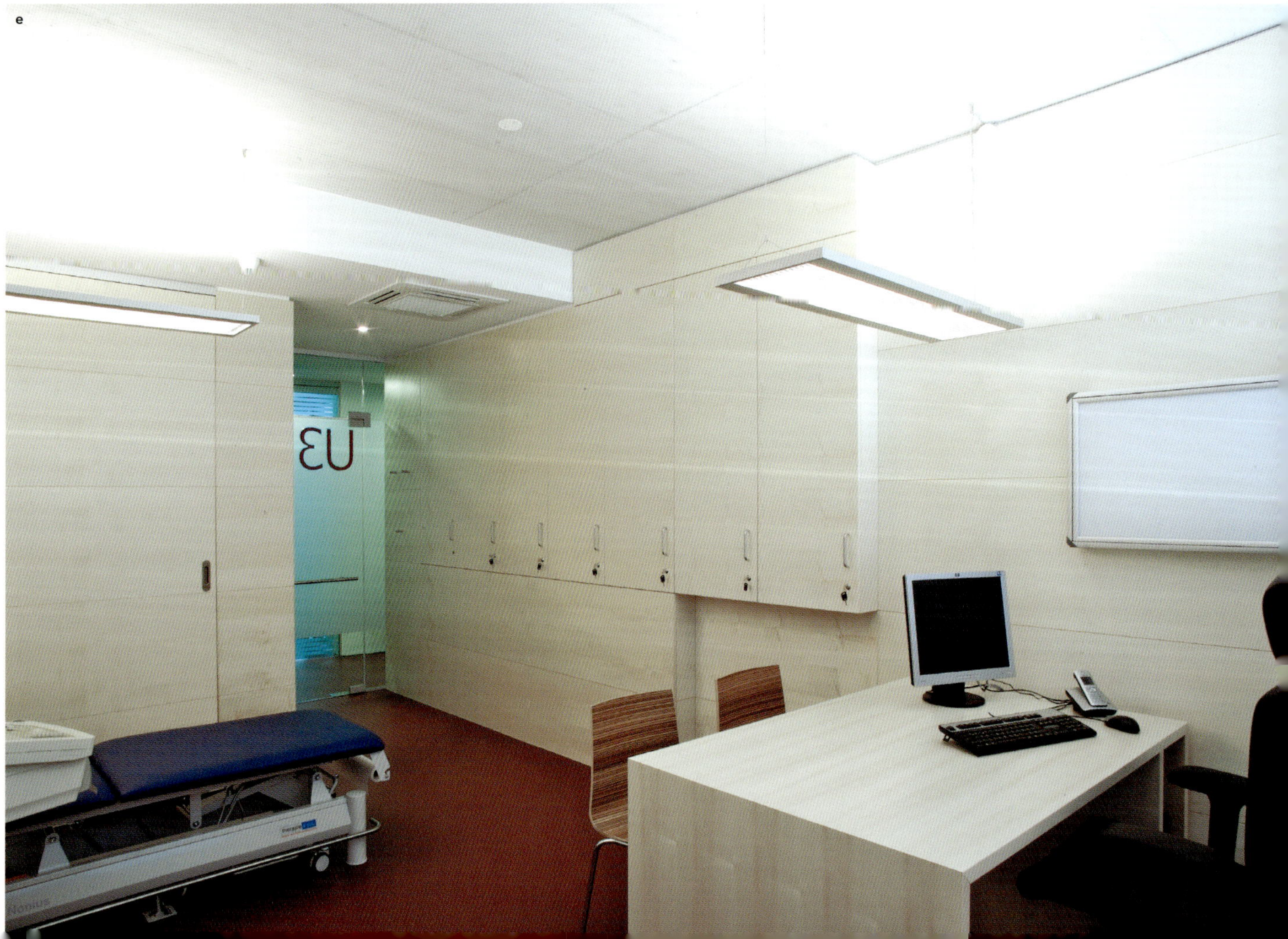

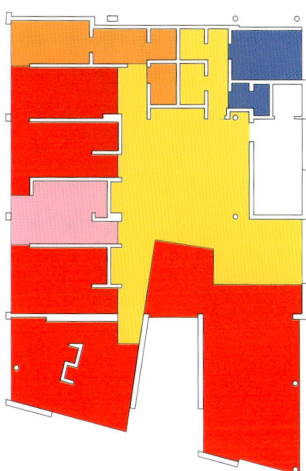

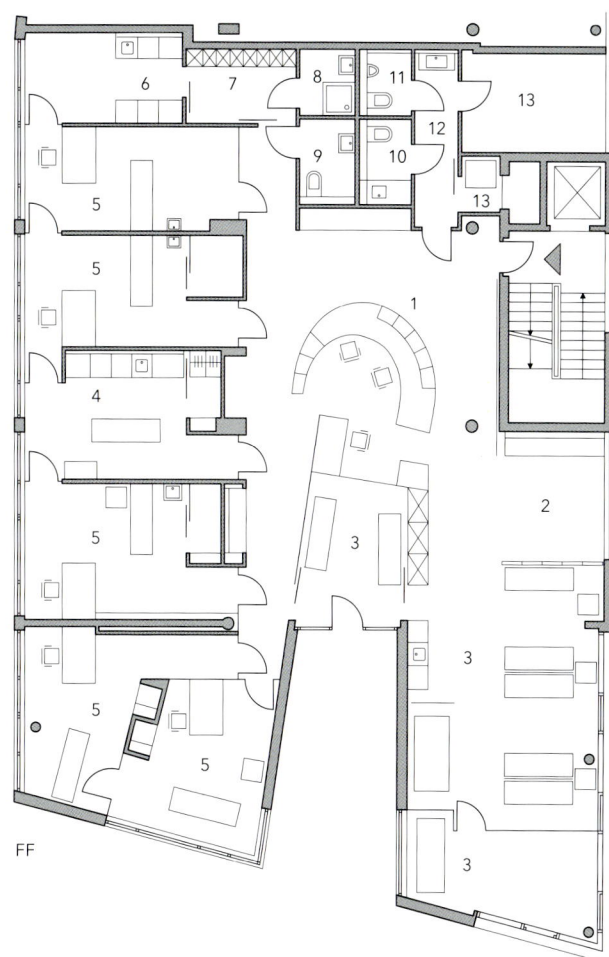

FF

Client | Operator	Dr. Thomas Reitinger
Planning time	02 2007 – 05 2007
Construction time	06 2007 – 08 2007
Usable floor space	332 sqm

a The semi-circular reception desk is free-standing and matches the glazed therapy room behind it.

b "Room boxes" with bright maple veneer are used as changing areas in the examination rooms.

c The therapy area can be divided into individual cubicles with curtains and sliding glass partition walls.

d Small waiting areas for patients are situated right next to the examination and treatment rooms.

e The friendly atmosphere of the examination rooms is defined by bright maple-veneer fittings and red flooring.

Diagrammatic plans, to scale 1:400
Floor plans, to scale 1:200

Floor plan layout

1	Reception	**6**	Staff lounge		disabled
2	Waiting area	**7**	Staff changing	**10**	Patient toilet L
3	Therapy		cubicle	**11**	Patient toilet G
4	Procedure room	**8**	Staff shower	**12**	Toilet anteroom
5	Examination and	**9**	Toilet for the	**13**	Store room
	treatment room				

Patients at the multiple practice come straight from the stairs to the reception. Diagonally opposite is the visible waiting area which, together with the extremely transparent treatment rooms, provides natural light to the internal area. All the other examination and treatment rooms on the U-shaped floor plan also receive plenty of natural light.

Usable floor spaces

Patient rooms	**yellow**	100 sqm	30 %
Examination |			
Treatment rooms	**red**	171 sqm	51 %
Specialist rooms	**pink**	20 sqm	6 %
Offices | Staff rooms	**orange**	26 sqm	8 %
Plant rooms	**blue**	15 sqm	5 %
Total		332 sqm	100 %

Performance data

Outpatients per year	4,500 [25 % private]
Number of services per year	75,000
Services to other clinics	X-ray, MRI, CT
Clinic opening hours	5 days | 60 hours
Waiting time [with | without appointment]	0 – 60 min. | 0 – 120 min.
Type and number of staff	2 doctors
	12 full-time staff
	6 external therapists

The practice for general medicine, situated in tranquil Preding in the Austrian state of Styria, is expanded by a spectacular extension. Thanks to the ceiling-high windows in the existing building, the examination rooms housed there have plenty of natural light. For the extension, the architect used a small triangular open area at the steep wooded terrain edge near the white single-family house with saddleback roof, where the practice is situated – there was no further space available. The unusual style of the single-storey extension, built entirely from prefabricated wooden components, is explained by this unconventional floor plan shape. The newly-obtained area extends over the reception area, the waiting area and a small office with consultation table. From the outside the building looks simple but striking. Dark grey fibre cement slabs are alternated with extensive glazing. The undersides of the roof overhangs protruding over the down-to-floor window areas are painted bright red, and this also catches the eye in the interior of the building, the ceiling colour also being red.

Inside the clinic a bright, less subdued red has been chosen as the colour for individual accenting in the case of the seating and the built-in furniture, without eclipsing the bright birch veneer of the custom-made furniture.

ANDREAS KANZIAN

PRACTICE FOR GENERAL MEDICINE
PREDING | A

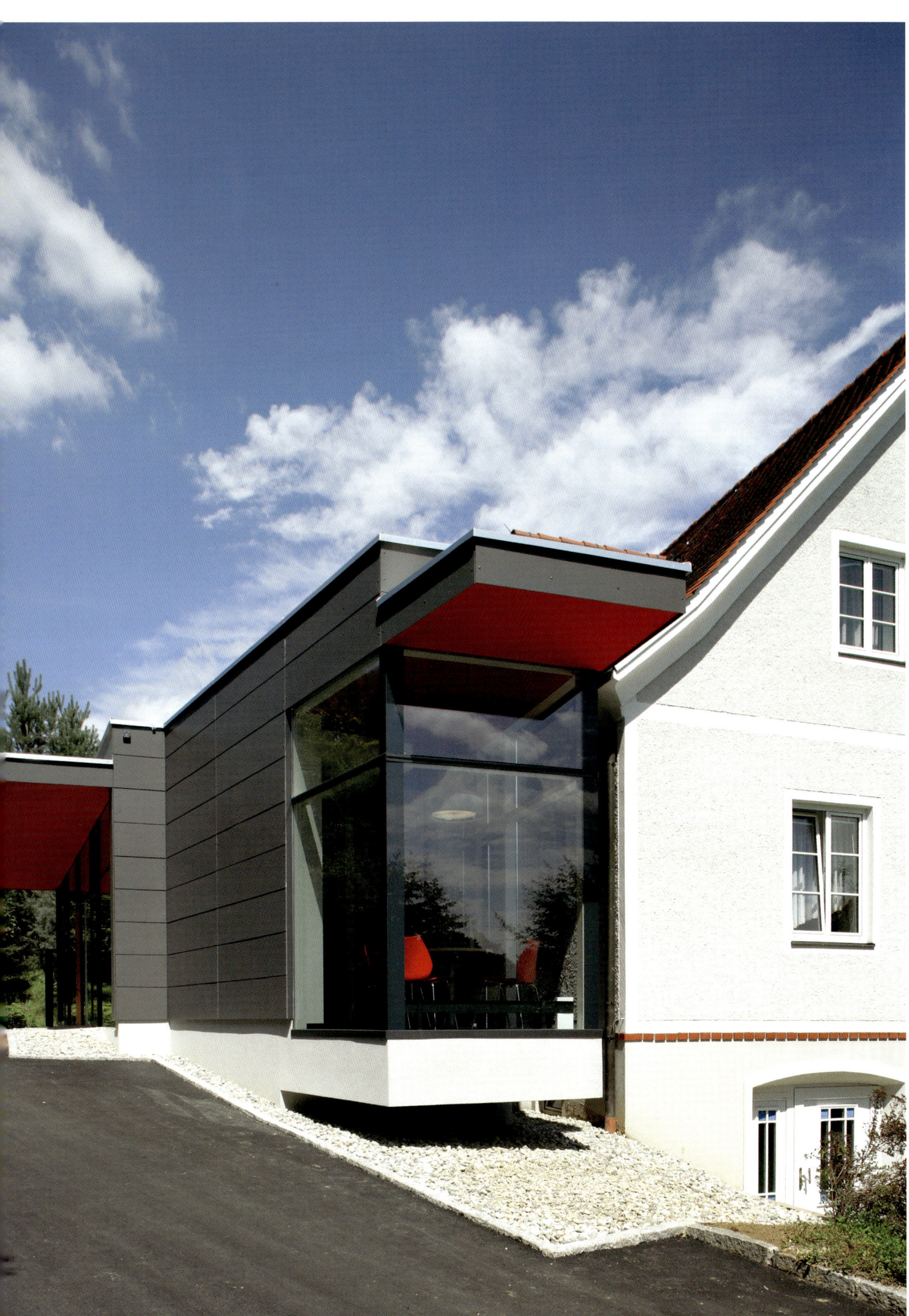

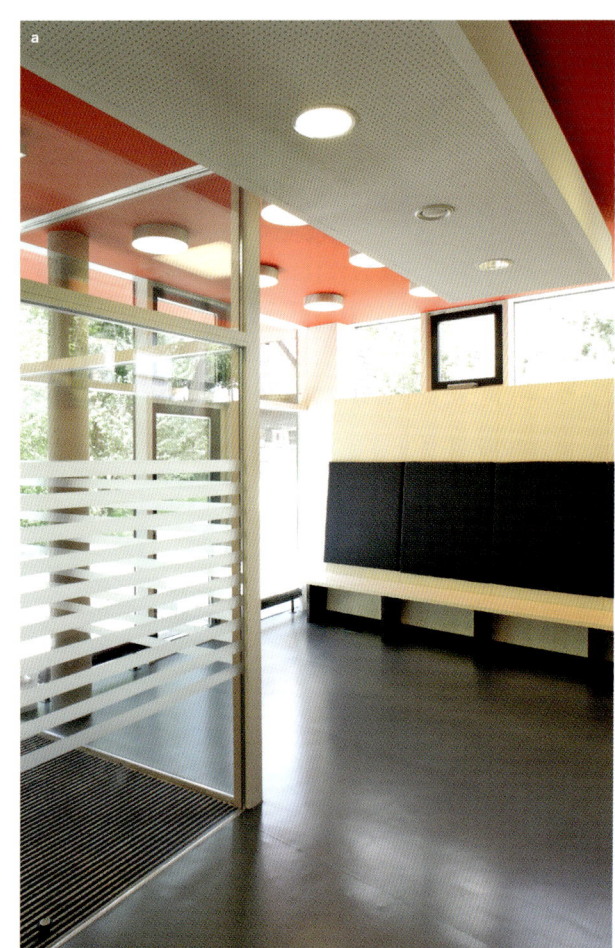

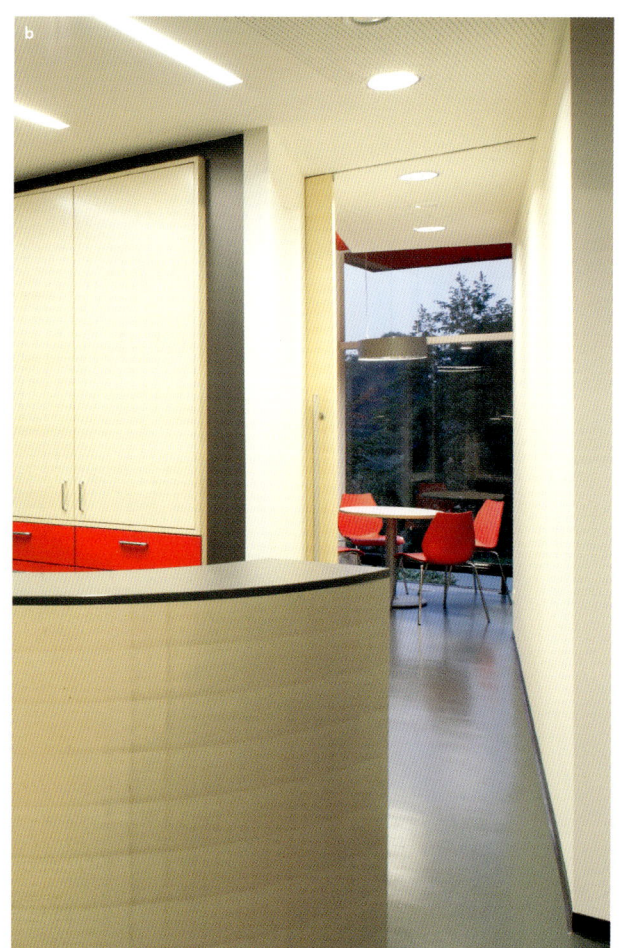

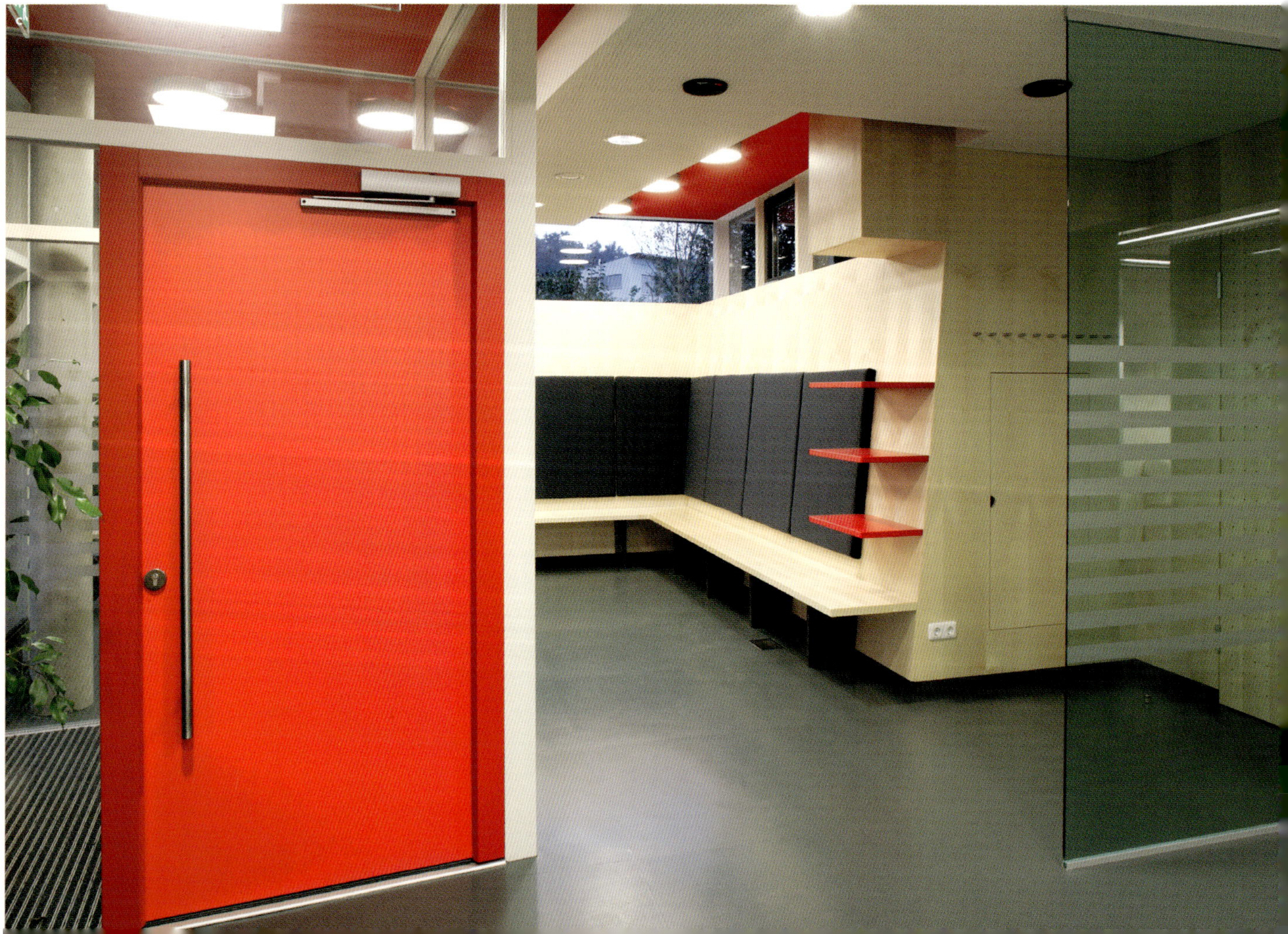

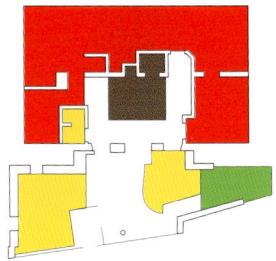

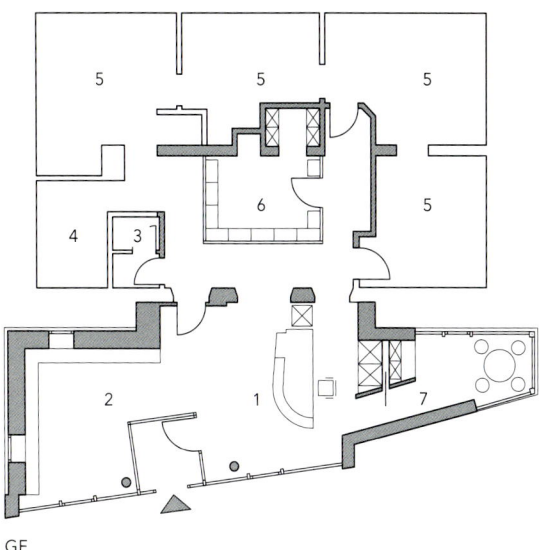

GF

**Client	Operator**	Dr. Wolfgang Geier
Planning time	09 2004 – 03 2005
Construction time	05 2005 – 07 2005
Usable floor space	111 sqm

a The open-plan waiting area goes directly into the spacious foyer.

b Thanks to these ceiling-high windows in the extension, the examination rooms housed in the existing building get plenty of light.

c Inside the clinic, bright red has been selected as the accentual colour for individual design elements.

Diagrammatic plans, to scale 1:400
Floor plans, to scale 1:200

Floor plan layout

1 Reception	4 Laboratory	6 Pharmacy
2 Waiting area	5 Examination	7 Consultation room
3 Patient toilet		

Taking into consideration local conditions, the porch, via which the patients access the spacious reception and waiting area in the single-doctor practice, is very welcome. The extension opens up the present examination and treatment rooms both of which receive natural light, in the best possible way.

Usable floor spaces

Patient rooms	**yellow**	26 sqm	23 %
Examination			
Treatment rooms	**red**	67 sqm	61 %
Administrative rooms	**green**	8 sqm	7 %
Supply	Waste disposal	**brown**	10 sqm	9 %
Total		111 sqm	100 %

Performance data

Outpatients per year	6,000
Number and type of services per year	Ultrasound [480]
	ECG [720]
	Pulmonary function [720]
	Sports medical diagnostics [240]
Clinic opening hours	5 days	40 hours
Waiting time [with	without appointment]	15 – 20 min.	60 – 90 min.
Type and number of staff	1 doctor [+ 1 doctor in training]
	2 full-time, 1 part-time

Strong red accents characterise the part-conversion of the old building practice in Graz. In addition to restructuring the organisation of the current rooms, the exceptional character of the old apartment dating from the turn of the 19th century needed to be brought to life. For this reason, the old room sizes have been restored to some extent.

Reception and waiting area are open-plan, in order to encourage and emphasise personal contact with the patient. The waiting area, furnished with high-quality geometric parquet flooring, is resplendent in all its former glory. The red waiting-room chairs are casually grouped in front of the plain white walls, with the central area left free. The room gives the impression of being spacious and inviting, thanks to its high ceilings and minimum seating; and patients who tend to be on edge are able to wait for their appointment in peace and quiet, in a pleasant atmosphere. Large folding doors open into adjoining rooms on both sides. The defining aspect of the design concept – the colour red – is unmistakably eye-catching. The ECG and endoscopy technical medical equipment is housed in "accessible furniture" in the examination rooms. Ceiling-high room dividers covered with horizontal wooden panels mark out the individual areas. Bright red eye-catching elements such as curtains, couches and seating furniture reflect the new interior design concept.

ANDREAS KANZIAN

PRACTICE FOR INTERNAL MEDICINE
GRAZ | A

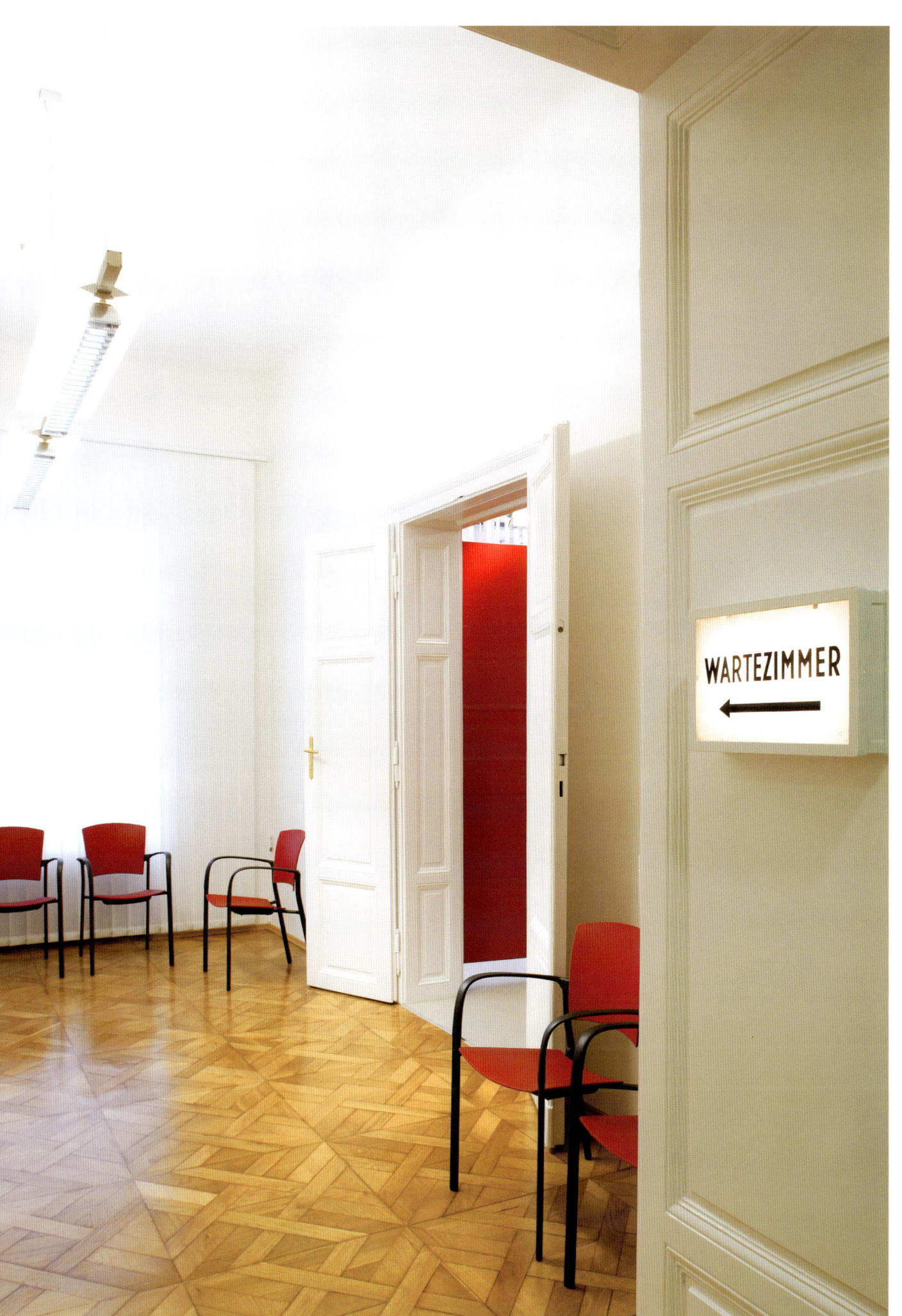

WARTEZIMMER

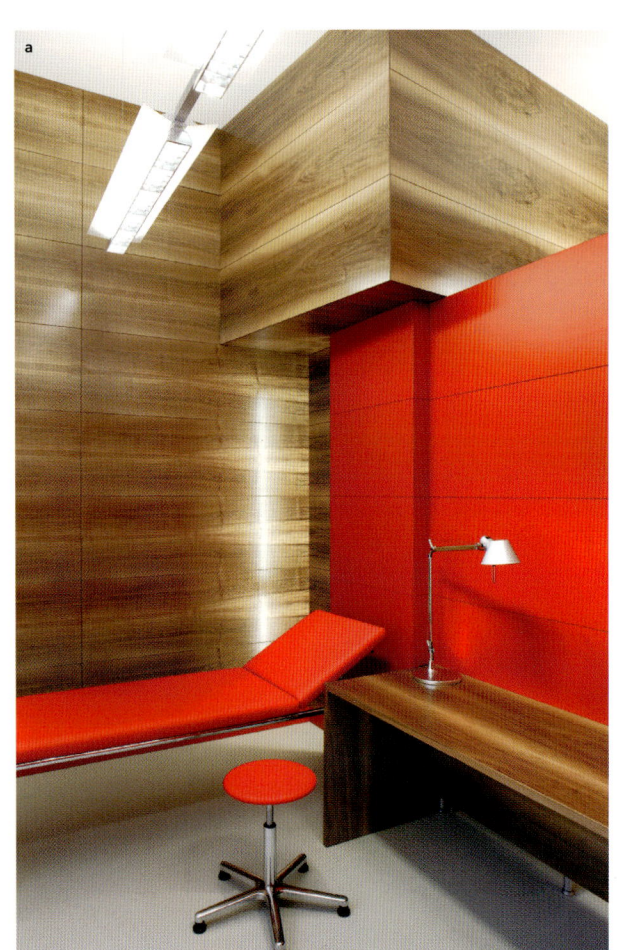

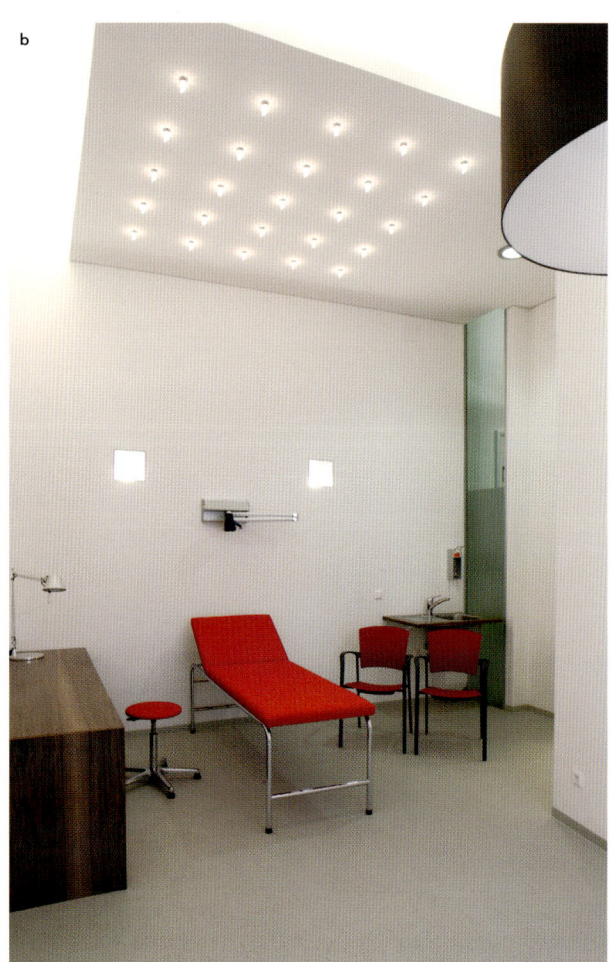

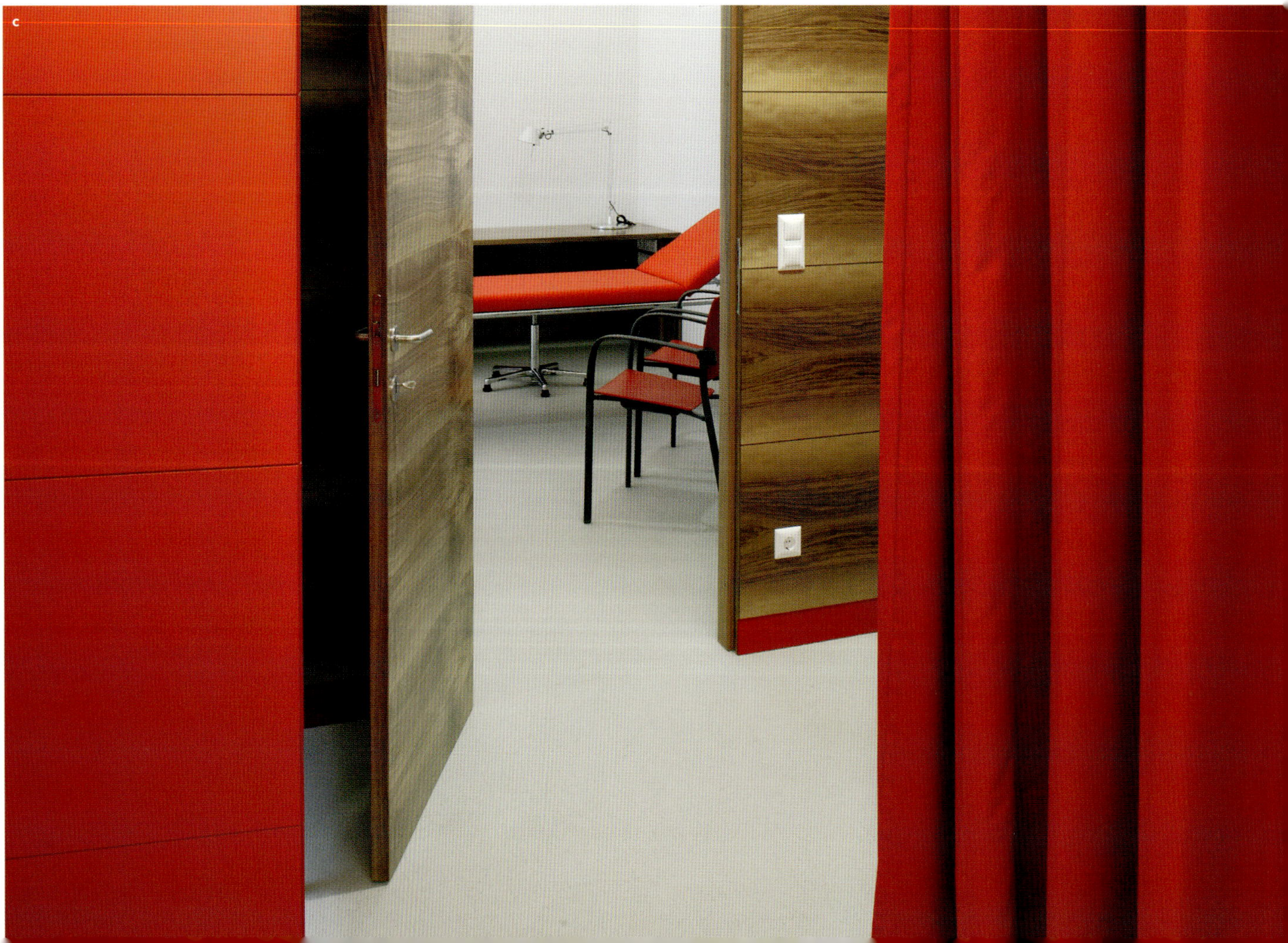

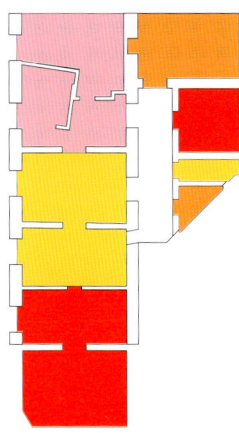

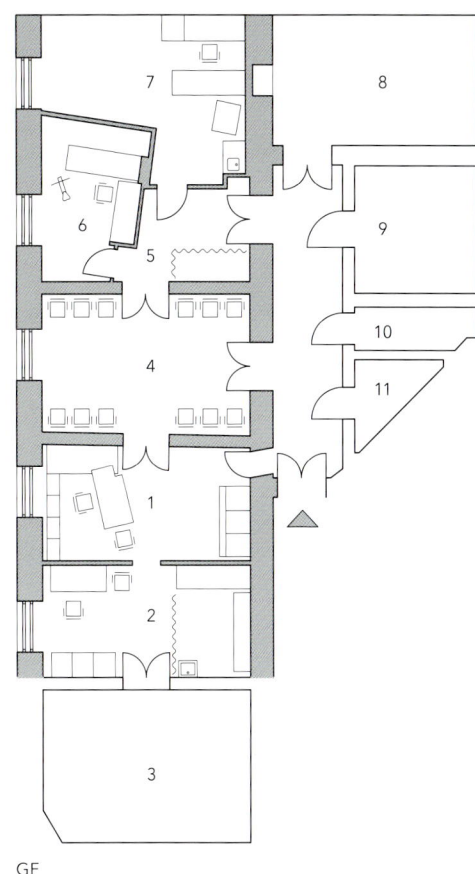

GF

Client | Operator   Dr. Andreas Mahr
Planning time   02 2003 – 06 2003
Construction time   07 2004
Usable floor space   181 sqm

a   ECG and endoscopy equipment is housed in "accessible furniture".

b   The defining aspect of the design concept – the colour red – is unmistakably eye-catching in the examination room.

c   Ceiling-high room dividers covered with horizontal wooden panels mark out the individual areas.

Diagrammatic plans, to scale 1:400
Floor plans, to scale 1:200

Floor plan layout

1	Reception	**5**	Anteroom	**8**	Lounge
2	Blood sample	**6**	Examination ECG	**9**	Laboratory
3	Treatment room	**7**	Examination	**10**	Patient toilet
4	Waiting area		endoscopy	**11**	Staff toilet

Patients access the reception room in this practice via the spacious waiting area. From there they can access the examination and treatment rooms on both sides, all benefiting from natural light.

Usable floor spaces

Patient rooms	**yellow**	50 sqm	28 %
Examination | Treatment rooms	**red**	59 sqm	32 %
Specialist rooms	**pink**	45 sqm	25 %
Offices | Staff rooms	**orange**	27 sqm	15 %
Total		181 sqm	100 %

Performance data

Outpatients per year	6,000
Number and type of services per year	Gastroscopy [400]
	ECG [3,000]
	Laboratory [400]
	Ergometry [1,300]
	Upper abdomen ultrasound [1,000]
	Pulmonary function [1,400]
Services to other clinics	CT and MRI [70],
	Colonoscopies [100],
	Cardiac catheter [50]
	X-ray [500], Scintigraphies of the thyroid glands [50]
	24-hour ECG [150]
Clinic opening hours	5 days | 22 hours
Waiting time [with | without appointment]	10 – 40 min. | 120 min.
Type and number of staff	1 doctor
	3 full-time staff
	2 part-time staff

The "edelweiss" dental practice, whose unusual name was not inspired by the mountain flower, rather by the snow-white furnishings adopted in the premises, is situated in the centre of Berlin, far away from mountains and alpine pastures. Nevertheless, the whitish gleam also appears to have been modelled on the bracts of the plant. Snow-white walls, cubic furniture and warm natural colours are predominant in the clinic interior; only the majestically dark leather-upholstered reception desk stands out. The rear wall, made of smooth velvety mineral-based fabric, is broken up with an undulating wooden relief. The microfibre velour-covered chairs and the sofa in the lounge-like waiting area, which is a harmonious grey-beige, are very inviting. The desk also offers somewhere to linger for those waiting who may not be quite so relaxed. All the furniture is classic and hand-made.

In the five treatment rooms, where patients are able to enjoy an impressive view over the city centre, white treatment units are embedded in the walls and oak- framed. The flooring consists of large ceramic tiles. One special feature is the innovative "video lights" examination light. This consists of a garland light over the workplace and a monitor window, on which the patients can view films as a distraction when undergoing lengthy treatment.

KLM ARCHITEKTEN HENRY SCHEIN DENTAL DEPOT

"EDELWEISS" DENTAL PRACTICE
BERLIN | G

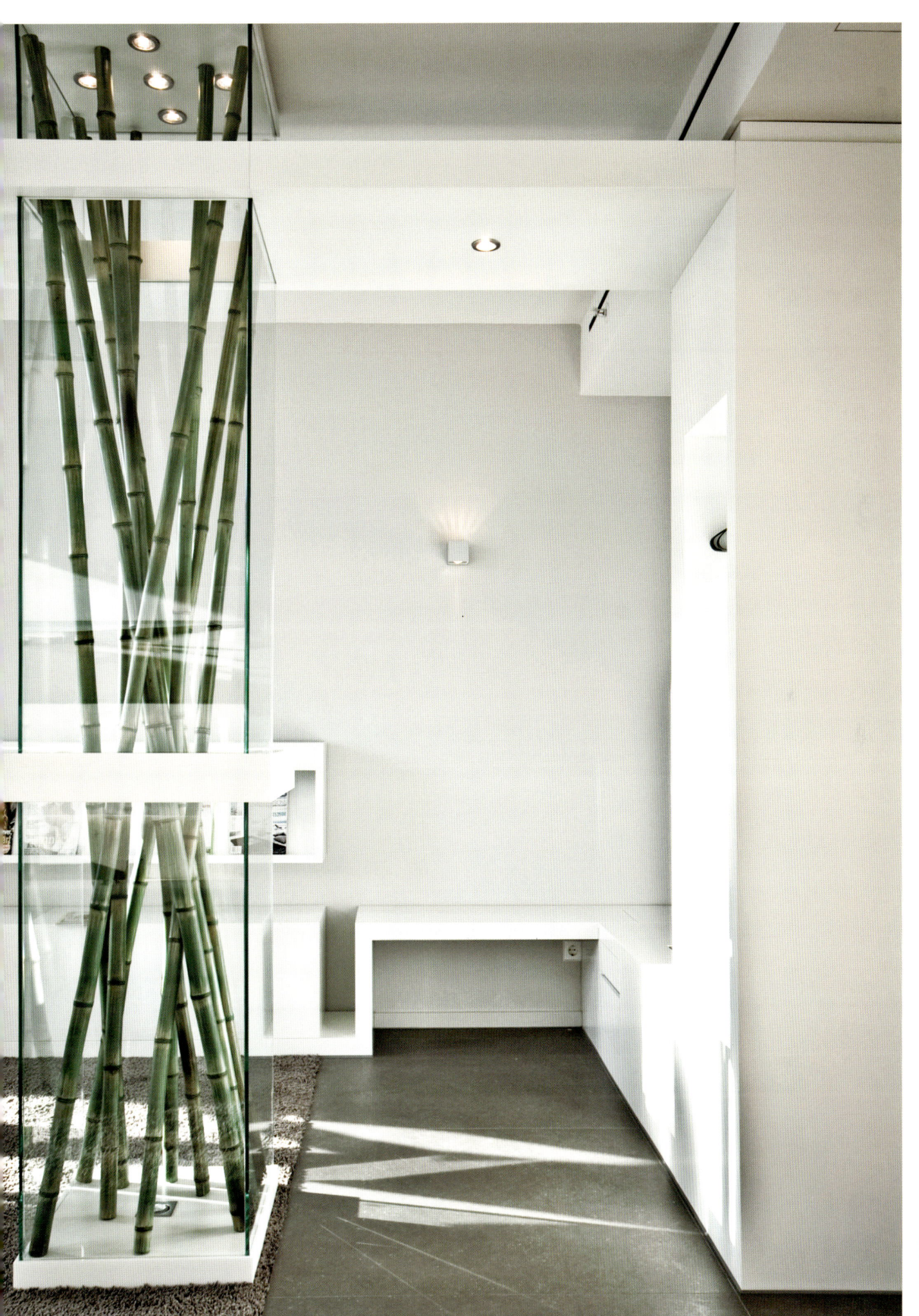

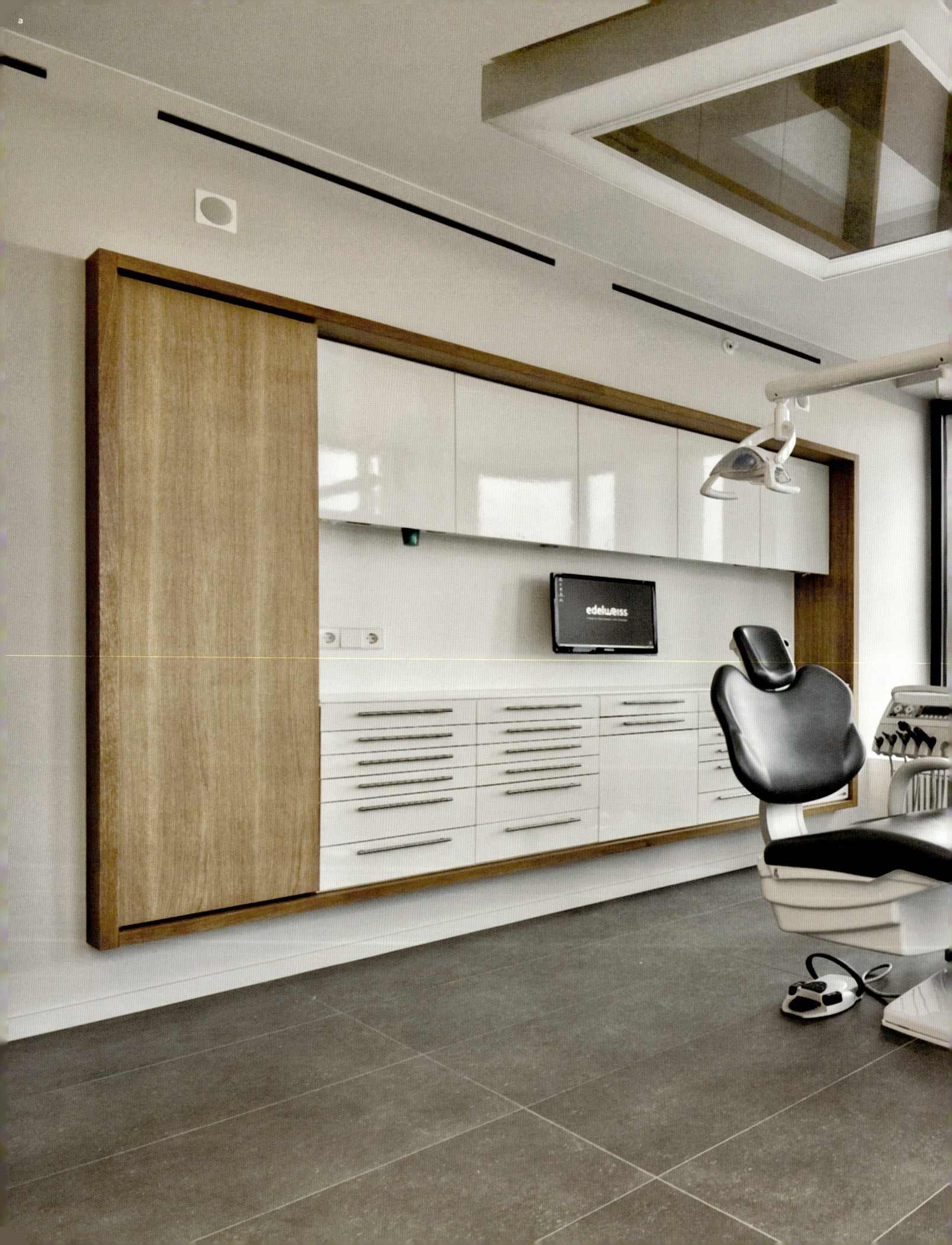

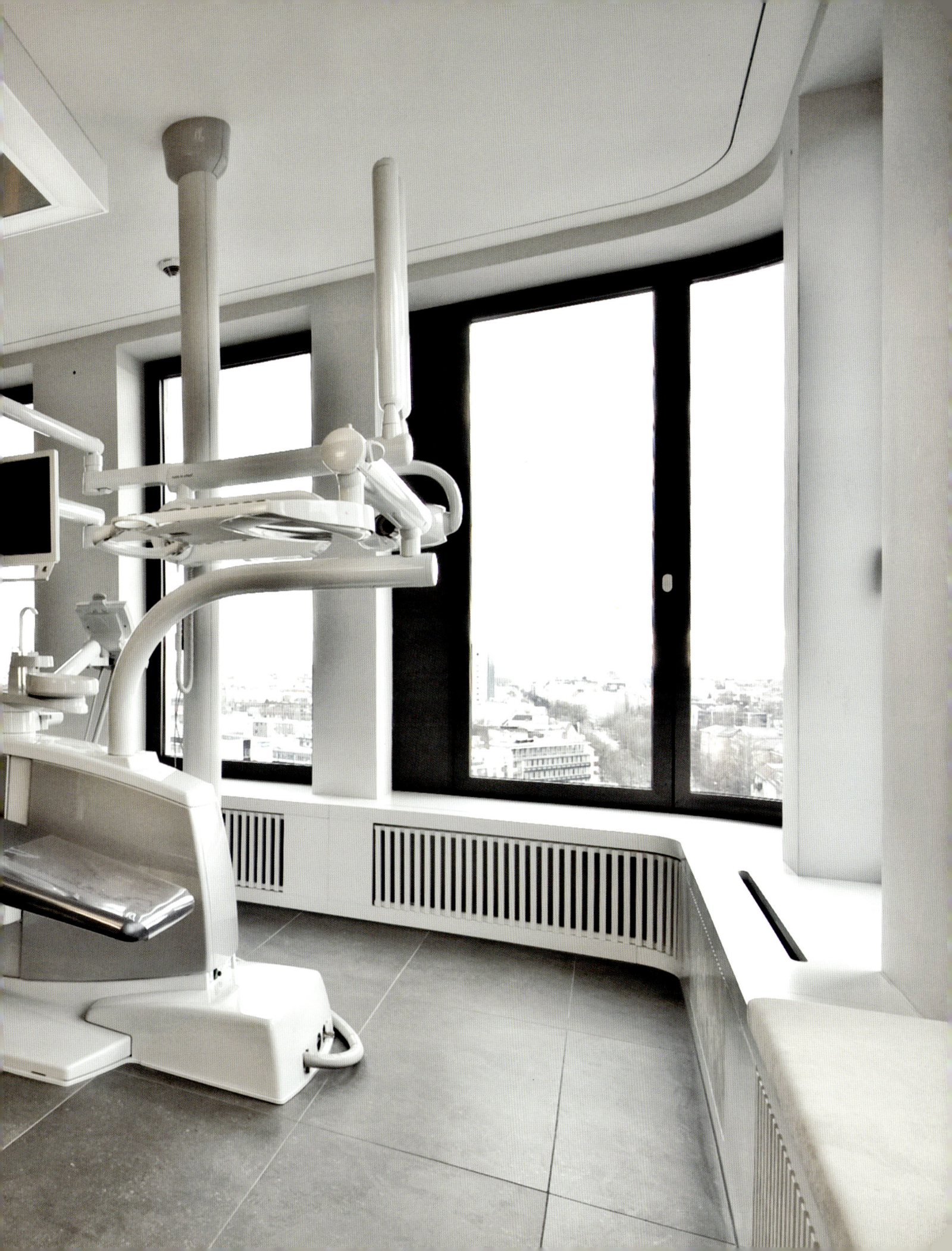

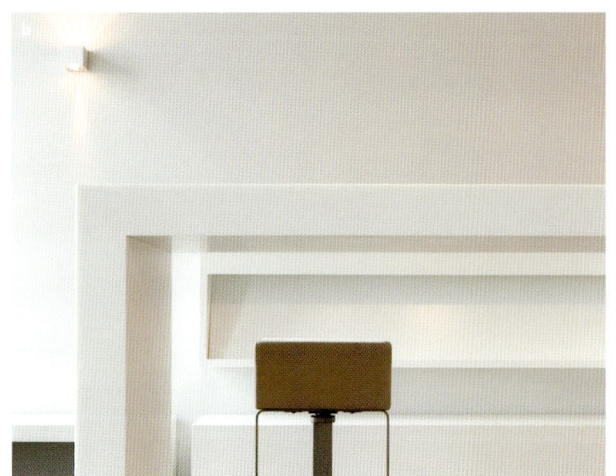

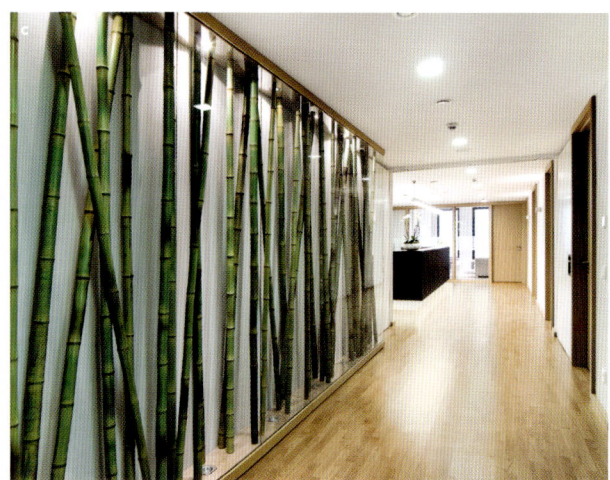

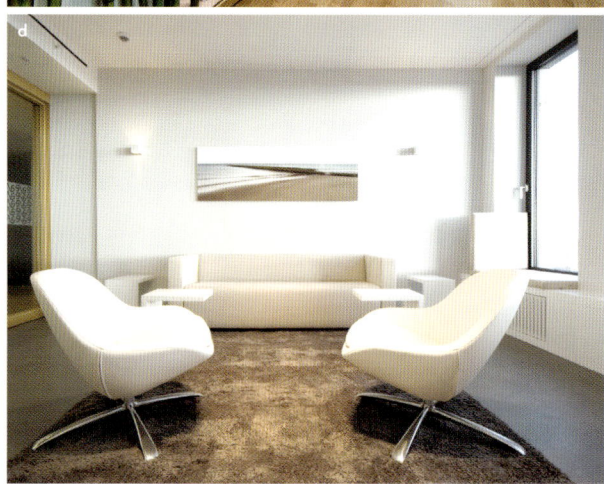

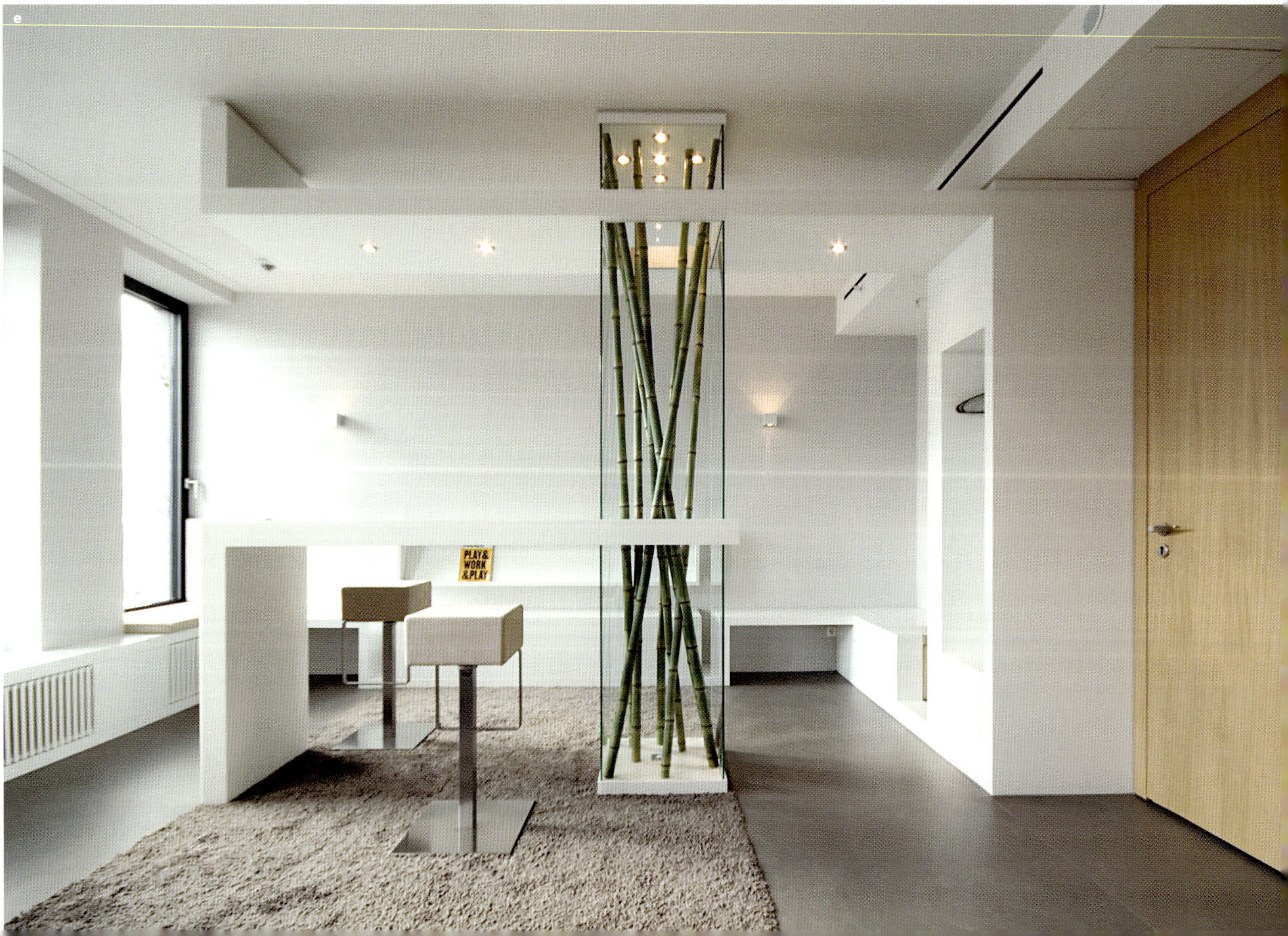

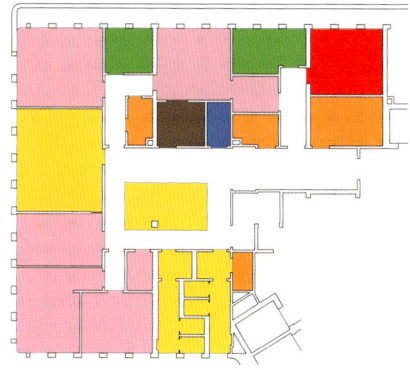

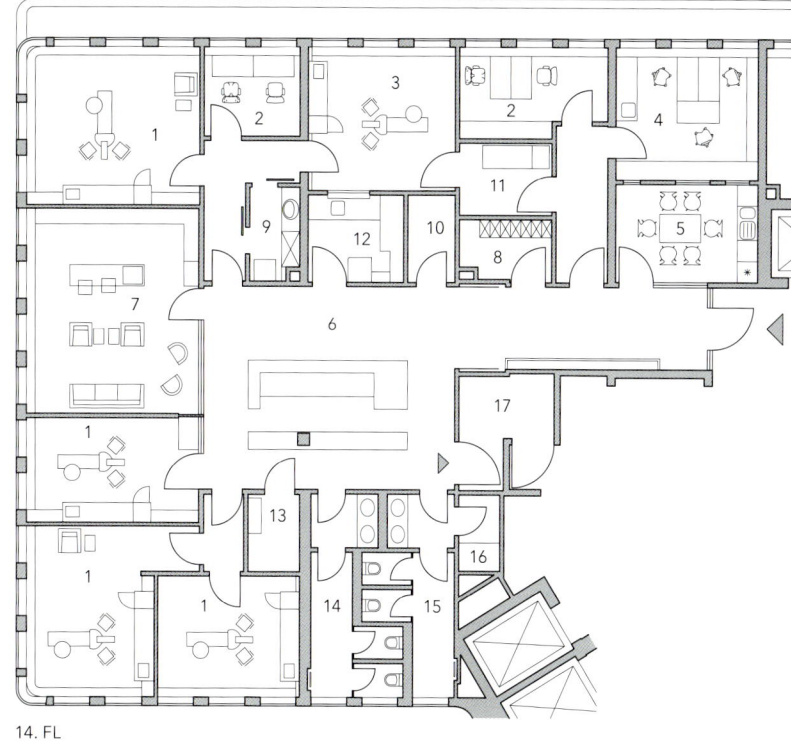

14. FL

Client	Dr. Simone Schauer
	Dr. Peter Kienzle
Operator	"Edelweiss"
	Dental Practice
Planning time	11 2007 – 05 2008
Construction time	06 2008 – 11 2008
Gross floor area	337 sqm
Usable floor space	227 sqm
Gross cubic capacity	910 cbm
Construction cost	350,000 EUR
Total cost	1,000,000 EUR

a Patients can enjoy an impressive view over the west part of Berlin city centre from the treatment rooms on the 14th floor of the Concorde building

b The design is an expression of the aesthetic demands of modern dentistry, with the desk in the waiting area made of white mineral-based fabric.

c The dark leather-upholstered reception desk and the illuminated display cabinet with the green bamboo poles stand out in the foyer.

d The lounge-like waiting area, with its warm natural colours, invites patients to tarry for a while.

e The edelweiss hand-made built-in pieces of furniture in the waiting area are well matched.

Diagrammatic plans, to scale 1:400
Floor plans, to scale 1:200

Floor plan layout

1	Treatment room	**7**	Waiting area	**11**	Quiet room
2	Office	**8**	Staff changing	**12**	Sterilisation room
3	Procedure room		cubicle	**13**	Examination X-ray
4	Laboratory	**9**	Doctor's shower	**14**	Toilet L
5	Staff lounge and		and changing	**15**	Toilet G
	small kitchen		cubicle	**16**	Staff shower
6	Reception	**10**	Installations room	**17**	Sluice emergency

Patients go directly past the reception and into the waiting area, which is easy to identity. By means of three short connecting corridors, all rooms, almost all of which receive natural light, are accessed from the central corridor.

Usable floor spaces

Patient rooms	**yellow**	63 sqm	28 %
Examination | Treatment rooms	**red**	16 sqm	7 %
Specialist rooms	**pink**	98 sqm	43 %
Administrative rooms	**green**	17 sqm	8 %
Offices | Staff rooms	**orange**	23 sqm	10 %
Supply | Waste disposal	**brown**	7 sqm	3 %
Plant rooms	**blue**	3 sqm	1 %
Total		227 sqm	100 %

Performance data

Number and type of services per year	Aesthetic dentistry Implantology, Oral surgery Prophylaxis, Bleaching Treatment under anaesthesia
Services to other clinics	Orthodontics
Clinic opening hours	5 days | 50 hours
Waiting time [with | without appointment]	0 – 15 min. | 15 – 60 min.
Type and number of staff	1 dentist
	1 dentist | oral surgeon
	2 prophylaxis assistants
	4 ZMF, 1 ZMV, 1 ZMV external
Clinic planning advice	1 additional treatment, extend range of laboratory equipment

In converting the physiotherapy practice, the usable floor space has been expanded thanks to the inclusion of an adjacent storage space. Thus a modern practice has been created, divided into different wings for physiotherapy and osteopathy.

The design focused on transforming the once cool, almost sterile atmosphere of the unmanageable rooms, which were divided into small sections, into an open structure with a bright, friendly ambience, without ignoring the important functions. The visual surfaces in the practice are characterised by the use of natural materials – colour-changing natural stone flooring, bright parquet flooring and cherrywood furniture. On entering the reception and waiting area, patients are taken aback by the impression of a spacious room and the extraordinary view of the therapy pool. The partition wall made of special-purpose glass, which separates the pool from the foyer, is useful both as clear glass and also as a sight screen during therapy. The translucent effect can be switched into an illumination of changing colour. The wall also creates illusion, as its warm orange and red colours make the walls appear like cubatures placed in the room. Additional windows and built-in dome lights bring natural light into the now large, high rooms.

**RALF KRAUSE
MARC BRUNE**

"SANITAS" THERAPY CENTRE
WILDESHAUSEN | G

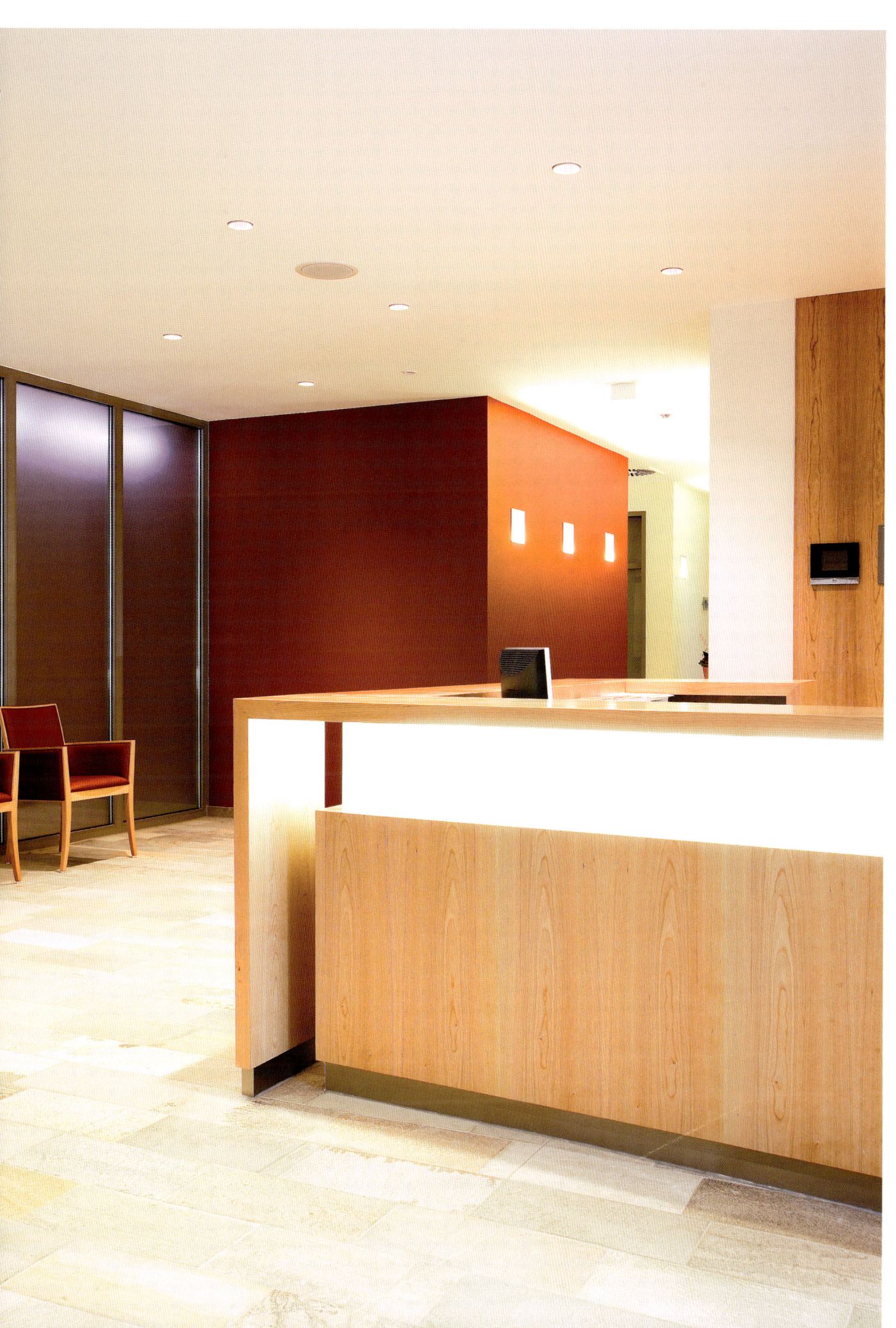

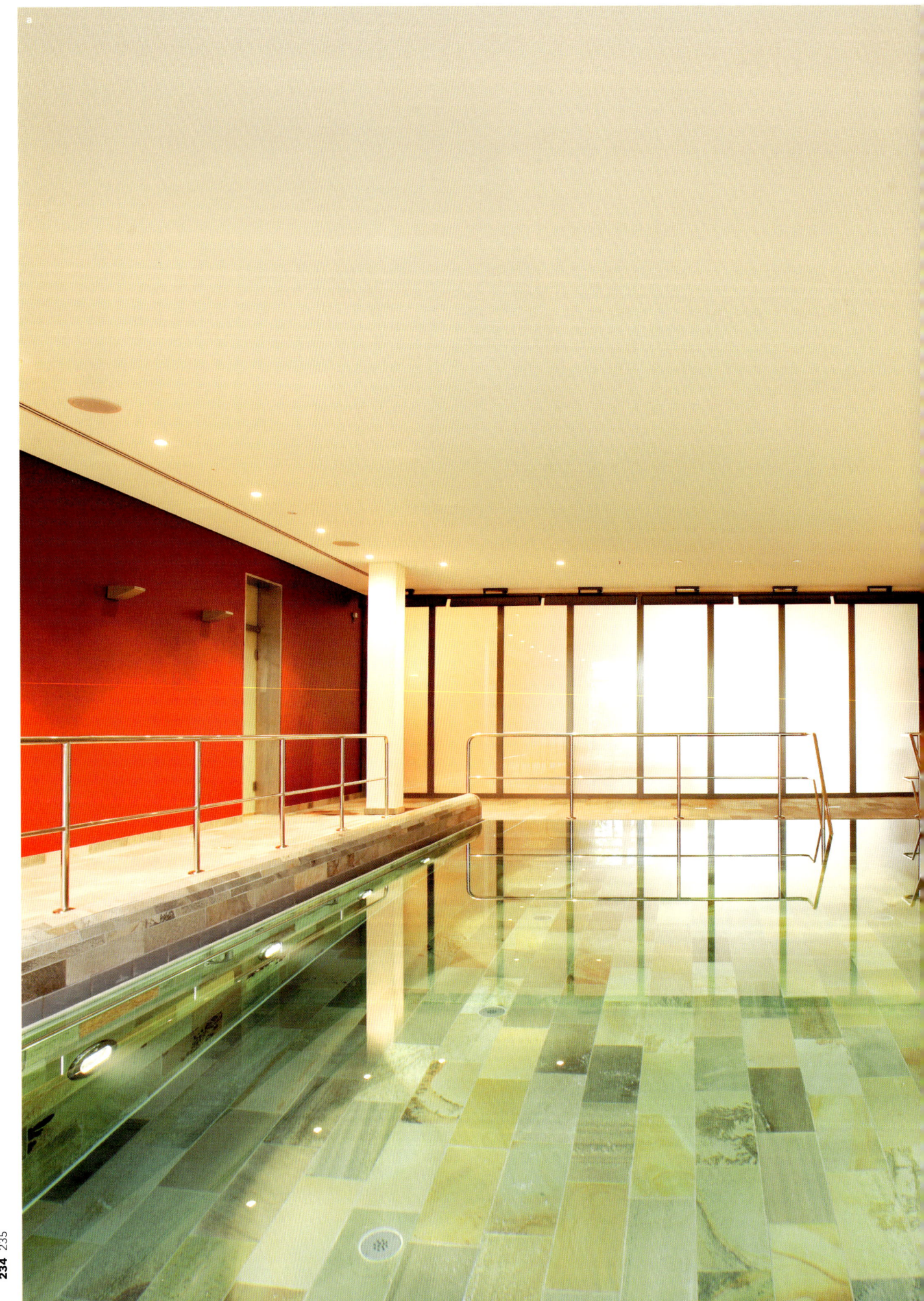

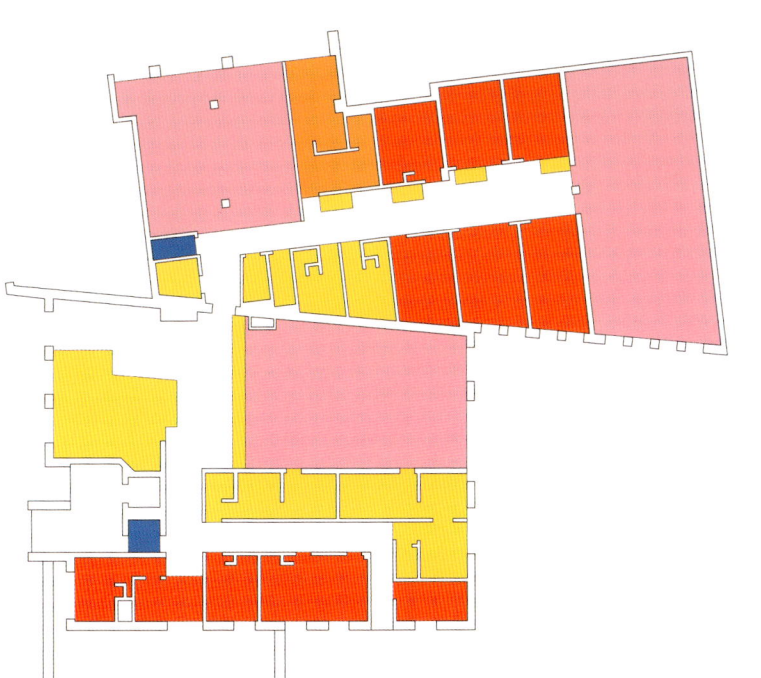

1 Waiting area
2 Reception
3 Therapy
4 Patient changing
  cubicle L
5 Patient toilet L
6 Treatment room
7 Patient shower L
8 Patient shower G
9 Patient changing
  cubicle G
10 Patient toilet G
11 Installations room
12 Toilet for the disabled
13 Diagnostics
14 Staff lounge
15 Staff changing cubicle
16 Staff toilet
17 Fitness room
18 Movement

Diagrammatic plans, to scale 1:400
Floor plans, to scale 1:200

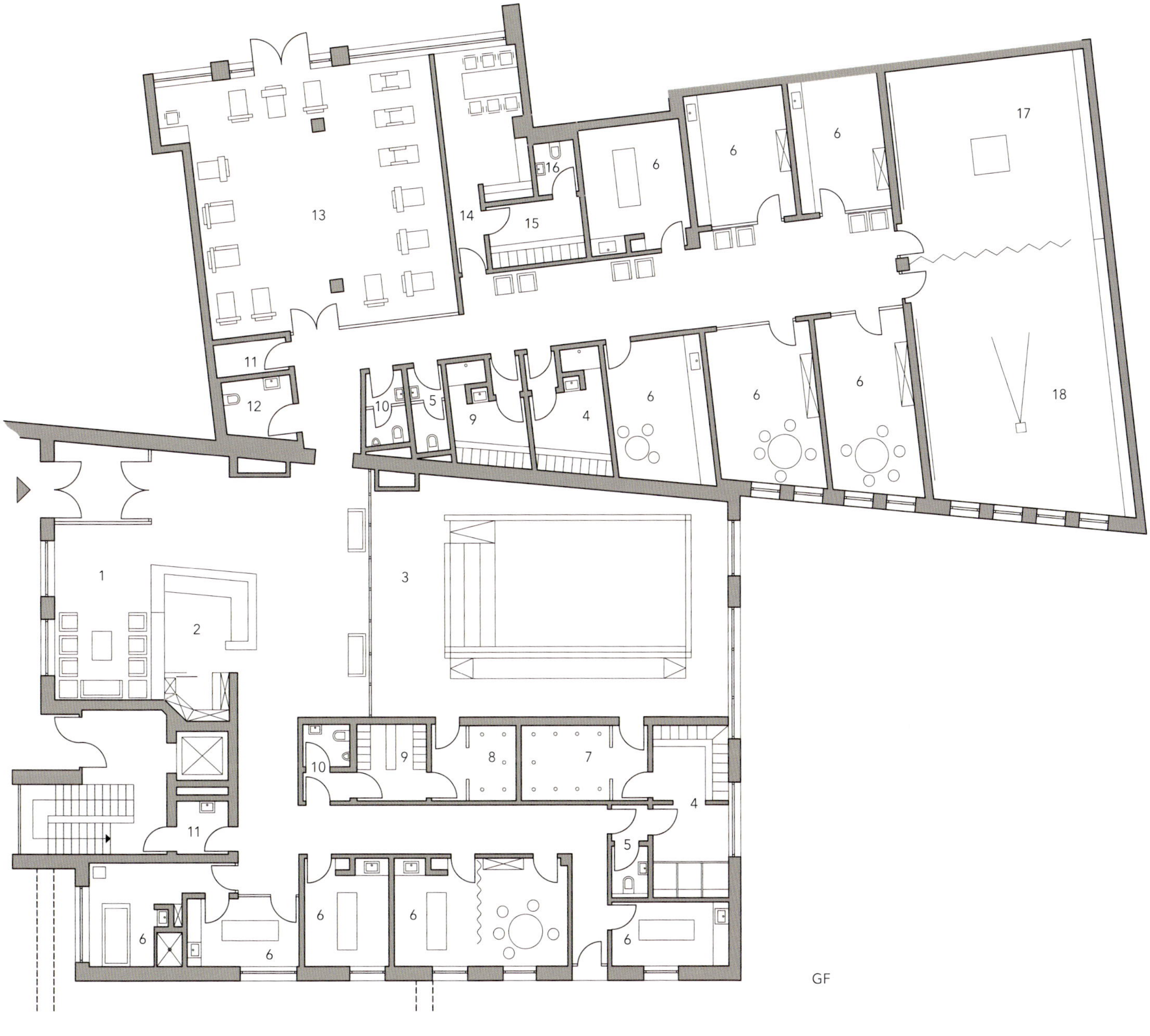

GF

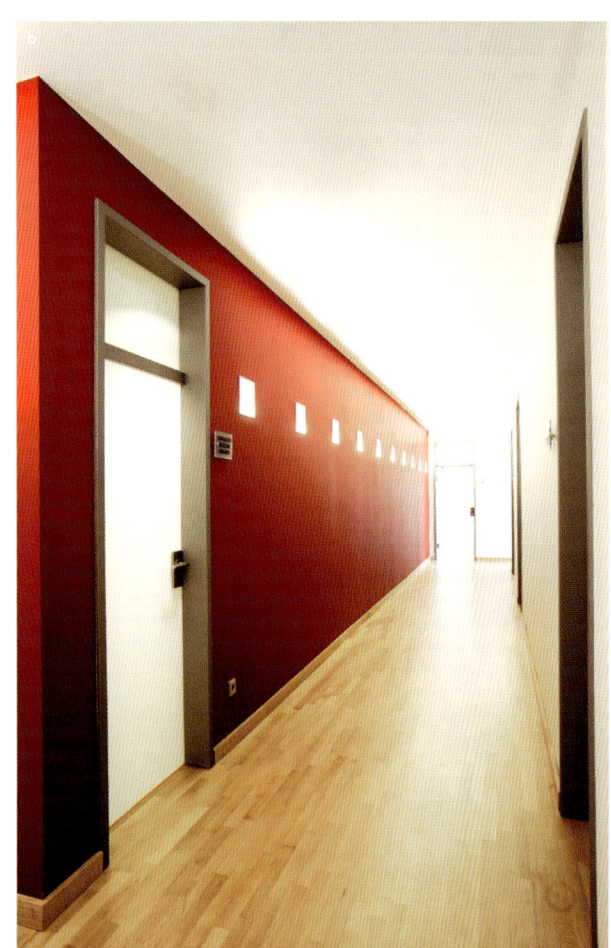

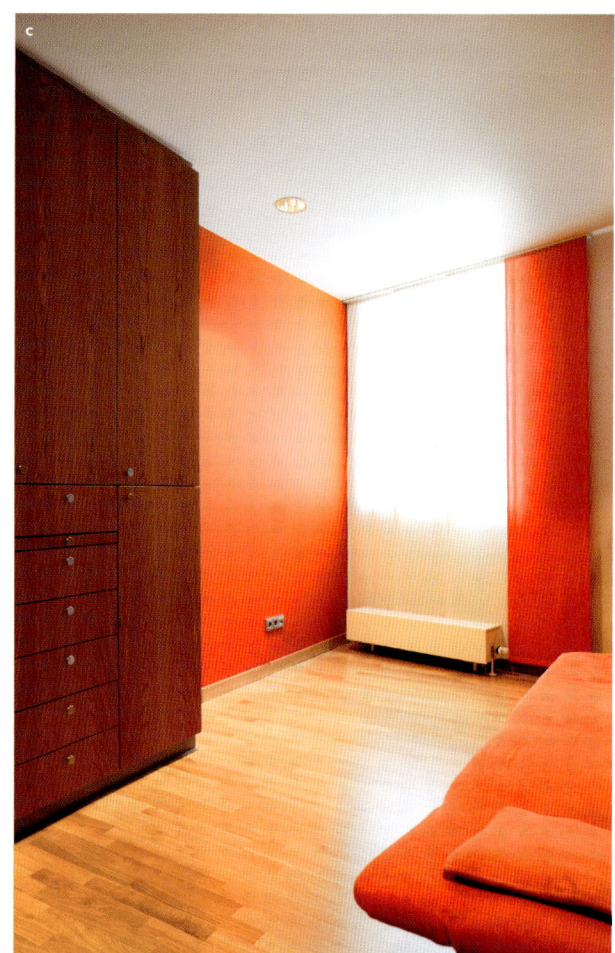

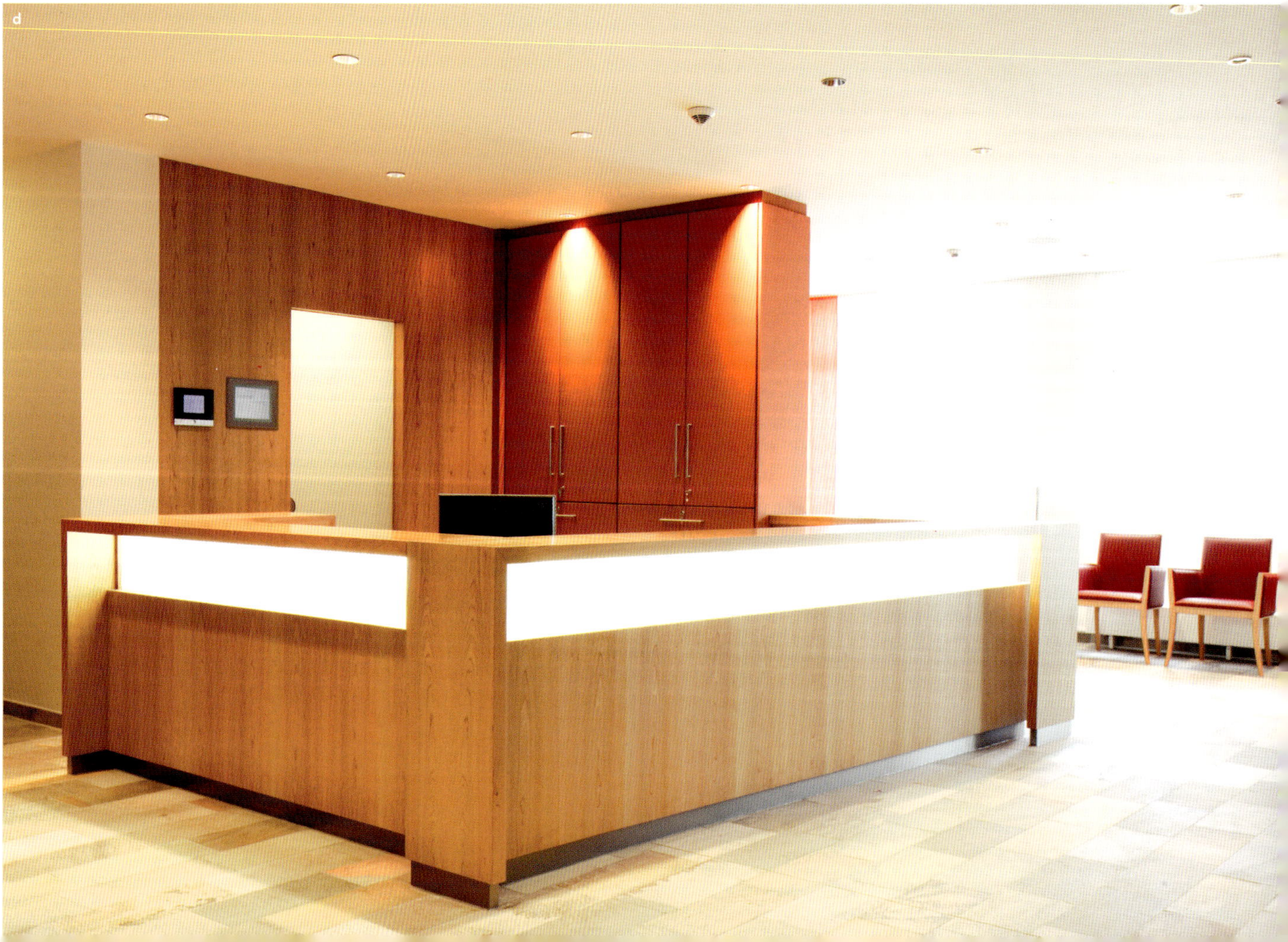

Client	Detlef Knechtel
Operator	"Sanitas"
	Therapy Centre
Planning time	08 2006 – 11 2006
Construction time	12 2006 – 04 2007
Gross floor area	930 sqm
Usable floor space	633 sqm
Gross cubic capacity	2,700 cbm

a   The therapy pool is separated from the
    foyer by a partition wall made of special-
    purpose glass.
b   Warm orange and red colours make the
    walls appear like cubatures placed in the
    room.
c   The visual surfaces in the practice are
    characterised by natural materials –
    colour-changing natural stone flooring,
    bright parquet flooring and cherrywood
    furniture.
d   On entering the therapy centre, patients
    are taken aback at the spacious impres-
    sion they get of the reception and the
    waiting area.

Floor plan layout

The highly-structured floor plan for the multiple practice enables clear
guidance for the patients, who are able to access both wings of the building from a central waiting area via the reception. Four treatment rooms
do not receive natural light. Unfortunately only one of the large treatment
rooms exits directly to the outside. No dedicated areas have been provided
for administration, stock, supplies or cleaning.

Usable floor spaces

Patient rooms	**yellow**	129 sqm	20 %
Examination |			
Treatment rooms	**red**	173 sqm	27 %
Specialist rooms	**pink**	297 sqm	47 %
Offices | Staff rooms	**orange**	28 sqm	5 %
Plant rooms	**blue**	6 sqm	1 %
Total		633 sqm	100 %

In the listed "Schranne", the former grain storehouse of the city of Mindelheim, an extensive, open-plan dental practice has been created which spans the whole storey.

The loft-like room, not supported by any pillars, is structured with the aid of freestanding room sculptures placed in its different functional areas — reception, waiting area and treatment unit — accentuating the room's effect. The deliberate absence of colour blurs the transitions between furniture, walls and ceiling and condenses them to the point where they overlap. The unbroken unity of the room is effectively supported by the jointless, dark grey Pandomo stone flooring. The organic design concept of the furniture is continued in the illuminated ceiling which spans the whole room. An innovative lighting concept with changeable light colours for different moods hides the ceiling panels hanging behind. The rooms intended for patients are almost all open-plan, while office and staff rooms and the laboratory are designed to be self-contained. The idea behind the unconventional interior design of the large treatment room is to minimise the distances for the attending physicians and to make it easy for patients to move around.

**LANDAU +
KINDELBACHER**

ORTHODONTIC CLINIC
MINDELHEIM | G

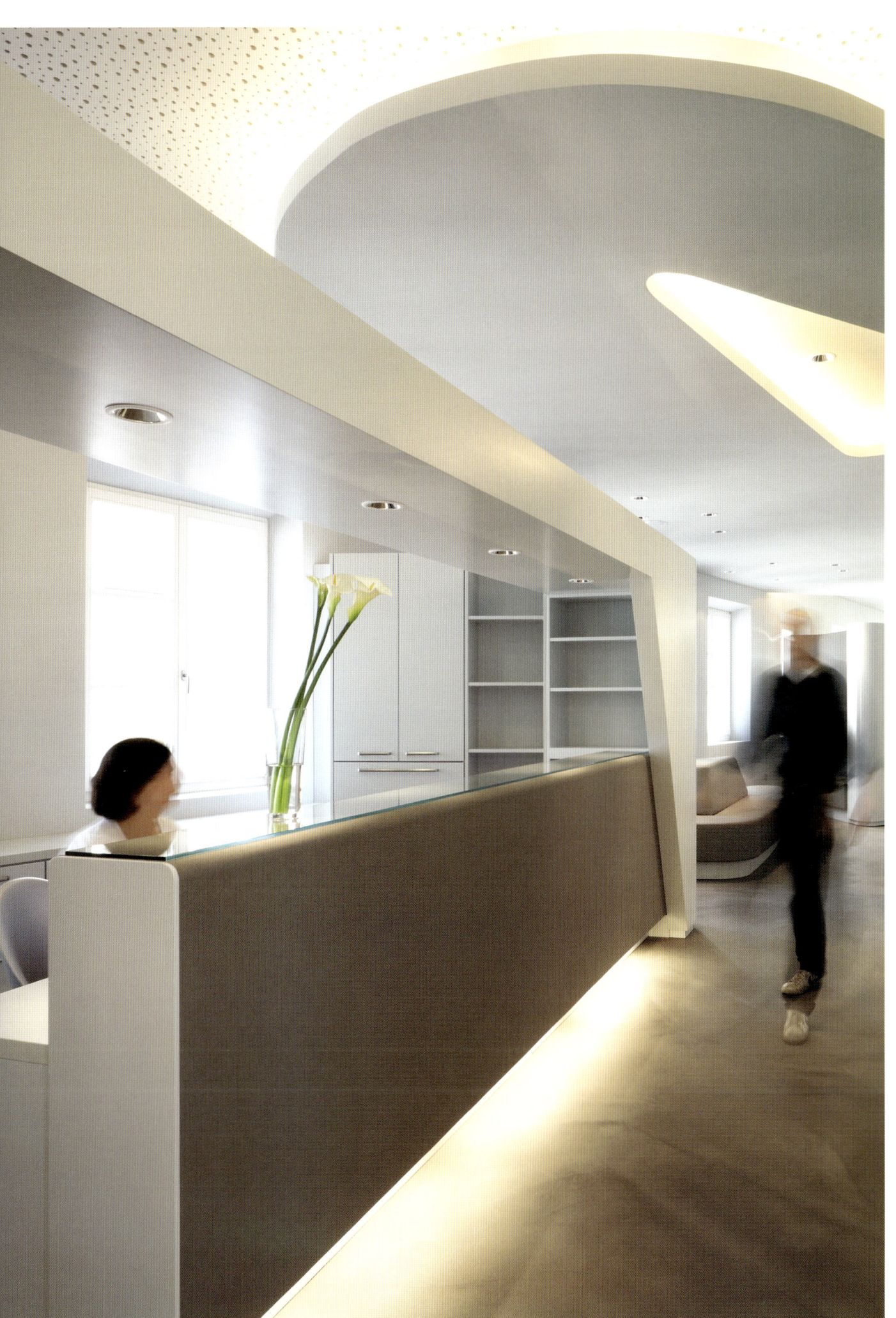

a

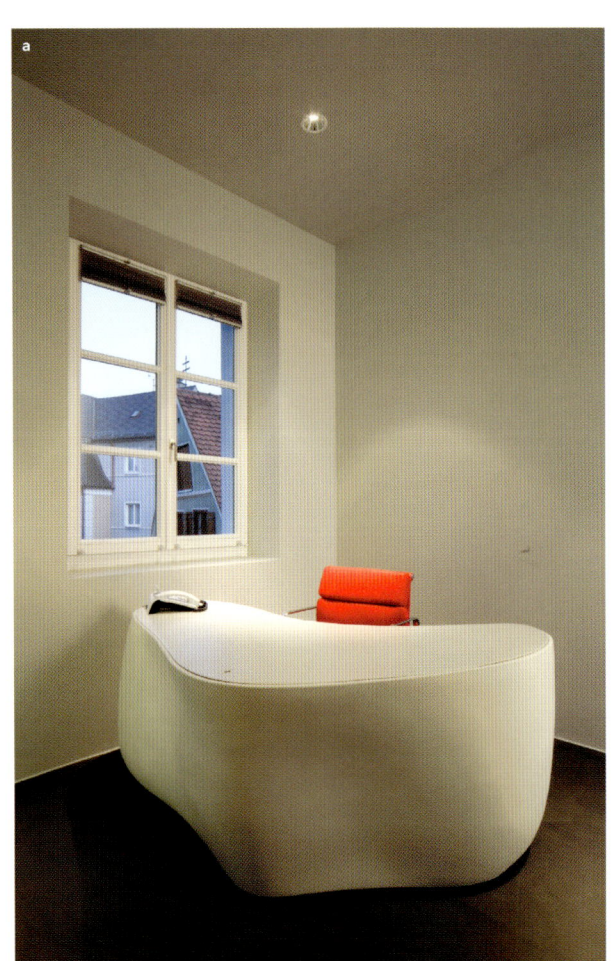

b

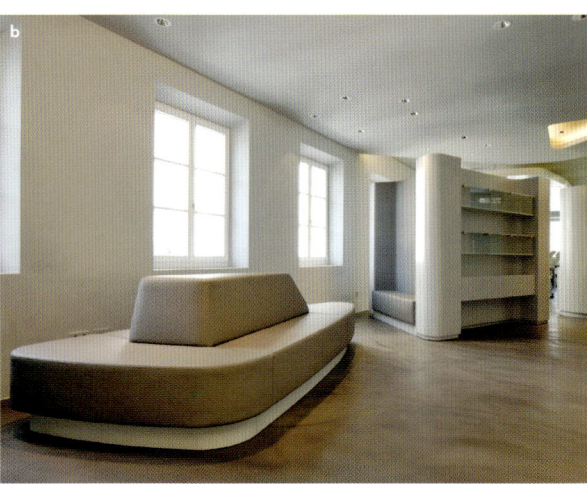

c

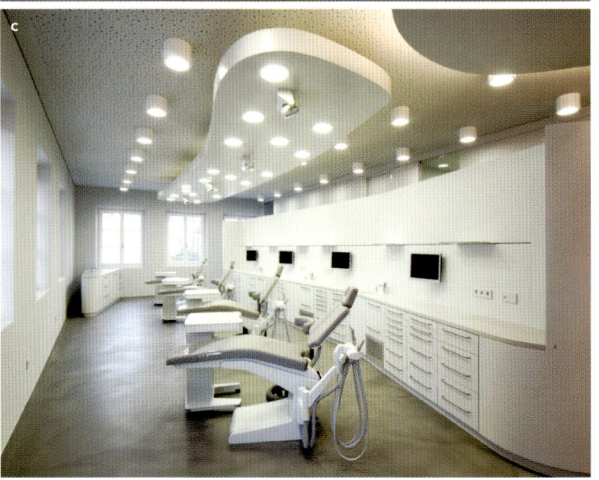

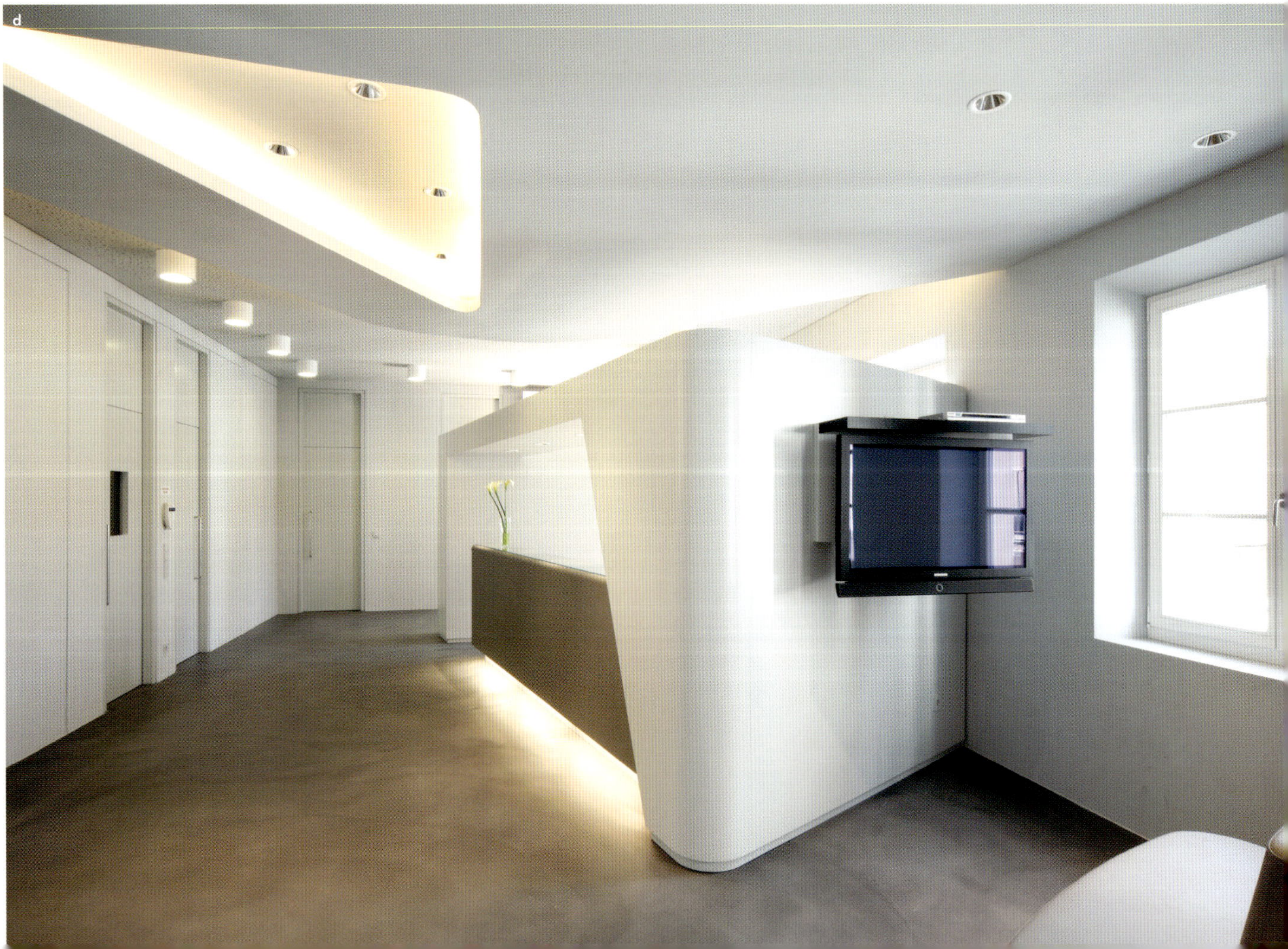

d

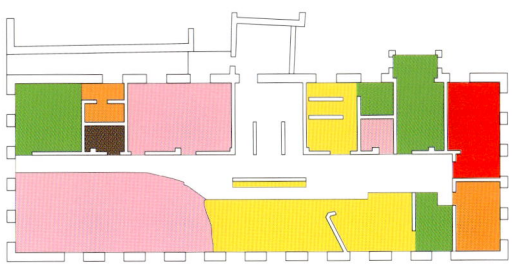

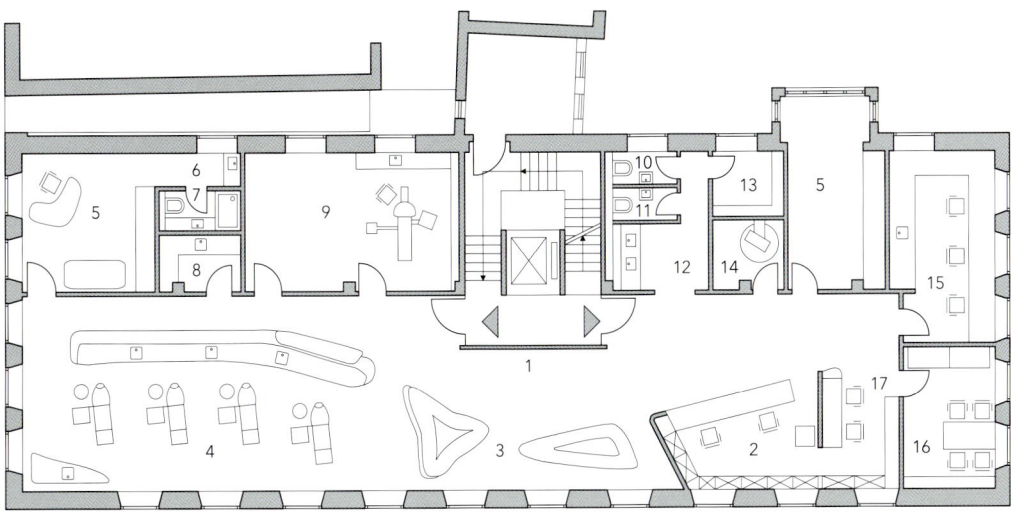

GF

Client	Operator	Dr. Eleni Stylianidou
Planning time	09 2005 – 04 2007
Construction time	10 2006 – 04 2007
Usable floor space	197 sqm
Total cost	600,000 EUR

a The absence of colour – apart from the red office chair which acts as an eye-catcher – blurs the transitions between furniture, walls and ceiling and condenses them to the point where they overlap.

b The loft-like reception and waiting area is structured with the aid of freestanding room sculptures, which accentuate the room's effect.

c The four side-by-side treatment units mean shorter journeys for the doctors, but the open layout may seem rather unusual for the patients.

d The unbroken unity of the room is impressively supported by the jointless Pandomo stone flooring.

Diagrammatic plans, to scale 1:400
Floor plans, to scale 1:200

Floor plan layout

1 Coat-rack
2 Reception
3 Waiting area
4 Treatment room
5 Office
6 Small kitchen
7 Staff toilet

and shower
8 Sterilisation room
9 Consultation and
   treatment room
10 Patient toilet G
11 Patient toilet L
12 Hygiene

13 Filing room
14 Examination X-ray
15 Laboratory
16 Staff lounge and
   small kitchen
17 Office

Patients access a large area, occupying almost the entire length of the floor plan, via the entrance situated in the centre of the long rectangular floor plan of this single-doctor practice. All the rooms in the medical practice can be accessed from this room. The layout means that almost all the rooms receive natural light, but it does make it necessary to walk long distances and might bring a certain turmoil to the open-plan treatment rooms.

Usable floor spaces

Patient rooms	**yellow**	50 sqm	25 %
Examination | Treatment rooms	**red**	16 sqm	8 %
Specialist rooms	**pink**	80 sqm	41 %
Administrative rooms	**green**	31 sqm	16 %
Offices | Staff rooms	**orange**	16 sqm	8 %
Supply | Waste disposal	**brown**	4 sqm	2 %
Total		197 sqm	100 %

Performance data

Outpatients per year	800
Services to other clinics	Dental treatments Orthodontic interventions
Clinic opening hours	5 days | 35 hours
Waiting time	10 – 30 min.
Number of staff	11

An ostentatious glass extension encloses one of the narrow sides of the listed house dating from the turn of the 19th century, where a dental practice is situated over the space of two floors. During planning, the architects were confronted by many challenges as the structure of the floor plan needed to be maintained.

In order to create an open and pleasant atmosphere in the room, the partition walls to the corridor have been removed in the reception and waiting-room area and a light glass wall was installed to the staircase. The fact that the examination and treatment rooms are interconnected means that there is unhindered passage for doctors and staff on both floors. The material used is bright and friendly, giving expanse and clarity to the rooms. European maple, satin stainless steel, etched glass, white Resopal and bright linoleum flooring have been used in their natural colours and textures and can therefore be experienced in all their haptic quality. While the furnishings in the foyer are made of maple, the pieces of furniture in the functional units present a white Resopal surface. One characteristic design feature in the practice is the illuminated orientation system, which replaces the need for normal door signs.

LANDAU + KINDELBACHER

DENTAL PRACTICE
ALTENBURG | G

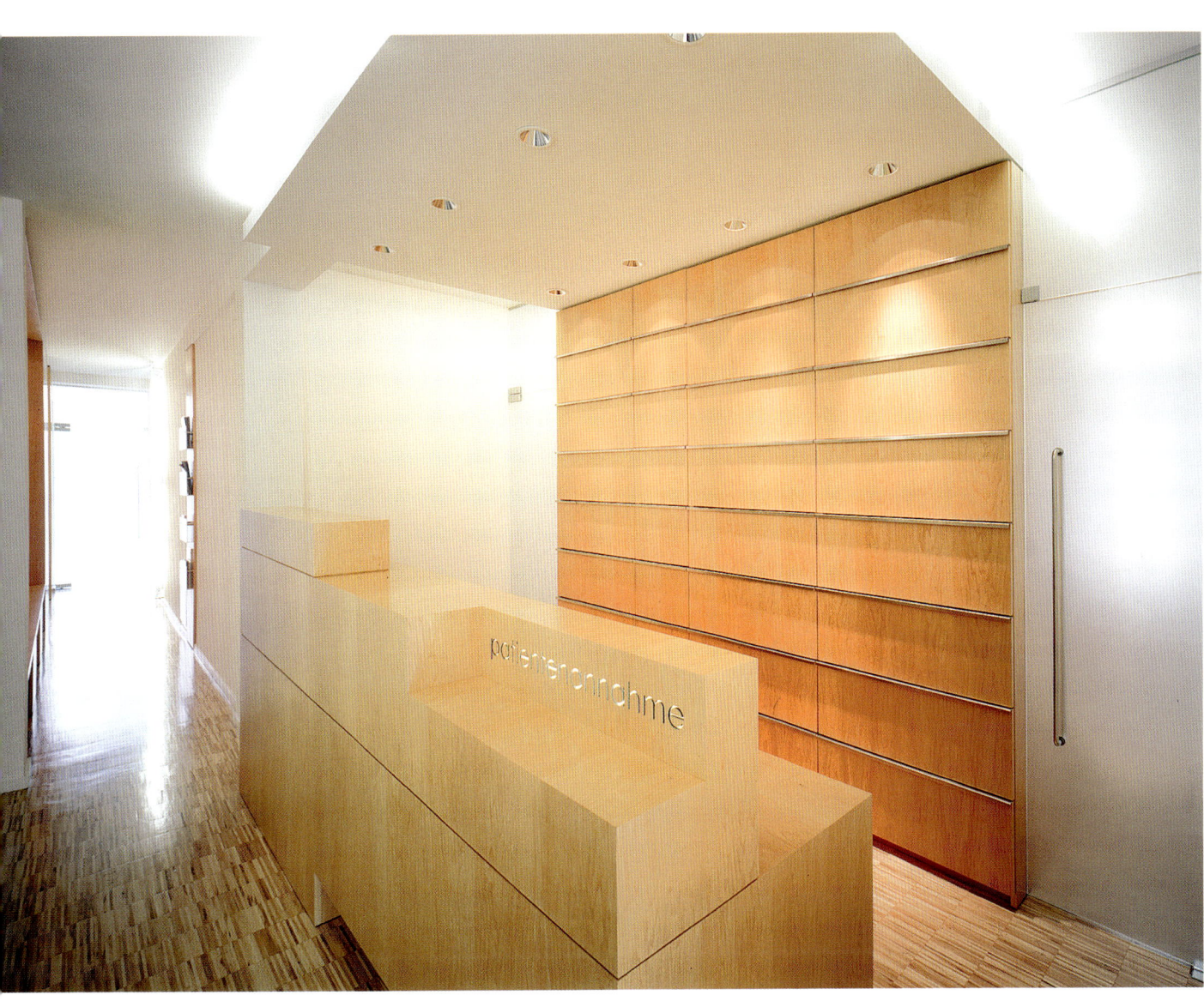

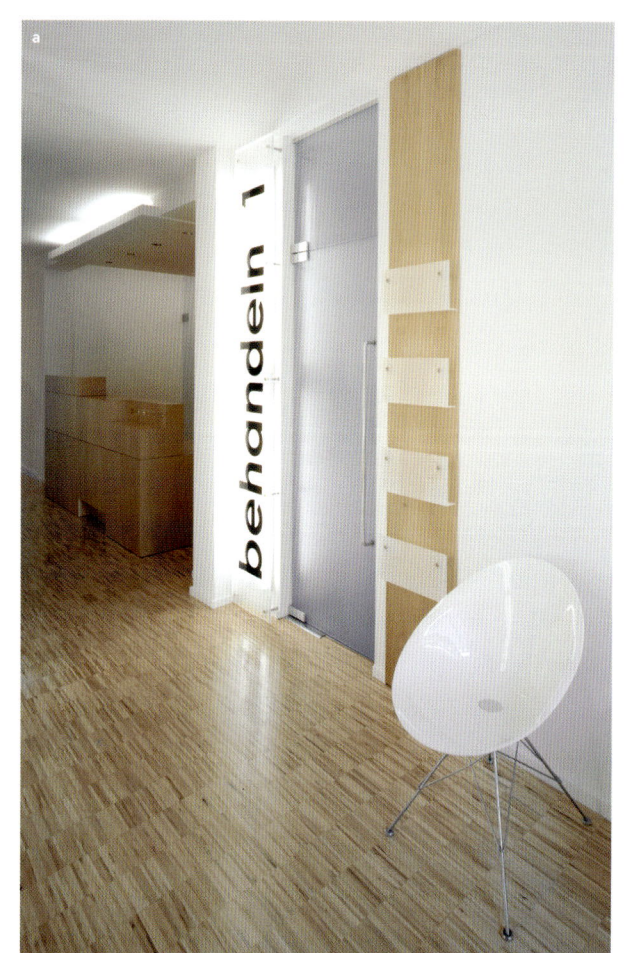

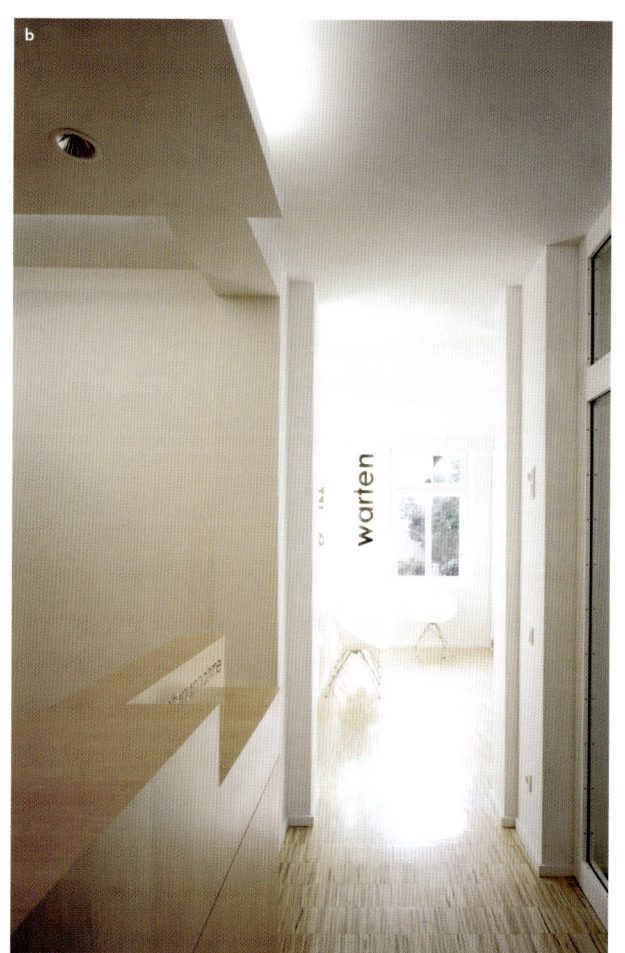

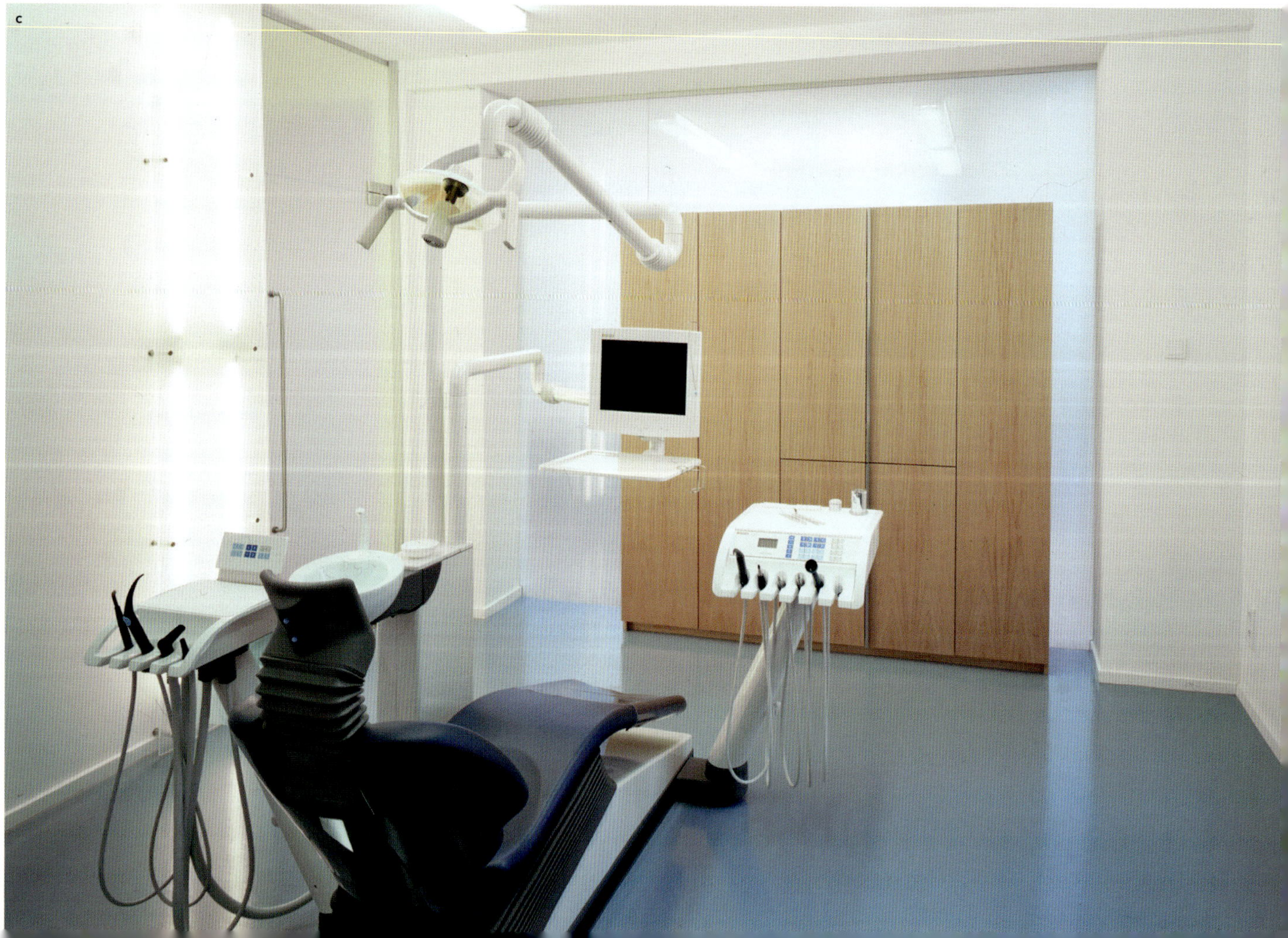

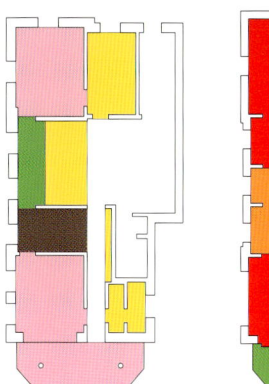
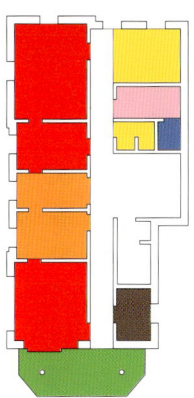

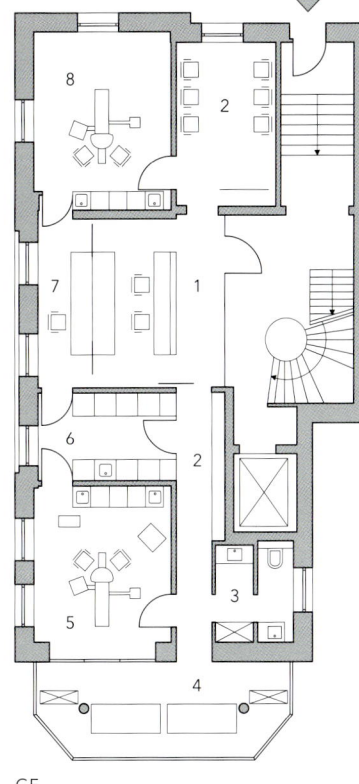

GF

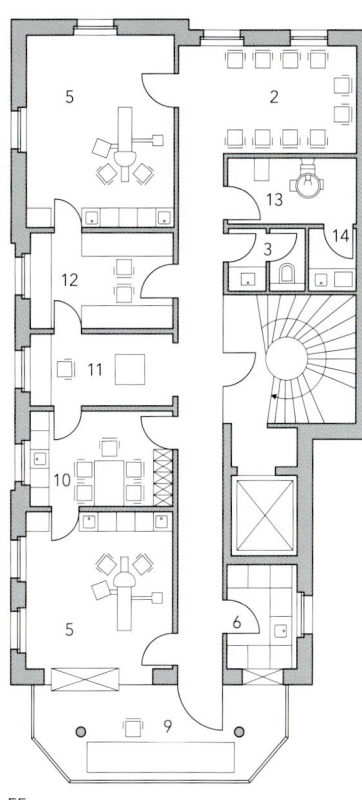

FF

Client	Operator	Dr. Steffen Dietel
	Dr. Ellen Dietel
Planning time	2003
Construction time	2003
Usable floor space	234 sqm

a A graphic, backlit orientation system does the job that door signs normally do.

b The waiting area has no doors, so as to convey an open, pleasant atmosphere.

c The use of bright, friendly material gives a sense of expanse and clarity to the treatment rooms.

Diagrammatic plans, to scale 1:400
Floor plans, to scale 1:200

Floor plan layout

1	Reception	**7**	Office	**11**	Office
2	Waiting area	**8**	Treatment room	**12**	Laboratory
3	Patient toilet		prevention	**13**	Examination X-ray
4	Recovery room	**9**	Office	**14**	Developing room
5	Examination	**10**	Staff lounge and		
6	Sterilisation room		changing cubicle		

At one corner of the long floor plan of this partnership practice, several steps take patients to the reception room with waiting area on the side. There are two treatment rooms on the ground floor, and three others with waiting area on the upper floor, which the patients can access via the central staircase or the lift. The central corridors on both floors make it easy for patients to find their way. All rooms receive natural light.

Usable floor spaces

Patient rooms	**yellow**	49 sqm	21 %
Examination			
Treatment rooms	**red**	56 sqm	24 %
Specialist rooms	**pink**	65 sqm	28 %
Administrative rooms	**green**	26 sqm	11 %
Offices	Staff rooms	**orange**	20 sqm	8 %
Supply	Waste disposal	**brown**	16 sqm	7 %
Plant rooms	**blue**	2 sqm	1 %
Total		234 sqm	100 %

Performance data

Outpatients per year	4,000 – 5,000
Services to other clinics	Orthodontics [200]
Clinic opening hours	5 days	50 hours
Waiting time [with	without appointment]	10 – 20 min.
	30 – 45 min.
Type and number of staff	2 doctors
	6 full-time staff
	2 trainees

Precision, professionalism and individuality, caution and confidence, care and cure, beauty and perfection, as we know them in nature, are all welcome aspects in this new dental clinic, appreciated by patients and staff alike.

Gently curved walls conduct patients and members of staff through the extensive rooms; light strips embedded in the ceiling emphasise the routing system dynamics. Opposite the spacious reception area is a lounge-like waiting area. Wall ornaments, reminiscent of young blades of grass, transform the open-plan waiting area into a place of contemplation. A pink corridor interlinks both practice wings. Different colour schemes help divide the premises into dental treatment, operation, oral hygiene and supply sections. Design features and materials point to nature and are metaphors for aspects like wellness, health and perfection. Abstract graphics of teeth are more evocative floral ornaments or water droplets. Unostentatious treatment rooms, which inspire a certain approachability and sense of protection, are situated within this area of creative interaction. Colourful eye-catching features – a yellow treatment chair for example – have the effect of playfully relaxing the atmosphere.

ANNETTE LIPPMANN

DENTAL CLINIC
SINDELFINGEN | G

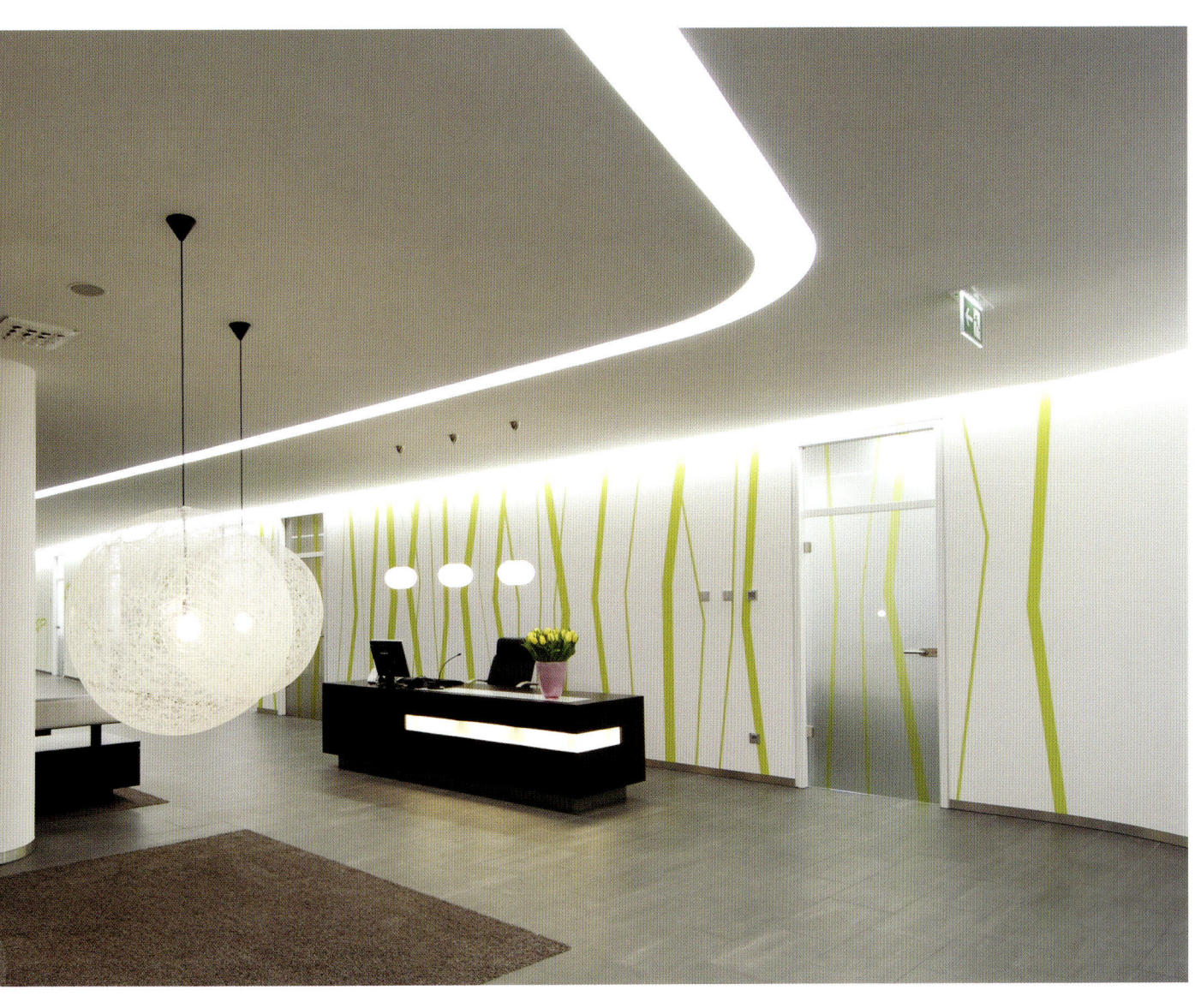

a

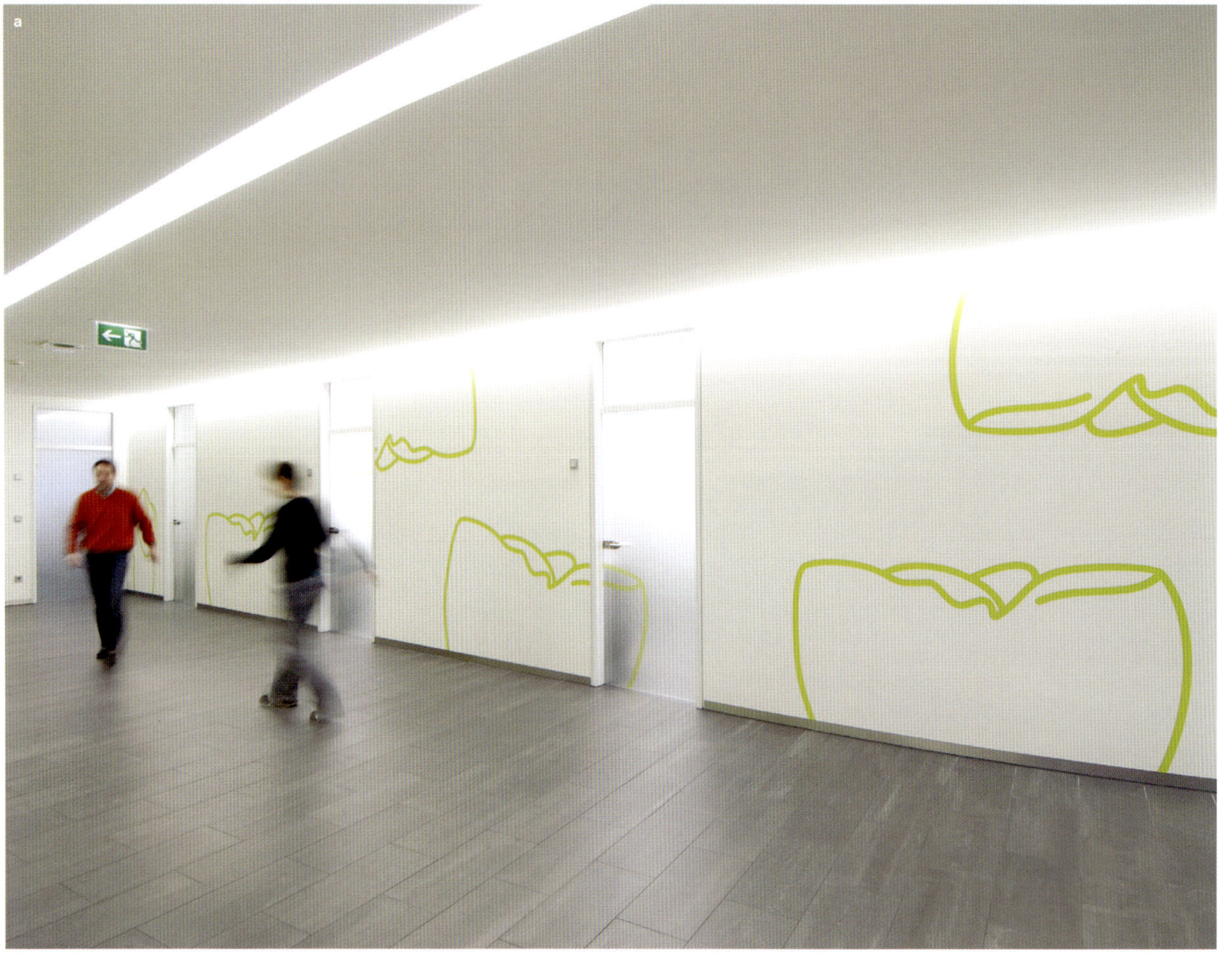

b

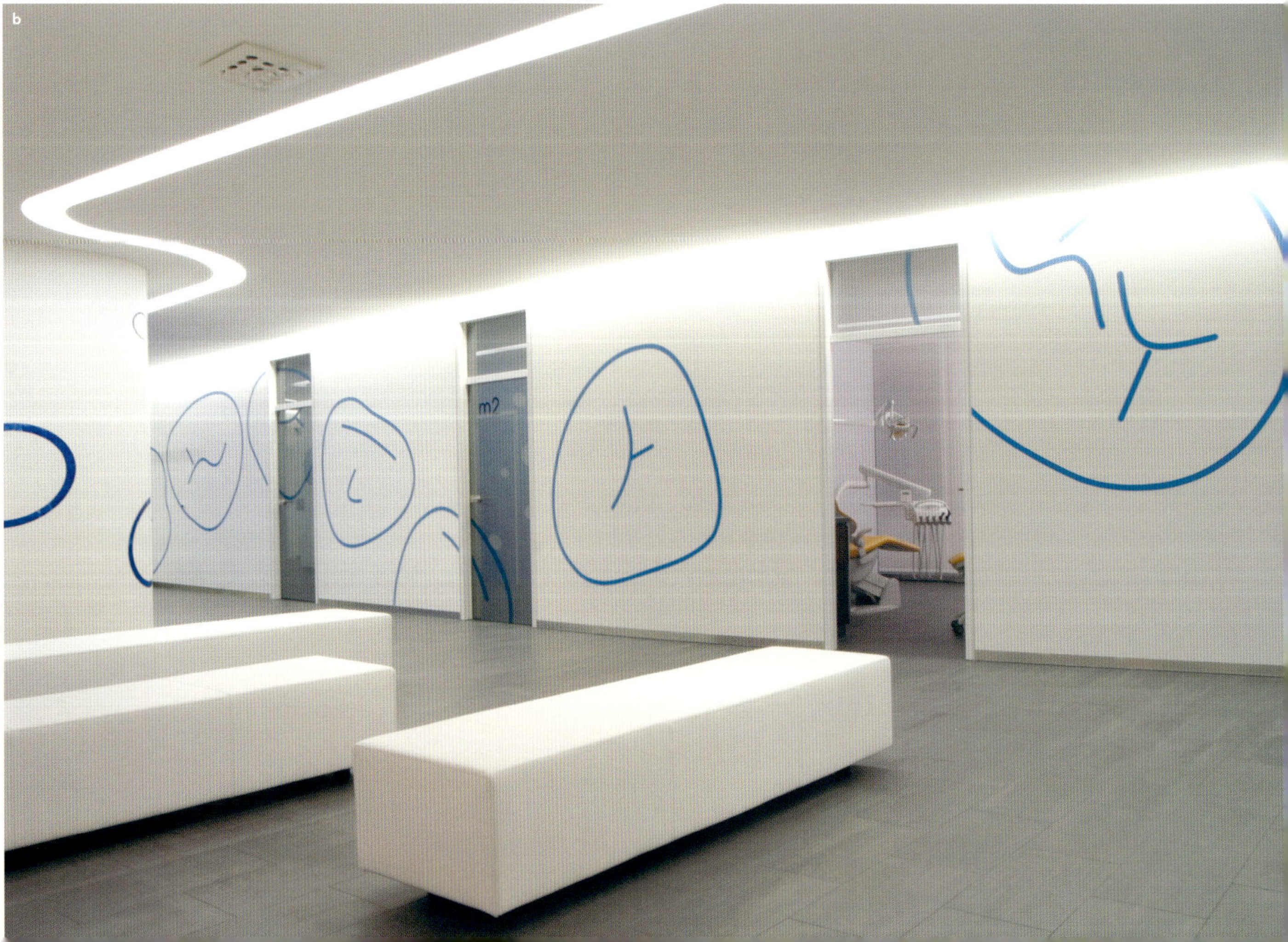

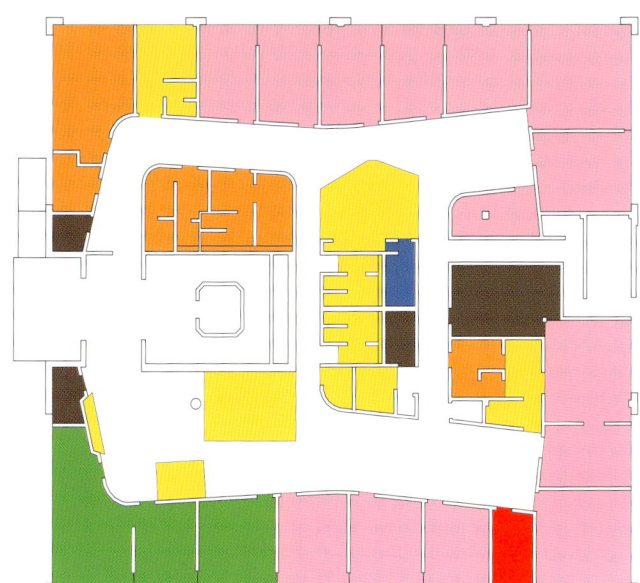

1 Waiting area
2 Reception
3 Office
4 Coat-rack
5 Store room
6 Nurses' office
7 Staff lounge
8 Hospital room
9 Treatment room
   oral hygiene
10 Treatment room
11 Examination X-ray
12 Sterilisation room
13 Staff changing
   cubicle
14 Patient sluice
15 Patient changing
   cubicle
16 Operating theatre
17 Recovery room
18 Laboratory
19 Consultation room
20 Staff shower
21 Staff changing
   cubicle G
22 Staff toilet G
23 Staff toilet L
24 Staff changing
   cubicle L
25 Patient toilet G
26 Patient toilet L
27 Installations room
28 Toilet for the
   disabled
29 Refreshment room

Diagrammatic plans, to scale 1:400
Floor plans, to scale 1:200

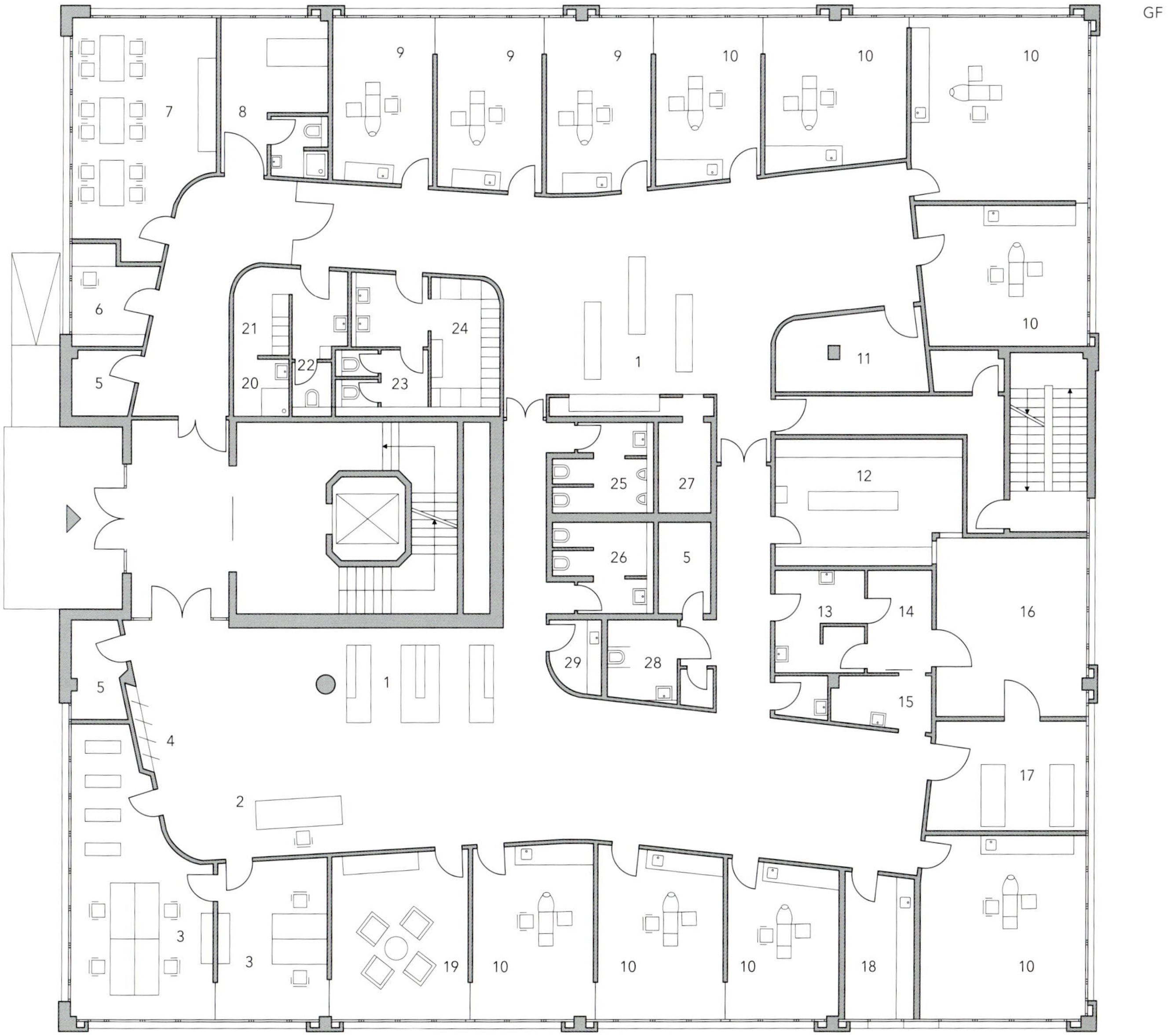

GF

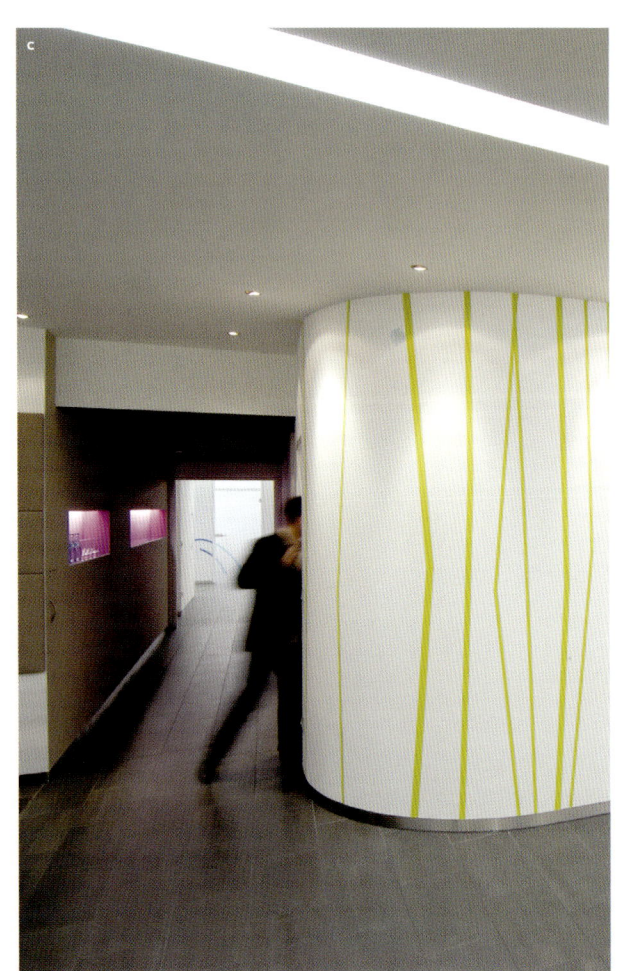

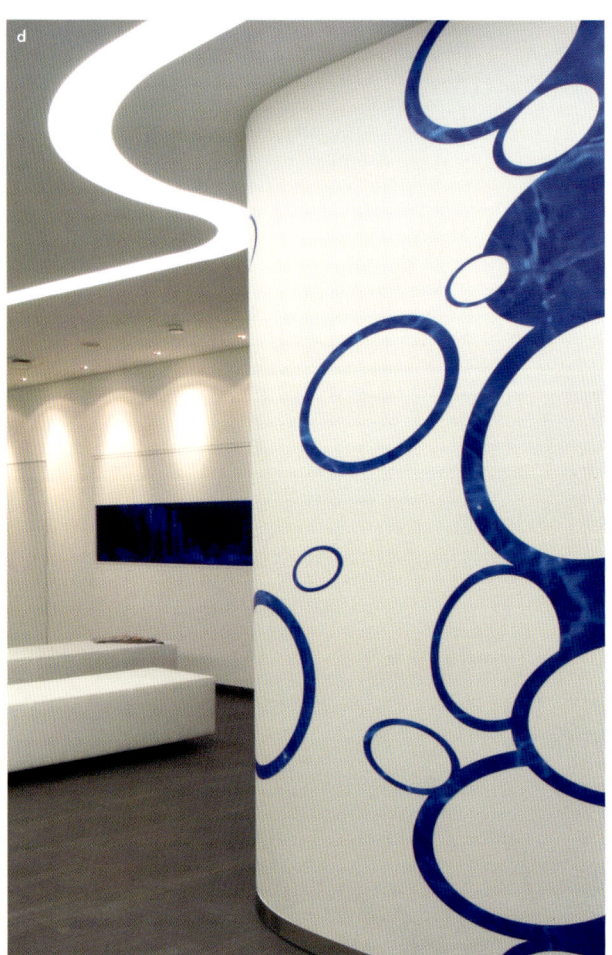

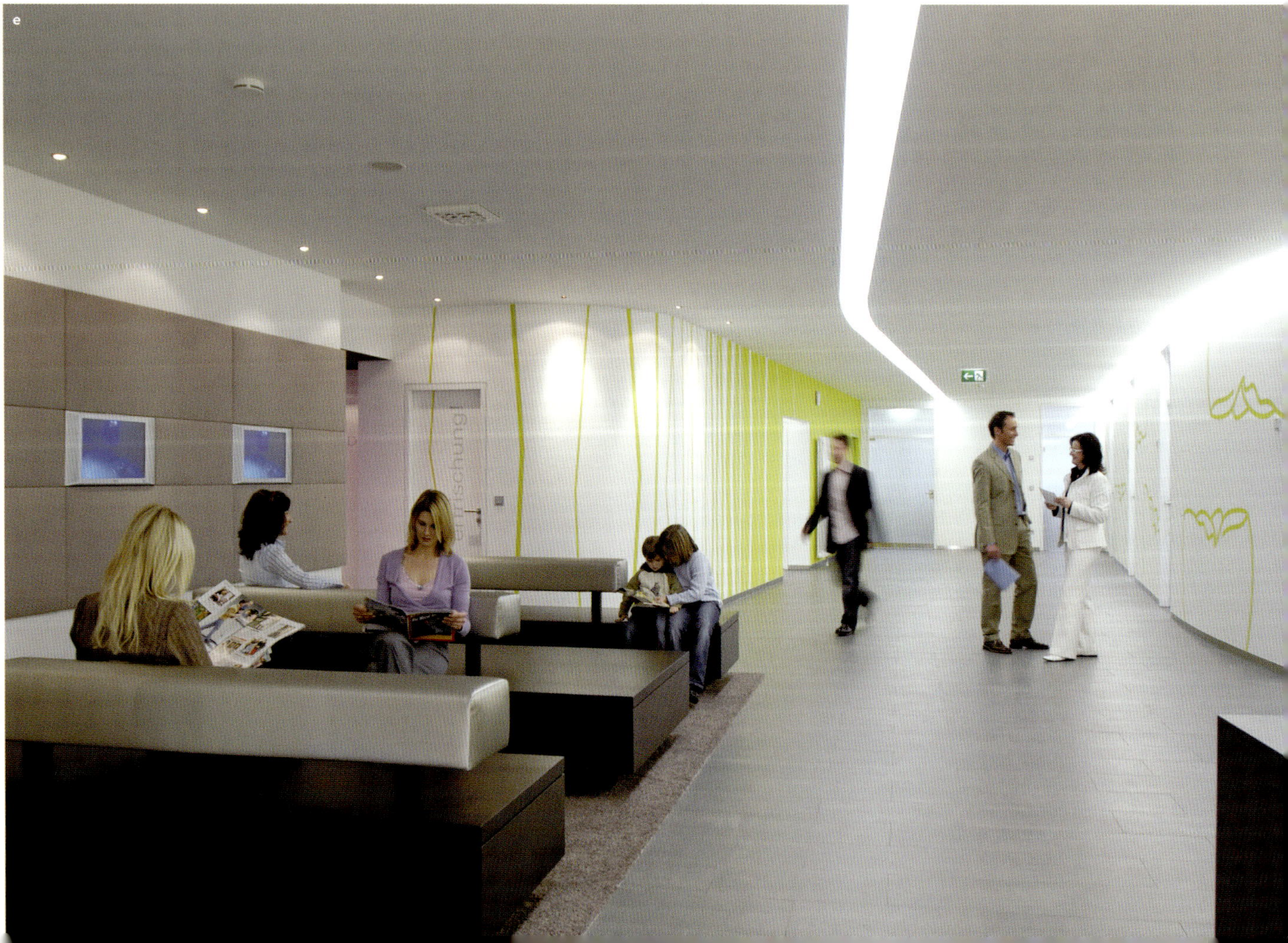

Client	Operator	Dr. Wolfgang Dinkelacker
	Dr. Oliver Brendel
Planning time	02 2005 – 07 2005
Construction time	07 2005 – 12 2005
Gross floor area	1,020 sqm
Usable floor space	645 sqm
Gross cubic capacity	3,519 cbm
Construction cost	741,846 EUR
Total cost	1,394,941 EUR

a Pictures and details of human molars adorn the walls, resembling water droplets and flower ornaments.

b Different colour schemes help divide the clinic into dental treatment, operation, oral hygiene and supply sections.

c Wall ornaments, reminiscent of young blades of grass, transform the open-plan waiting area into a place of calming contemplation.

d Gently curved walls and light bands in the ceiling conduct patients and employees through the extensive rooms.

e The lounge-like waiting area is connected to the spacious reception area.

Floor plan layout

The access point on the square floor plan of this multiple practice and clinic with two wide, curved corridors is in the centre of one of the sides of the square; the somewhat wider of the two doors points towards the reception. Diagonally opposite is one of the waiting areas, which is easy to identify; the second waiting area is accessed via a passage. The walking distances, due to the size of the floor plan, are justifiable on account of its square shape. The rooms without natural light are not absolutely dependent on it.

Usable floor spaces

Patient rooms	**yellow**	109 sqm	17 %
Examination |			
Treatment rooms	**red**	11 sqm	2 %
Specialist rooms	**pink**	312 sqm	48 %
Administrative rooms	**green**	79 sqm	12 %
Offices | Staff rooms	**orange**	87 sqm	14 %
Supply | Waste disposal	**brown**	41 sqm	6 %
Plant rooms	**blue**	6 sqm	1 %
Total		645 sqm	100 %

Performance data

Outpatients per year	20,000
Services to other clinics	DNA bacteria test
	Histology
	Oral surgery
	[2,000]
Clinic opening hours	5 – 6 days
	60 – 70 hours
Waiting time	10 min.
Type and number of staff	4 doctors
	20 full-time staff
	2 part-time staff
	1 trainee

An open-plan, transparent and extremely communicative practice has been created in the alleyway of a Biedermeier house in Josefstadt Vienna, notwithstanding the small space available.

This has been achieved thanks to the use of a limited number of colours and materials: The whole floor including the seating furniture in the waiting, play and therapy area, are covered with light green rubber, as if they were all of a piece, and the walls gleam with the same delicate lime green throughout. The whole practice consists of two larger rooms facing the street and a small kitchen facing the courtyard. The necessary transparency between both main rooms, which are subdivided into several areas, is provided by an aperture. At ground level facing the street are the entrance with coat-rack and parking area for prams. The combined waiting and play area is situated behind a bench with integrated storage space. The vibrant red of the wall-mounted backrest and the cube seat creates an interesting eye-catching feature. The ophthalmologist's workplace is situated in the second room: a large sliding door can easily turn it into a self-contained space, creating a sense of intimacy. The consultation area with classical side table and Thonet chairs forms an appealing contrast to the streamlined, modern design of the rest of the practice.

LOOPING ARCHITECTURE

CHILDREN'S EYE CENTRE
VIENNA | A

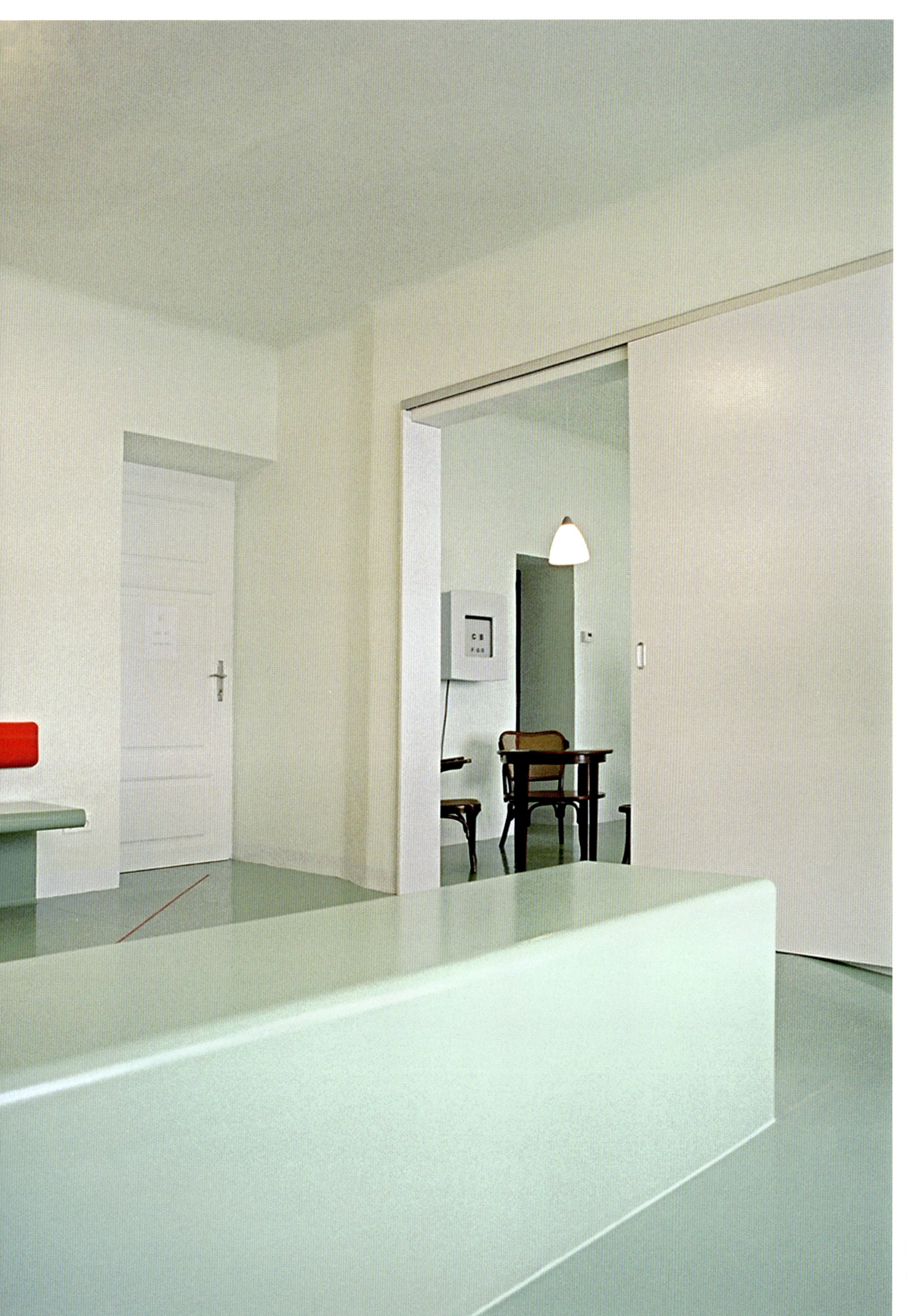

a

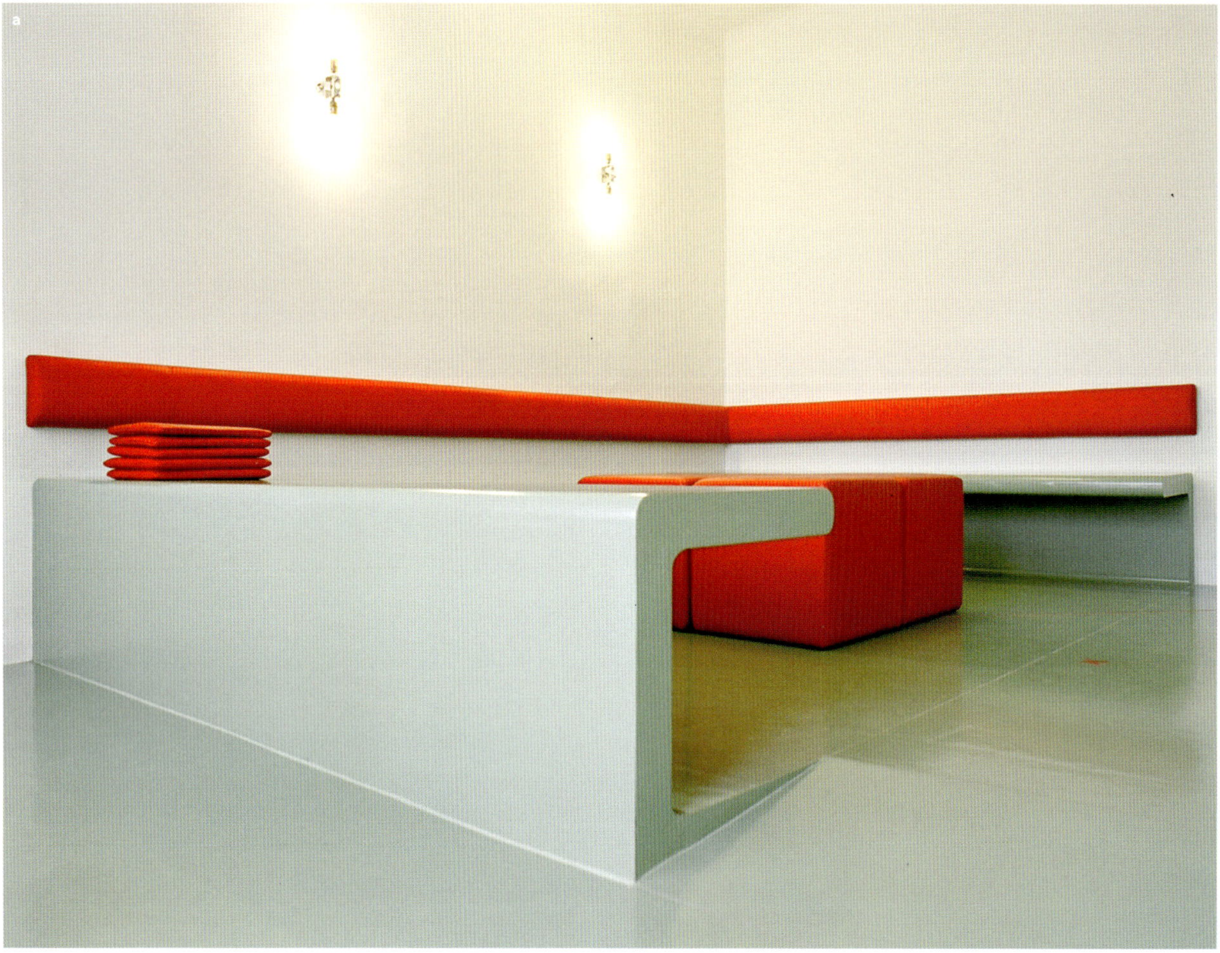

b

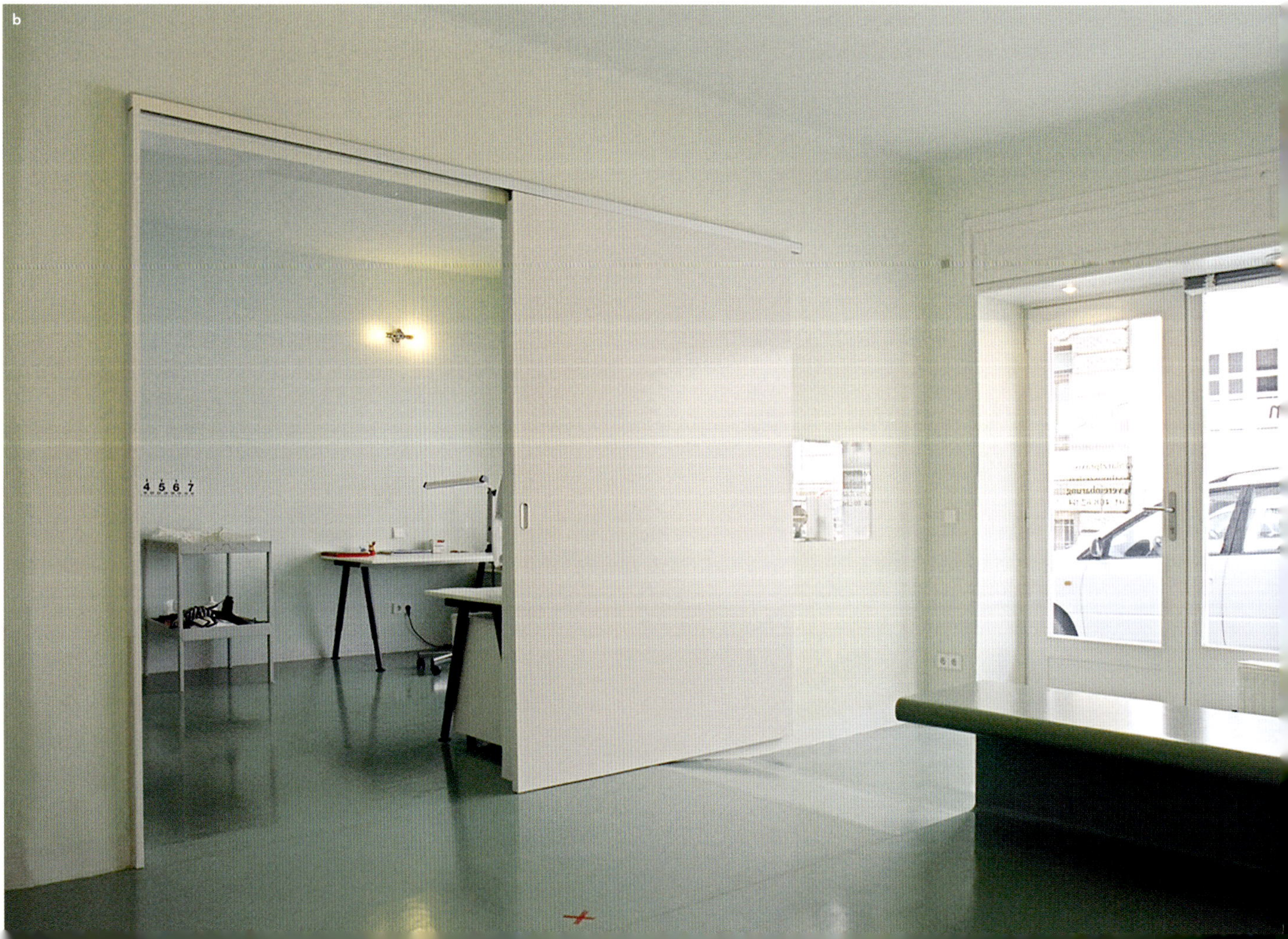

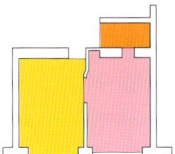

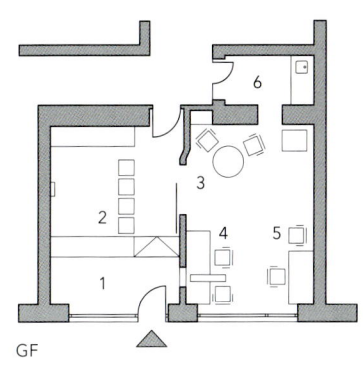

GF

Client	Prof. Dr. Andrea
	Müllner-Eidenböck
	Christine Weinzierl
Operator	Prof. Dr. Andrea
	Müllner-Eidenböck
Planning time	04 2005 – 05 2005
Construction time	05 2005 – 06 2005
Usable floor space	45 sqm
Gross cubic capacity	135 cbm
Construction cost	29,000 EUR

a The whole floor, and the seating furniture in the waiting, play and therapy areas, are covered with light green rubber to create a unified look.

b A large sliding door allows the ophthalmologist's working zone to be partitioned off from the waiting area.

Diagrammatic plans, to scale 1:400
Floor plans, to scale 1:200

Floor plan layout

1 Coat-rack **4** Workplace therapy
2 Lounge **5** Workplace **6** Small kitchen
3 Consultation room

This single-doctor practice only has three rooms, located quite near the entrance. Except for the waiting area and the small kitchen, all medical functions requiring a usable floor space are concentrated in one room. Both larger rooms have natural light, the small kitchen receives light through the doors. The toilet for patients and for staff is located in the corridor of the Biedermeier house.

Usable floor spaces

Patient rooms	**yellow**	21 sqm	47 %
Specialist rooms	**pink**	20 sqm	44 %
Offices | Staff rooms	**orange**	4 sqm	9 %
Total		45 sqm	100 %

Performance data

Outpatients per year	800
Clinic opening hours	2 days | 5 – 10 hours
Waiting time	none
Number of staff	1 – 2

Next to the turbulent Frankfurt "Fressgass", the practice clinic at the old opera provides a place of peace and tranquillity. An aesthetically appealing and individual practice for plastic surgery has been created on the upper floor of the new building.

In its simple elegance, far from resembling a conventional and sterile medical supply space, the reception boast a puristically austere desk, made of Wenge-coloured wood, which evokes that of a prestigious hotel. Specially-designed stone walls made of anthracite-coloured artificial stone attract the attention. Thanks to the bright, light-toned walls and the warm shade of the "Ipé-Lapacho" parquet [Brazilian walnut], the corridor appears exceptionally elegant. The consultation and treatment rooms are situated behind ceiling-high wooden doors. On the other side of the building is the surgical wing, with recovery room, patient rooms, sterile and social rooms. The operating room is equipped with state-of-the-art technology and a clean-air ceiling. Both patient rooms – as is the case for the whole practice – are equipped to a high standard and furnished like elegant hotel rooms, with the cosy design hiding sophisticated technology. The large roundarched windows in the practice rooms exude a special charm. In addition to these windows, the wide pools of ceiling light provides atmospheric illumination.

EVA LOREY

PRACTICE CLINIC AT THE OLD OPERA
FRANKFURT ON THE MAIN | G

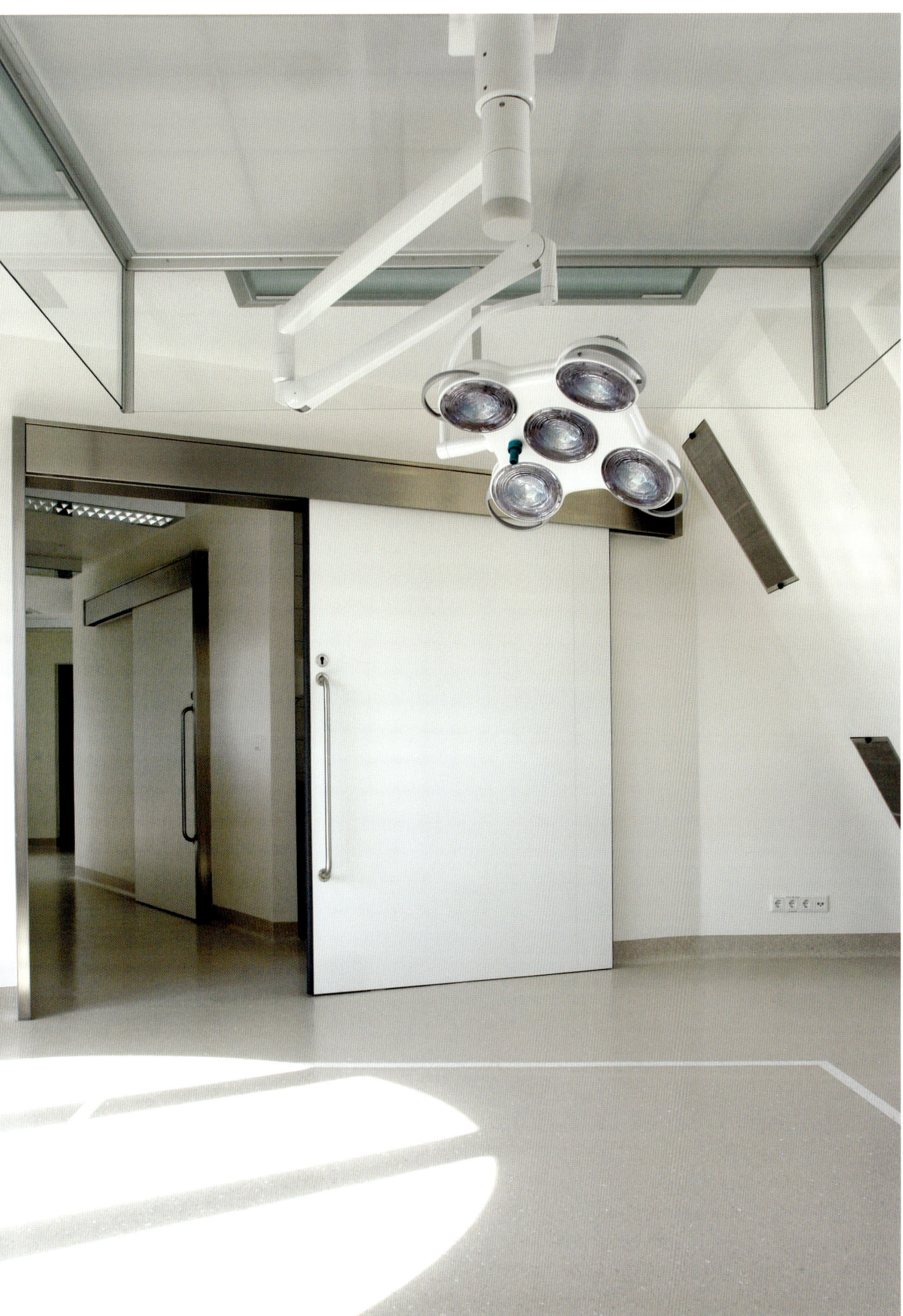

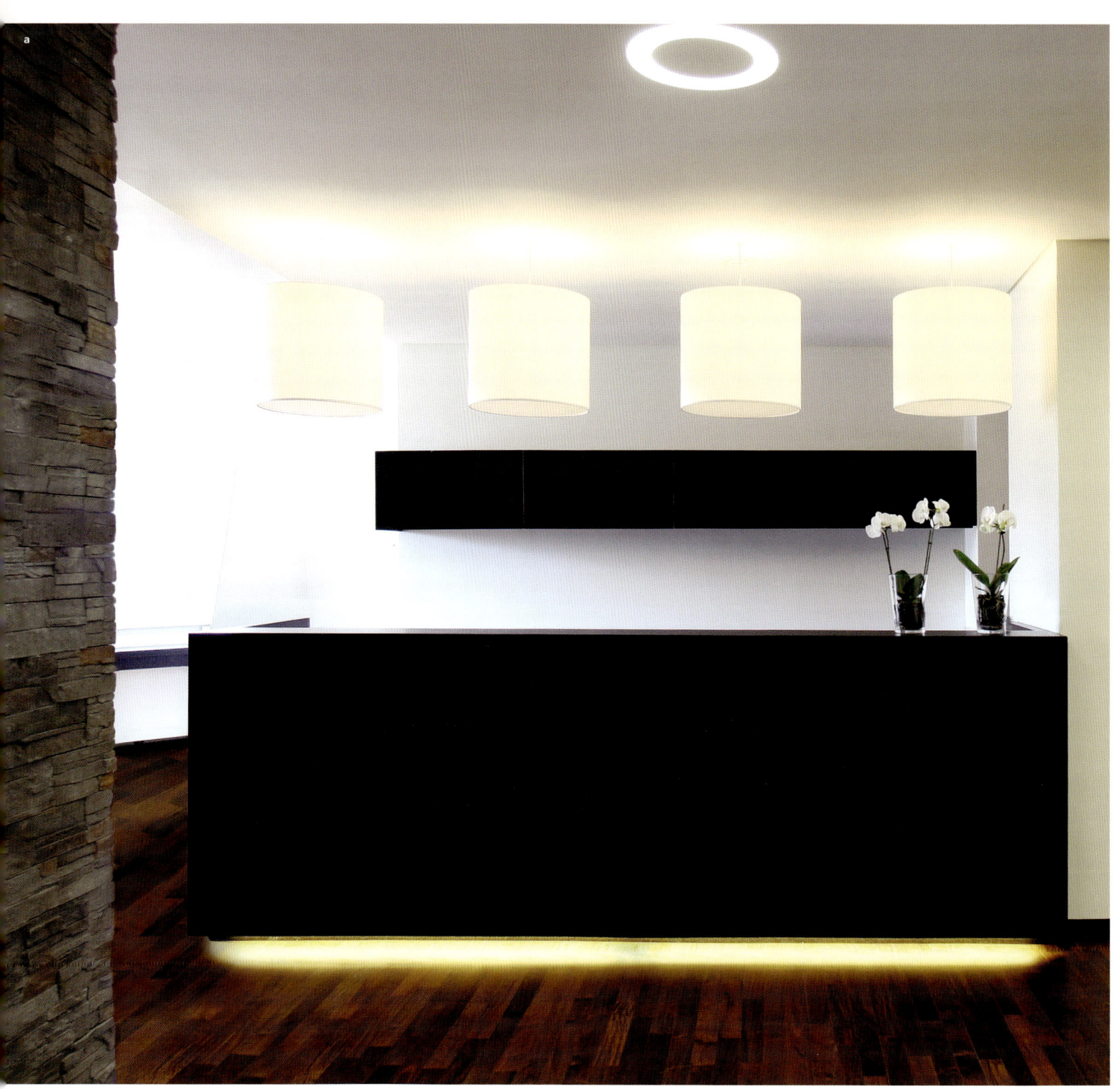

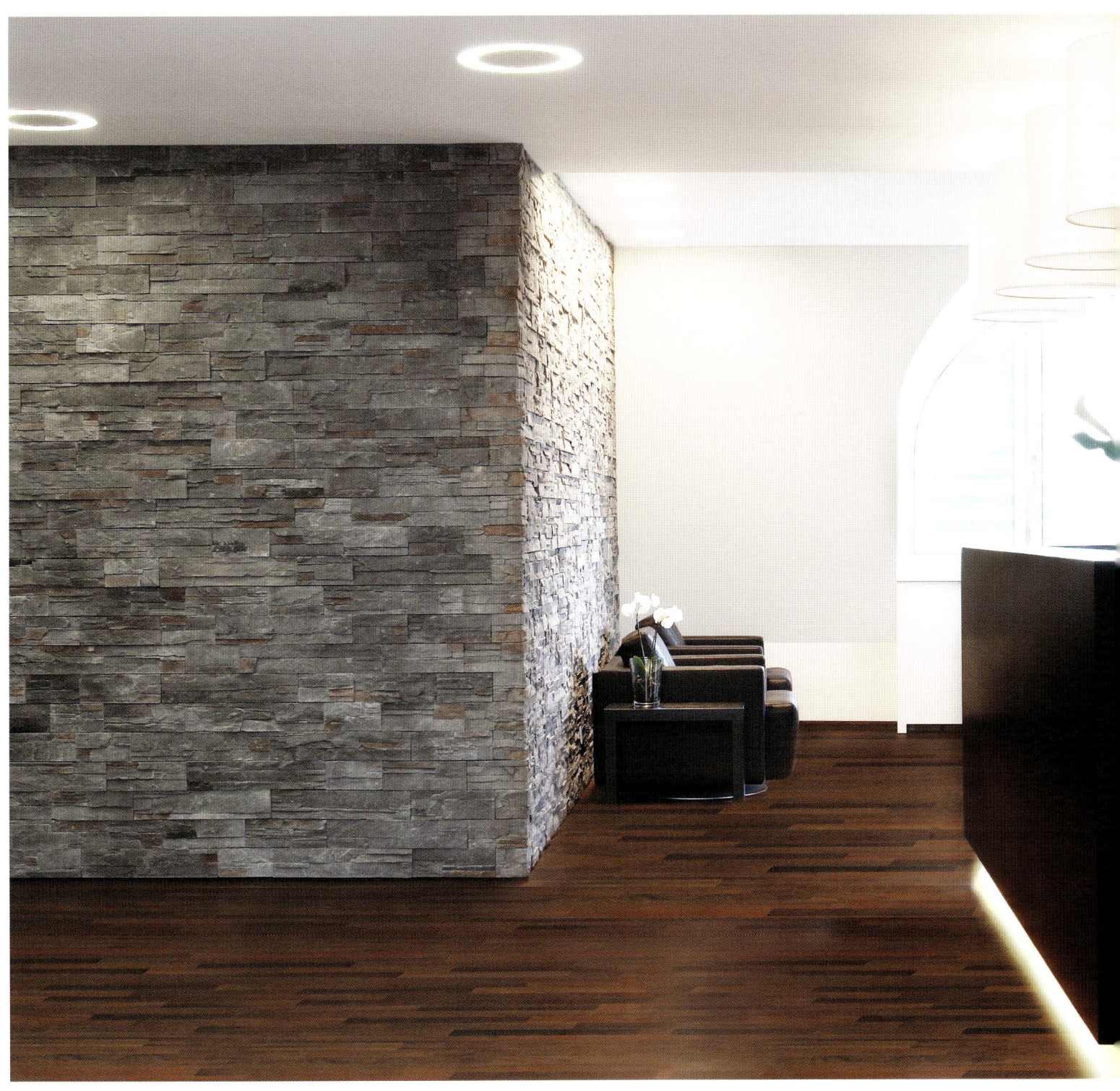

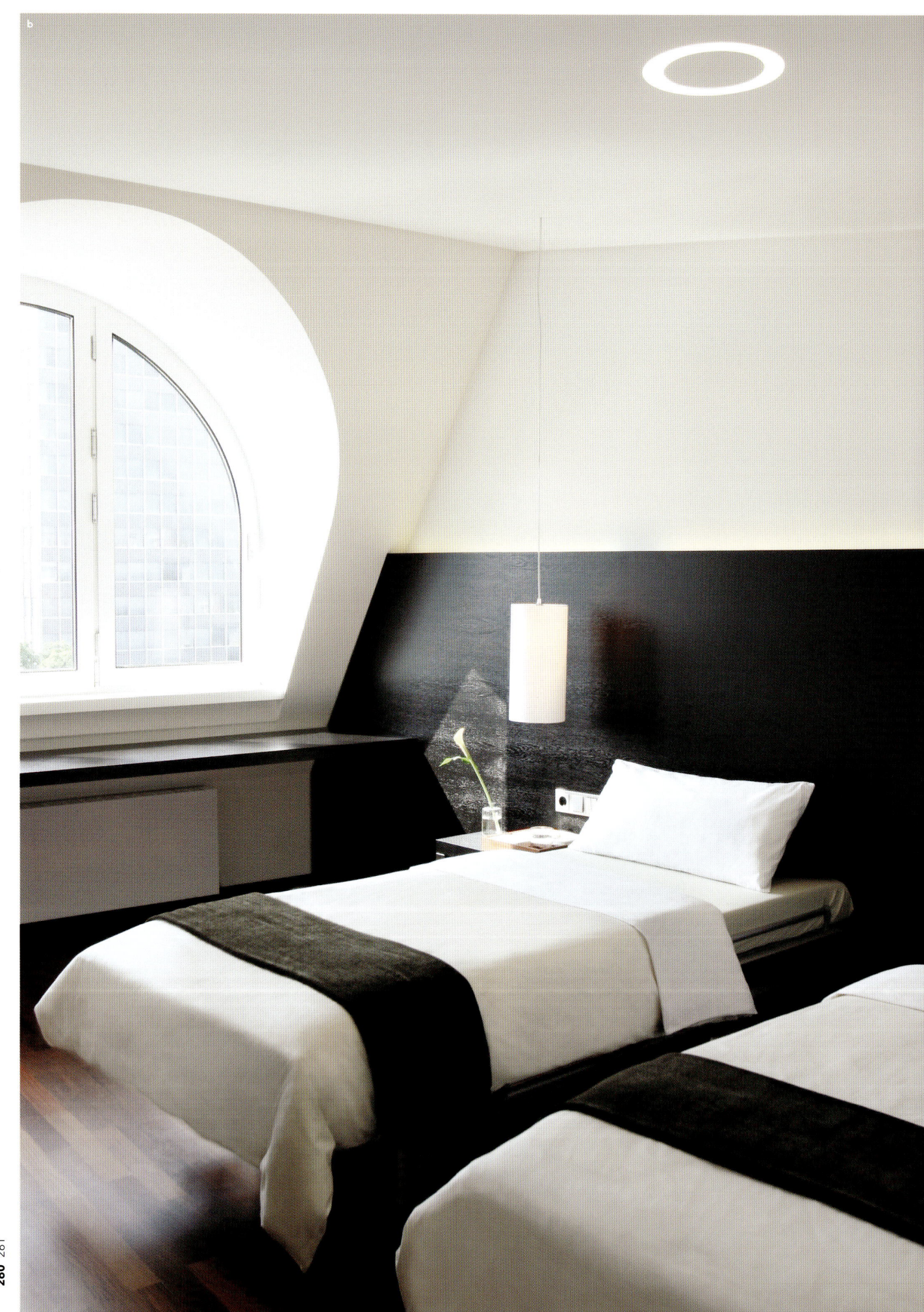

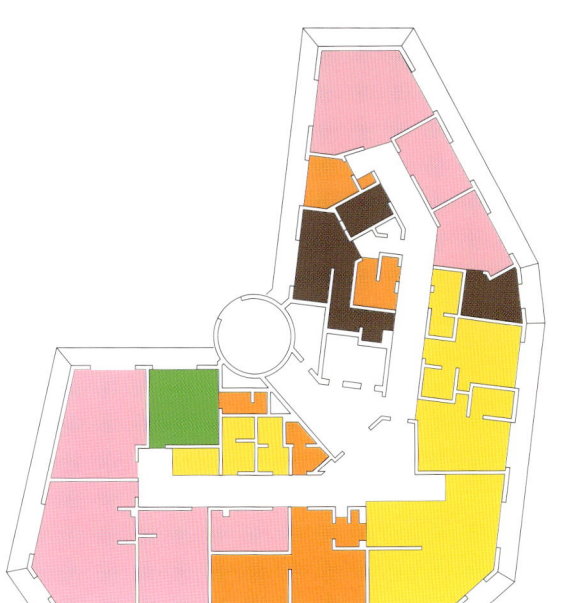

1	Reception	**10**	Staff toilet and shower
2	Waiting area	**11**	Patient toilet L
3	Coat-rack	**12**	Patient toilet G
4	Staff room and small kitchen	**13**	Staff toilet
5	Prep room	**14**	OP-Trakt
6	Nurses' office	**15**	Single room
7	Treatment room laser	**16**	Patient toilet and shower
8	Treatment room	**17**	Double room
9	Office		

Diagrammatic plans, to scale 1:400
Floor plans, to scale 1:200

TP

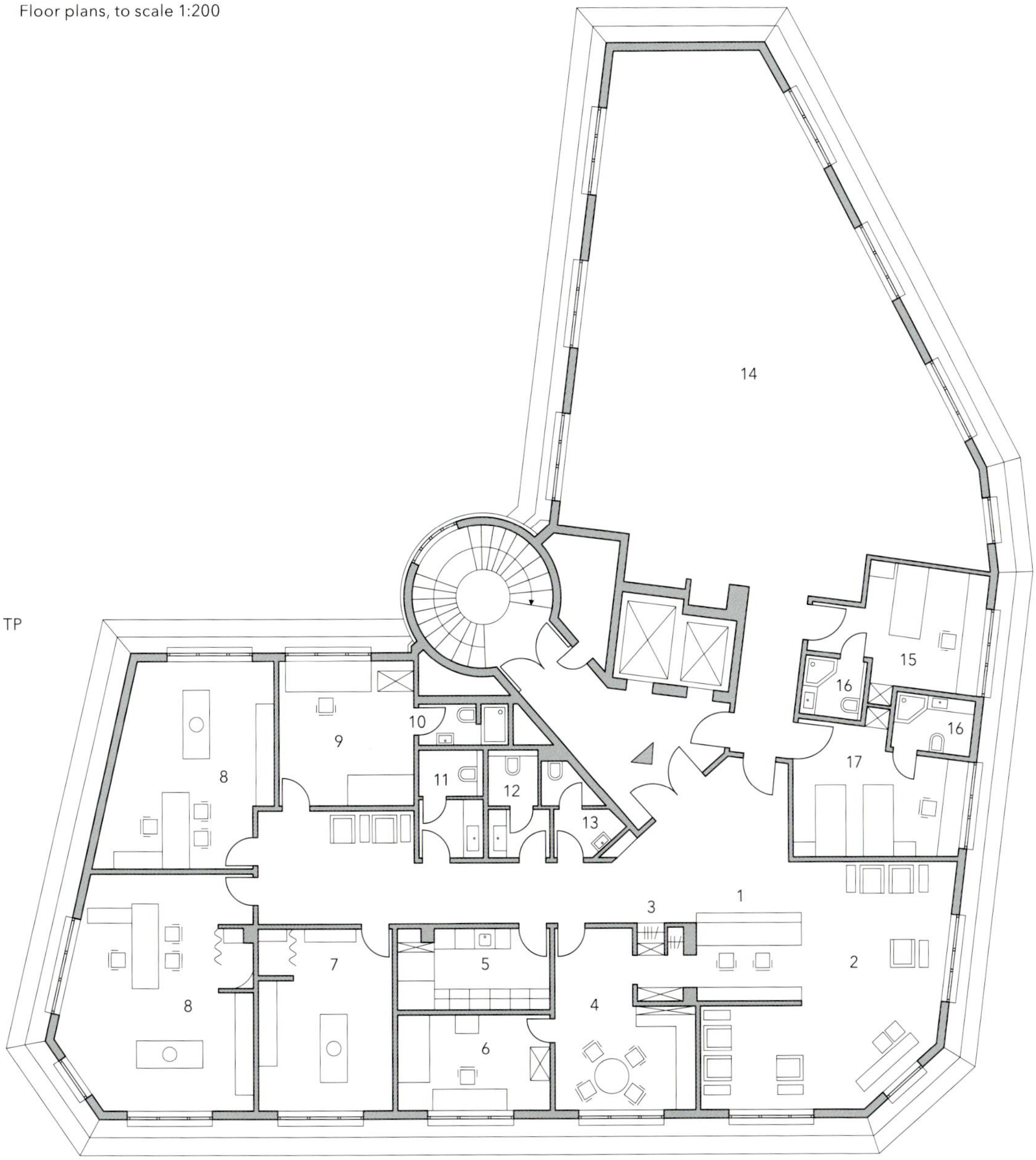

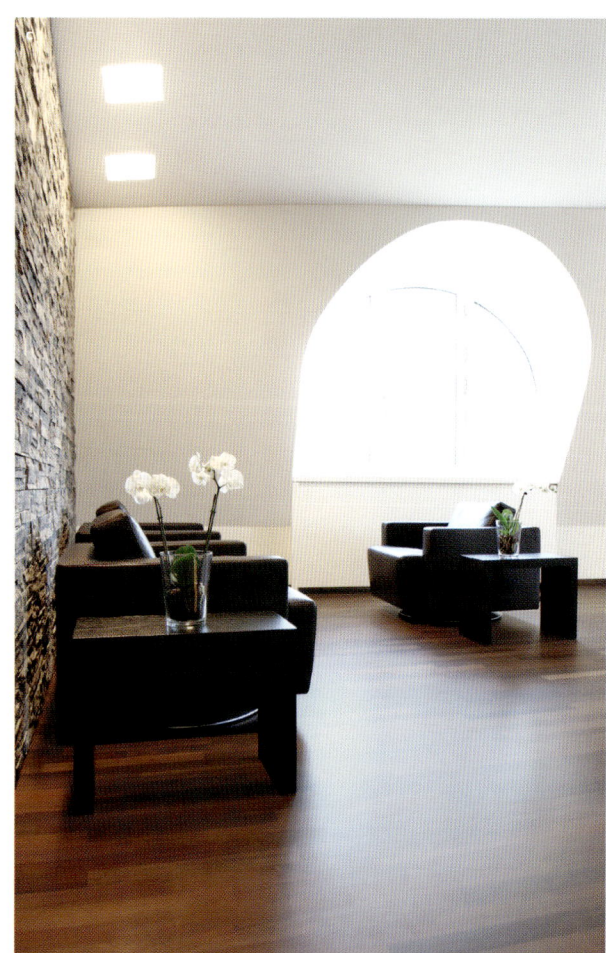

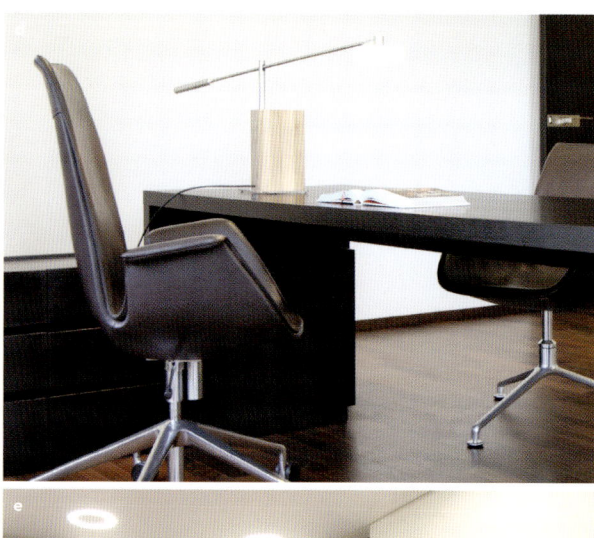

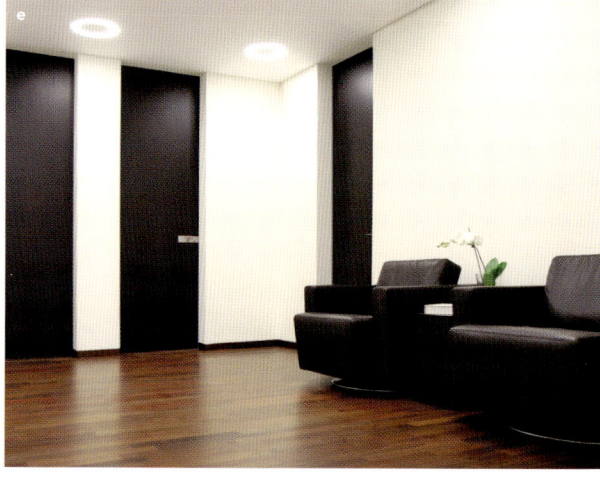

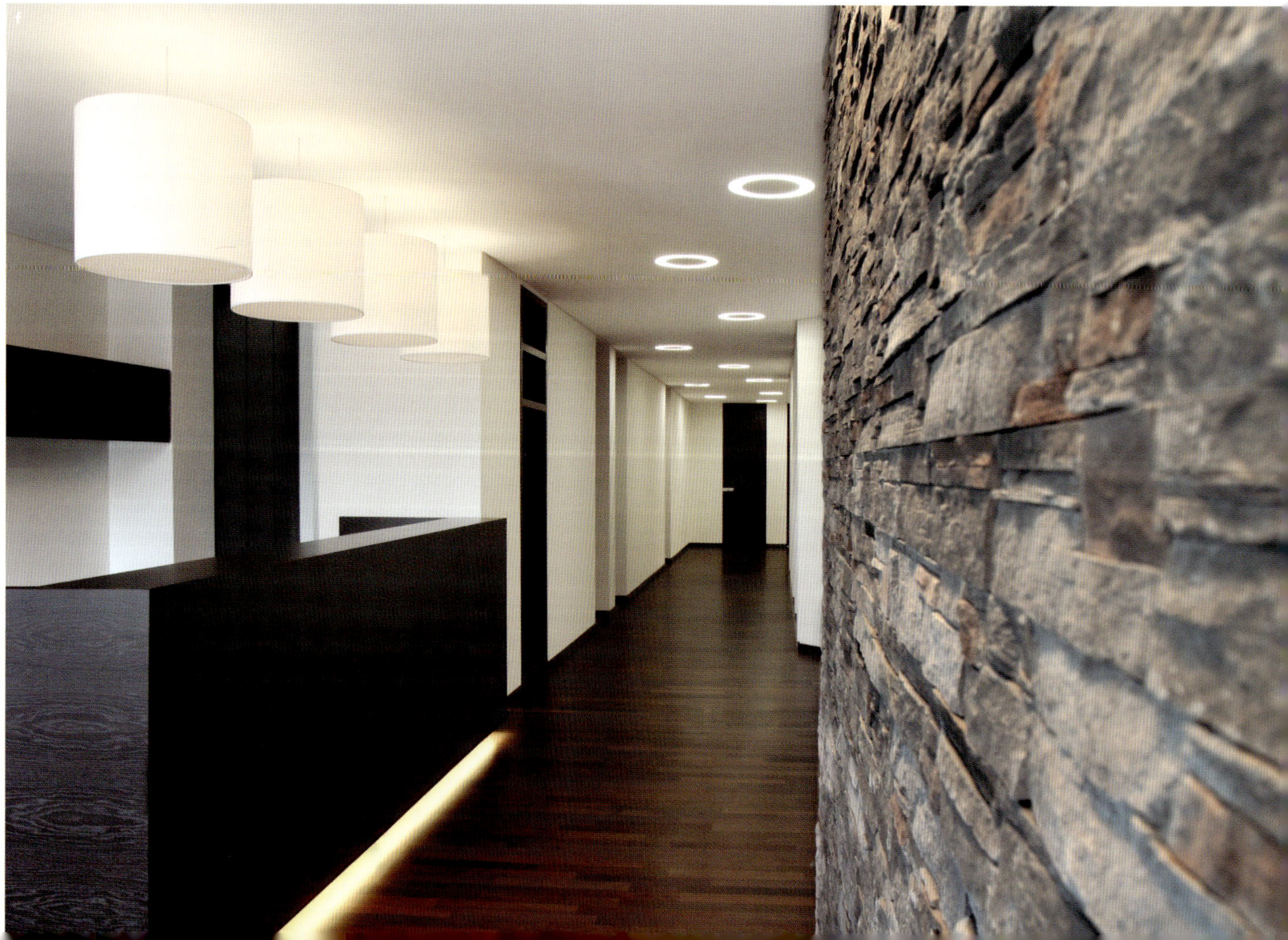

**Client	Operator**	Dr. Marcus Tammer
Planning time	02 2005 – 09 2005
Construction time	09 2005 – 04 2006
Gross floor area	470 sqm
Usable floor space	390 sqm
Gross cubic capacity	1,100 cbm

a Puristic austerity in the foyer: the elegant reception desk is made of Wenge-coloured wood with four cylindrical lights.

b The cosy double-bedded room offers a comfortable inpatient stay.

c Large round-arched windows lend a special charm to the practice rooms.

d View into one of the elegant consultation and treatment rooms.

e Ceiling-high wooden doors provide structure to the corridor along its length.

f The specially-designed wall made of anthracite-coloured artificial stone sets natural accents.

Floor plan layout

Patients can directly access the reception and the waiting area of this multiple practice with clinic and operating area via its central hub area, which is equipped with stairs and two lifts. From the intersection of the two almost right-angled corridors, on one side they can reach the consultation and treatment rooms and on the other side, via sluices, the surgical wing. Only the not-so-important rooms receive no natural light.

Usable floor spaces

Patient rooms	**yellow**	111 sqm	28 %
Specialist rooms	**pink**	155 sqm	40 %
Administrative rooms	**green**	18 sqm	5 %
Offices	Staff rooms	**orange**	73 sqm	19 %
Supply	Waste disposal	**brown**	33 sqm	8 %
Total		390 sqm	100 %

In order to meet future requirements in health care, the new Stuttgart dermatologists' practice needed a floor plan that was as flexible as possible. For this reason a cosmetic studio that functions entirely independently has been factored into the planning.

The operationally-separate, but visually-matching, areas in the medical practice and the cosmetic studio can be accessed via a shared anteroom with seating. A bright sunshine-yellow room box, which is situated between anteroom, cosmetic studio and the practice, is used as an examination room for UV therapy; on the outside it provides a seating arrangement for the patients. The centre-point of the dermatological practice is the long reception desk, which stands out with its cosy, bright and cheerful presence in front of the polychrome cabinet feature. From there patients have a good overview of all the rooms. In order to give the whole practice a uniform look and to accentuate the basic structure of the rooms, the ceiling is universally made of polished exposed concrete.

**MIKROPOLIS
ULRIKE MANSFELD
TILMAN HELLER**

DERMATOLOGICAL PRACTICE
STUTTGART | G

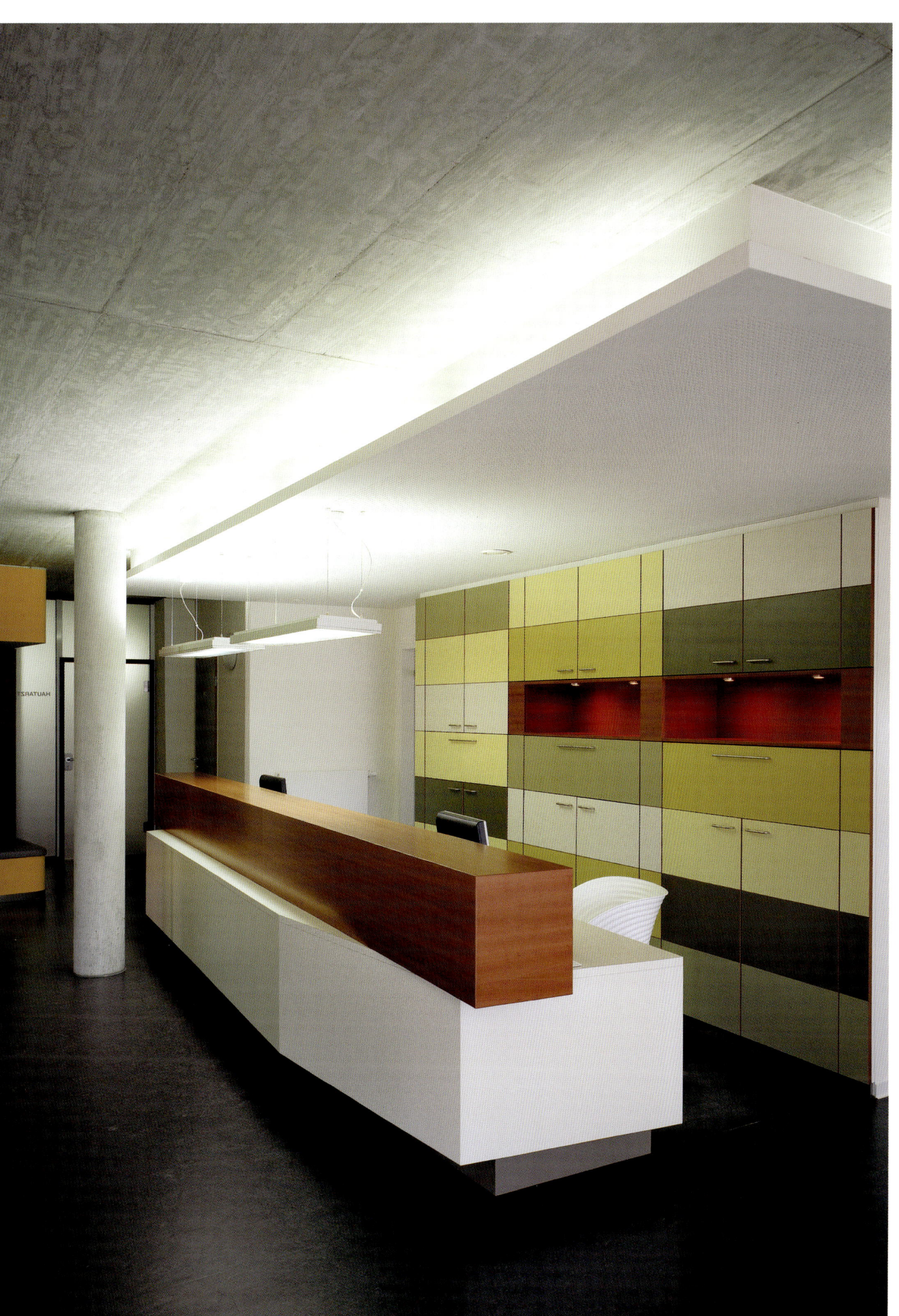

a
LICHTTHERAPIE

b

c
KOSMETIK

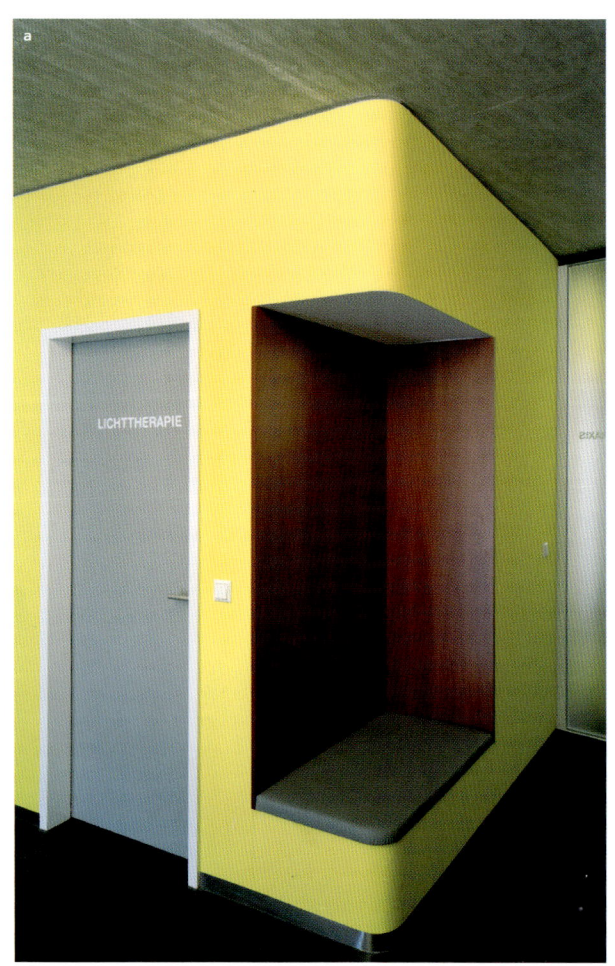

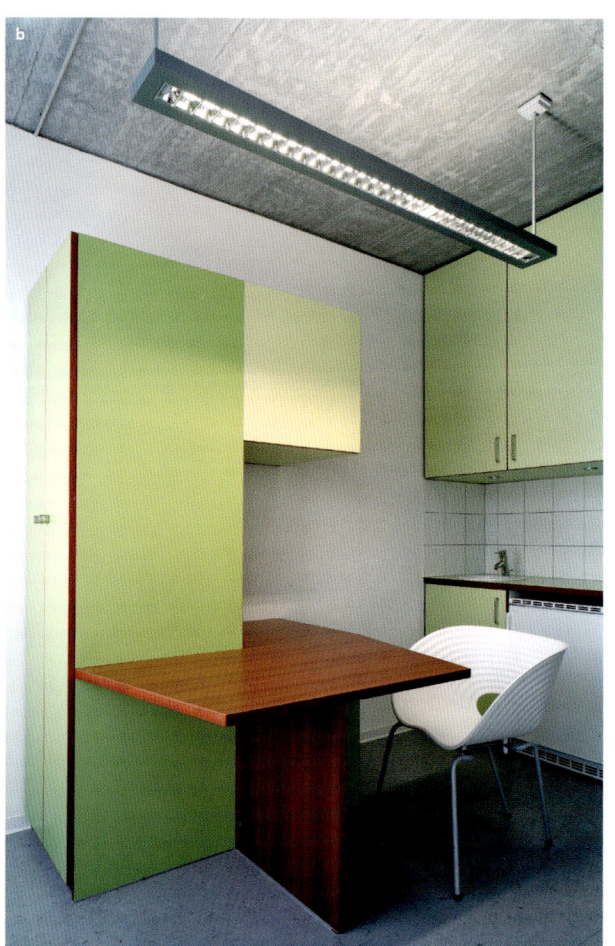

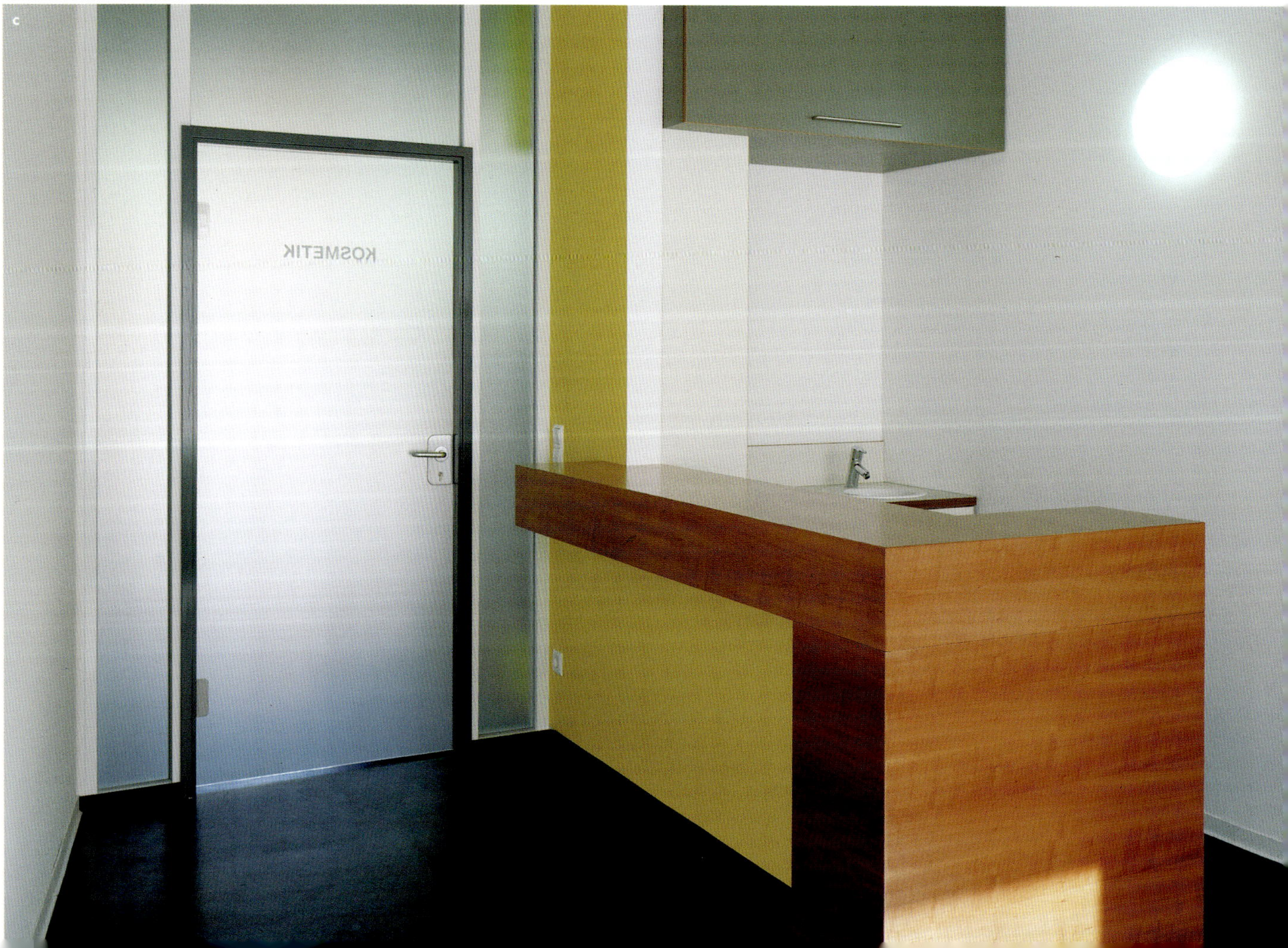

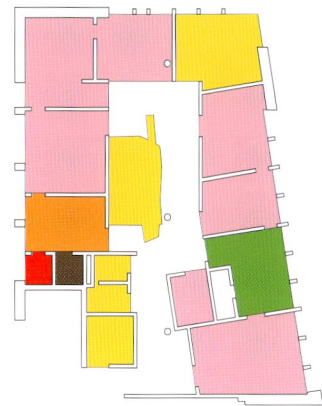

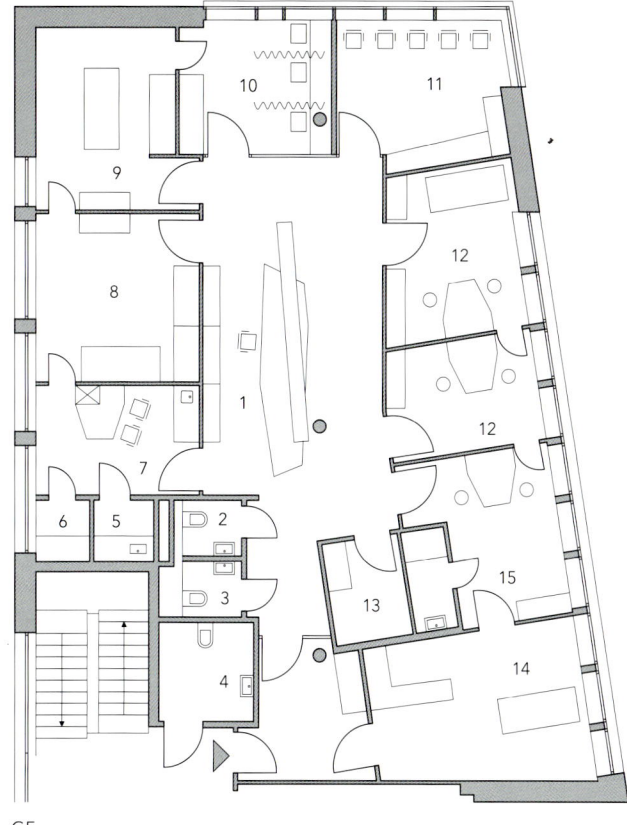

GF

Client | Operator   Dr. Michael Schliz
Construction time   2005
Usable floor space   219 sqm
Gross cubic capacity 520 cbm

a The sunshine-yellow room box reflects various functional requirements: UV therapy
   examination room and seating arrangement
   for patients who are waiting.
b The ceilings are universally made of polished
   exposed concrete, in order to give the different working areas a uniform look.
c In order to meet future requirements in
   health care, a cosmetic studio that functions
   entirely independently has been planned.

Diagrammatic plans, to scale 1:400
Floor plans, to scale 1:200

Floor plan layout

1 Reception	**7** Staff lounge	treatment room
2 Patient toilet G	**8** Treatment room	**13** Examination
3 Patient toilet L	**9** Procedure room	UV therapy
4 Toilet for the disabled	**10** Examination	**14** Treatment room
5 Cleaning room	**11** Waiting area	cosmetics
6 Laboratory	**12** Examination and	**15** Office

The access point of the conical rectangular floor plan for this single-doctor
practice is approximately in the centre of the wider narrow side. Patients
access the large central room with reception via an anteroom. All the rooms in
the practice, predominantly supplied with natural light, are grouped around
this space.

Usable floor spaces

Patient rooms	**yellow**	51 sqm	24 %
Examination			
Treatment rooms	**red**	3 sqm	1 %
Specialist rooms	**pink**	129 sqm	59 %
Administrative rooms	**green**	18 sqm	8 %
Offices	Staff rooms	**orange**	15 sqm	7 %
Supply	Waste disposal	**brown**	3 sqm	1 %
Total		219 sqm	100 %

Performance data

Outpatients per year	6,000
Type of services per year	Conservative and operative dermatology
Services to other clinics	Surgical procedures which make inpatient stay necessary.
Clinic opening hours	5 days	40 hours
Waiting time [with	without appointment]	0–10 min.	0–60 min.
Type and number of staff	1 doctor
	1 full-time staff
	1 trainee

Dark oak parquet flooring and bright built-in furniture are in harmonious contrast to one another in the new ORL Clinic in the House of Health medical services centre in Feuerbach, Stuttgart.

As soon as patients enter, their gaze is drawn to a pleasantly tranquil, functional room partition with a white, high-gloss coating. Narrow green jointing accentuates the materiality of the panels, while a more durable matt beige coating has been selected for the usable floor spaces. The wall unit, which dominates the room, is more than just a nice eye-catching feature: It combines a wide variety of functions such as reception desk, shelving, cupboards and seating areas, and partitions off the rear areas from the public, hiding from view a small kitchen and a room for allergy testing. Patient, doctor and staff zones are visually separate, however they are functionally linked and they give structure to the floor plan of this practice. Opposite the reception, behind two translucent glass elements, are the two examination and treatment rooms and the friendly waiting area. The curtain, decorated with abstract floral motifs, and the chair cushions, which are in the same green, set colourful accents in the otherwise almost entirely white practice.

MIKROPOLIS ULRIKE MANSFELD

OTORHINOLARYNGOLOGY [ORL] CLINIC STUTTGART | G

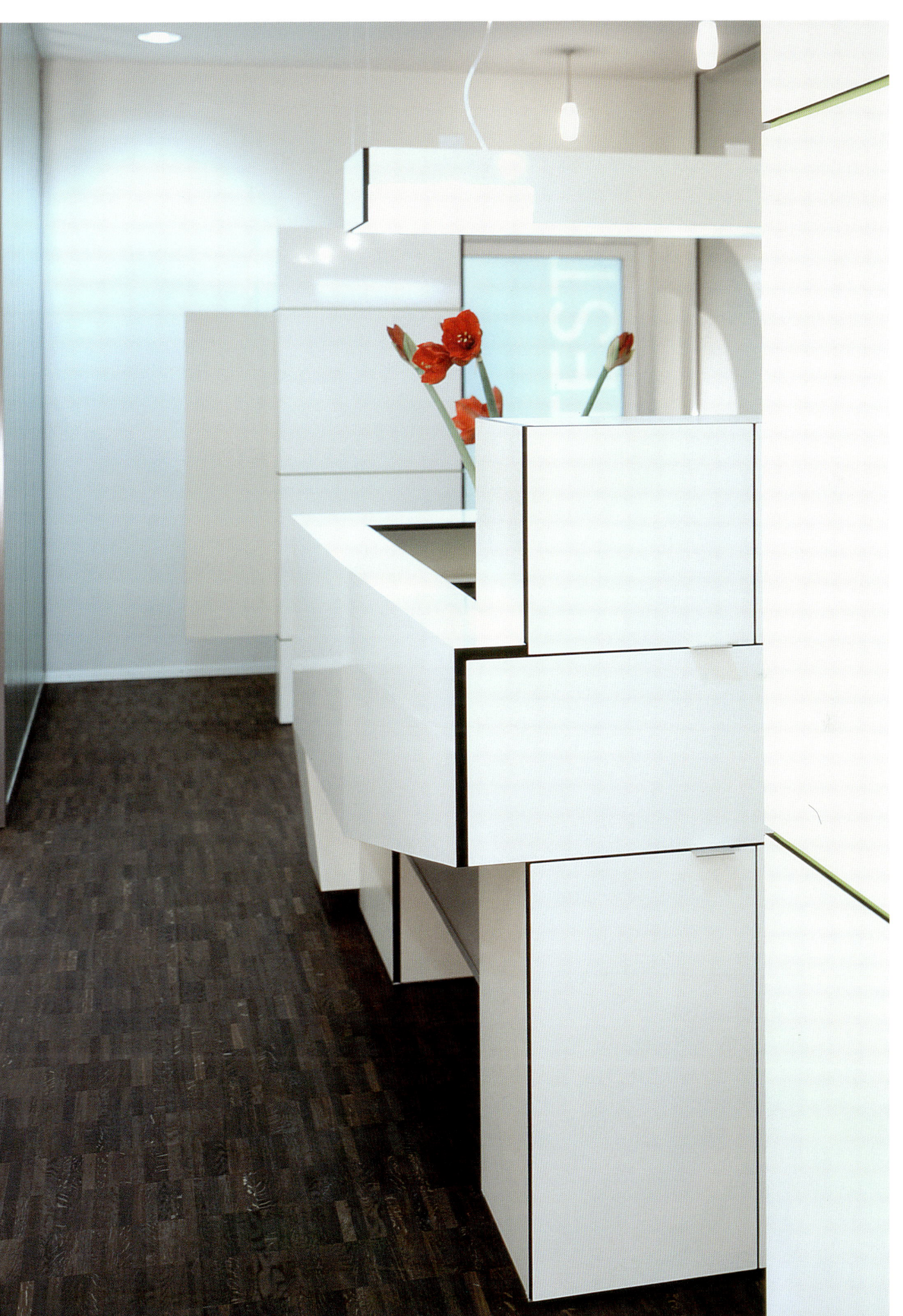

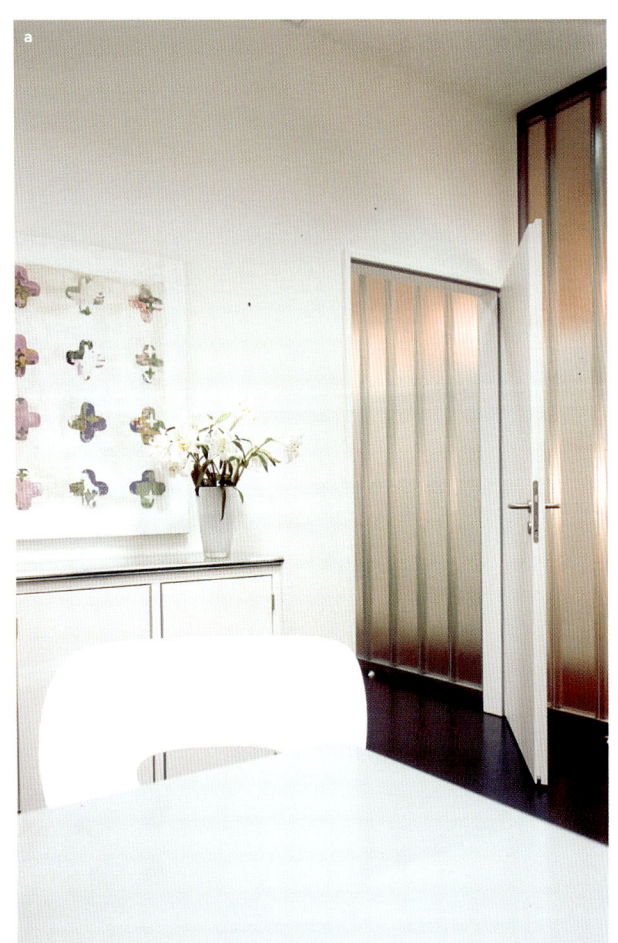
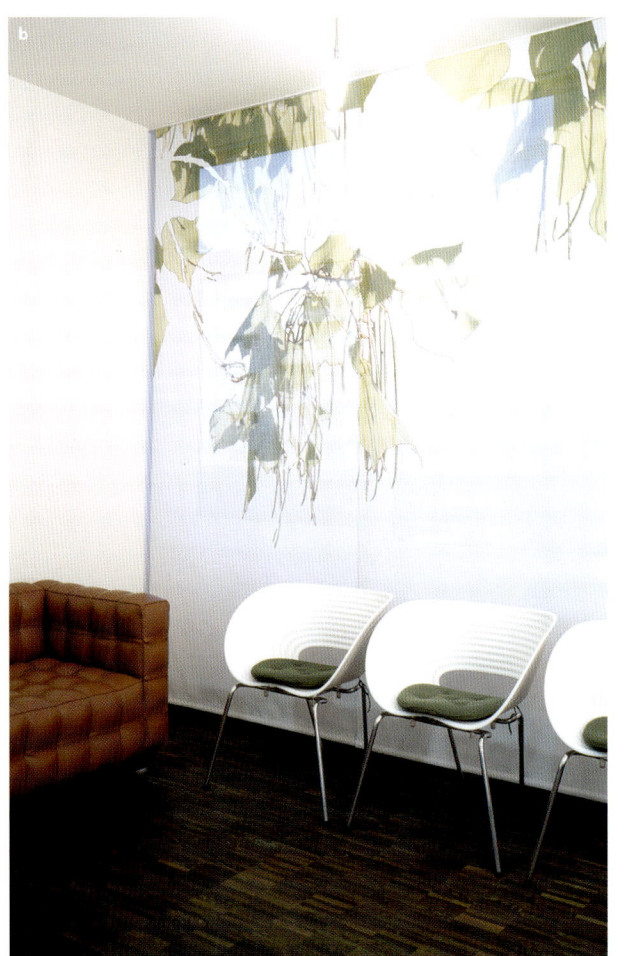

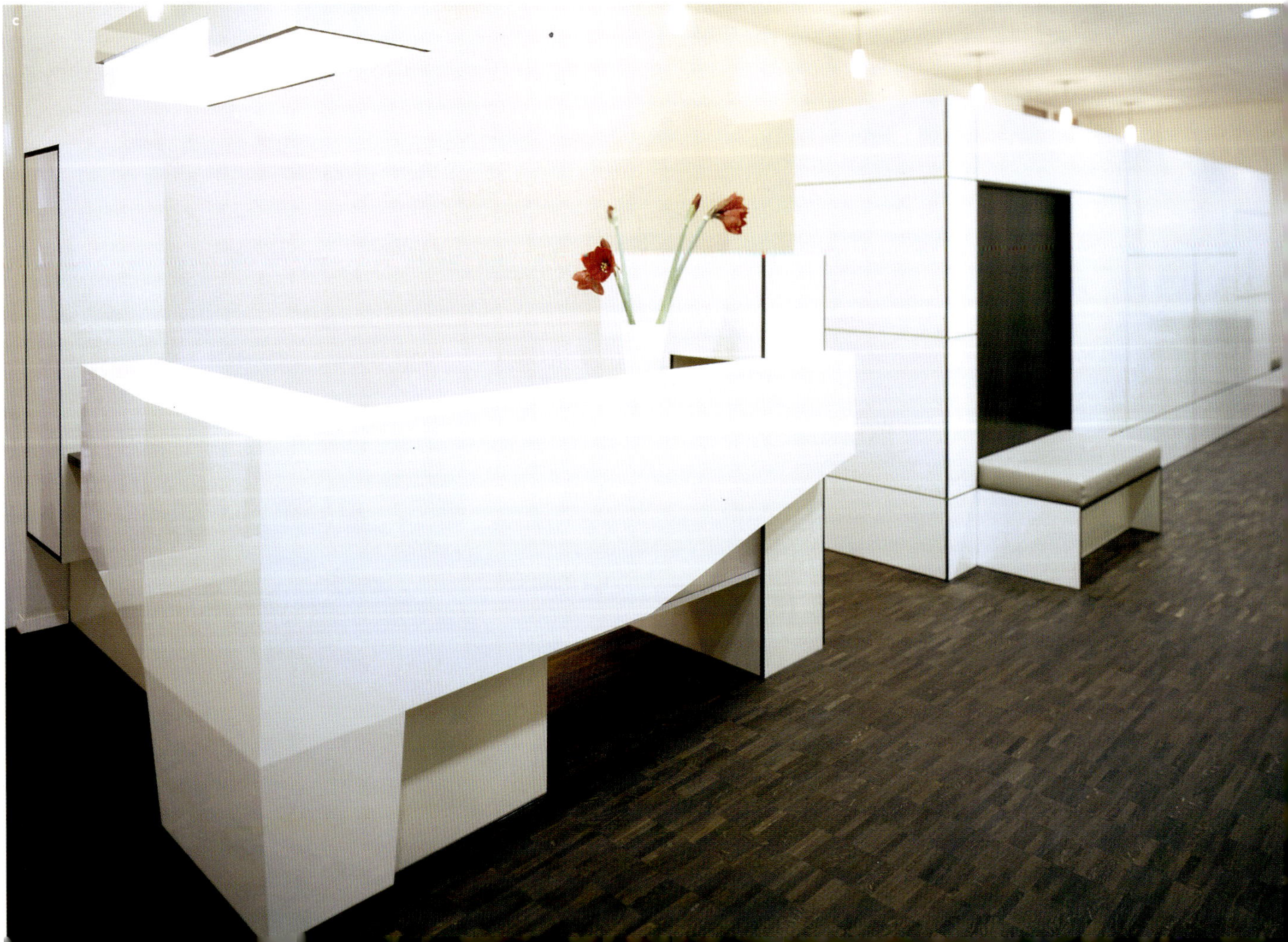

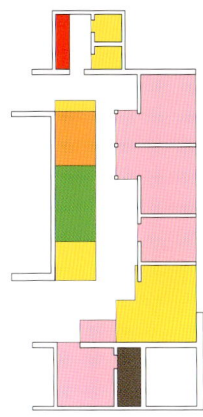

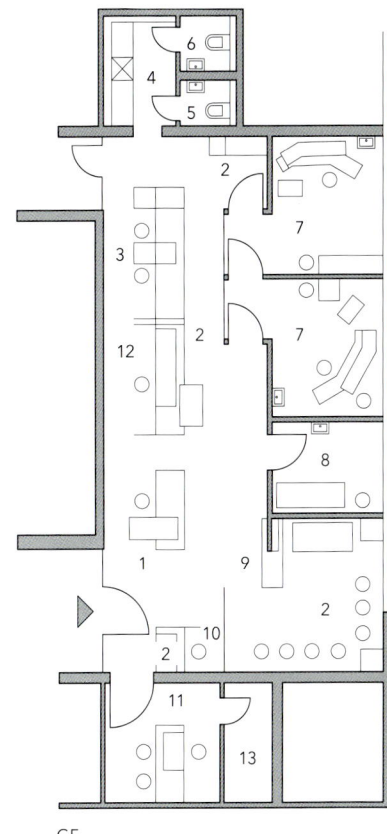

GF

Client	Dr. Peter Avelini
Operator	Dr. Peter Avelini
	Dr. Oliver Weise
Construction time	2004
Usable floor space	107 sqm

a The treatment rooms are situated behind a translucent partition wall.

b The floral motifs and the seat cushions, which are in the same green, in the waiting area set colourful accents in the otherwise almost entirely white practice.

c More than just a nice eye-catching feature, the room partition combines a wide variety of functions such as reception desk, shelving, cupboards and a seating arrangement.

Diagrammatic plans, to scale 1:400
Floor plans, to scale 1:200

Floor plan layout

1	Reception	**7**	Examination and treatment room	**11**	Examination
2	Waiting area			**12**	Office
3	Small kitchen	**8**	Treatment room infusion	**13**	Store room and filing room
4	Laboratory				
5	Patient toilet G	**9**	Coat-rack		
6	Patient toilet L	**10**	Treatment room		

Usable floor spaces

Patient rooms	**yellow**	29 sqm	27 %
Examination | Treatment rooms	**red**	3 sqm	3 %
Specialist rooms	**pink**	53 sqm	50 %
Administrative rooms	**green**	10 sqm	9 %
Offices | Staff rooms	**orange**	7 sqm	6 %
Supply | Waste disposal	**brown**	5 sqm	5 %
Total		107 sqm	100 %

Performance data

Outpatients per year	8,000
Clinic opening hours	5 days | 40 hours
Waiting time [with | without appointment]	0 – 30 min. | 0 – 60 min.

The conceptual idea for the newly-designed rooms at the orthopaedic practice is based on the essence of orthopaedics. The area of interaction, inherent in the treatment of the human musculoskeletal system, between movement and posture, modern and traditional, is conveyed by the architecture of the rooms.

The curved reception desk with the portrayal of an athletic body is shaped like a spinal column. A colour scheme underlies the design of the practice, which concentrates on three areas. The largest area with corridor, reception, waiting and therapy area is orange. This colour has a warming, bright, communicative effect; it can also be found on letterheads and visiting cards. In order to make it easier for patients to find their way around the practice, the intensity of the orange increases from the reception up to the centre of the practice and decreases again in the same way from the centre out. The four treatment cubicles are also in orange shades which vary in intensity, so that the cubicle can be selected according to the patient's treatment duration. In the two consulting rooms, however, a predominant pastel-green combined with a cherry blossom motif creates a rather more cheerful, carefree and calming atmosphere. An airy, cool, light blue tone prevails in the sanitary rooms. One element connecting the three areas is a recurrent dark brown shade, both in the furniture and the wall elements and in the parquet flooring.

MATEJA MIKULANDRA-MACKAT

ORTHOPAEDIC CLINIC IN ADLERSHOF HEALTH CENTRE
BERLIN | G

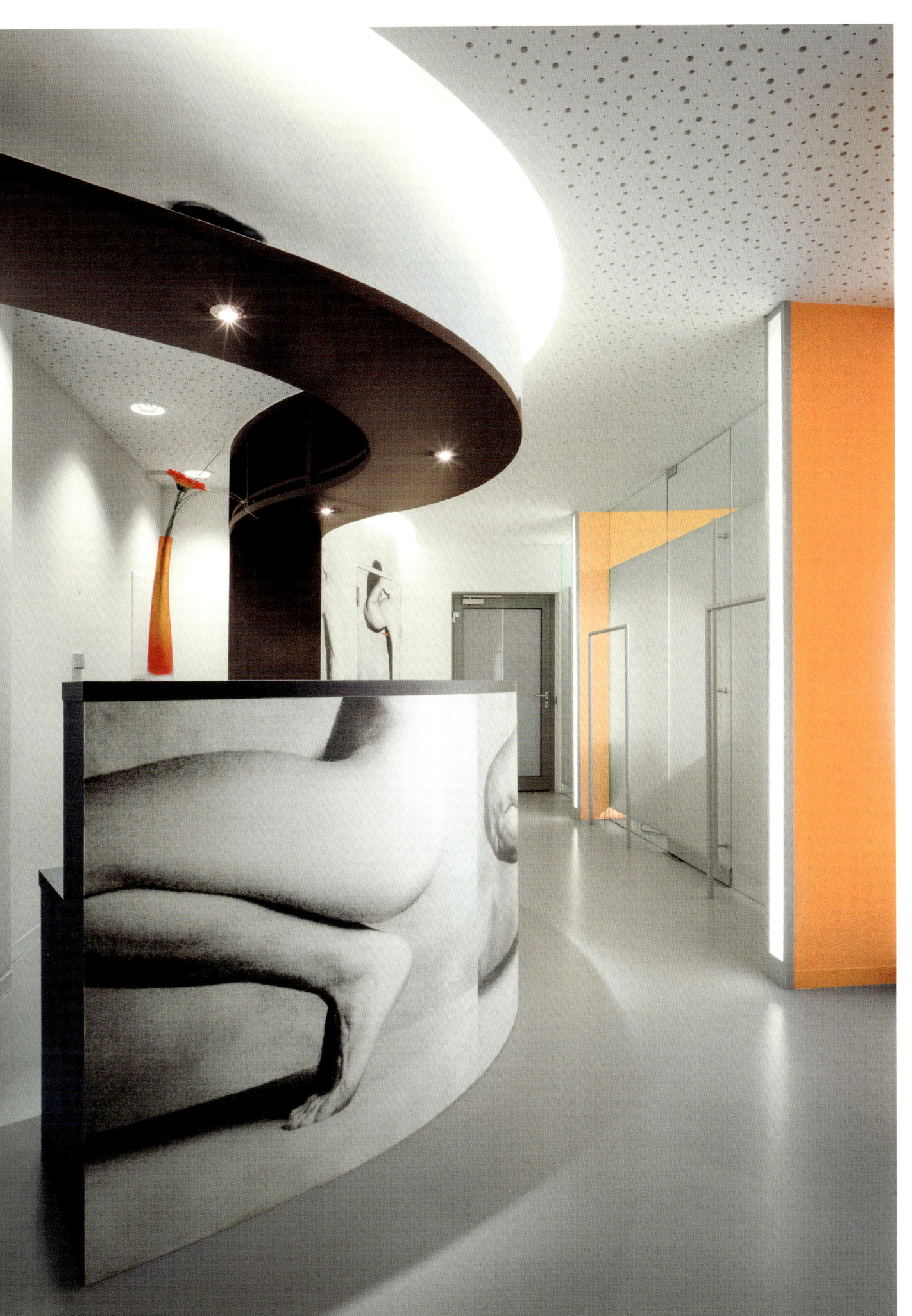

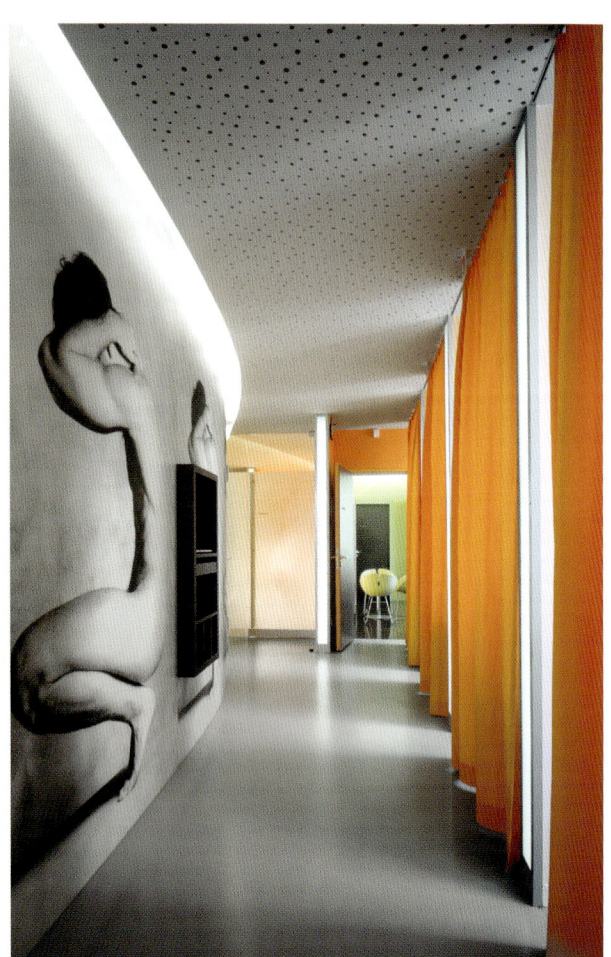

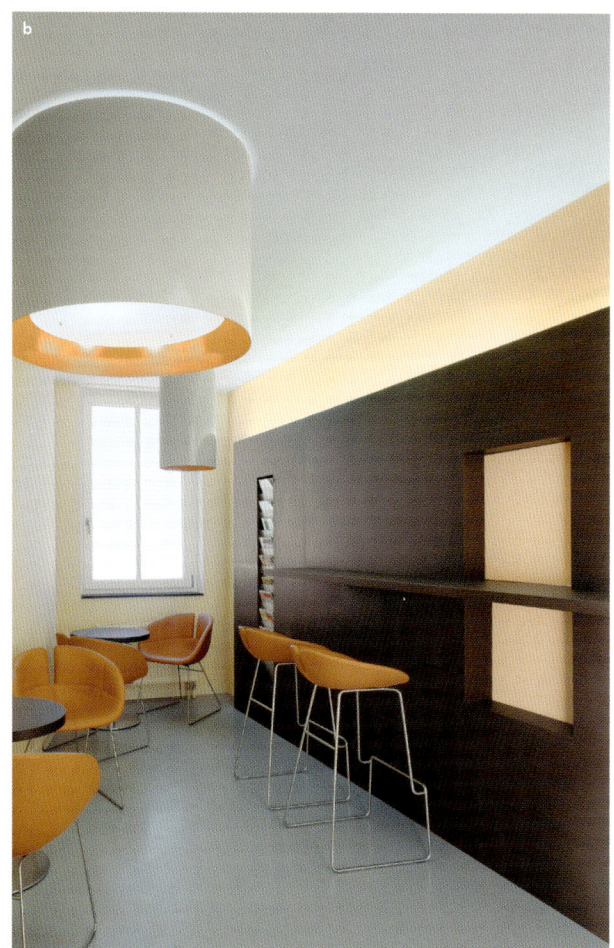

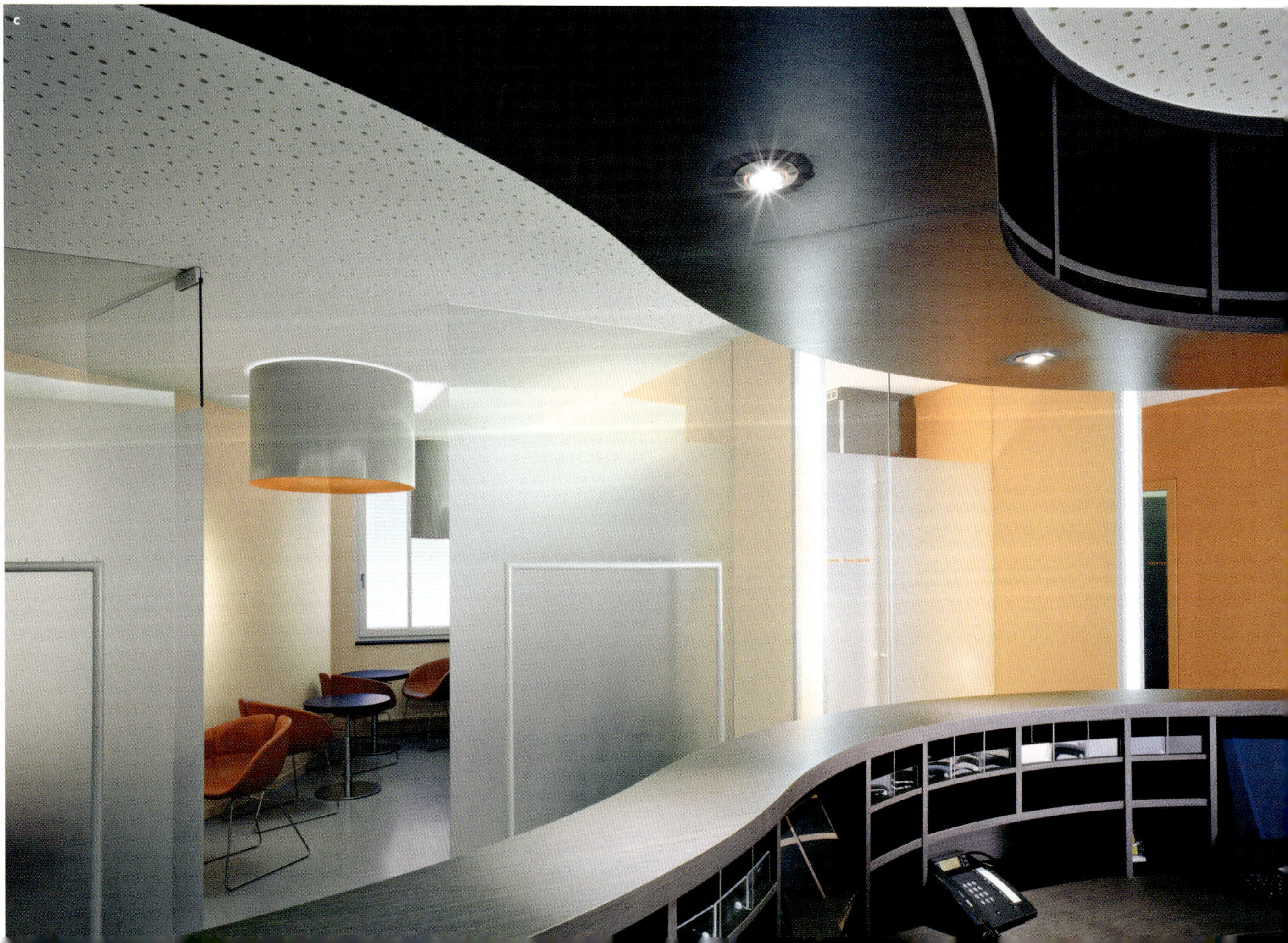

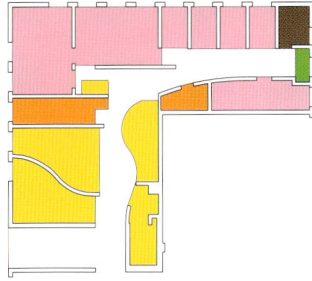

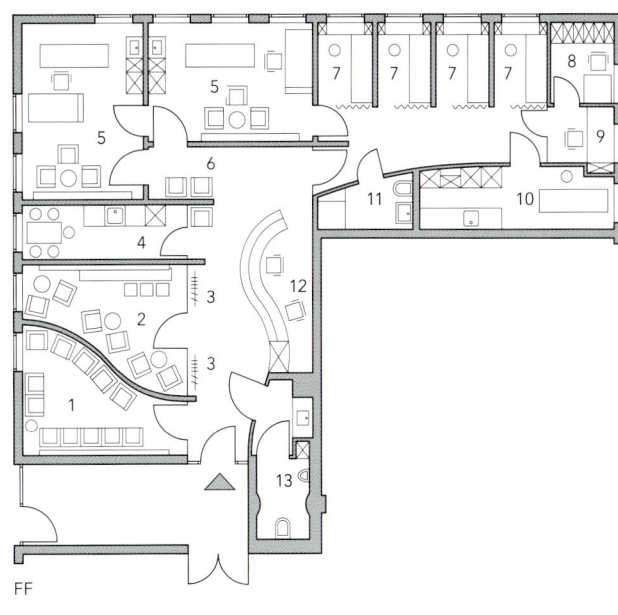

FF

Client	Dr. Matthias Finkelstein
Operator	Dr. Matthias Finkelstein
	Dr. Carl Neisser
Planning time	11 2003 – 05 2004
Construction time	06 2004 – 01 2005
Gross floor area	179 sqm
Usable floor space	122 sqm
Gross cubic capacity	492 cbm
Construction cost	190,000 EUR

a In order to make it easier for patients to find their way around, the intensity of the orange increases from the reception towards the centre of the practice and decreases again in the same way from the centre out.

b Private patient waiting area: vibrant warm orange combined with a brown colour, recurrent in furniture and wall elements.

c The curved reception desk is shaped like a spinal column.

Diagrammatic plans, to scale 1:400
Floor plans, to scale 1:200

Floor plan layout

1	Panel patient' waiting area	**5**	Examination and treatment room	**10**	Multi-purpose room
2	Private patients' waiting area	**6**	Lounge	**11**	Staff toilet and shower
3	Coat-rack	**7**	Treatment room	**12**	Reception
4	Staff lounge	**8**	Store room	**13**	Patient toilet
		9	Office		

The angular compact floor plan of this partnership practice with a similarly-shaped corridor means that the rooms are accessible without having to walk far. From an entrance situated in the centre of one branch of the building, patients directly access the reception with the two separate waiting areas for national health and private patients.

Usable floor spaces

Patient rooms	**yellow**	44 sqm	36 %
Examination | Specialist rooms	**pink**	60 sqm	49 %
Administrative rooms	**green**	2 sqm	2 %
Offices | Staff rooms	**orange**	12 sqm	10 %
Supply | Waste disposal	**brown**	4 sqm	3 %
Total		122 sqm	100 %

When upgrading and converting the former rural medical practice to a group practice for four doctors, the defining themes were views of the interior of the practice and of the outside. The grey, exposed concrete cube lined with window strips and apertures has been built around the existing structure and an extension from the 1970s and, with its defiant architecture, deliberately contrasts with the rural type of construction. The architect designates his construction positively as "stone" or "rock", which represents the "traction" and "heaviness" of the old-established practice.

The large reception and waiting area is used jointly for the entrance, the office and the toilet facilities. Ample window strips afford a fantastic panoramic view over the wooded Tyrolean mountains, thus integrating the modern building with its idyllic surroundings. The clear interior design concept forms a delightful contrast to traditional customary local construction. Green benches, which are combined to form a seating unit on a low platform, are more reminiscent of a waiting area than a rural medical practice. The basement in the three-storey extension houses the dental treatment rooms and the ground floor accommodates the premises for general medicine, internal medicine, X-ray and laboratory. On the upper floor there is even space for a small flat with a roof terrace.

GERHARD MITTERBERGER

MATREI HEALTH CENTRE
MATREI | A

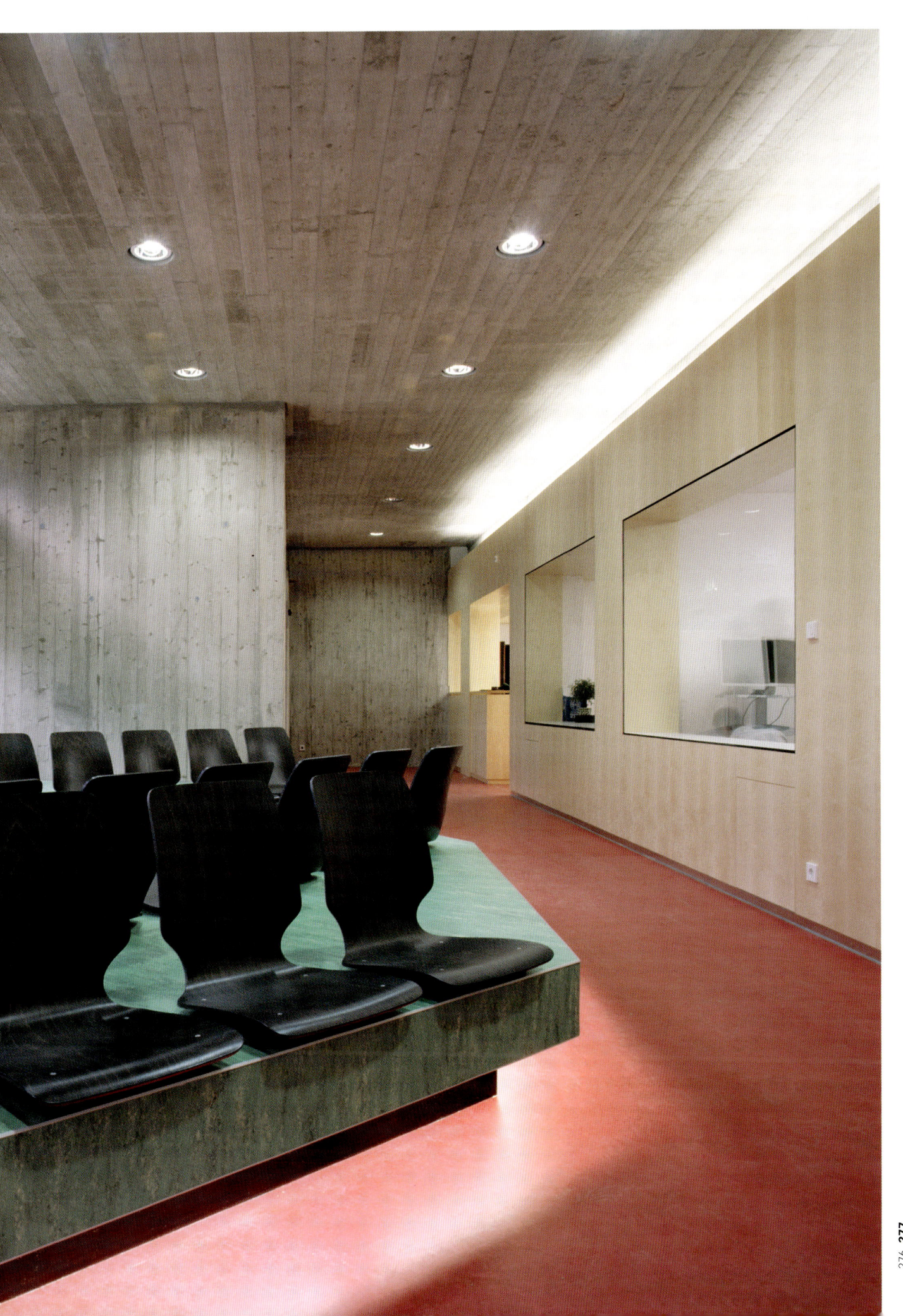

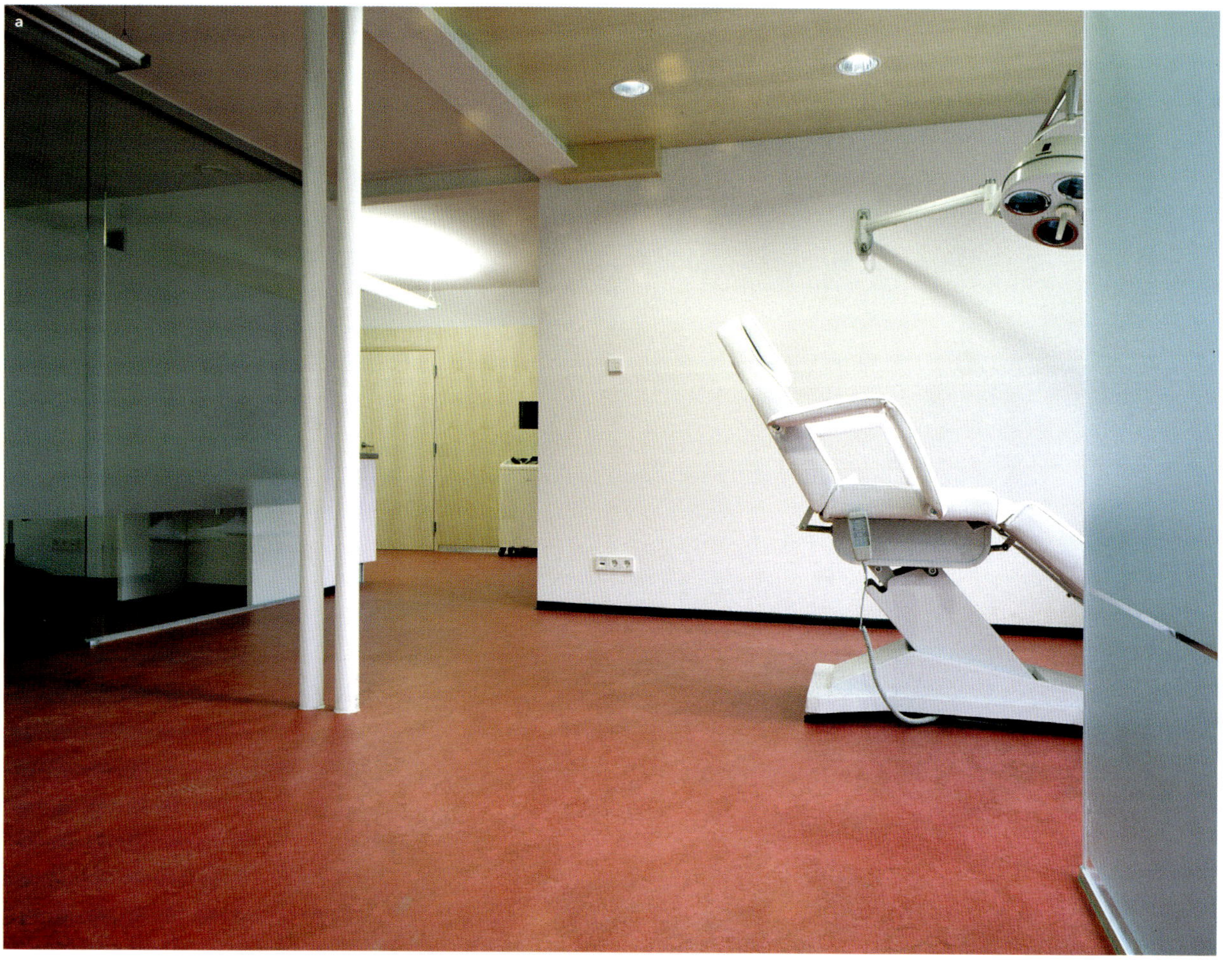

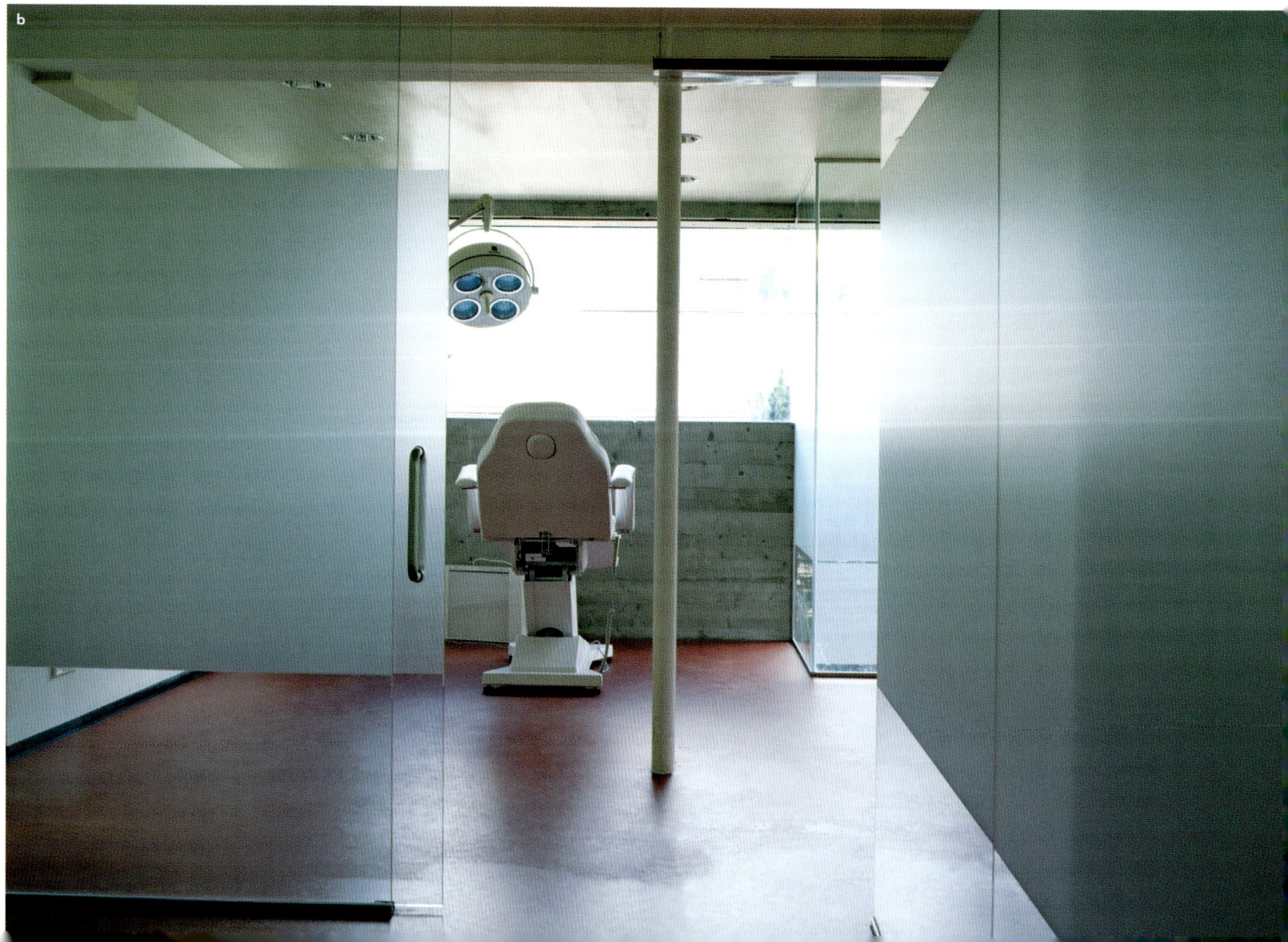

a

b

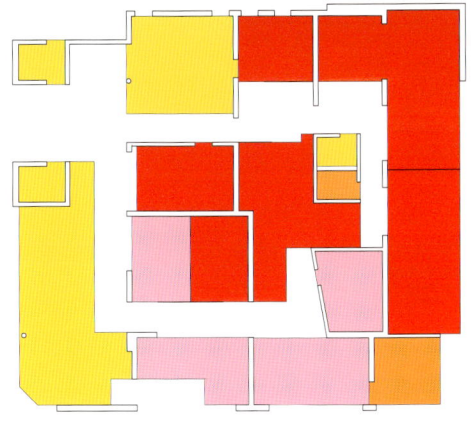

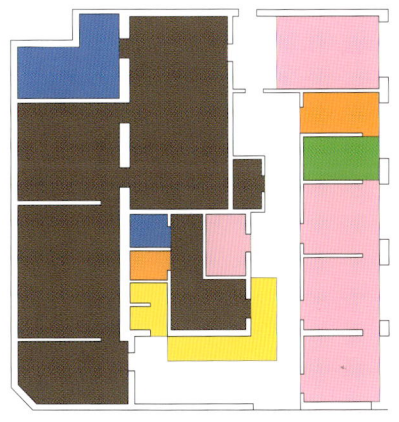

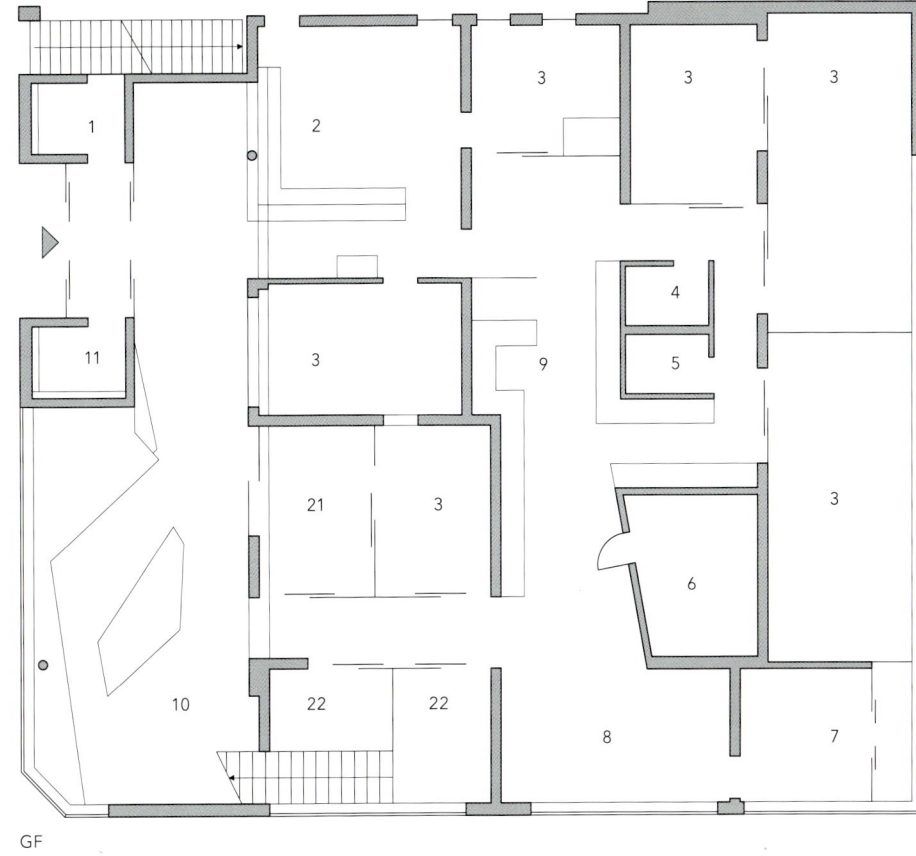

GF

Diagrammatic plans, to scale 1:400
Floor plans, to scale 1:200

1   Patient toilet L
2   Reception
3   Examination
4   Patient toilet
5   Staff shower
6   Examination X-ray
7   Staff lounge
8   Treatment room
    infusion
9   Laboratory
10 Waiting area
11 Patient toilet G
12 Store room
13 Installations room
14 Prosthetic dentistry
15 Small kitchen
16 Office
17 Dental treatment
    room
18 Sterilisation room
19 Staff toilet
20 Toilet anteroom
21 Examination
    sonography
22 Examination ENT

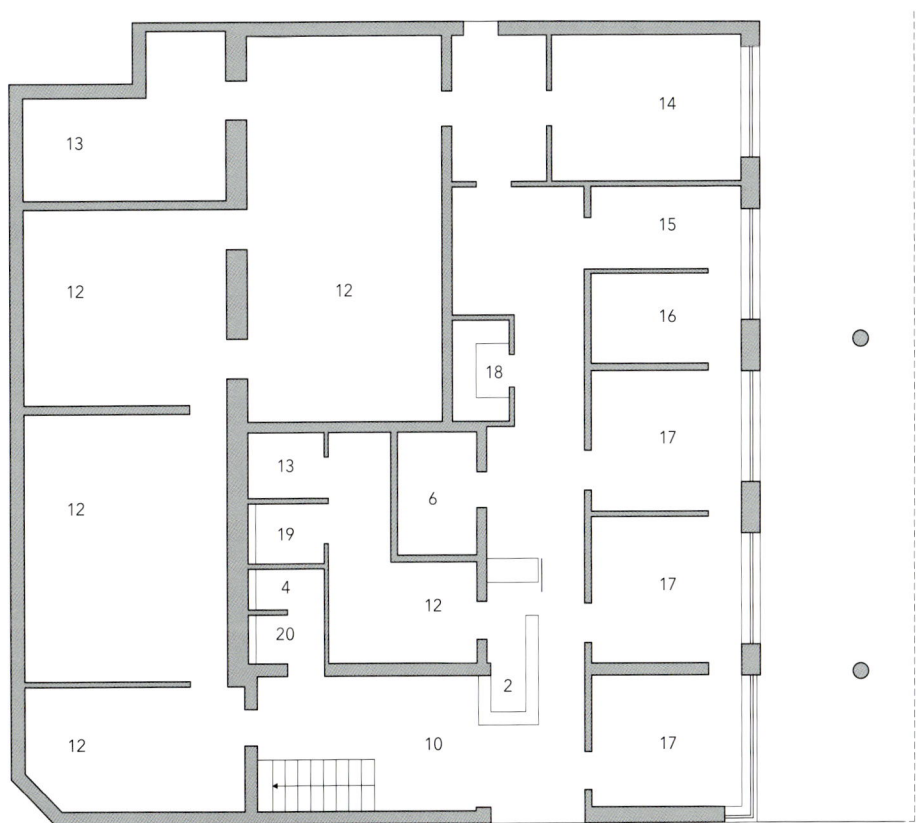

BSMT

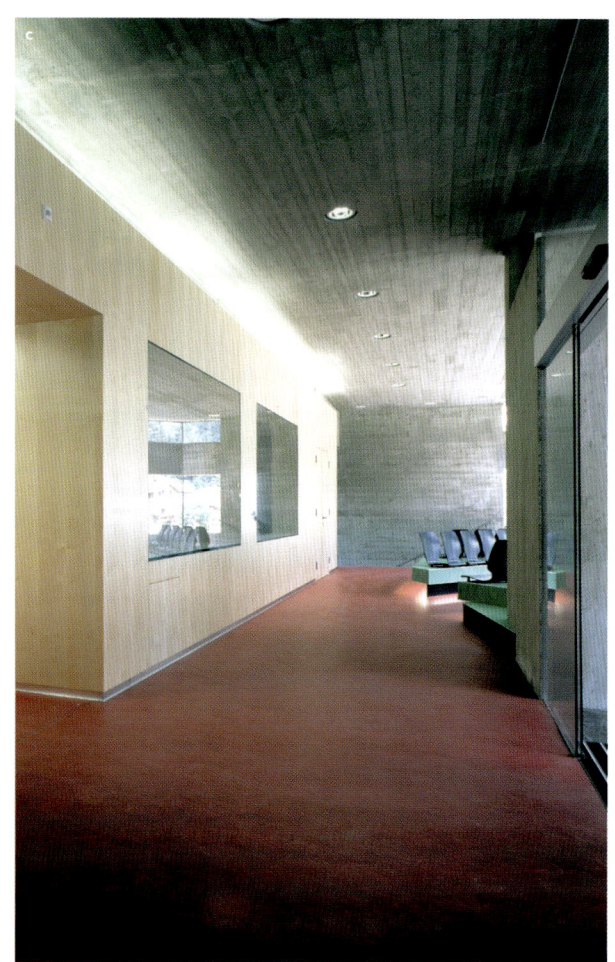

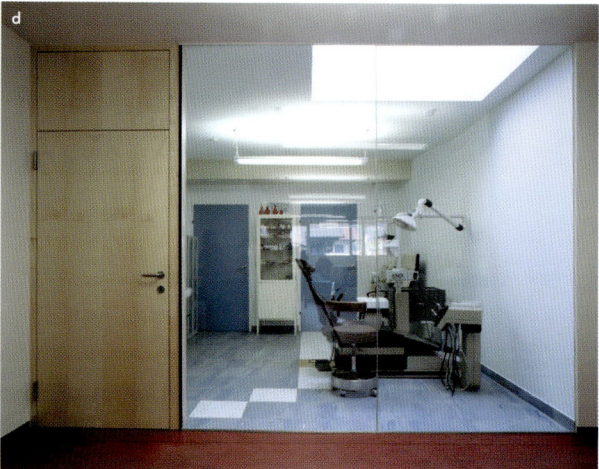

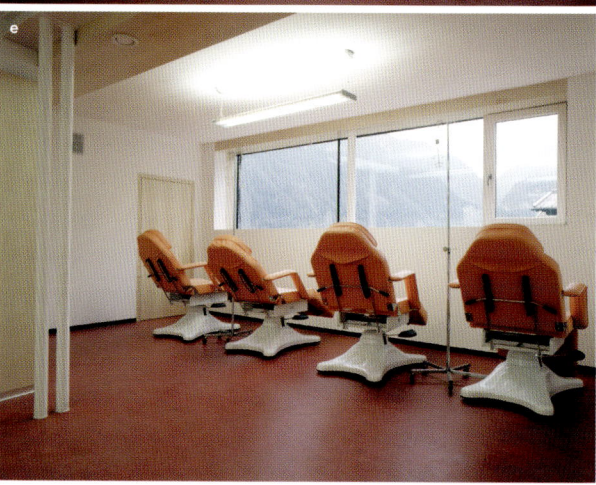

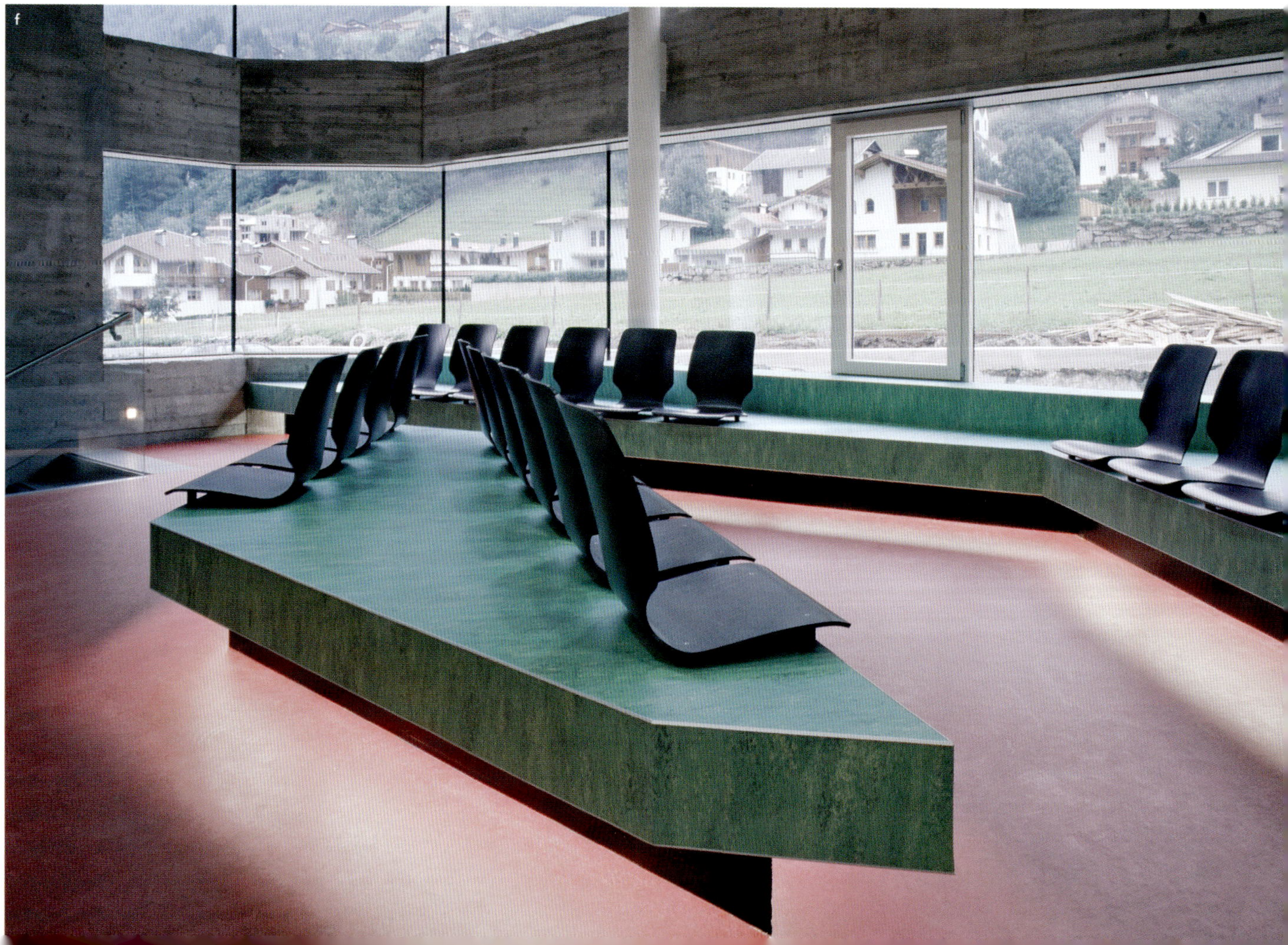

**Client	Operator**	Dr. Gerhard Gamper
	Dr. Cornelia Gamper
	Dr. Isabella Troyer
	Dr. Johann Trojer
	Nikolaus Trojer
Planning time	2003 – 2004
Construction time	2004 – 2005
Usable floor space	735 sqm
Gross cubic capacity	1,587 cbm
Construction cost	917,500 EUR
Total cost	1,000,000 EUR

a The ENT examination room is simple and unpretentious.

b Defining design principles, when converting this group practice, were views within the practice and outside.

c Rough materiality of the exposed concrete cube is also present everywhere.

d Superior transparency: this "glass" examination room is additionally illuminated by an ample skylight.

e The red linoleum, laid almost everywhere, makes the practice rooms seem cosy.

f Generous window strips in the joint waiting and reception area offer a panoramic view.

Floor plan layout

This multiple practice is spread over two levels; most examination and treatment rooms are on the ground floor due to the requirement for natural light. In the basement, the rooms are easy to reach from the waiting area which is situated at the stairwell. On the ground floor, with spacious reception and waiting area, patients are called directly by the doctor.

Usable floor spaces

Patient rooms	**yellow**	129 sqm	17 %
Examination			
Treatment rooms	**red**	184 sqm	25 %
Specialist rooms	**pink**	162 sqm	22 %
Administrative rooms	**green**	11 sqm	1 %
Offices	Staff rooms	**orange**	34 sqm	5 %
Supply	Waste disposal	**brown**	189 sqm	26 %
Plant rooms	**blue**	26 sqm	4 %
Total		735 sqm	100 %

Performance data

Outpatients per year	12,000
Clinic opening hours	5 days	40 hours
Waiting time [with	without appointment]	10 min.	up to 60 min.
Type and number of staff	5 doctors 10 clerical staff

"Oft kroch ein Käfer kribbelkrab | am hübschen Blümlein auf und ab" – the poem "Sie war ein Blümlein hübsch und fein" by Wilhelm Busch is the underlying conceptual idea for the conversion of this paediatric practice.

Little bugs and grasshoppers point the way to the examination rooms, where each wall is adorned with appropriate lines of verse. Young people need nature and animals, as well as generally elementary things like water and sufficient space to play. In designing the practice, a lot of emphasis was placed on the natural elements to bring nature to life in the form of a playroom. The design of the paediatric practice concentrates on the wellbeing of its young patients. It's not just about the acute healing of illnesses, but it's also about the long-term health of the children. The central image of the interior decoration is a summer meadow: structures that have a natural order, child-oriented designs with appropriate horizons, friendly pastel colours in green and blue. However, the summer meadow does not only represent this cheerful practice in a figurative sense, it is also found in the epoxy resin-moulded grasses on the backlit panels at the reception. Small glades and surfaces of water are embedded as areas of blue rubber amidst the otherwise uniform solid wood – a light blue lampshade provides extra light. Overall in this practice the architecture makes nature come alive.

NULL2ELF

PAEDIATRIC PRACTICE
HAAN | G

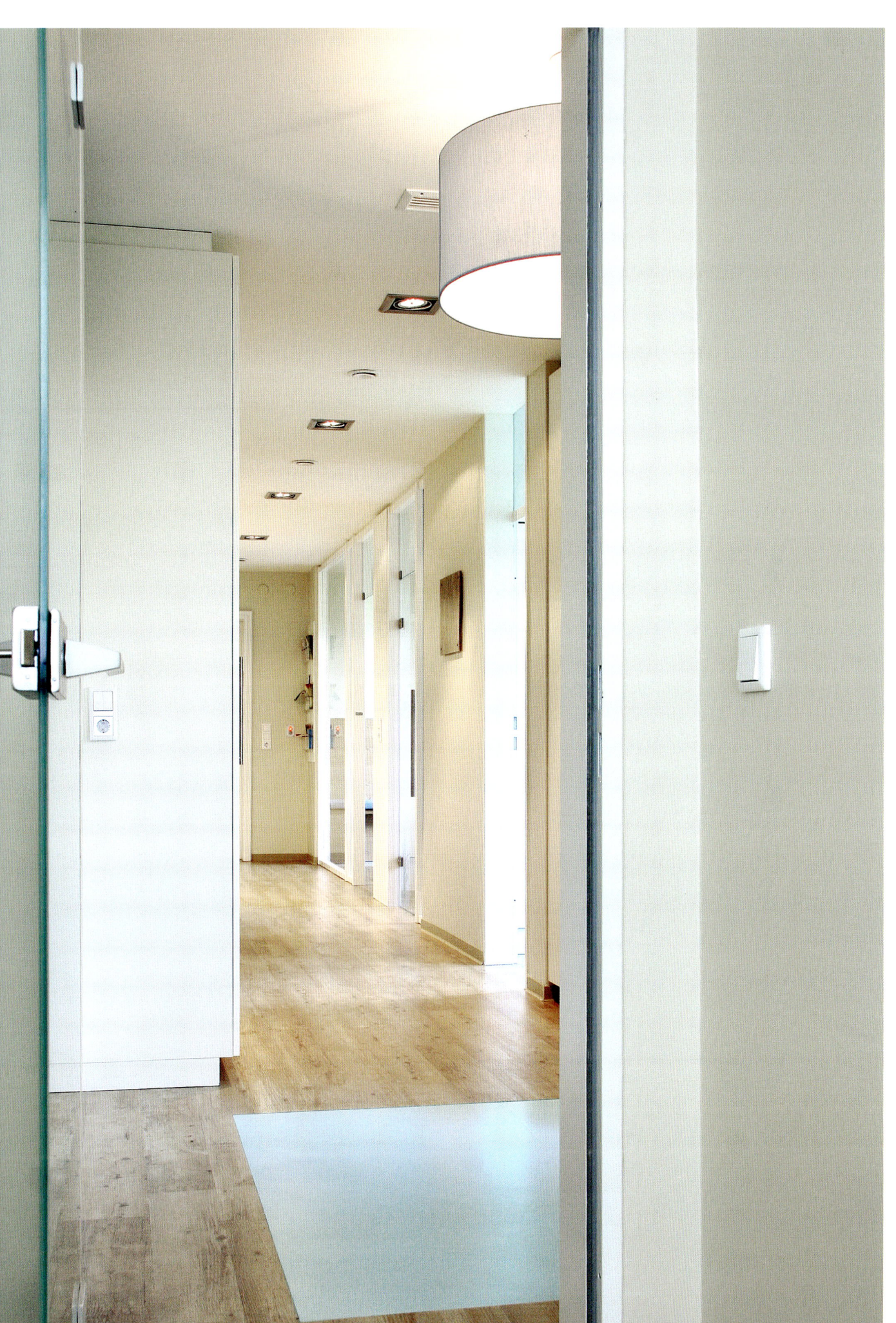

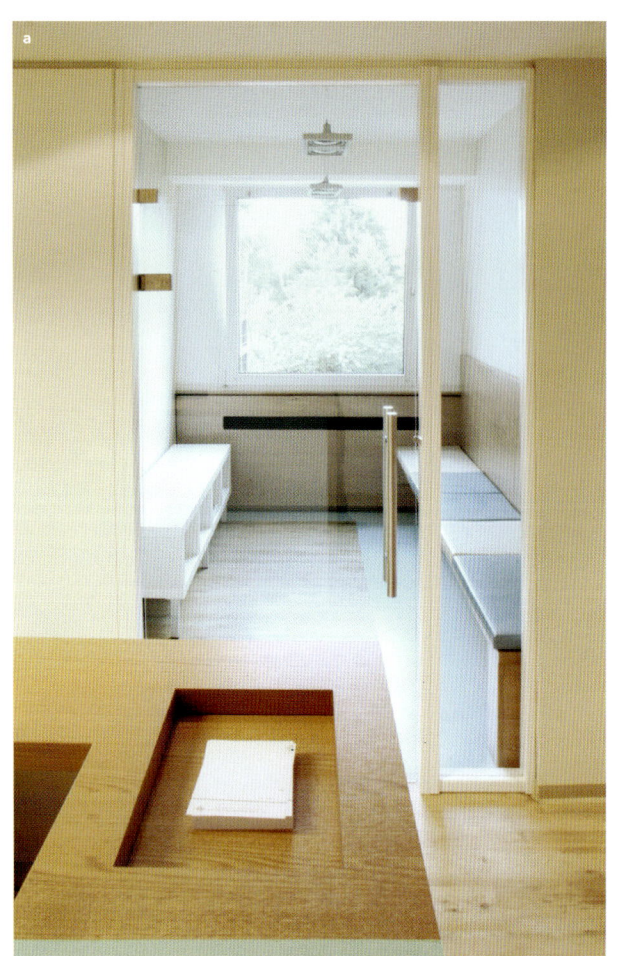
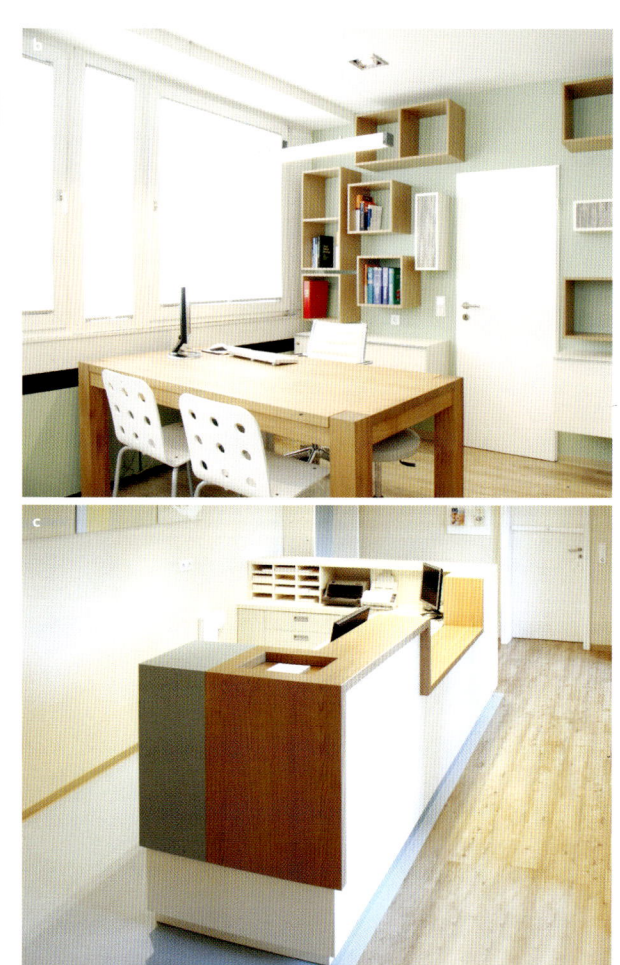

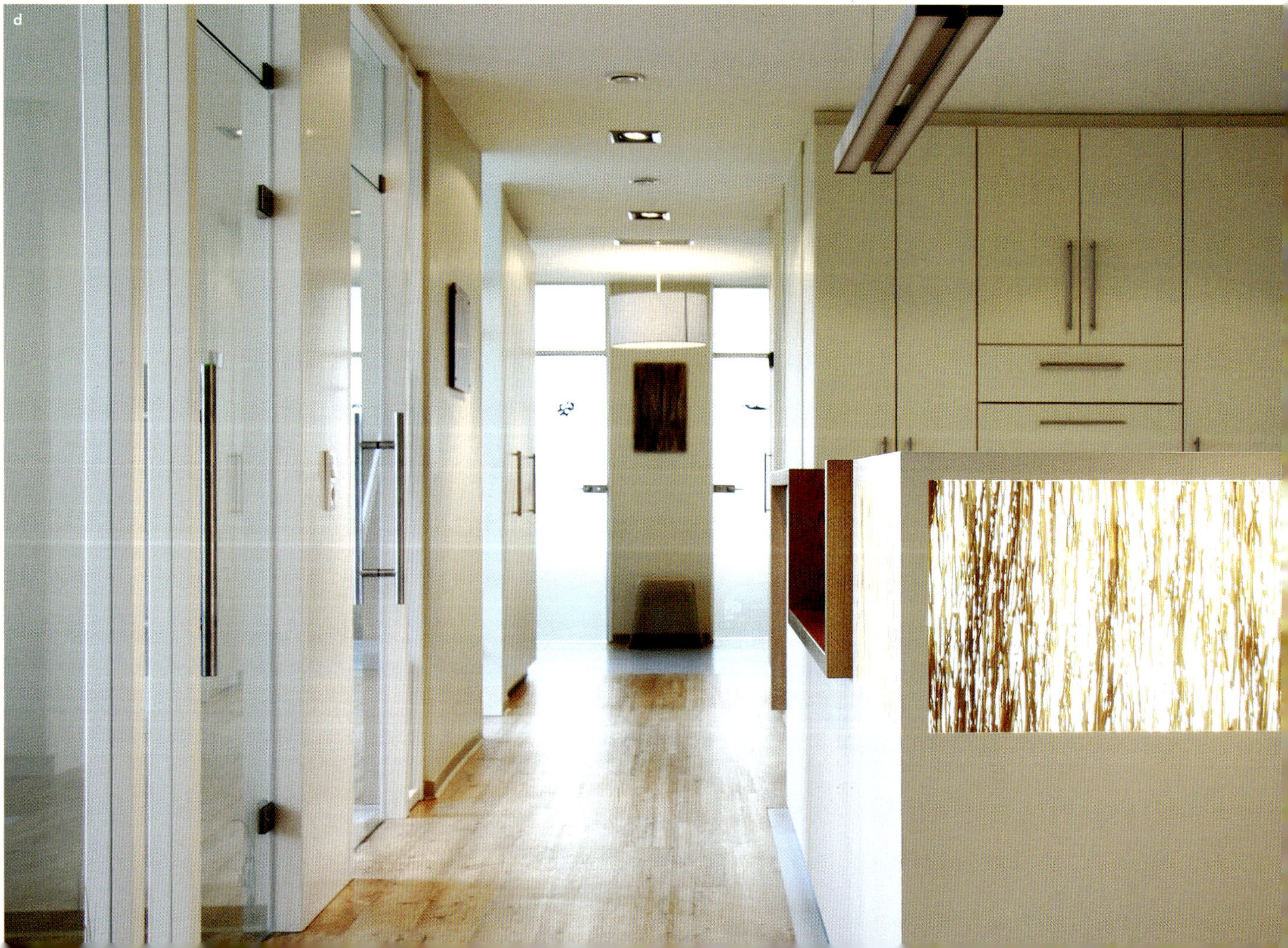

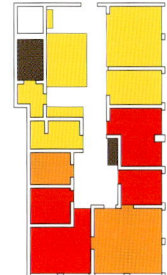

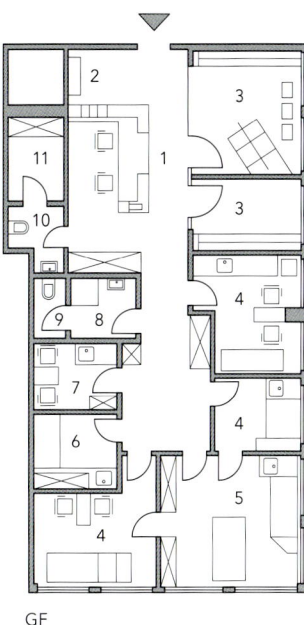

GF

**Client	Operator**	Dr. Gabriela Warbanow	
Planning time	02 2007– 04 2007	
Construction time	04 2007– 05 2007	
Gross floor area	105 sqm	
Usable floor space	87 sqm	
Gross cubic capacity	289 cbm	
Construction cost	70,000 EUR	
Total cost	75,000 EUR	

a   The waiting area, which is easy to spot from the reception, is bright and friendly.

b   In the examination room, the central design concept of the summer meadow is expressed in pastel-green walls.

c   The reception desk, at two different heights, is designed to be suitable for children.

d   The PVC floor covering in a natural wood look is continually relieved by contrasting areas of rubber.

Diagrammatic plans, to scale 1:400
Floor plans, to scale 1:200

Floor plan layout

1	Reception	**5**	Doctor's office	**9**	Patient toilet L
2	Coat-rack	**6**	Laboratory	**10**	Patient toilet G
3	Waiting area	**7**	Staff lounge	**11**	Cleaning room
4	Examination	**8**	Winding space		

With this single-doctor practice, arranged on a long rectangle, the planner has made good use of the space available. There is one central corridor, the breadth of which alters where this is needed, and this leads to the reception and waiting area and also all the other rooms.

Usable floor spaces

Patient rooms	**yellow**	34 sqm	39 %
Examination			
Treatment rooms	**red**	29 sqm	33 %
Offices	Staff rooms	**orange**	19 sqm	22 %
Supply	Waste disposal	**brown**	5 sqm	6 %
Total		87 sqm	100 %

"Naturally good!" – This is the motto of the Krefeld dental practice, specialising in traditional Chinese medicine. The dandelion motif is used throughout the practice as a recurring decorative element. The patient is conducted through the rooms based on drawings showing the plants throughout their lifecycle. The central feature is the white reception desk with the office cube behind it – a continuous, painted band picks up on the dark shade of the floor and forms a stark contrast to the light furnishings. Desk and cube are accentuated by indirect cove lighting and appear to float above the floor. In order to optimise workflow, and as interesting detail, the counter top, used for admitting patient cards, is slotted in layers. Dandelion motifs painted on the wall point the way to the transparent waiting area, which is furnished with inviting, dark leather chairs, and to the four treatment rooms, whose floors have a look of slate and whose white built-in furniture with Wenge wood worktops convey a warm, calming atmosphere.

In keeping with this interior design concept, visiting cards, flyers and website have been developed to guarantee a high degree of recognition and to gain confidence in the medical services by using the practice brand.

NULL2ELF

DENTAL PRACTICE
KREFELD | G

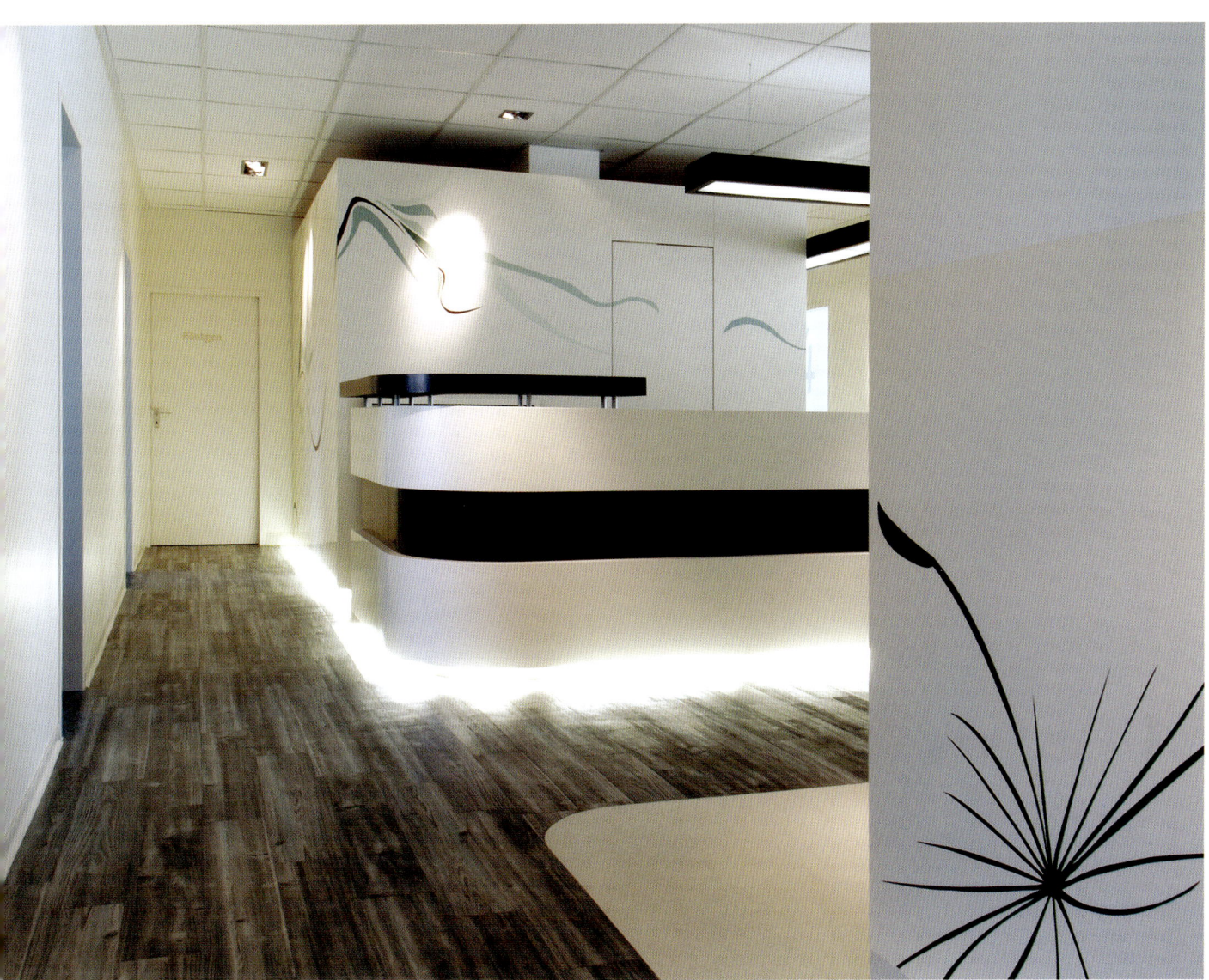

a

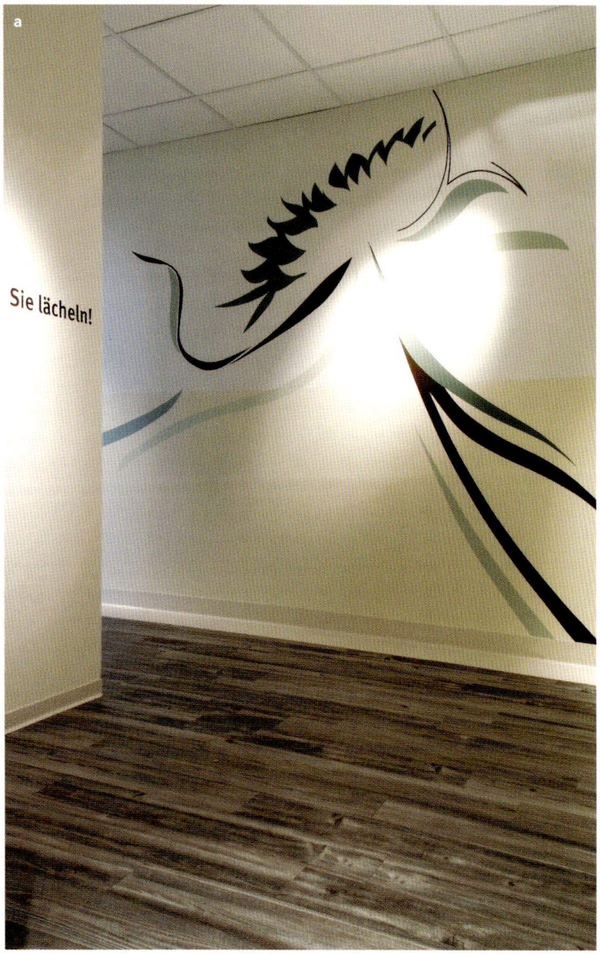

b

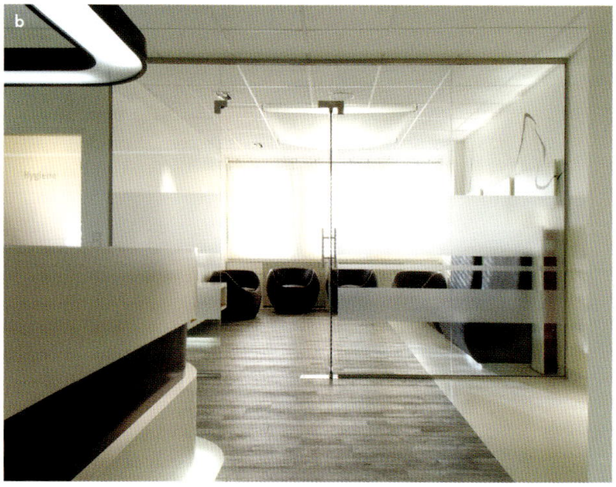

c

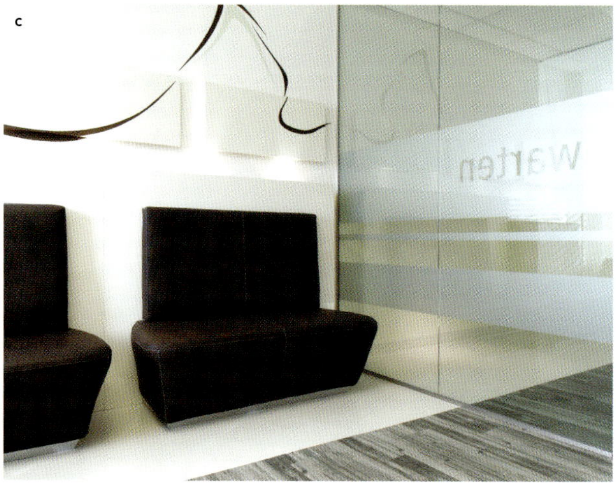

d

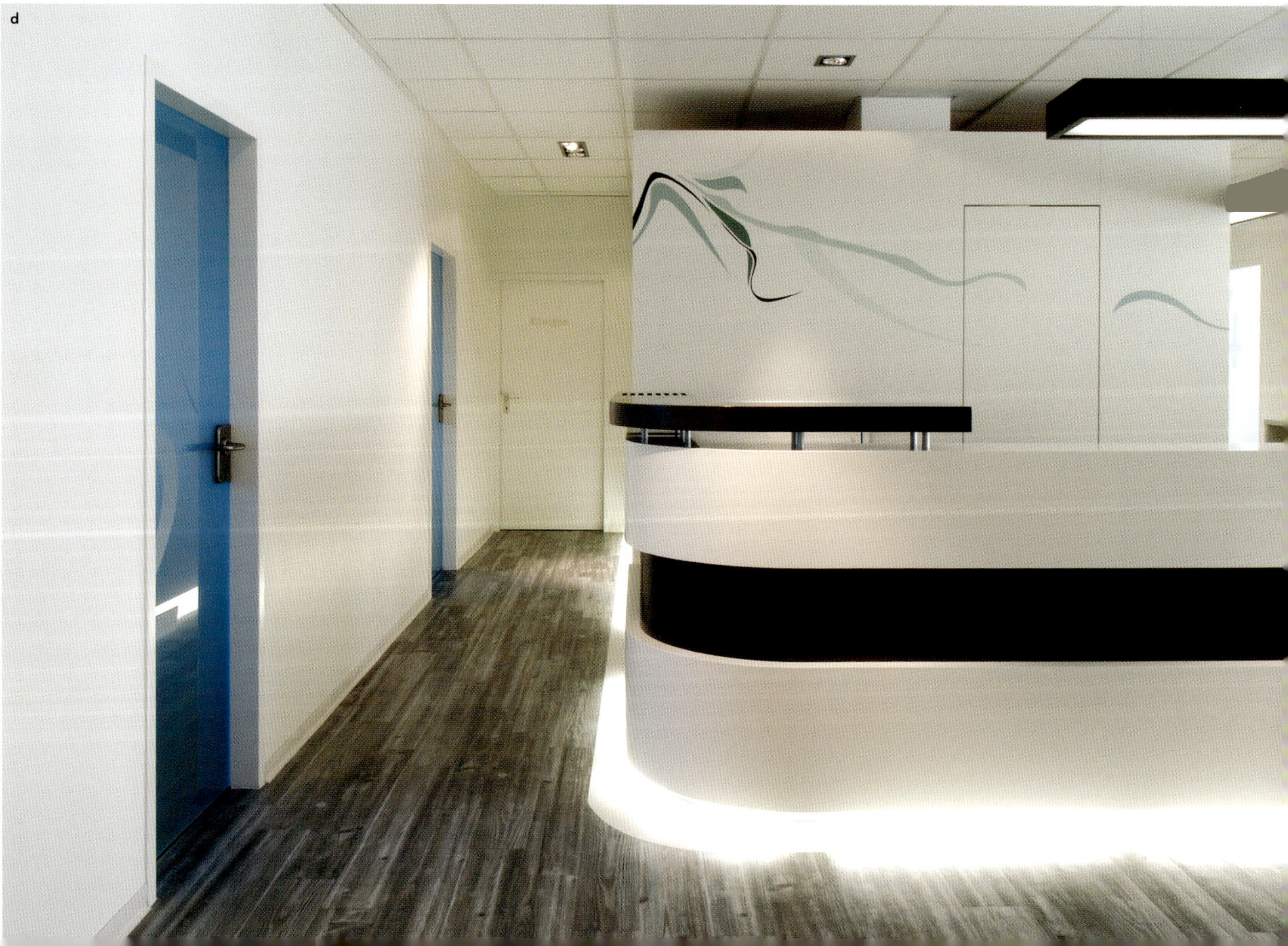

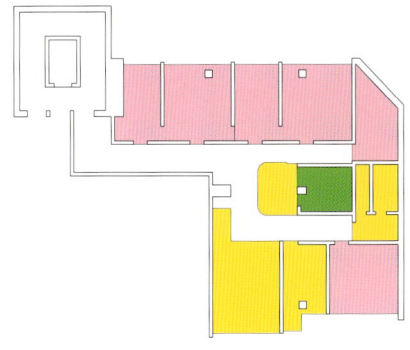

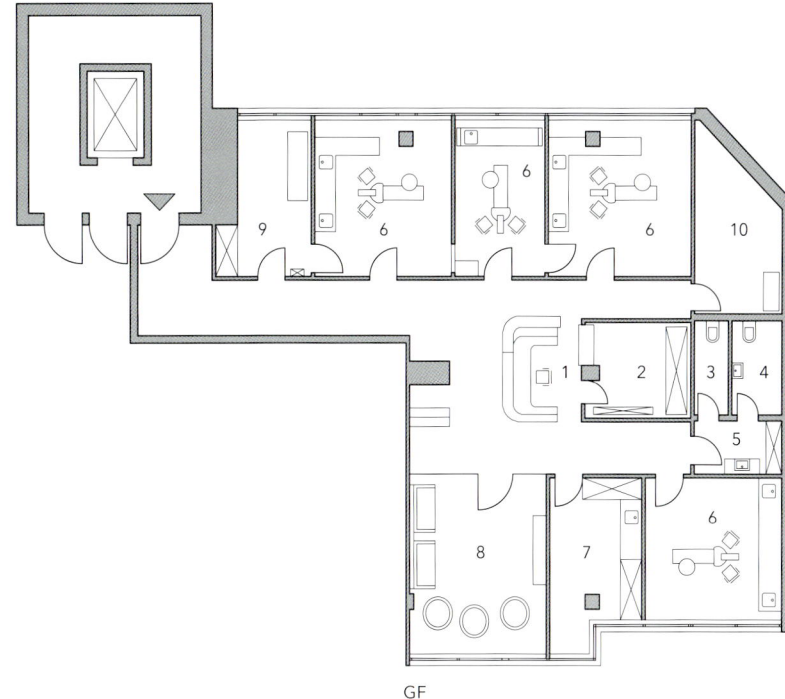

GF

Client | Operator   Ewa Ruschke
                          Wojciech Goral
Planning time   07 2005 – 10 2005
Construction time   09 2005 – 10 2005
Usable floor space   142 sqm
Gross cubic capacity 450 cbm
Construction cost   80,000 EUR
Total cost   120,000 EUR

a The dandelion motif is used as a recurring
   decorative element throughout the practice.
b The transparent waiting area is furnished with
   dark leather chairs.
c Areas of rubber set into the floor show the
   patients the way.
d The reception desk and the office cube behind
   it are accentuated by the cove lighting and
   appear to float above the floor.

Diagrammatic plans, to scale 1:400
Floor plans, to scale 1:200

Floor plan layout

1 Reception	**5** Toilet anteroom	**9** Treatment room
2 Office	**6** Treatment room	**10** Examination X-ray
3 Patient toilet G	**7** Hygiene	
4 Patient toilet L	**8** Waiting area	

Patients access the reception, situated in the centre of this multiple practice,
and the waiting area diagonally opposite, via an angled piece of corridor. Two
short corridors, clearly laid out, lead to the treatment rooms. Apart from the
office, all other rooms requiring natural light have windows.

Usable floor spaces

Patient rooms	**yellow**	50 sqm	35 %
Specialist rooms	**pink**	84 sqm	59 %
Administrative rooms	**green**	8 sqm	6 %
Total		142 sqm	100 %

Performance data

Outpatients per year	7,000
Number and type of services per year	Filling [3,000]
	Root canal treatment [1,500]
	Crown [4,000]
	Prothese [1,000]
	Implant [60]
Services to other clinics	Wisdom teeth extraction [800]
	Bone grafting [50]
	Root end resection [600]
	Gum grafting [50]
Clinic opening hours	5 days	60 hours
Waiting time [with	without appointment]	0 – 45 min.	0 – 120 min.
Type and number of staff	4 doctors
	4 full-time staff
	3 trainees
Clinic planning advice	additional:
	Treatment room
	Digitalisation
	Infrared cameras
	Laser
	Milling machine

"Travel healthily" – the newly-established "medical + dental suite" at Cologne Bonn Airport has succeeded in promoting itself with this slogan. In the centre of the terminal, at the transition to the underground long-distance railway station, a joint general medicine and dentistry practice has been created.

The centrepiece of the interior design is a 25-metre long wall, extending across the practice, whose curved shape is reminiscent of the wing of an aircraft. Many other details also evoke associations with aviation: the apertures in the waiting area, round-shaped like aircraft doors, the spotlights on the walls, resembling the marker lights of a runway, or the nose-shaped reception desk, which is clearly reminiscent of a cockpit on the floor plan. Except for the waiting area, which is laid with dark parquet flooring of Wenge wood, a brownish-coloured concrete floor has been chosen for the entire practice. One fine detail is a 25-centimeter wide stainless steel strip, which clads the aperture to the waiting area, matches the greyish paint of the curved wall. The absolute highlight of this exceptional, extremely dynamic practice, however, is the breathtaking view of what's going on at the airport. Behind Terminal D, which you view from the waiting and treatment area, you can watch aircrafts taking off and landing and forget that you are actually at a medical facility.

PD RAUMPLAN

MEDICAL + DENTAL SUITE AT COLOGNE BONN AIRPORT
COLOGNE | G

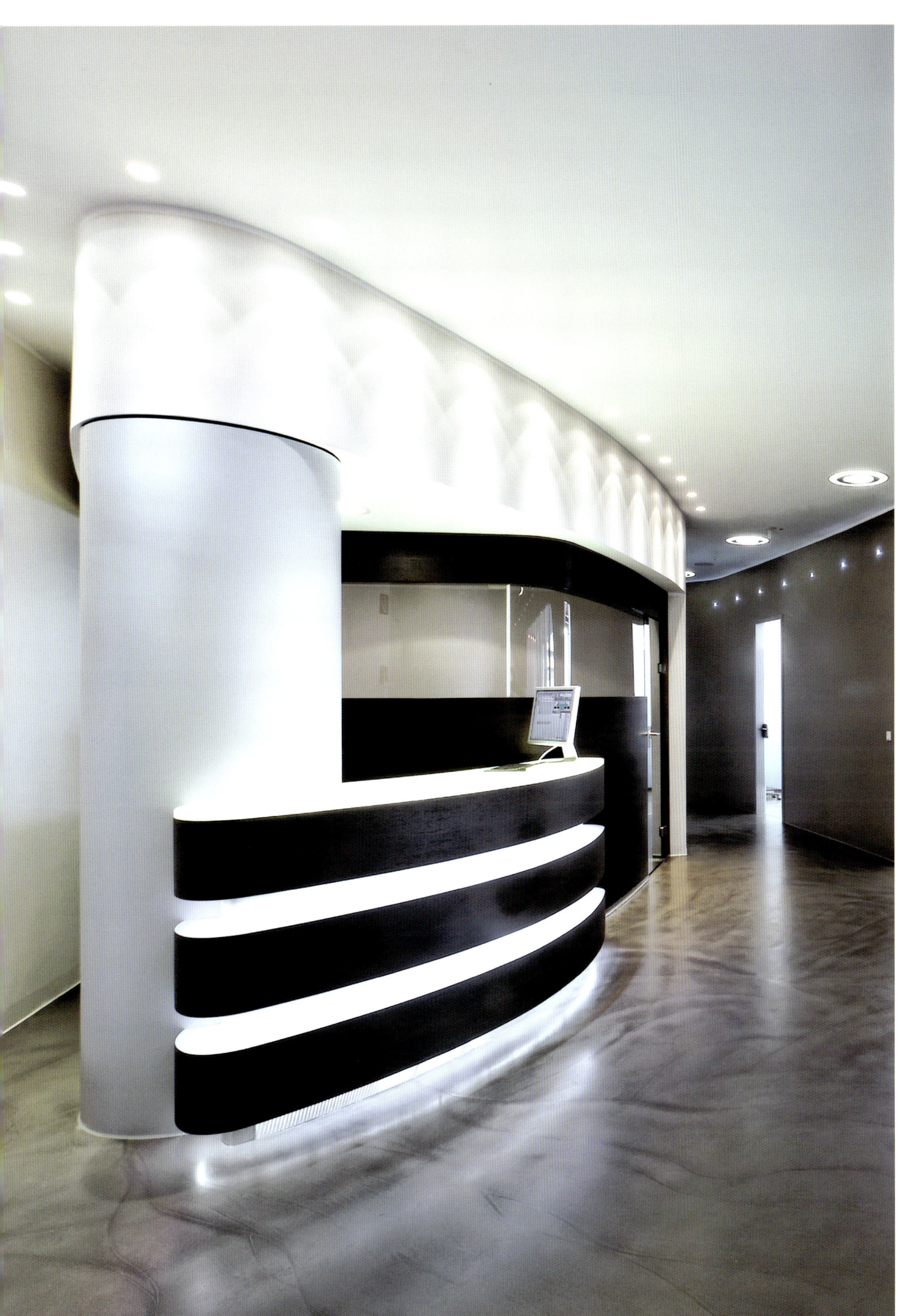

a

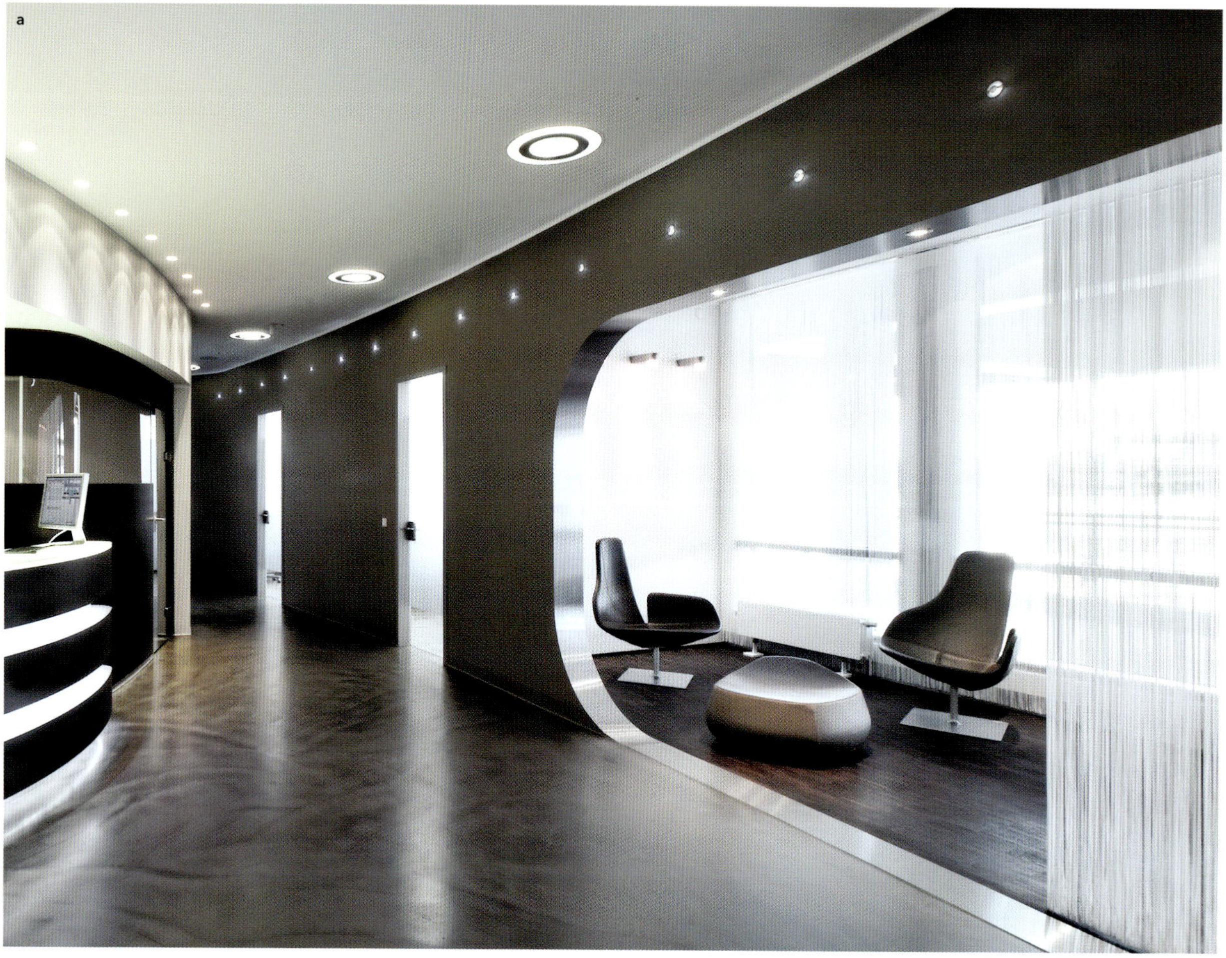

b

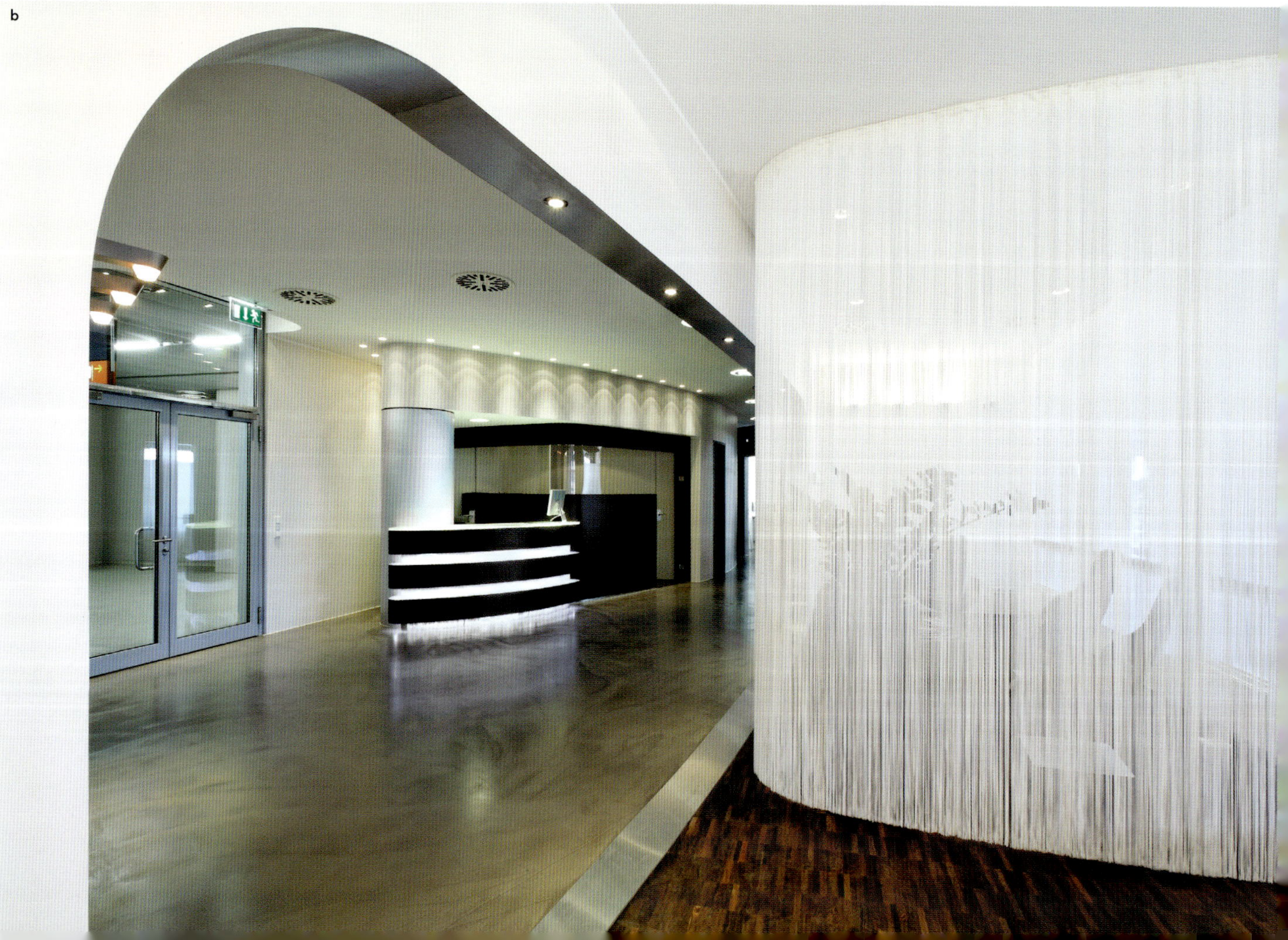

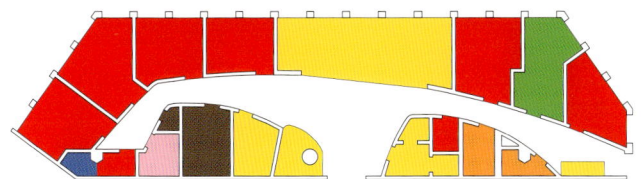

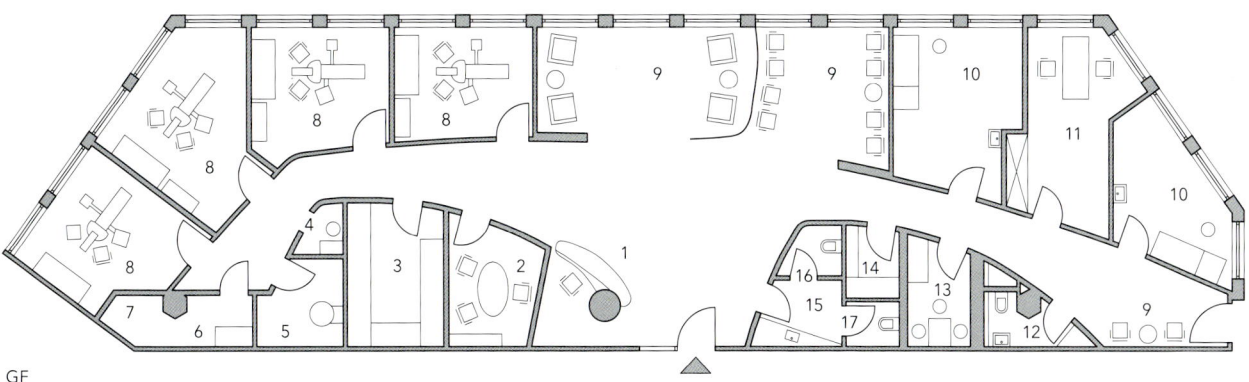

GF

Client	Jochem Heibach
Operator	Jochem Heibach
	Dr. Jens Knitter
Planning time	11 2006 – 03 2007
Construction time	04 2007 – 07 2007
Gross floor area	240 sqm
Usable floor space	202 sqm
Construction cost	300,000 EUR

a Small details evoke the world of aviation: the apertures in the waiting area, round-shaped like aircraft doors, the spotlights on the walls, which look like marker lights on a runway …

b … or the nose-shaped reception desk, which is reminiscent of a cockpit on the floor plan.

Diagrammatic plans, to scale 1:400
Floor plans, to scale 1:200

Floor plan layout

1	Reception	6	Laboratory	12	Staff toilet
2	Consultation room	7	Installations room	13	Staff lounge
3	Sterilisation room	8	Treatment room	14	Laboratory
4	Cleaning room and store room	9	Waiting area	15	Toilet anteroom
5	Examination X-ray	10	Examination	16	Patient toilet L
		11	Office	17	Patient toilet G

In the centre of the long polygonal floor plan is the entrance to this multiple practice, and from there the visible reception and waiting areas can be accessed directly. The suite of rooms opposite the entrance is fully equipped with natural light. The rooms at the side of the entrance, including the staff lounge, have to make do without natural light.

Usable floor spaces

Patient rooms	**yellow**	63 sqm	31 %
Examination | Treatment rooms	**red**	94 sqm	47 %
Specialist rooms	**pink**	5 sqm	3 %
Administrative rooms	**green**	16 sqm	8 %
Offices | Staff rooms	**orange**	9 sqm	4 %
Supply | Waste disposal	**brown**	13 sqm	6 %
Plant rooms	**blue**	2 sqm	1 %
Total		202 sqm	100 %

Performance data

Outpatients per year	18,000
Services to other clinics	Dental laboratory [2,500]
Clinic opening hours	7 days | 70 hours
Waiting time [with | without appointment]	5 – 15 min.
	15 – 45 min.
Type and number of staff	4 doctors
	4 full-time staff
	1 trainee

Ornamental patterns are the central motif of the interior design of this surgical practice clinic in Goethestraße, Frankfurt. Historical gobelins are used for the floral decoration and can also be found in the wall tapestry in the waiting areas. Particularly evident is the winding vines design on the white reception desk in the foyer, where the ornamentation is etched into the twelve millimetre thick, mineral-filled panel. The remaining three millimetres are so translucent, that, illuminated from behind, they create a wonderful effect — similar to a silhouette. In contrast with this somewhat whimsical pattern for the other areas of the practice it has been adopted a rather more modest, slightly curved line with rounded corners, whose design concept is reminiscent of the architecture of the 1970s. Illuminated wall niches, partly glazed, are used in the corridor area for the presentation of cosmetic products, as well in the examination rooms for accommodating medical preparations. Patients can relax while reading Goethe quotations inscribed on the corridor walls, if they so wish.

The whole practice exudes an atmosphere of elegant restraint, which is also supported by the elected choice of floral decorations and fine materials, like the Wenge solid wood parquet in the treatment rooms.

PD RAUMPLAN

"GOETHE 10" PRACTICE CLINIC
FRANKFURT ON THE MAIN | G

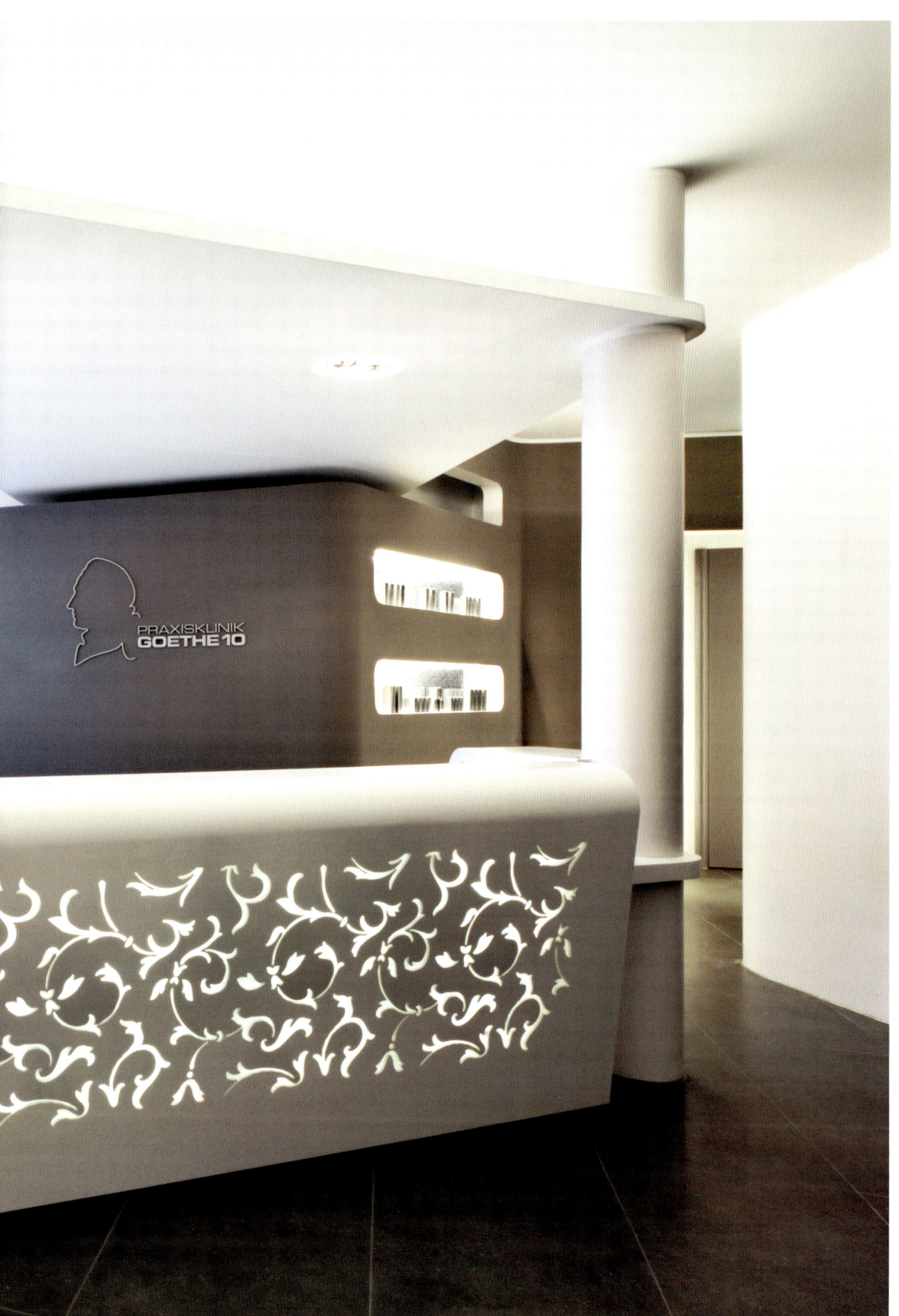

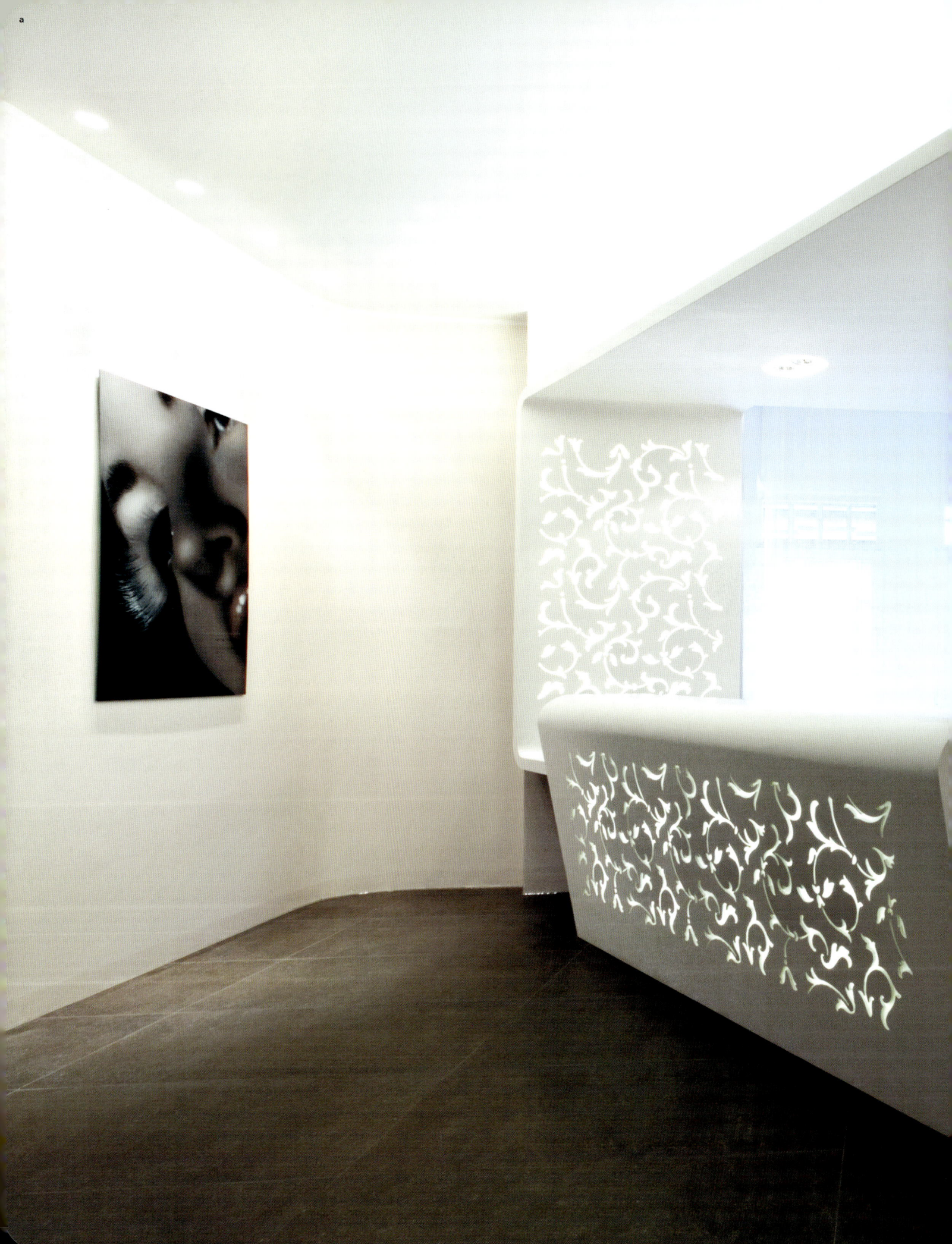

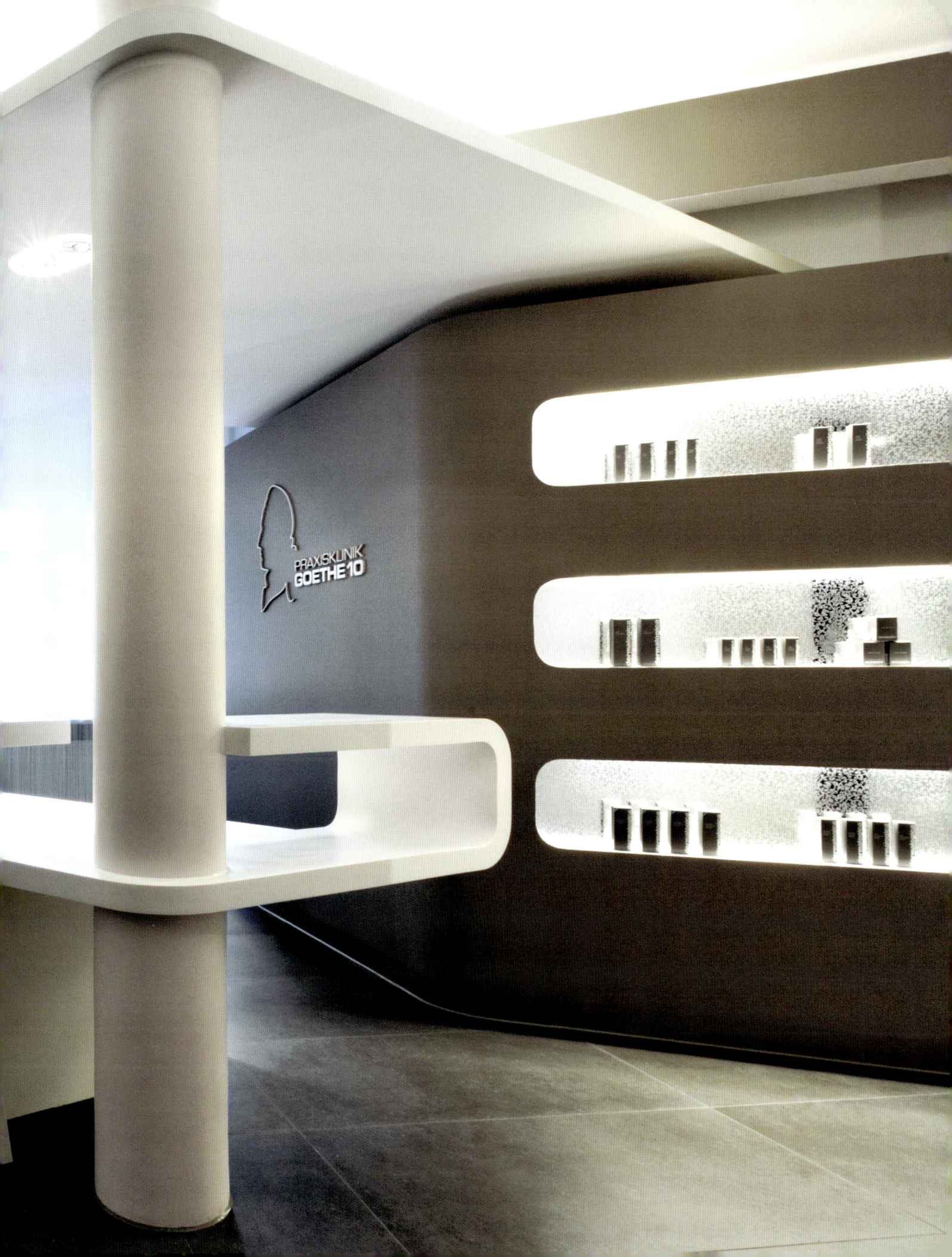

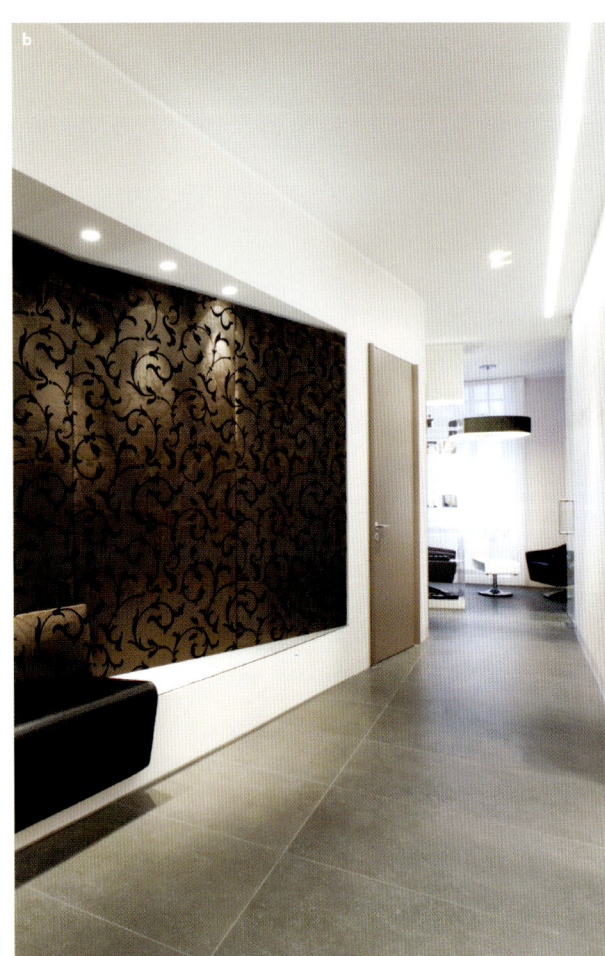

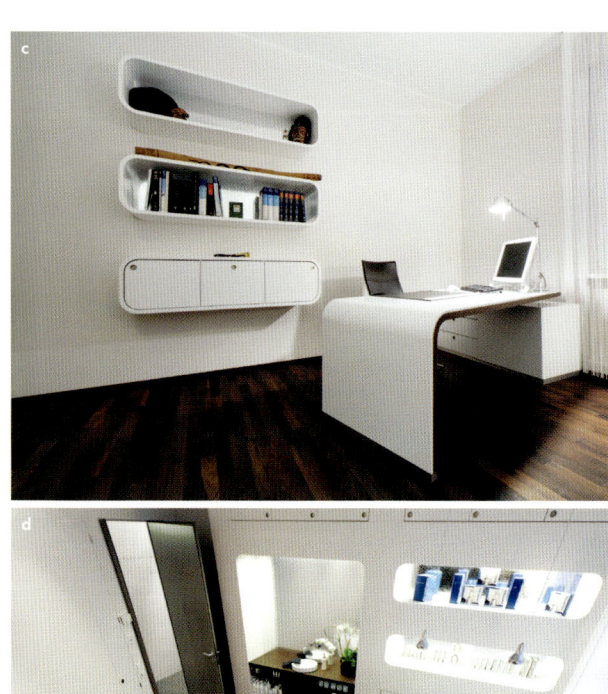

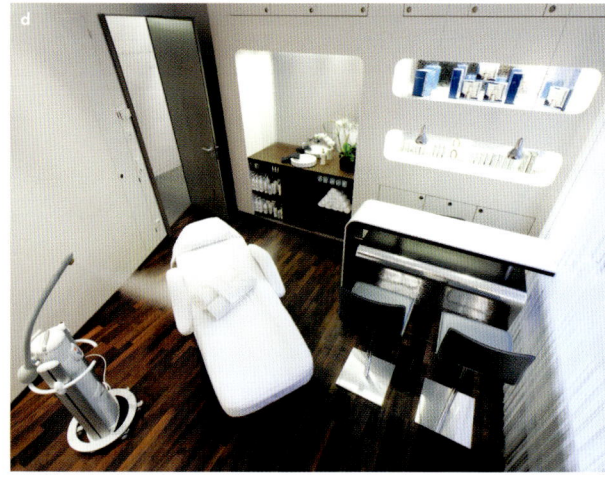

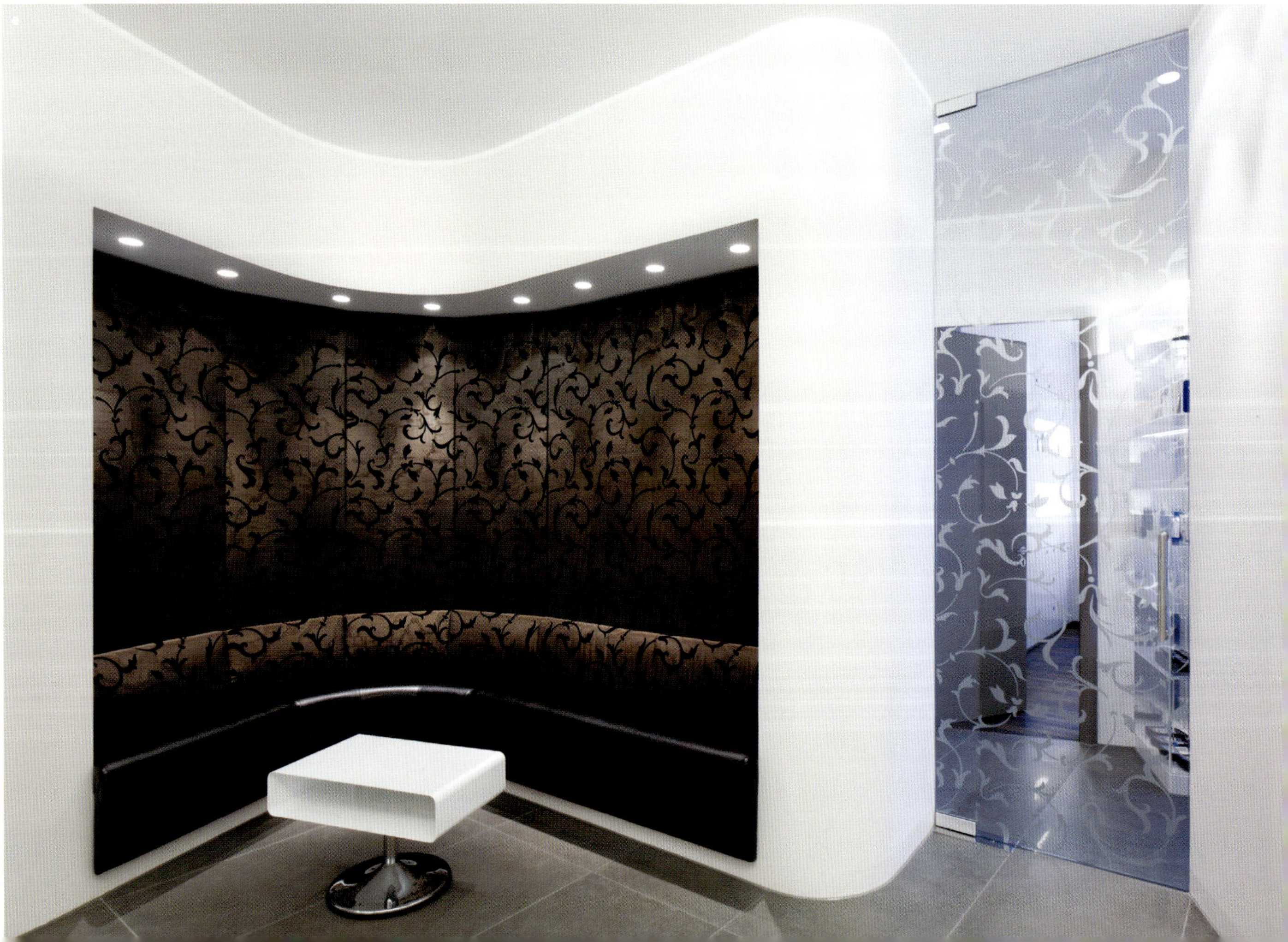

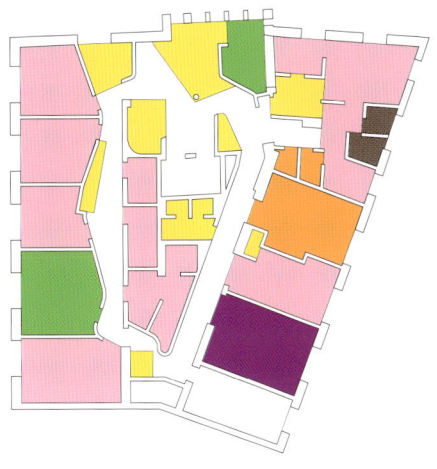

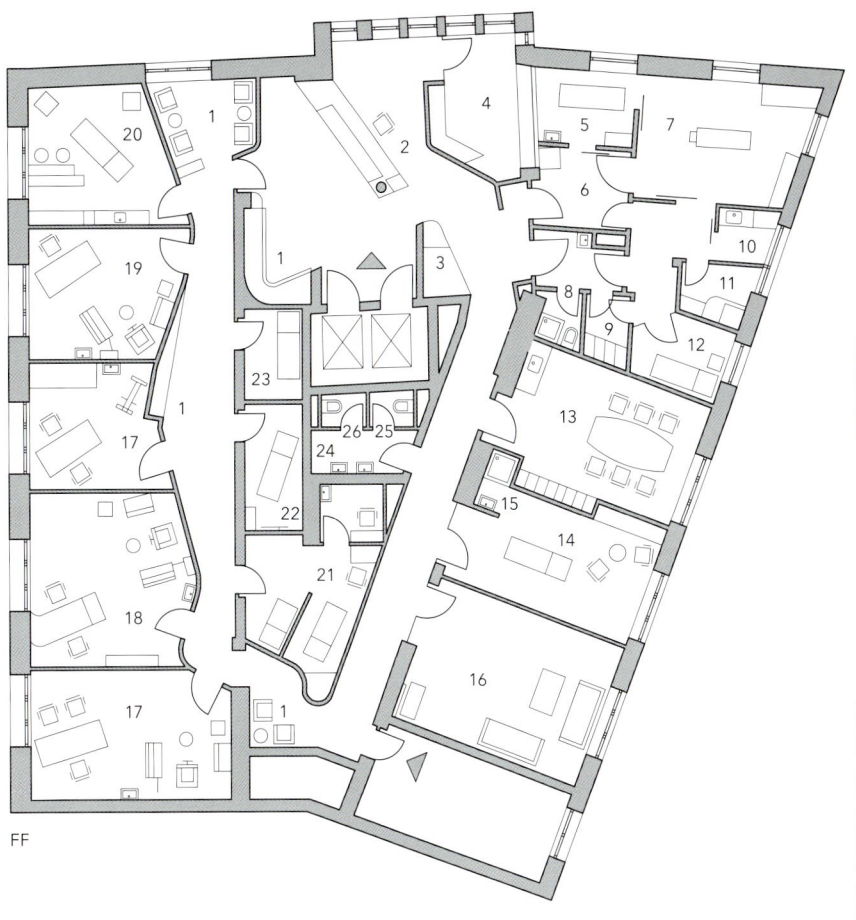

FF

Client	Operator	Dr. Thomas Fischer
Planning time	07 2006 – 09 2006
Construction time	09 2006 – 01 2007
Gross floor area	360 sqm
Usable floor space	273 sqm
Construction cost	425,000 EUR

a The ornamentation on the white reception desk is etched into the twelve millimetre thick, mineral-filled panel.

b Vine patterns modelled on historic gobelins can also be found on the wall tapestry in the waiting areas.

c In contrast with the somewhat whimsical pattern, dominating the reception and waiting areas, in the rest of the practice have been adopted more modest, slightly curved lines.

d The dark Wenge wood parquet flooring imparts a cosy, yet elegant atmosphere to the treatment rooms.

e Floral predominance: In the waiting area, the patients are surrounded by extremely elaborate vine patterns.

Diagrammatic plans, to scale 1:400
Floor plans, to scale 1:200

Floor plan layout

1	Waiting area	**11**	Sterilisation room sterile
2	Reception		
3	Coat-rack	**12**	Recovery room
4	Accounts office	**13**	Staff lounge and staff changing cubicle
5	Prep room		
6	Patient changing cubicle	**14**	Massage room
		15	Patient shower
7	Procedure room	**16**	Seminar and refreshment room
8	Staff toilet and shower		
		17	Treatment room dermatology
9	Staff changing cubicle		
		18	Office ENT
10	Sterilisation room unsterile	**19**	Examination and

treatment ENT	
20	Treatment room cosmetics
21	Examination otoneurology
22	Treatment room infusion
23	Examination sonography
24	Toilet anteroom
25	Patient toilet L
26	Patient toilet G

Patients come straight from a group of lifts to the reception of this multiple practice, which is designed on a polygonal floor plan with a corridor running around a concentric group of rooms. There are waiting areas at four points, only one of which is visible from the reception. The rooms located in the core group receive no natural light, while rooms at the outer front have windows.

Usable floor spaces

Patient rooms	**yellow**	47 sqm	17 %
Specialist rooms	**pink**	141 sqm	52 %
Administrative rooms	**green**	30 sqm	11 %
Offices	Staff rooms	**orange**	25 sqm	9 %
Supply	Waste disposal	**brown**	6 sqm	2 %
Training rooms	**violet**	24 sqm	9 %
Total		273 sqm	100 %

Performance data

Outpatients per year	5,000
Inpatients per year	80 – 90 day-patient
Clinic opening hours	5 days	55 hours
Waiting time [with	without appointment]	10 – 15 min.	10 – 30 min.
Type and number of staff	2 – 3 doctors
	4 full-time staff
	1 part-time staff

With the Vitalicum, another practice has been implemented in the building at Opernplatz in Frankfurt. The floor plan is identical, the material is similar and the design concept deliberately draws heavily on the "A1" Dental Practice [see pages 310 to 315], in order to appeal to the same patient collective. Technically, however, this private practice should be more dynamic.

The unusually-curved partition wall in the foyer, which also acts as a transition to one of the waiting areas, expresses this requirement very effectively. Reflectors are integrated into the white wall panels, which throw light indirectly onto the ceiling and illuminate the area behind. On the opposite side, behind an aluminium-panelled wall, is another waiting area. The corporate identity of this private medical group practice is represented by the "Vitalicum" lettering on this wall in twenty-millimetre thick stainless steel letters. A headwall gleams in red at the end of the corridor. The horizontally-backlit, staggered frosted pane strips, made additional ceiling lights redundant and therefore they were not adopted in this area. The dark-smoked oak parquet flooring combined with the bright interior imparts a refined, yet lively, atmosphere to the whole practice.

PD RAUMPLAN

VITALICUM
FRANKFURT ON THE MAIN | G

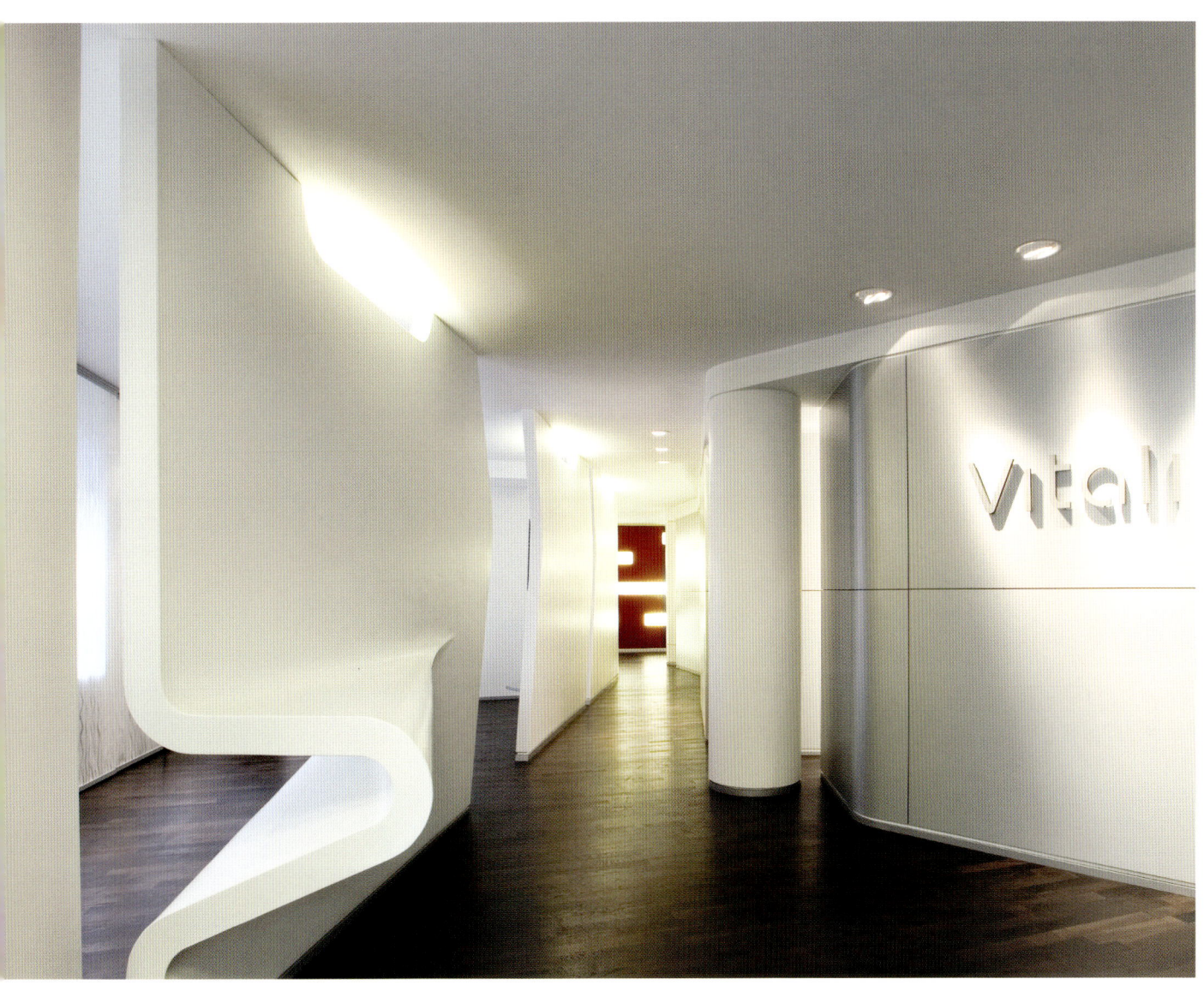

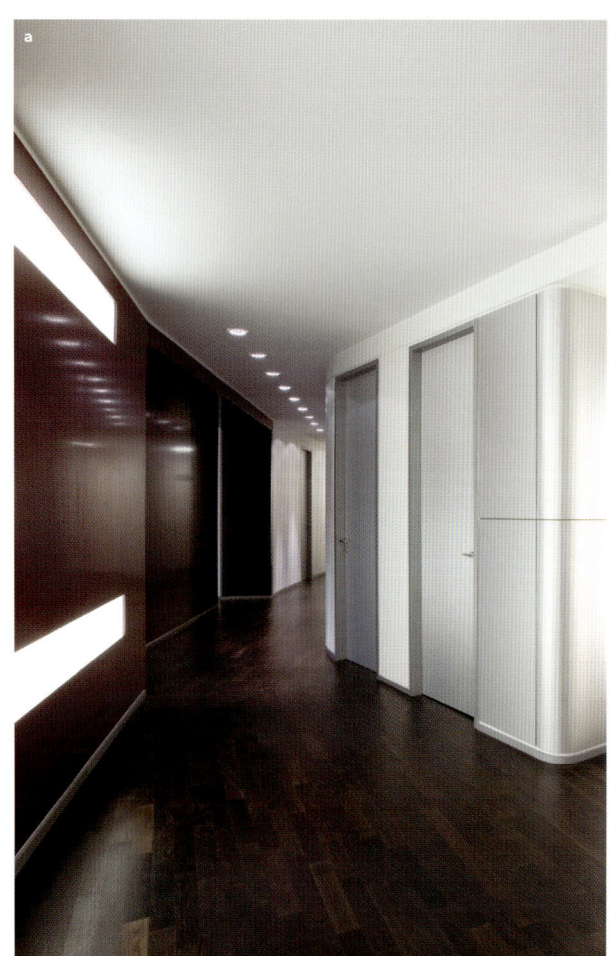

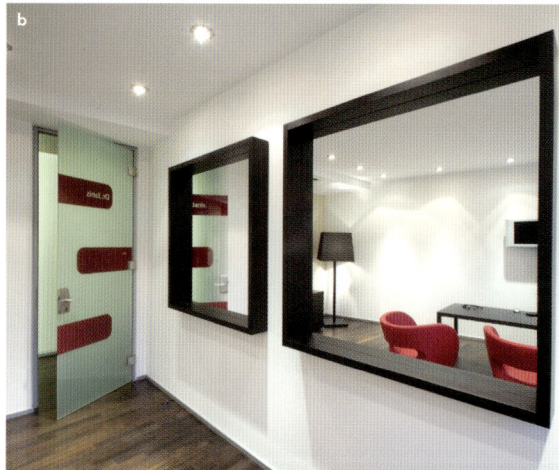

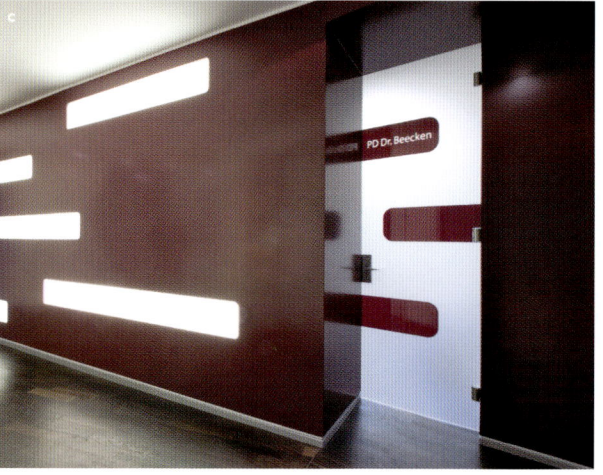

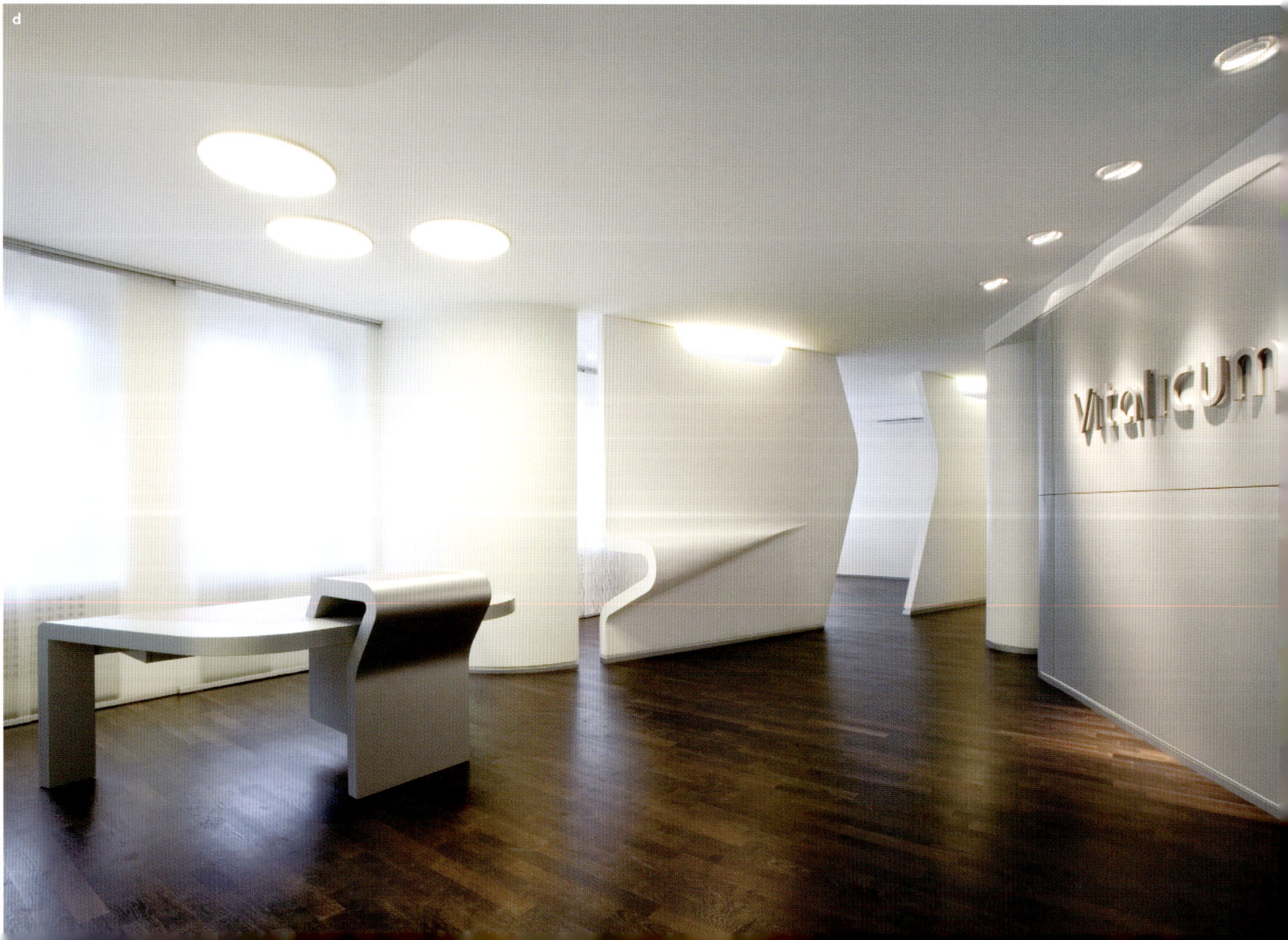

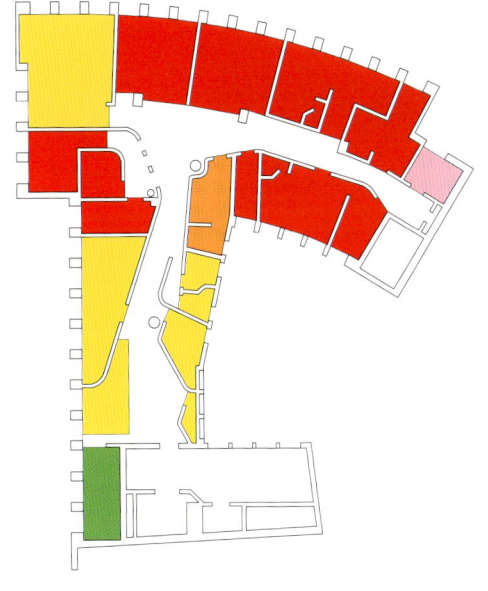

Diagrammatic plans, to scale 1:400
Floor plans, to scale 1:200

FF

1 Reception
2 Waiting area
3 Examination
4 Consultation room
5 Examination and
   treatment room
6 Laboratory
7 Store room
8 Staff lounge
9 Staff toilet
   and shower
10 Patient toilet L
11 Patient toilet G
12 Coat-rack
13 Administration
   and store room

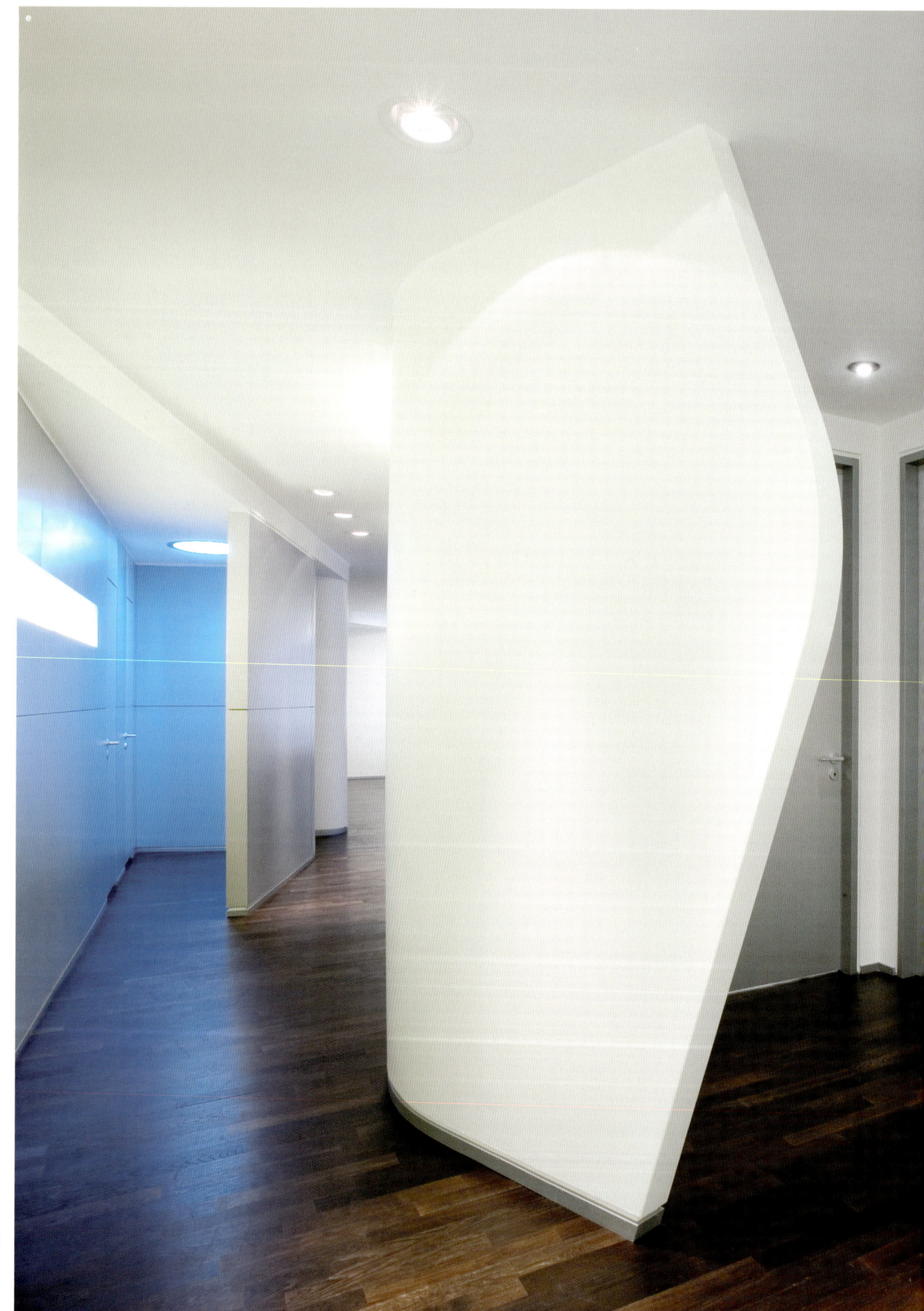

Client	Operator	Dr. Wolf-D. Beeken
	Dr. Michael Janis
Planning time	05 2005 – 06 2005
Construction time	06 2005 – 09 2005
Gross floor area	350 sqm
Usable floor space	247 sqm
Construction cost	480,000 EUR

a Dark-smoked oak parquet flooring imparts a refined, yet lively, atmosphere to the whole practice.

b View into one of the examination and treatment rooms.

c Thanks to the horizontally-backlit, staggered satinised pane strips, additional ceiling lights were not needed in the corridor.

d One of the waiting areas is situated behind the unusually-curved partition wall in the foyer.

e The dynamic lines of the walls impressively reflect the formal design concept.

Floor plan layout

The slightly modified T-shaped floor plan for this multiple practice contains a uniform corridor, likewise modified, where the top beam appears on the one side only as an intimation. From the foot of the T with the reception and waiting areas, the patients access all rooms in the practice, which, with the exception of a small examination room, benefit from natural light.

Usable floor spaces

Patient rooms	**yellow**	80 sqm	32 %
Examination | Treatment rooms	**red**	139 sqm	56 %
Specialist rooms	**pink**	6 sqm	2 %
Administrative rooms	**green**	11 sqm	5 %
Offices | Staff rooms	**orange**	11 sqm	5 %
Total		247 sqm	100 %

Performance data

Clinic opening hours	6 days | 72 hours
Waiting time [with | without appointment]	5 min. | 15 min.
Type and number of staff	6 doctors
	5 team assistants

This small dental practice, not far from the Arc de Triomphe in the centre of Paris, is characterised by aluminium panelling and an extensive use of glass. Before the conversion, the two-storey shop was occupied by a lighting manufacturer's showroom.

In a relatively small space a group practice with four treatment rooms has been created, in total harmony with the magnificent façade of the art nouveau building. In order to make best use of the natural light, which only comes in from the street frontage, the partition wall between the two adjacent treatment rooms and the wall between the treatment room on the left of the entrance and the corridor was built in frosted glass. The other wall surfaces are covered in aluminium panels. Only the wall to the staircase is furnished with Wenge-veneered panels to add some warmth to the dominant aluminium look. In the treatment rooms, the contemporary atmosphere in the foyer is toned down and warmth is added with panelling and maple-veneer fittings. After the extremely straight-line design of the entrance, softer lines and curves are introduced to lead patients into the rear part of the practice. With its trapezoidal shape, the backlit reception desk of aluminium laminate combines straight and round lines and is modestly integrated into the foyer. A water wall is mounted behind the desk: It serves as an object of art and at the same time contributes to create a pleasant atmosphere.

PD RAUMPLAN

"CENTRE D'ENDODONTIE"
ENDODONTOLOGY CLINIC
PARIS | F

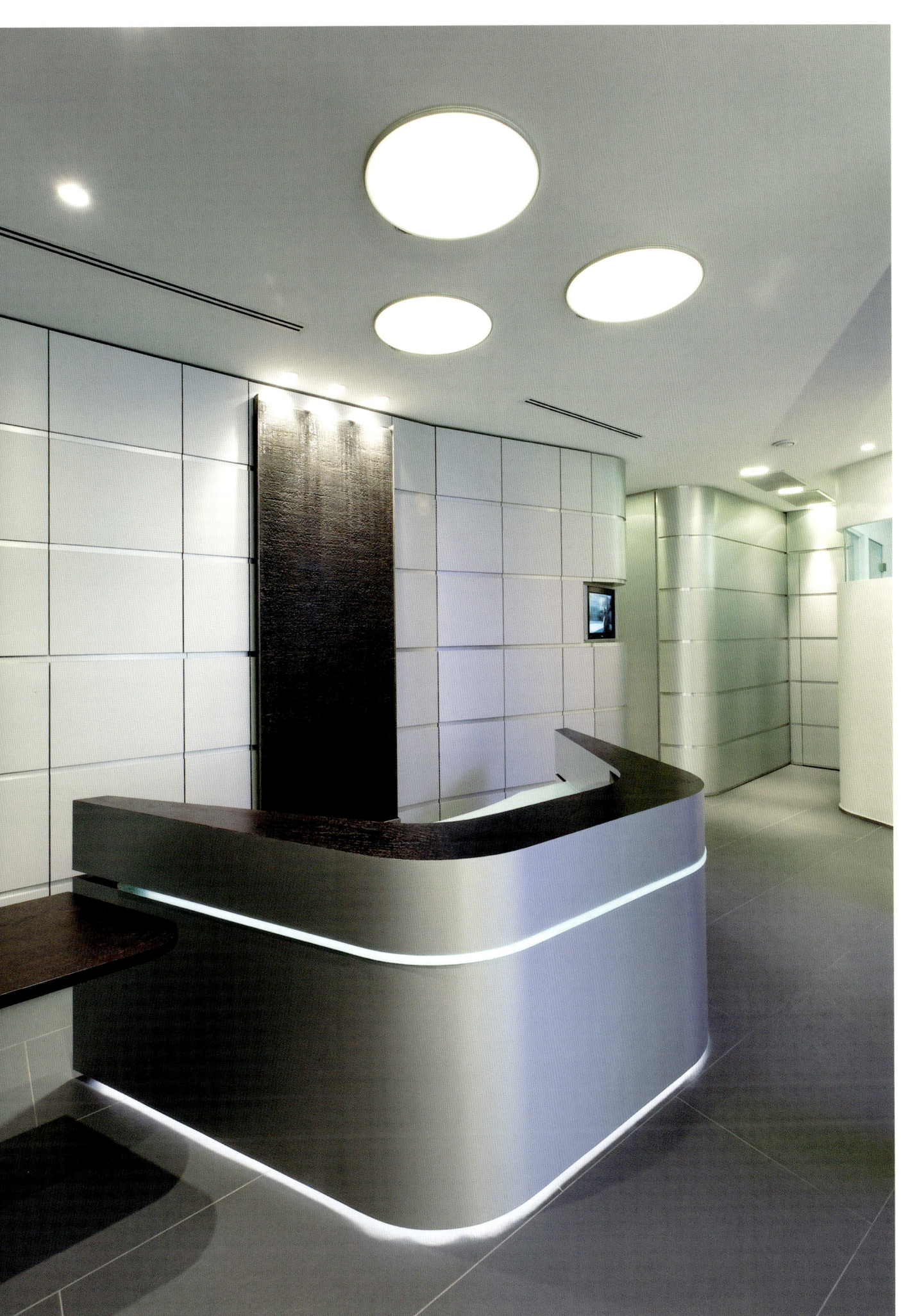

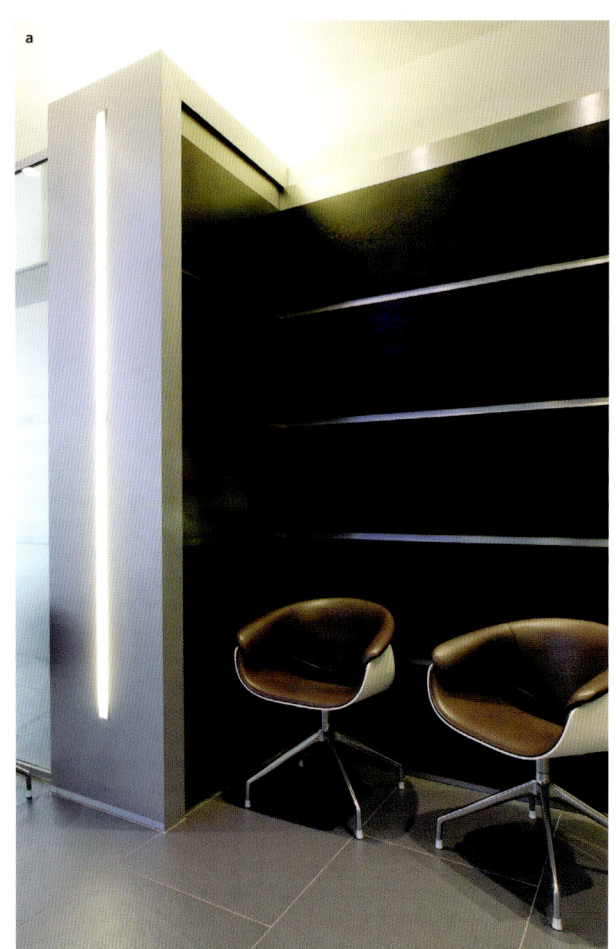

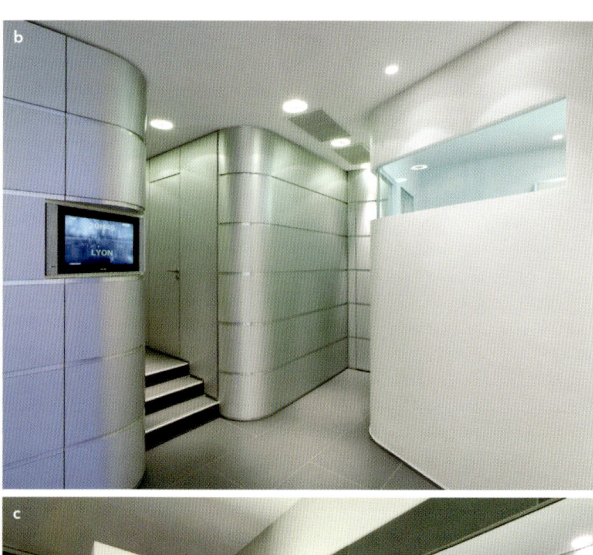

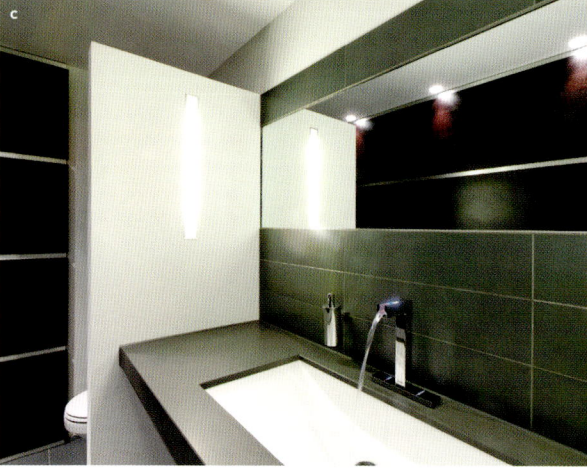

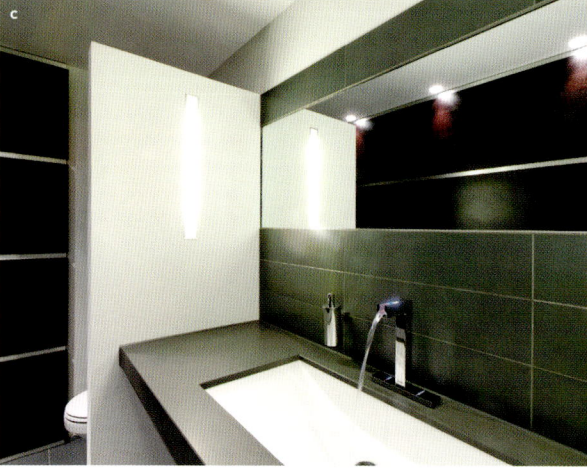

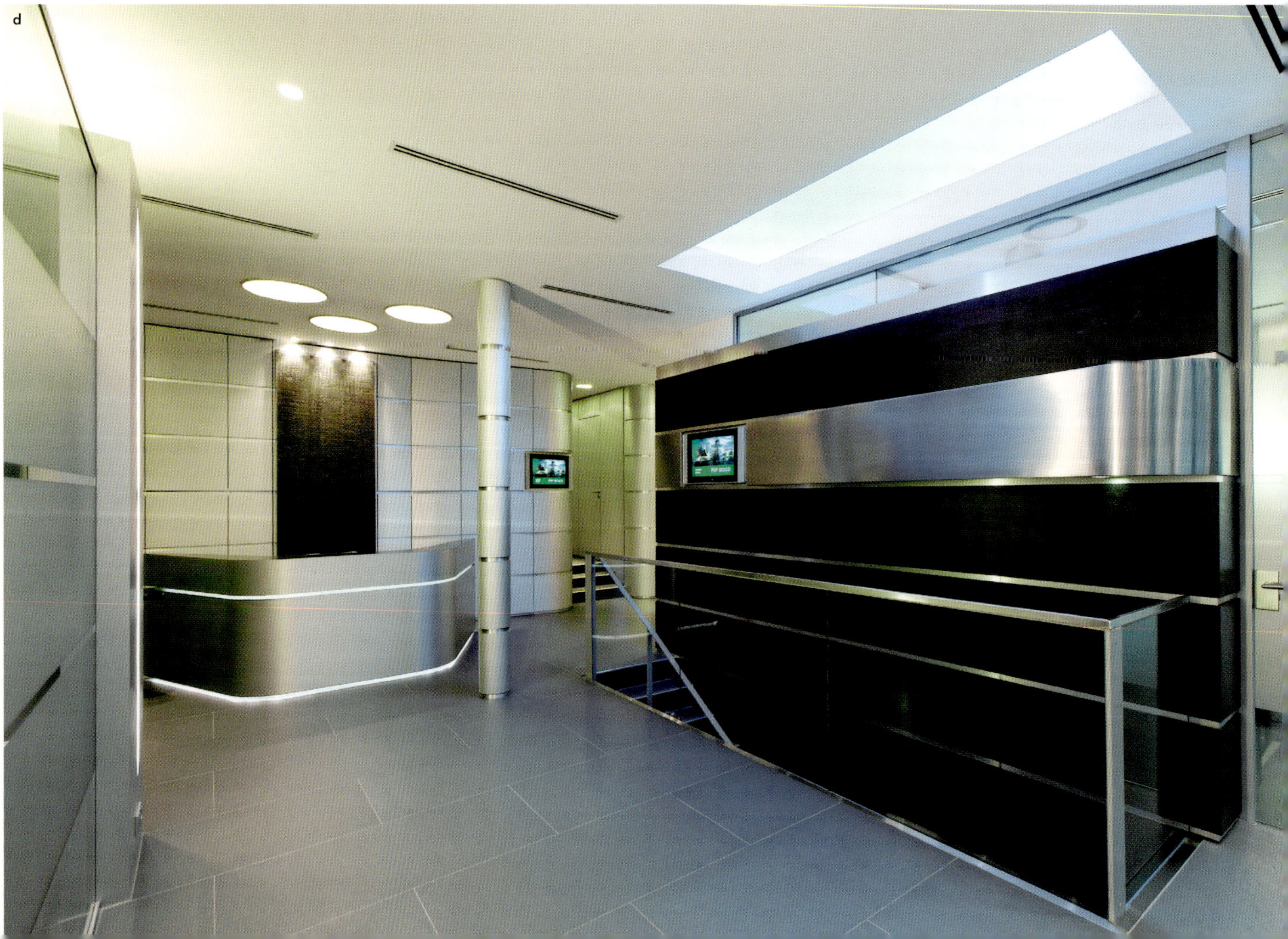

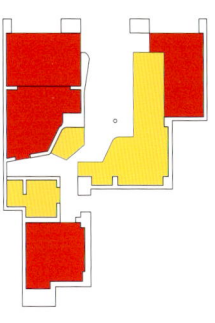

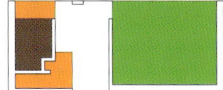

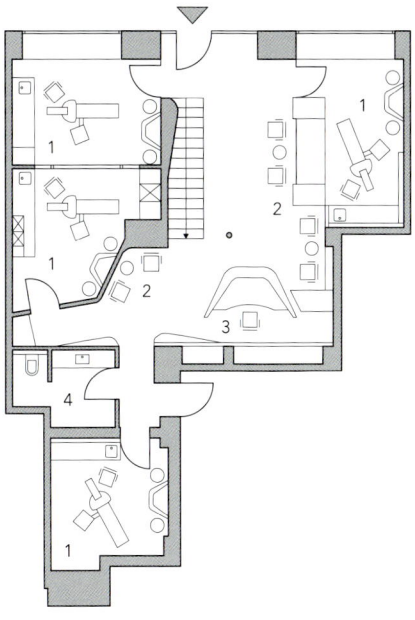

GF

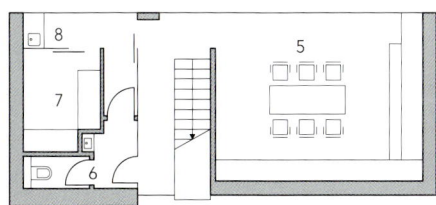

BSMT

Client	Operator	Dr. Jacob Amor
	Dr. David Bensoussan
	Dr. Herve Uzan
Planning time	05 2005 – 08 2005
Construction time	09 2005 – 12 2005
Gross floor area	160 sqm
Usable floor space	121 sqm
Construction cost	290,000 EUR

a The waiting area is furnished with Wenge-veneered panels, which add a touch of warmth to the cold aluminium look.

b The straight-line design is later replaced by curves, which escort patients into the rear section of the practice with a softer line.

c The patient toilet is elaborately designed.

d This trapezoid-shaped reception desk of aluminium laminate combines straight and curved lines and is modestly integrated into the foyer.

Diagrammatic plans, to scale 1:400
Floor plans, to scale 1:200

Floor plan layout

1	Treatment room	**4**	Patient toilet	**7**	Sterilisation room
2	Waiting area	**5**	Office	**8**	Small kitchen
3	Reception	**6**	Staff toilet		

Via the multiple practice entrance in the centre of the street frontage, the patients go straight past two treatment rooms and waiting area to the reception, whence two short connecting corridors lead to the remaining two treatment rooms. Rooms not found on the ground floor are accessed via a central, single flight of stairs. The large room there designated as an office may also be used as staff lounge.

Usable floor spaces

Patient rooms	**yellow**	29 sqm	24 %
Examination | Treatment rooms	**red**	51 sqm	42 %
Administrative rooms	**green**	29 sqm	24 %
Offices | Staff rooms	**orange**	6 sqm	5 %
Supply | Waste disposal	**brown**	6 sqm	5 %
Total		121 sqm	100 %

The reception area of the dental practice at Opernplatz exudes elegant spaciousness. The gaze of those entering the practice is involuntarily drawn to the treatment room in the rear with its opaque glass doors. The open-plan waiting area is visually separated off from the corridor by a transparent, undulating string curtain; a glass pane concealed behind it shields the patients who are waiting from the noise at the reception desk.

The spacious effect of the open-plan room concept is impressively aided by the smoked oak parquet flooring. In addition to the delicately-plastered wall surfaces, large aluminium wall panels, accentuating the straight-line objectivity of the practice, conflict with this cosy wooden component. Moreover, the reception desk, reminiscent of a spaceship cockpit, guarantees a "wow" effect with its backlit glass pane. By means of continuous ceiling lighting, patients are guided from the waiting area to the treatment rooms, where light steles take over, marking the way to the various rooms and providing extra light at the same time. The dark parquet flooring in the corridor is laid up one metre into the training rooms visually extending the corridor. Only then does the silver-coloured laminate flooring begin, offsetting the treatment furniture [specially designed for the practice].

PD RAUMPLAN

**"A1" DENTAL PRACTICE
AT OPERNPLATZ**
FRANKFURT ON THE MAIN | G

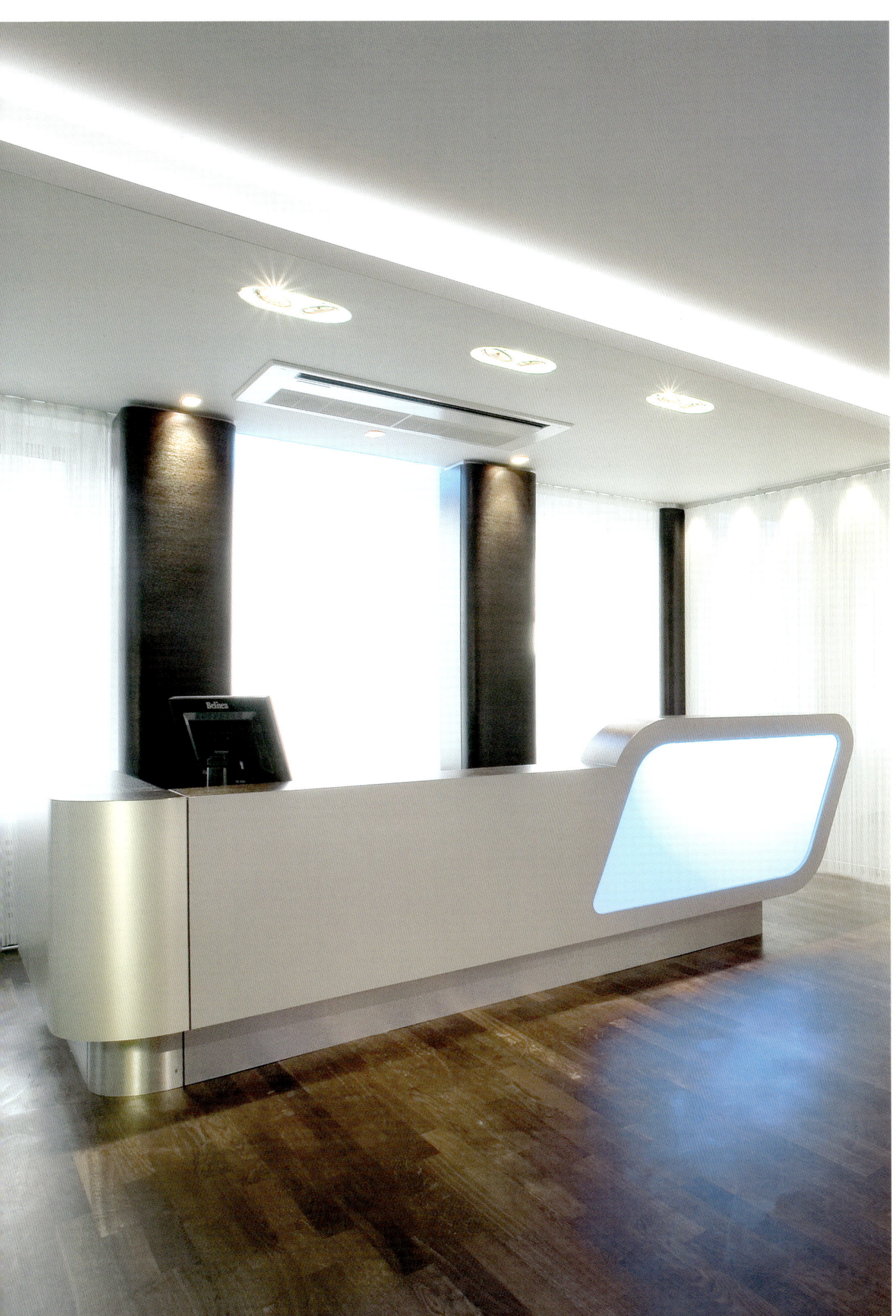

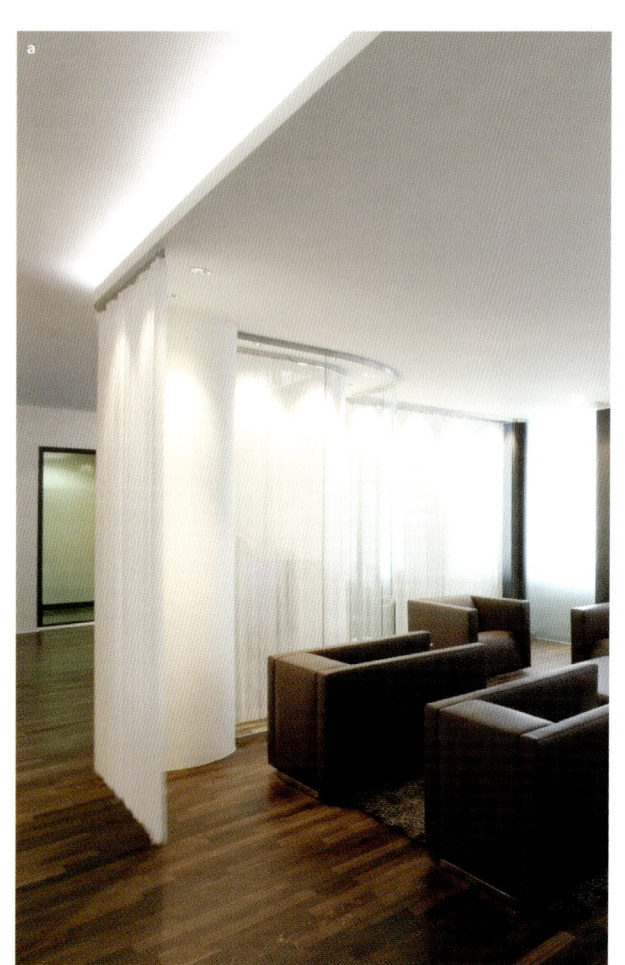

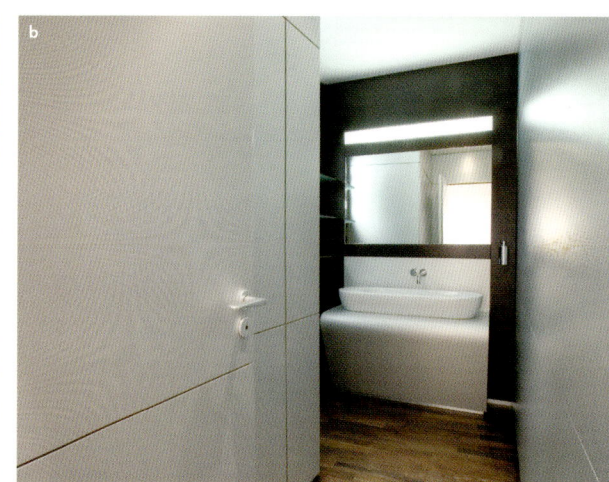

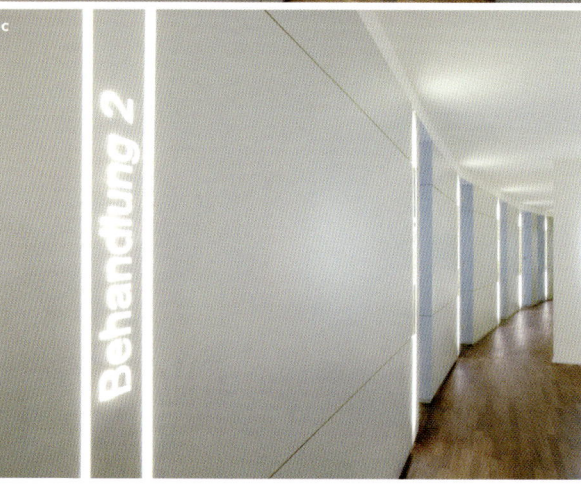

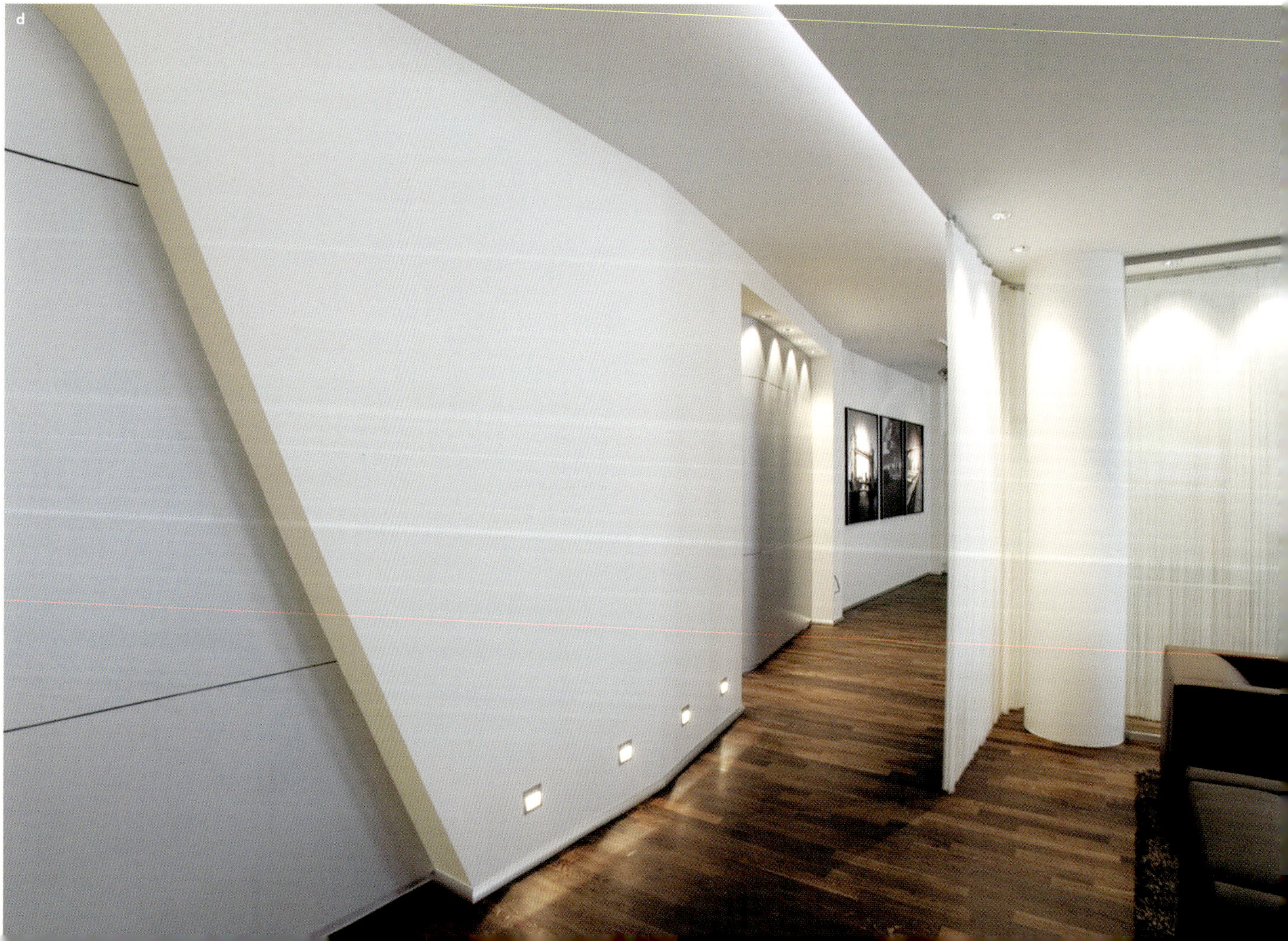

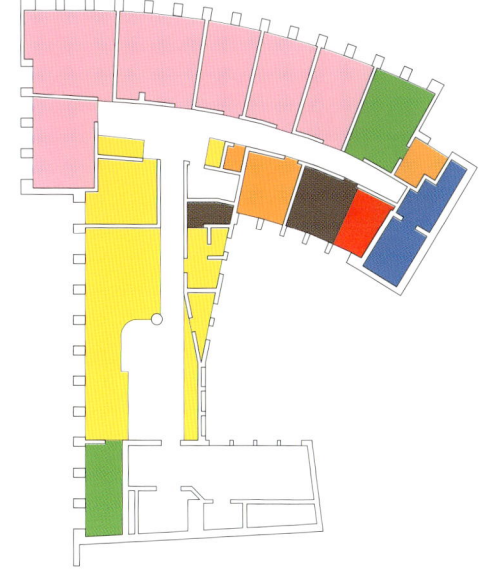

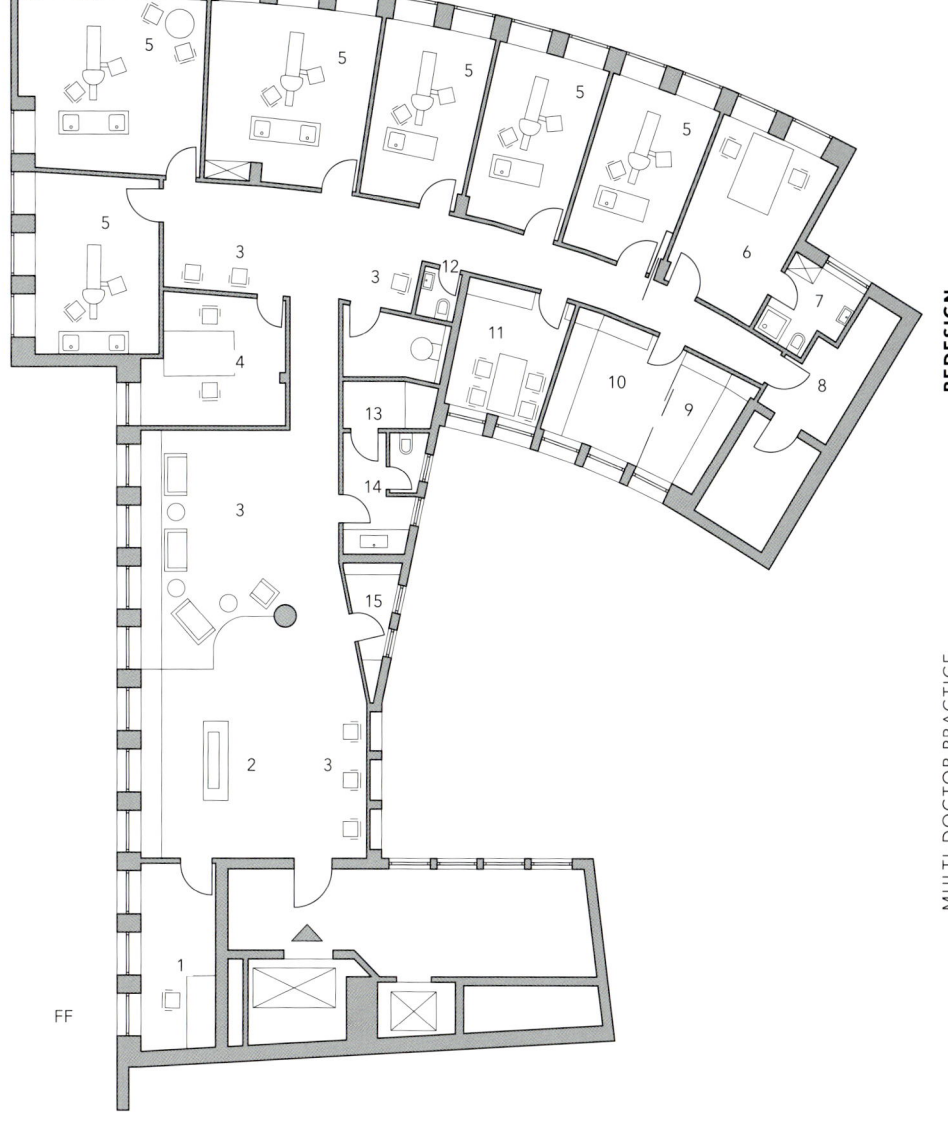

Diagrammatic plans, to scale 1:400
Floor plans, to scale 1:200

FF

1 Office
2 Reception
3 Waiting area
4 Consultation room
5 Treatment room
6 Office
7 Staff toilet
and shower
8 Installations room
9 Laboratory
10 Sterilisation room
and store room
11 Staff lounge
12 Staff toilet
13 Cleaning room
14 Patient toilet
15 Coat-rack

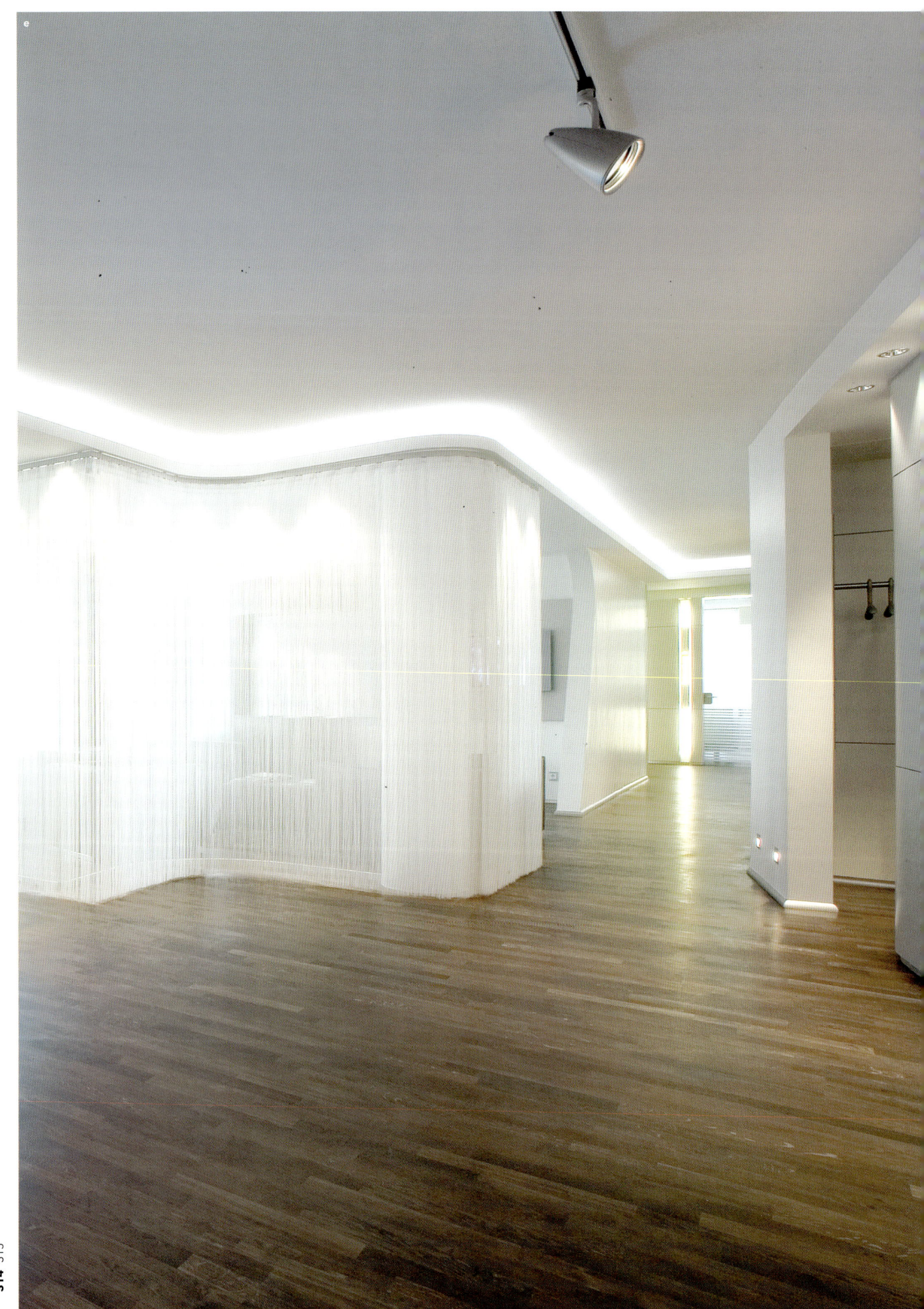

Client	Dr. Dietrich Fischer-Brocks
	Dr. Robert Weinreich
Operator	Dr. Robert Weinreich
Planning time	09 2004 – 12 2004
Construction time	01 2005 – 04 2005
Gross floor area	350 sqm
Usable floor space	267 sqm
Construction cost	420,000 EUR

a   The open-plan waiting area is separated off from the corridor visually by a transparent, undulating string curtain.

b   Aluminium wall panelling accentuates the straight-line objectivity of the practice.

c   Light steles show the way to the treatment rooms and provide extra light at the same time.

d   The sense of space of the open plan room is further enhanced by the light smoked oak parquet flooring.

e   By means of continuous ceiling lighting, the patient is escorted from the waiting area to the treatment rooms.

Floor plan layout

The entrance to the multiple practice is situated at one end of the T-shaped floor plan. From there the patients progress to the reception and waiting areas and to the examination and treatment rooms situated in the slightly-rounded corridor of the top T-beam, fully supplied with natural light.
This easily-manageable practice features all service areas, including the cleaning room which is nearly always omitted.

Usable floor spaces

Patient rooms	**yellow**	72 sqm	27 %
Examination | Treatment rooms	**red**	7 sqm	3 %
Specialist rooms	**pink**	112 sqm	42 %
Administrative rooms	**green**	29 sqm	11 %
Offices | Staff rooms	**orange**	18 sqm	7 %
Supply | Waste disposal	**brown**	14 sqm	5 %
Plant rooms	**blue**	15 sqm	5 %
Total		267 sqm	100 %

Performance data

Clinic opening hours	7 days | 91 hours
Waiting time	none
Number of staff	5 – 6

Lavender evokes images of the South of France, holidays, rest and relaxation. The lavender fragrance is calming and is, in many ways, healing and soothing for humans. All these positive associations have been included in the conversion of this practice: The Mediterranean plant is the authoritative motif here.

The typical lavender colour has been spread out into three tones. It livens up and accentuates individual walls and pieces of furniture – and stands out quite radiantly in front of the pure white background of the practice furnishings. The Lamiaceae motif is repeated on large-scale photos and as orientational feature on the frosted glass door to the examination room, where the elegant form of a very delicate flower stem has been lasered. As the practice occupies the whole ground floor of an art nouveau house dating to the year 1912, it was chosen to retrieve many original features of the building, in striking contrast with the contemporary, straight-line furniture. Softly gliding sliding doors create rooms in a practical and functional way, without taking up a lot of space, like in the treatment room, which houses three smaller cubicles. An elaborate media installation system allows all rooms to be filled with different sound, complementing the treatment in line with the practice guidelines. A large screen in the waiting area doubles up as training aid for staff as well as information point for patients, illustrating the range of services available in the practice.

RISCHKO ARCHITEKTEN

PRACTICE FOR GENERAL MEDICINE
REMSCHEID | G

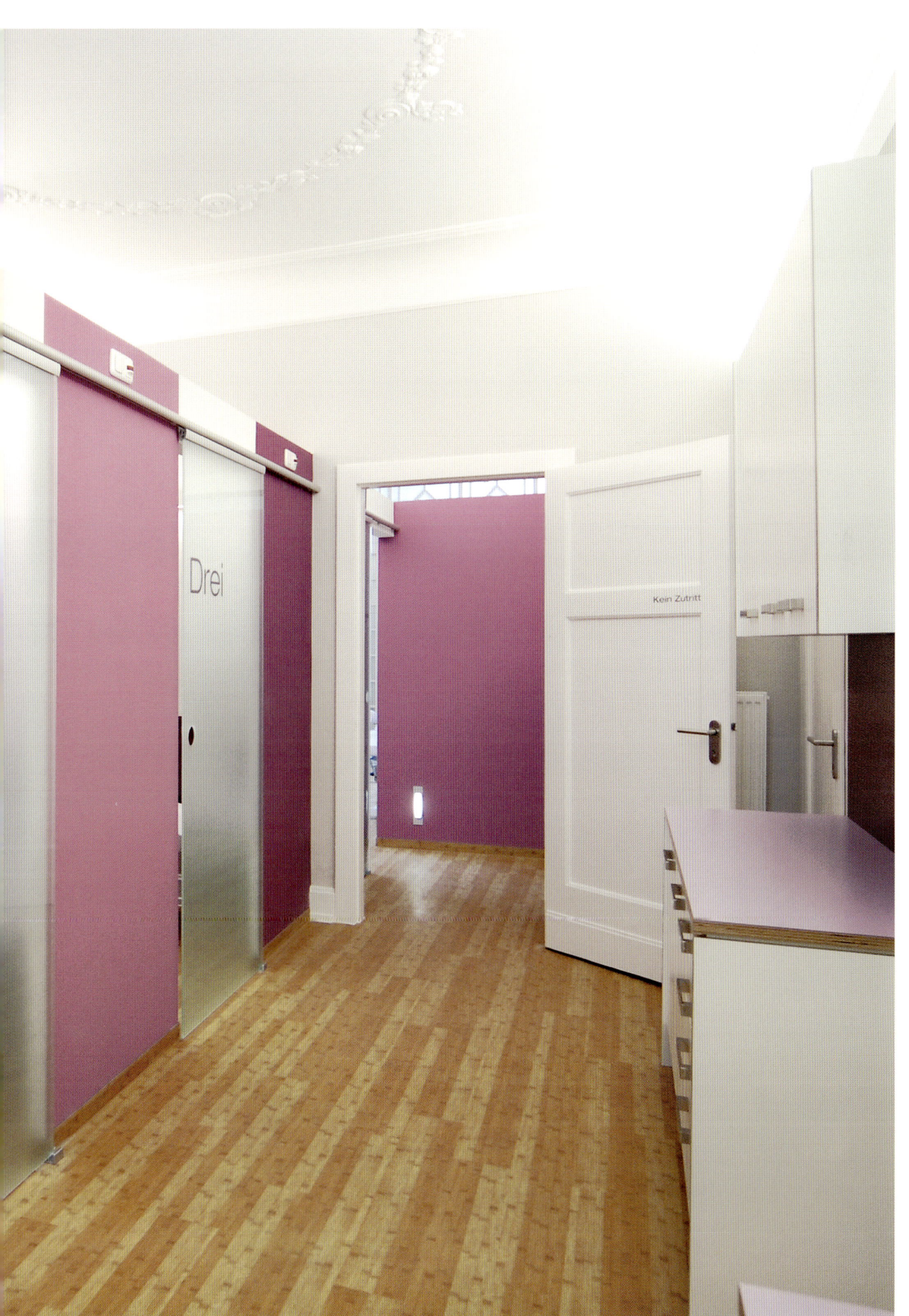

Drei

Kein Zutritt

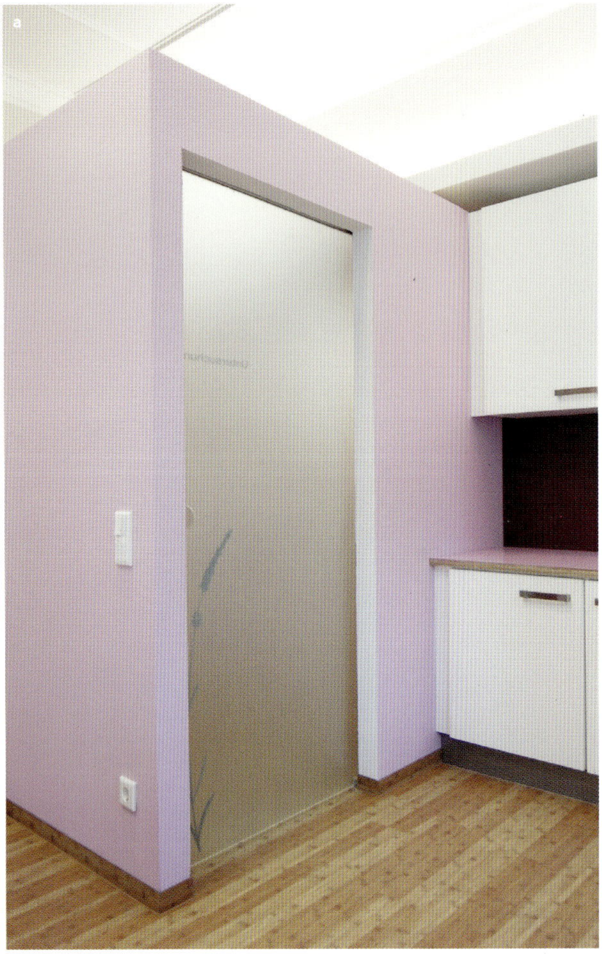
a

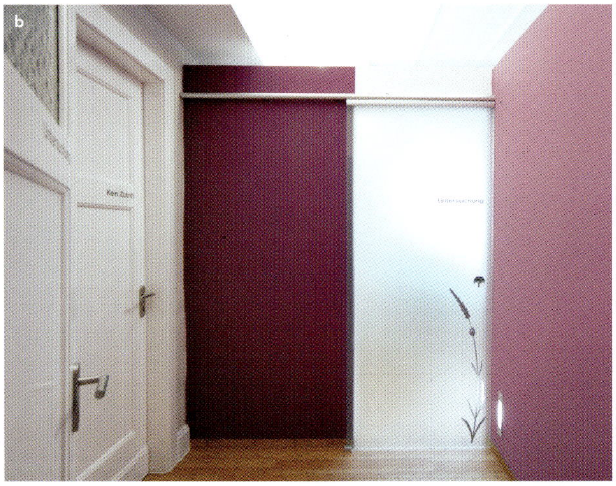
b

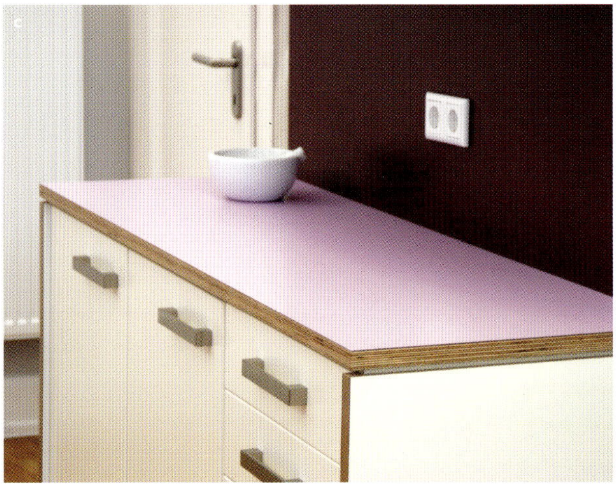
c

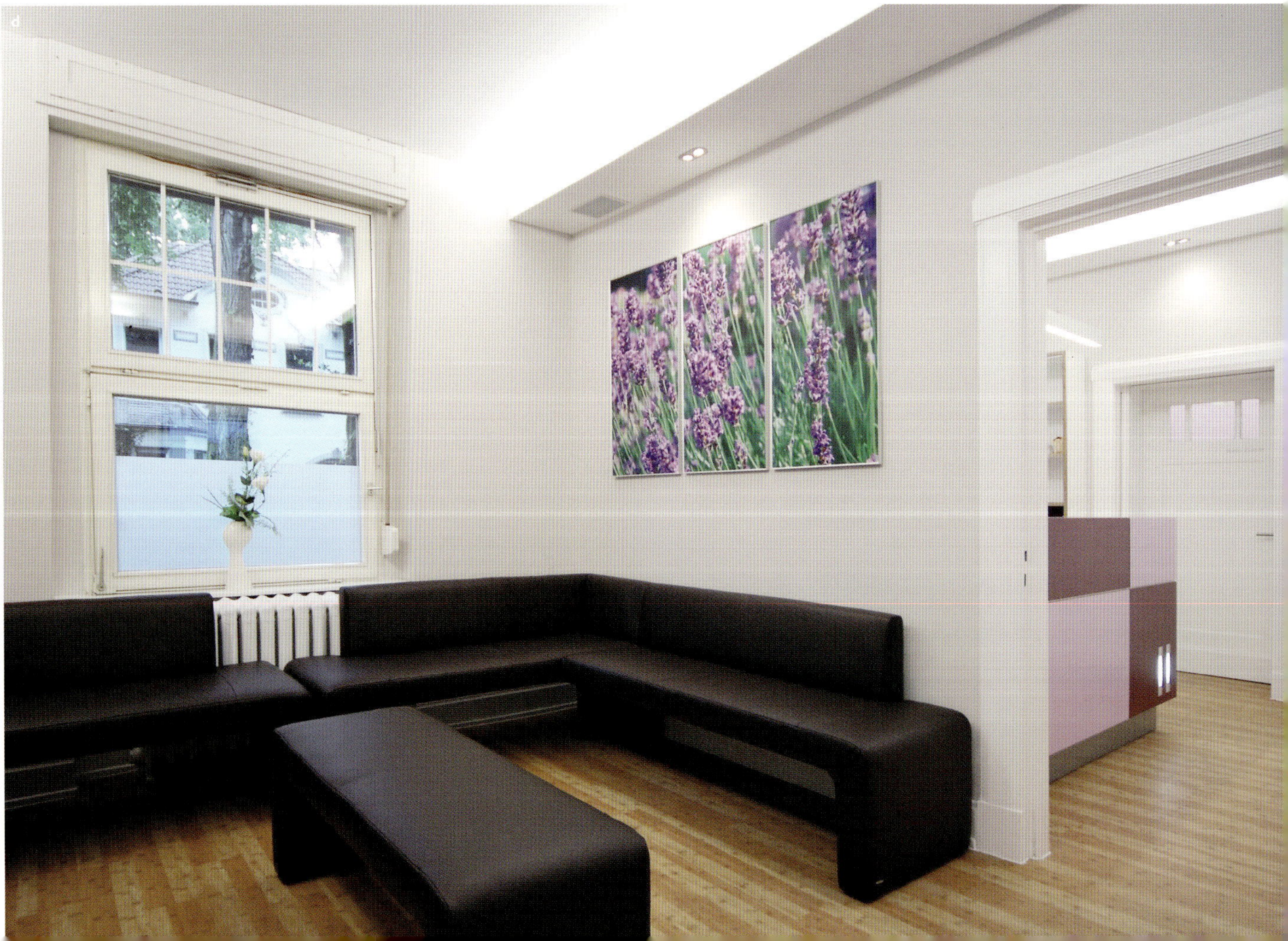
d

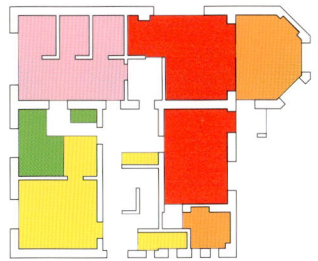

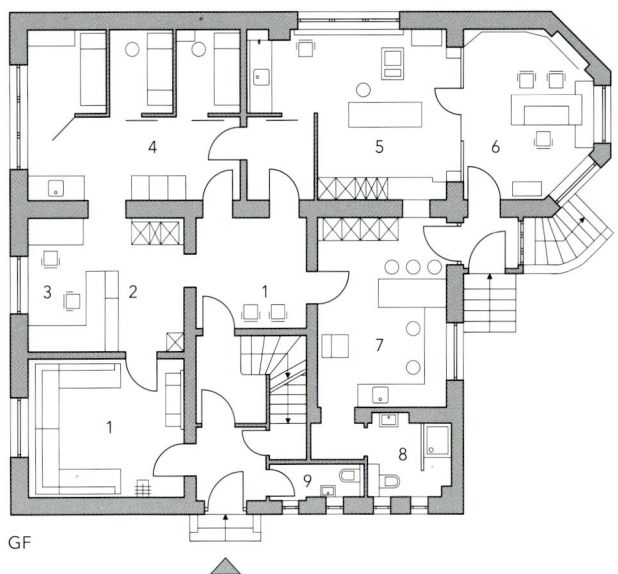

GF

Client | Operator Dr. Bettina
                        Stiel-Reifenrath
Construction time   2007
Gross floor area   150 sqm
Usable floor space 133 sqm
Gross cubic capacity 480 cbm
Construction cost   52,000 EUR
Total cost   89,000 EUR

a A delicate lavender stem has been lasered
   into the glass door of the examination room
   as an orientational feature.
b Softly gliding sliding doors separate the
   rooms without taking up a lot of space.
c The lavender colour is adopted throughout the practice in three tones to liven up
   individual walls and pieces of furniture.
d Elements of the old building have been
   retrieved in contrast to the straight-line
   furniture in the waiting area.

Diagrammatic plans, to scale 1:400
Floor plans, to scale 1:200

Floor plan layout

1 Waiting area		infusion	**8** Staff toilet
2 Reception		**5** Examination	and shower
3 Office		**6** Doctor's office	**9** Patient toilet
4 Treatment room		**7** Laboratory	

The predefined floor plan of this art nouveau mansion has been skilfully
used for the space required for a single-doctor practice. The waiting area is
right next to the entrance, and connects to the reception room. From there
patients can access the treatment and examination rooms, which all have
natural light, via an internal distribution room. The staff lounge, the storage
and cleaning rooms are situated in the basement

Usable floor spaces

Patient rooms	**yellow**	27 sqm	20 %
Examination			
Treatment rooms	**red**	45 sqm	34 %
Specialist rooms	**pink**	29 sqm	22 %
Administrative rooms	**green**	10 sqm	8 %
Offices	Staff rooms	**orange**	22 sqm	16 %
Total		133 sqm	100 %

Performance data

Outpatients per year	3,200 – 3,600
Clinic opening hours	5 days
Waiting time [with	without appointment]	0 – 20 min.	0 – 60 min.
Type and number of staff	1 doctor
	2 part-time staff
	1 trainee

The setting up of a group practice was the reason behind this conversion of the existing, single-handed surgical practice, which dates from the 1970s. An expanded room allocation plan and current requirements for outpatient operations meant that the premises had to be completely gutted and an entirely new room layout implemented.

All told, this practice is spread over two floors: The ground floor houses the reception and waiting area, examination and doctor's room; the basement contains further practice rooms and in the rear, a separate area, there is an operating theatre with the necessary ancillary rooms. The atmosphere in the practice rooms is bright and friendly. Colours and materials are limited to white walls and bright wooden parquet flooring. The ceiling-high door frames, made of solid oak, lend structure to the wall surfaces. Bright green corresponds to the corporate identity of the practice and is used for the routing and patient orientation system. Round, soft shapes, perfected in the "snail" shape of the spiral staircase, dominate the upper floor, from where all rooms of the practice exit. The complementary curve of a spiral staircase opens the waiting area up into the reception area; opposite this area is the staircase to the basement.

RISCHKO ARCHITEKTEN

SURGICAL CLINIC
MÖNCHENGLADBACH | G

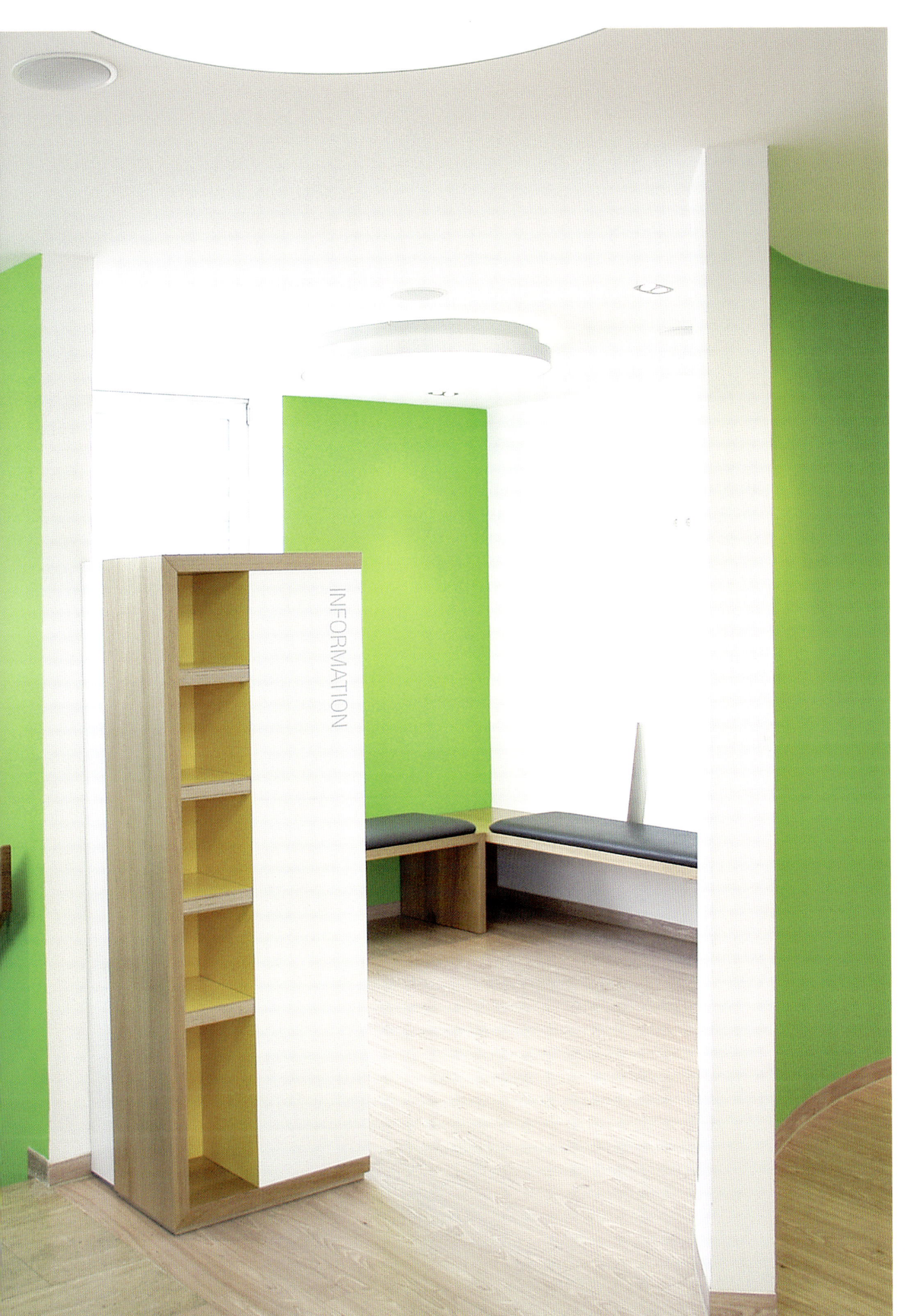

INFORMATION

a

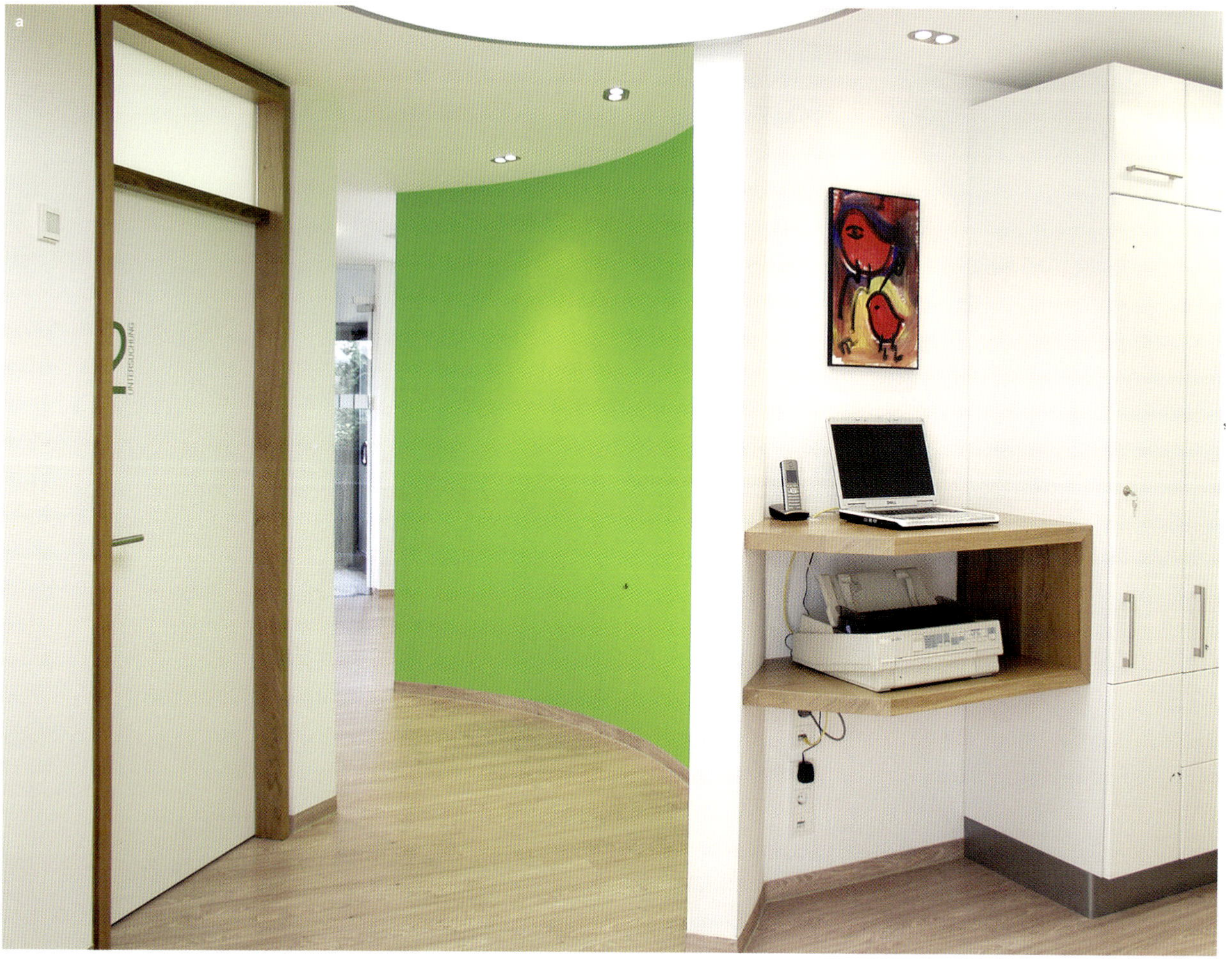

b

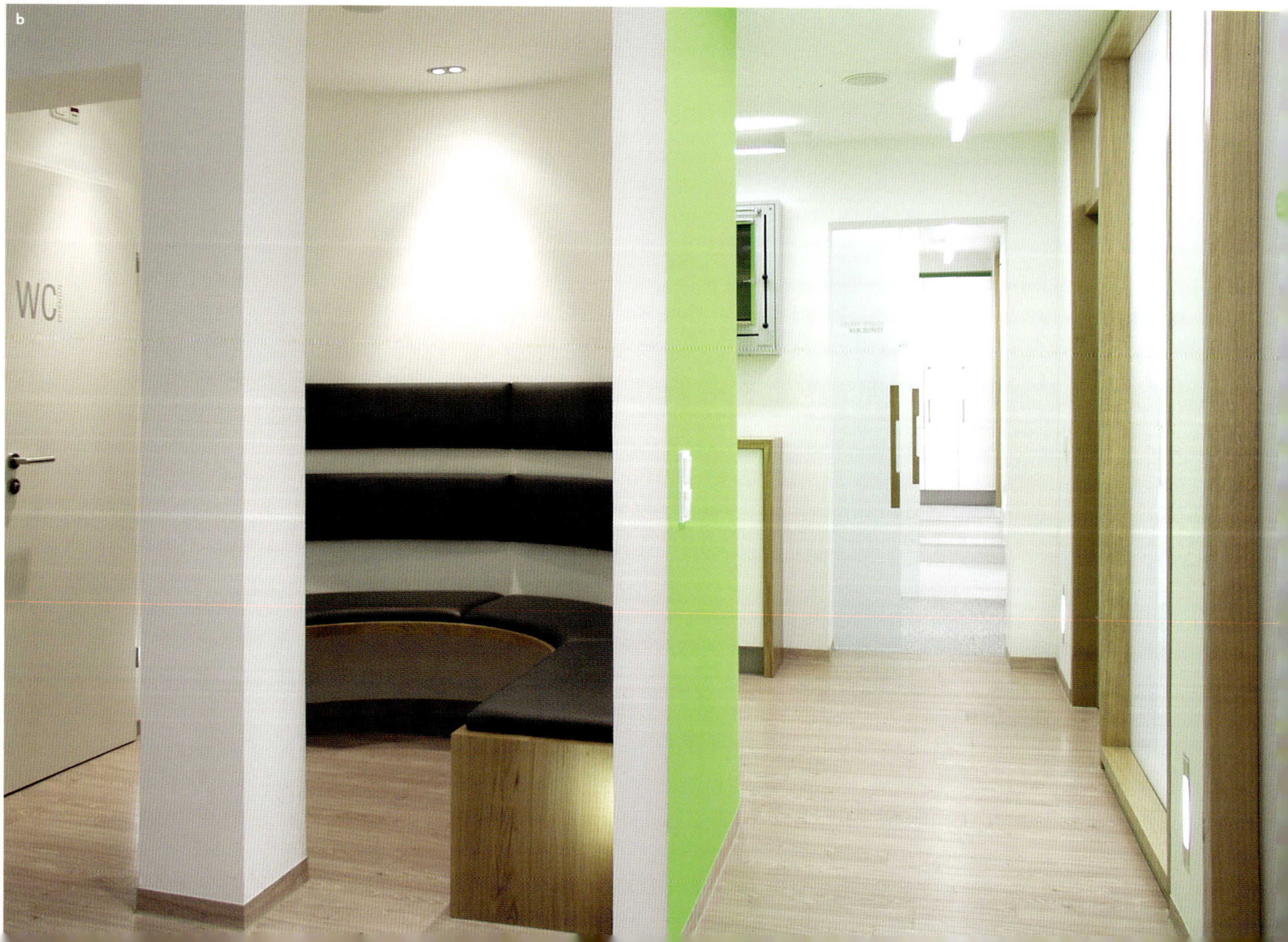

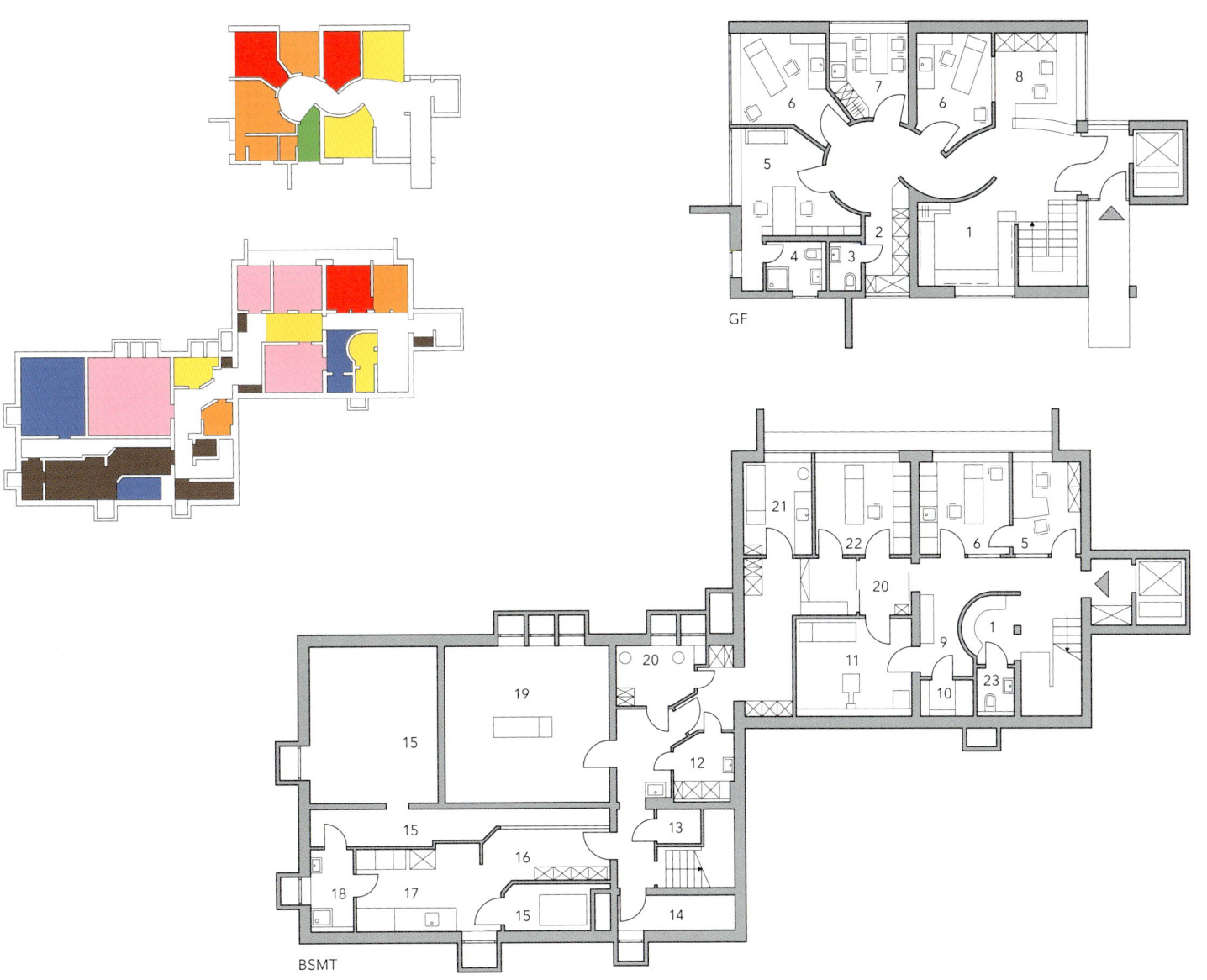

GF

BSMT

Diagrammatic plans, to scale 1:400
Floor plans, to scale 1:200

1 Waiting area
2 Filing room
3 Staff toilet
4 Doctor's toilet
   and shower
5 Doctor's office
6 Examination
7 Staff lounge
8 Reception
9 Switch room

10 Developing room
11 Examination X-ray
12 Staff sluice
13 Cleaning room
14 Waste and
    disposal room
15 Installations room
16 Sterile goods
    store room
17 Instrument

preparation room
18 Wash and
    drying room
19 Operating theatre
20 Patient sluice
21 Recovery room
22 Procedure room
23 Patient toilet

c

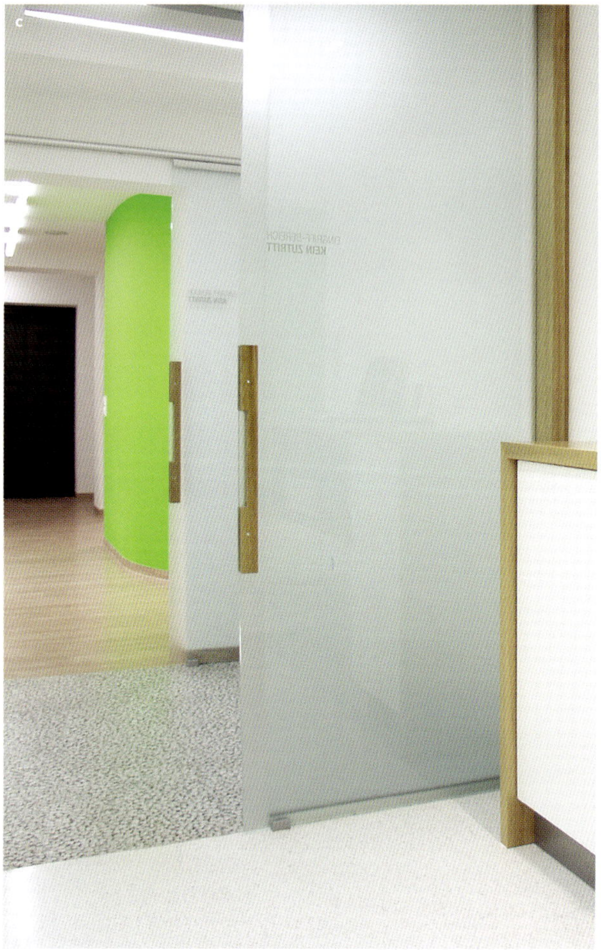

d

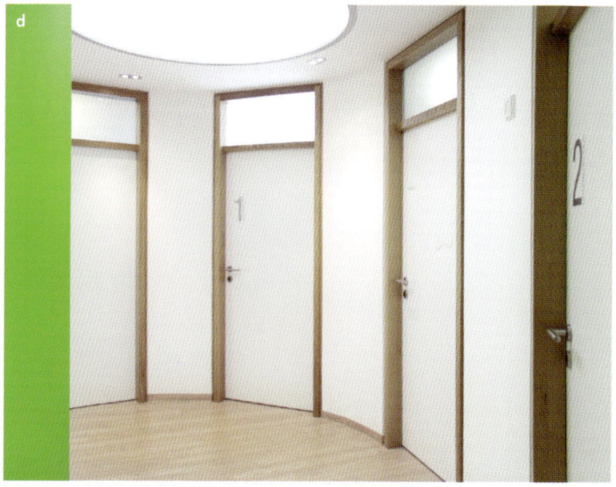

e

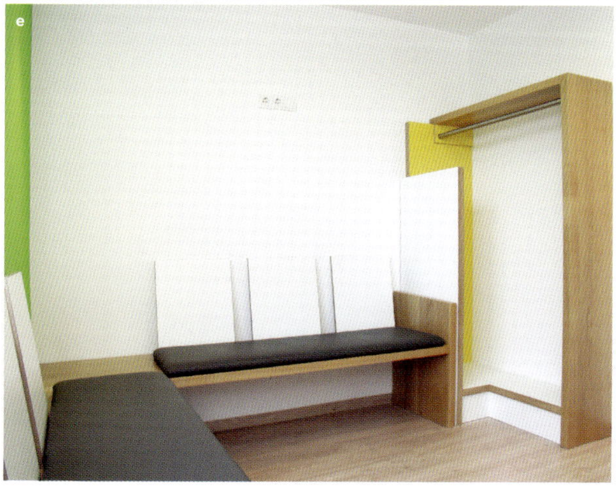

f

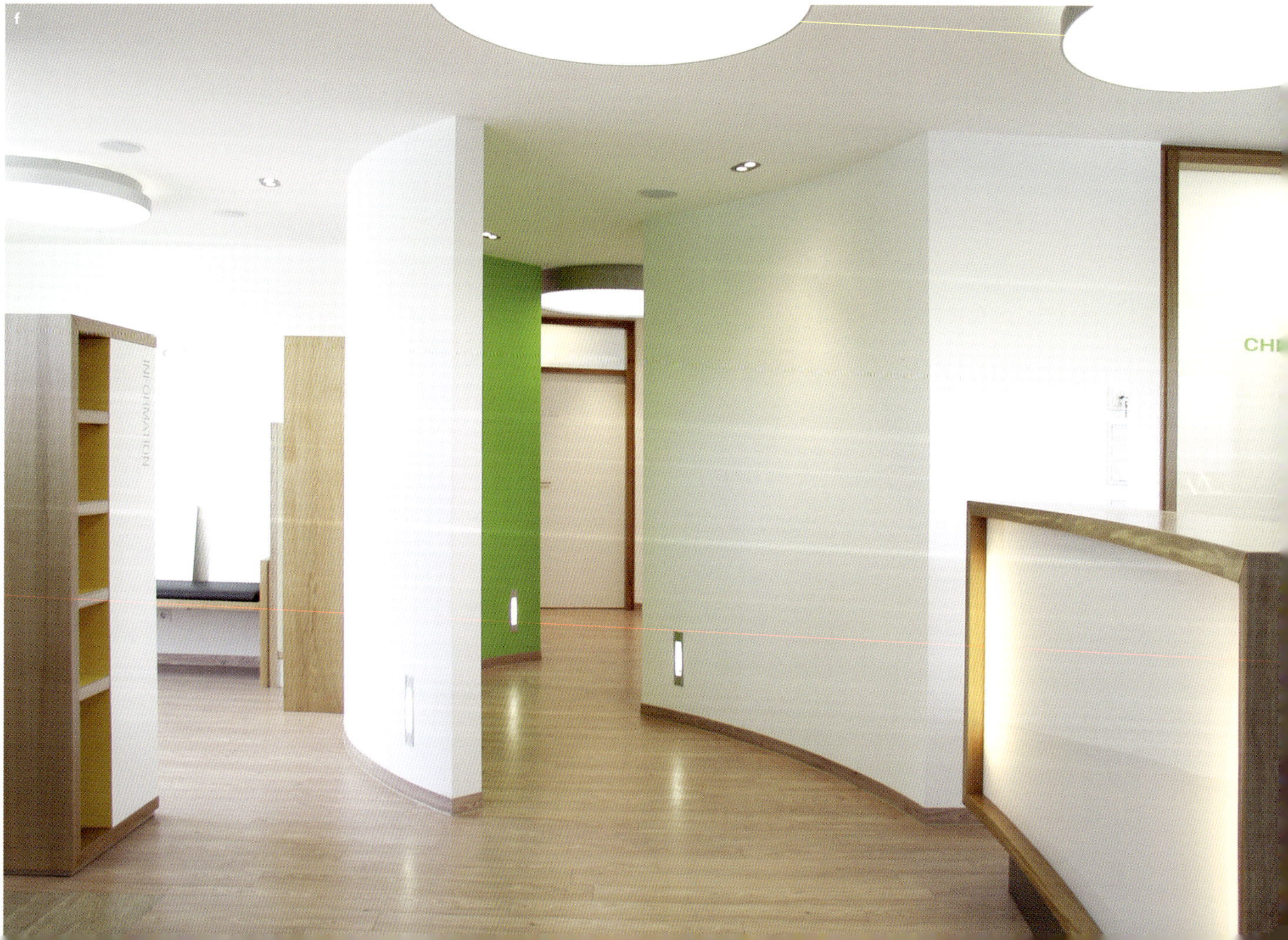

Client	Dr. Thomas Krings		
	Dr. Doris Krings		
Operator	Dr. Thomas Krings		
Construction time	10 2006 – 12 2006		
Gross floor area	260 sqm		
Usable floor space	242 sqm		
Gross cubic capacity	655 cbm		
Construction cost	156,000 EUR		

a The atmosphere in the practice rooms is bright and friendly.
b In the waiting area on the lower floor, architects chose a simple combination of bright green and white colours to complement the solid oak parquet flooring.
c On the upper floor round, soft shapes are predominant …
d … , which are perfected in the spiral staircase: all rooms in the rear area of the practice exit from here.
e The furniture and fittings in the waiting area are individually planned and are customised to the design concept.
f The complementary curve for the spiral staircase opens up the waiting area towards the reception area.

Floor plan layout

From the narrow side of this rectangular floor plan, the patients in this partnership practice access the reception and the waiting area. A rounded corridor leads to two examination rooms and the staff rooms. Via the stairs at the entrance [or via the lift], the patients access the basement, which is more than twice as large and houses a number of rooms which receive natural light only via cellar shafts. The unusual floor plan contains all necessary rooms, including a waste disposal room and a cleaning room.

Usable floor spaces

Patient rooms	**yellow**	39 sqm	16 %
Examination | Treatment rooms	**red**	29 sqm	12 %
Specialist rooms	**pink**	61 sqm	25 %
Administrative rooms	**green**	5 sqm	3 %
Offices | Staff rooms	**orange**	38 sqm	16 %
Supply | Waste disposal	**brown**	35 sqm	14 %
Plant rooms	**blue**	35 sqm	14 %
Total		242 sqm	100 %

Performance data

Outpatients per year	16,000
Number and type of services per year	X-ray examination [3,000]
	Outpatient operation [600]
Services to other clinics	Inpatient operation [300]
	CT | MRI [500]
Clinic opening hours	5 days | 47.5 hours
Waiting time [with | without appointment]	5 – 30 min. | 10 – 60 min.
Type and number of staff	2 doctors
	2 full-time staff
	2 part-time staff
	2 trainees

The practice for holistic medicine extends over two floors of a renovated town house in the centre of Brauweiler. Some architectural features of the building could not be altered, like the supporting structure, the position of the entrance and the internal distribution of space. Further constraints were posed by the relatively low ceilings and the limited number of windows on the ground floor and in the basement.

Bright wall colours and the warm shade of the Zebrano wood bring brightness and structure to the space. The core area on the ground floor is naturally illuminated thanks to the generously glazed integrity designed for enhanced sound insulation. Wooden frames surround the frosted glass surfaces adjacent to and above the doors and impart a straight-line structure to the large wall areas. One particular eye-catching feature is the aquarium, which is sunk into the wall to the two rear, large examination and treatment rooms and acts as a screen in conjunction with a small waiting bench. The basement, housing four therapy cubicles and doctor, staff and technical rooms, is accessed via an internal staircase. When redesigning the practice, particular attention was given to the furniture and fitting, which are individually planned, in line with the client's holistic philosophy. Grained Zebrano wood complements the white surfaces to achieve a uniform ambience and a serene atmosphere in all areas of the practice.

RISCHKO ARCHITEKTEN

PRACTICE FOR HOLISTIC MEDICINE
PULHEIM-BRAUWEILER | G

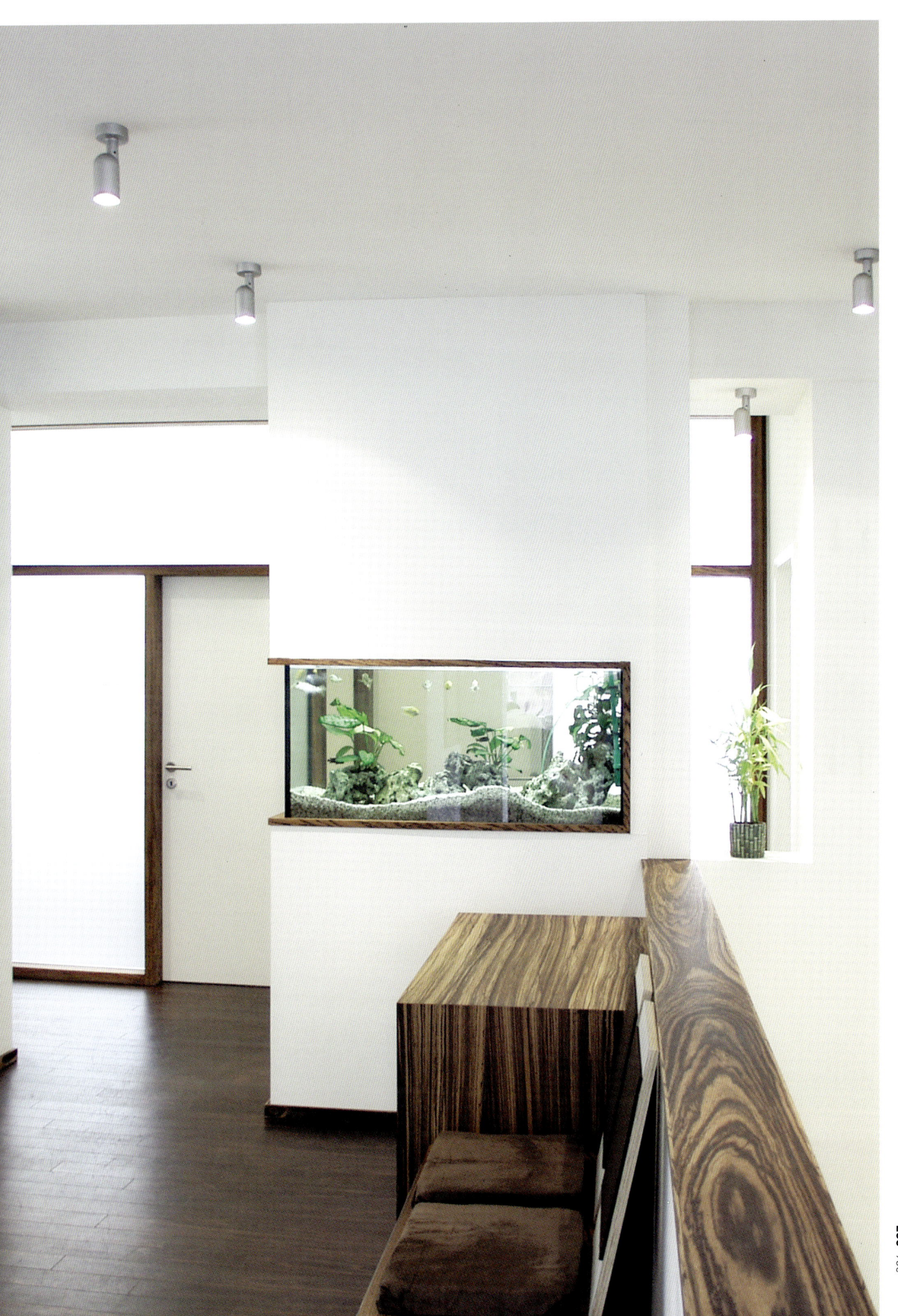

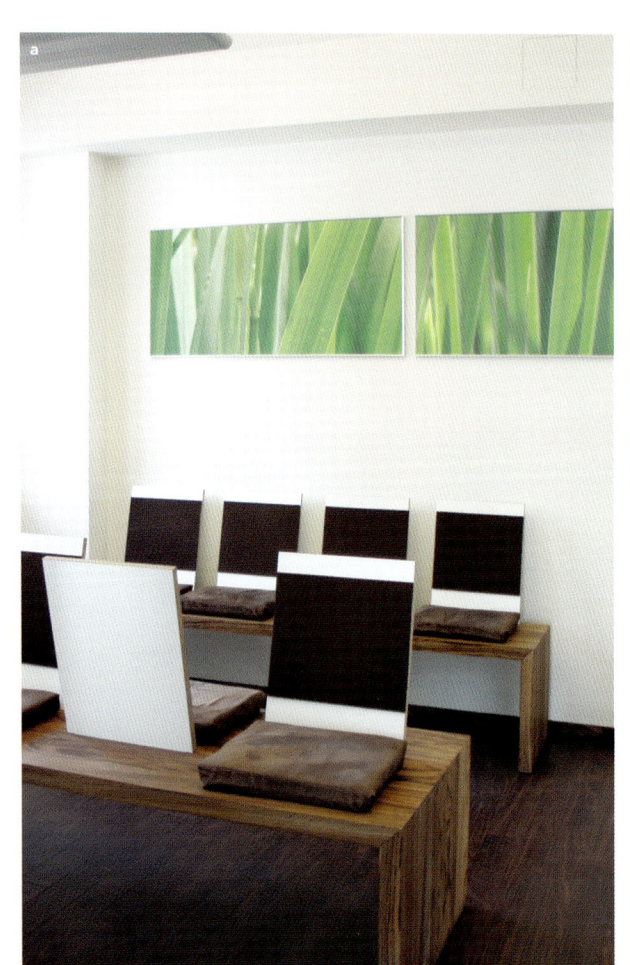

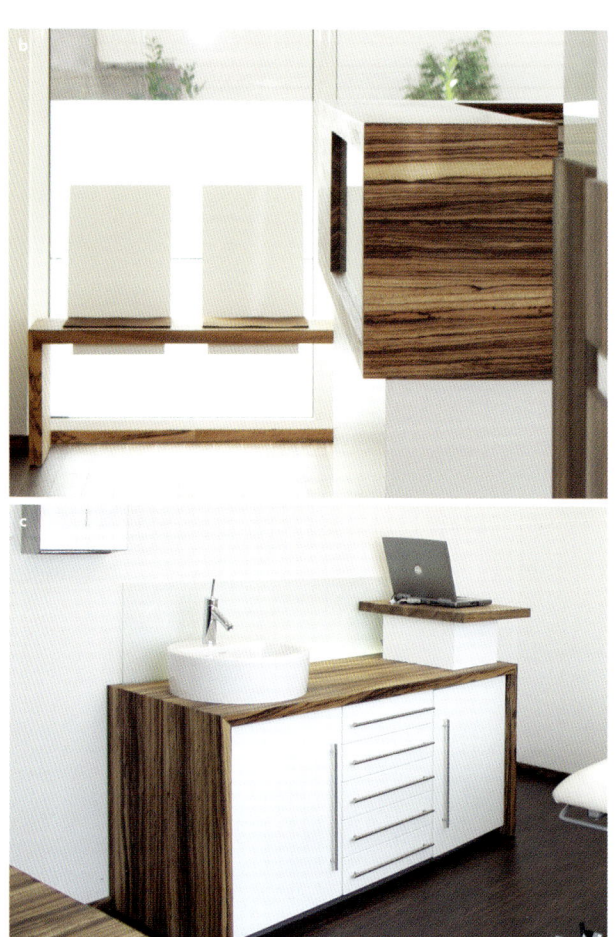

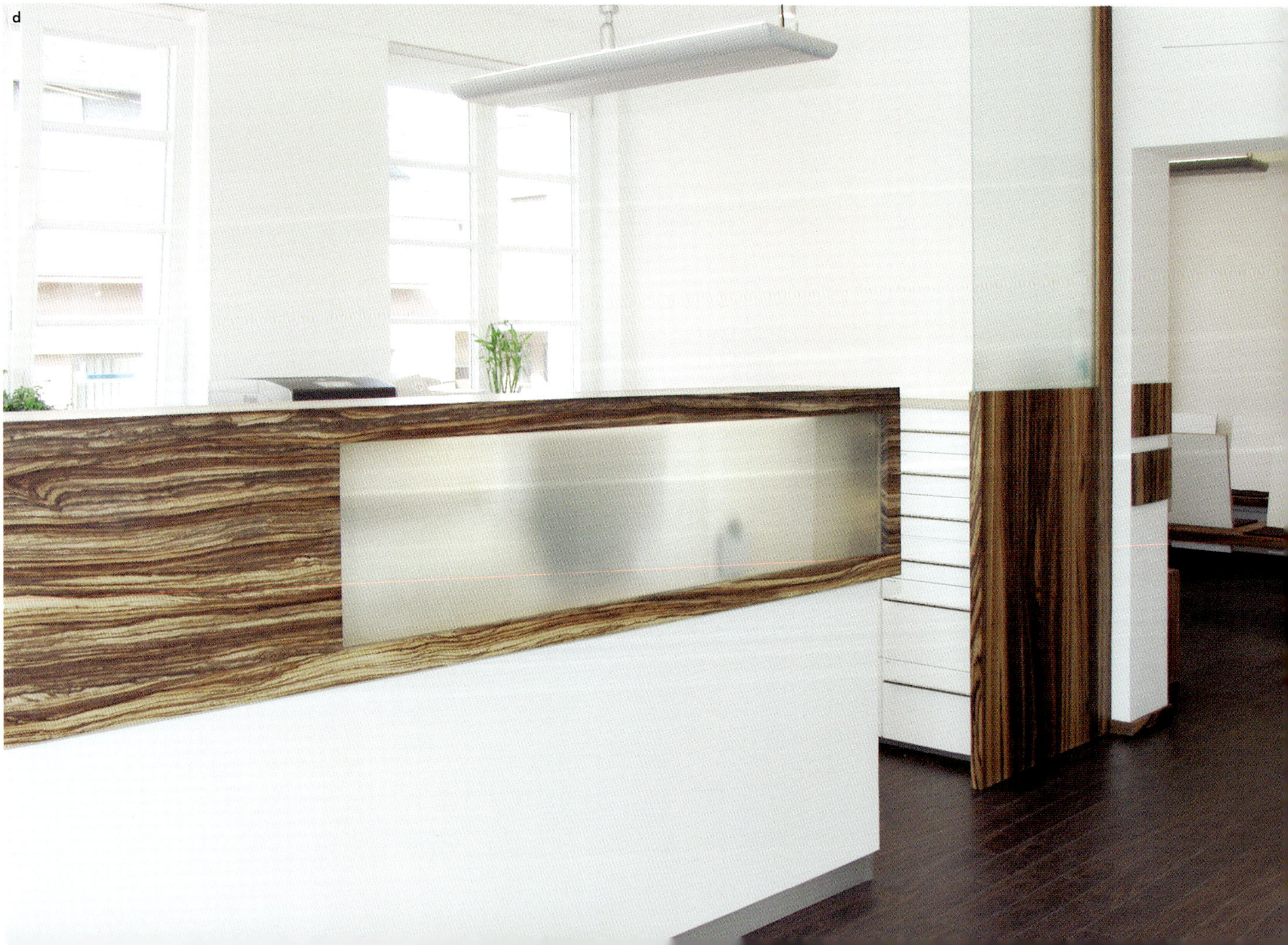

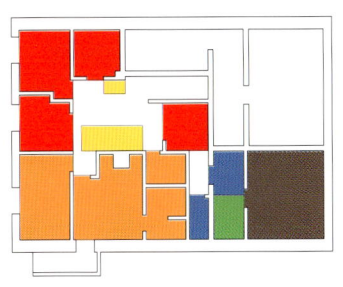

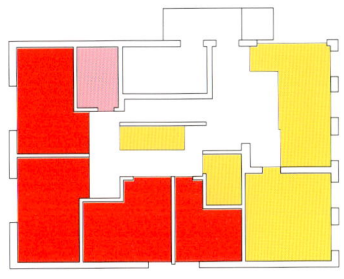

BSMT

GF

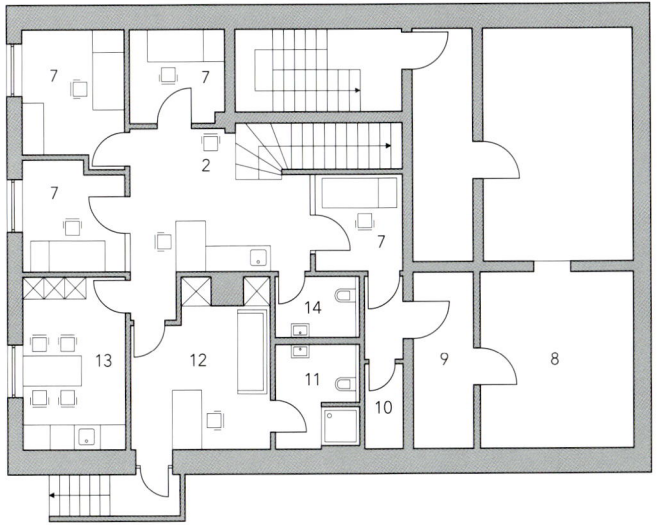

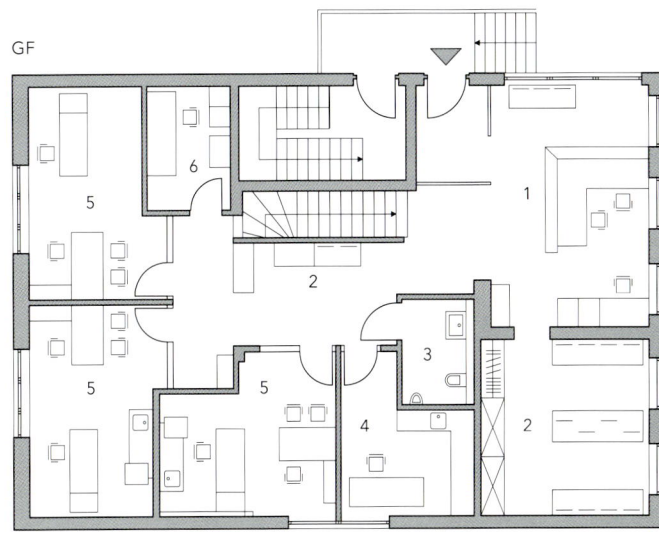

Client	Operator	Dr. Manuel M. Grahmann
Usable floor space	268 sqm
Gross cubic capacity	502 cbm
Construction cost	124,000 EUR
Total cost	186,000 EUR

a Furniture and fittings are individually planned and tailored to the client's holistic treatment concept.

b Maximum natural lighting is attained thanks to generously glazed integrity.

c Unobtrusive design with a few stylistic elements and colours characterise the treatment rooms of the practice.

d Bright wall colours and the warm shade of the Zebrano wood bring brightness and structure to the space.

Diagrammatic plans, to scale 1:400
Floor plans, to scale 1:200

Floor plan layout

1	Reception	**6**	Examination sonography	**10**	Installations room
2	Waiting area			**11**	Staff toilet and shower
3	Patient toilet	**7**	Treatment room		
4	Laboratory	**8**	Lavatory	**12**	Doctor's office
5	Examination and treatment room	**9**	Server room and filing room	**13**	Staff lounge
				14	Staff toilet

The predefined rectangular building structure and the unmodifiable internal development of the two-storey multiple practice with no lift are constraints that complicated the redesign of this practice. Nevertheless, there are good functional relationships between the rooms. With the exception of one room used for medical purposes on each floor, they all have natural light.

Usable floor spaces

Patient rooms	**yellow**	66 sqm	25 %
Examination | Treatment rooms	**red**	116 sqm	43 %
Specialist rooms	**pink**	9 sqm	3 %
Administrative rooms	**green**	4 sqm	2 %
Offices | Staff rooms	**orange**	43 sqm	16 %
Supply | Waste disposal	**brown**	22 sqm	8 %
Plant rooms	**blue**	8 sqm	3 %
Total		268 sqm	100 %

Performance data

Outpatients per year	4,000
Number and type of services per year	Gastroscopy [200]
	Ultrasound [1,000]
	Stress ECG [500]
	Long-term ECG [200]
	Colonoscopy [150]
Services to other clinics	
Clinic opening hours	5 days | 45 hours
Waiting time [mit Termin]	10 – 15 min.
Type and number of staff	4 doctors
	6 medical assistants

Transparency is the motto of this general medical practice, situated in the middle of a new residential area in the municipality of Alt-Erlaa in the south of Vienna. A large window frontage, a ground-level barrier-free access and a generous floor plan characterise the premises of this mixed use building. In order to achieve the desired effect of transparency and to make the practice an "open" point of contact for all patients, the General Practitioner called it Wiesenstadt Health Centre, anticipating extensions in other medical areas.

The practice occupies a T-shaped floor plan which runs for the whole depth of the building and presents a long display window frontage along the street, behind which are an open-plan reception and waiting area and large consultation room, protected from external onlookers by means of panel imprinted with medical logos. The desired openness is further achieved in the interior with a combination of light colours – from white to sand –, transparent or satinised glass and a sophisticated lighting system. One particularly attractive feature is the "roulette" in the waiting area: Illuminated by a large lighting system in the ceiling, the round rotating table capture the attention while acting as newspaper storage.

ROCHUSKAHR ARCHITEKTUR

WIESENSTADT HEALTH CENTRE
VIENNA | A

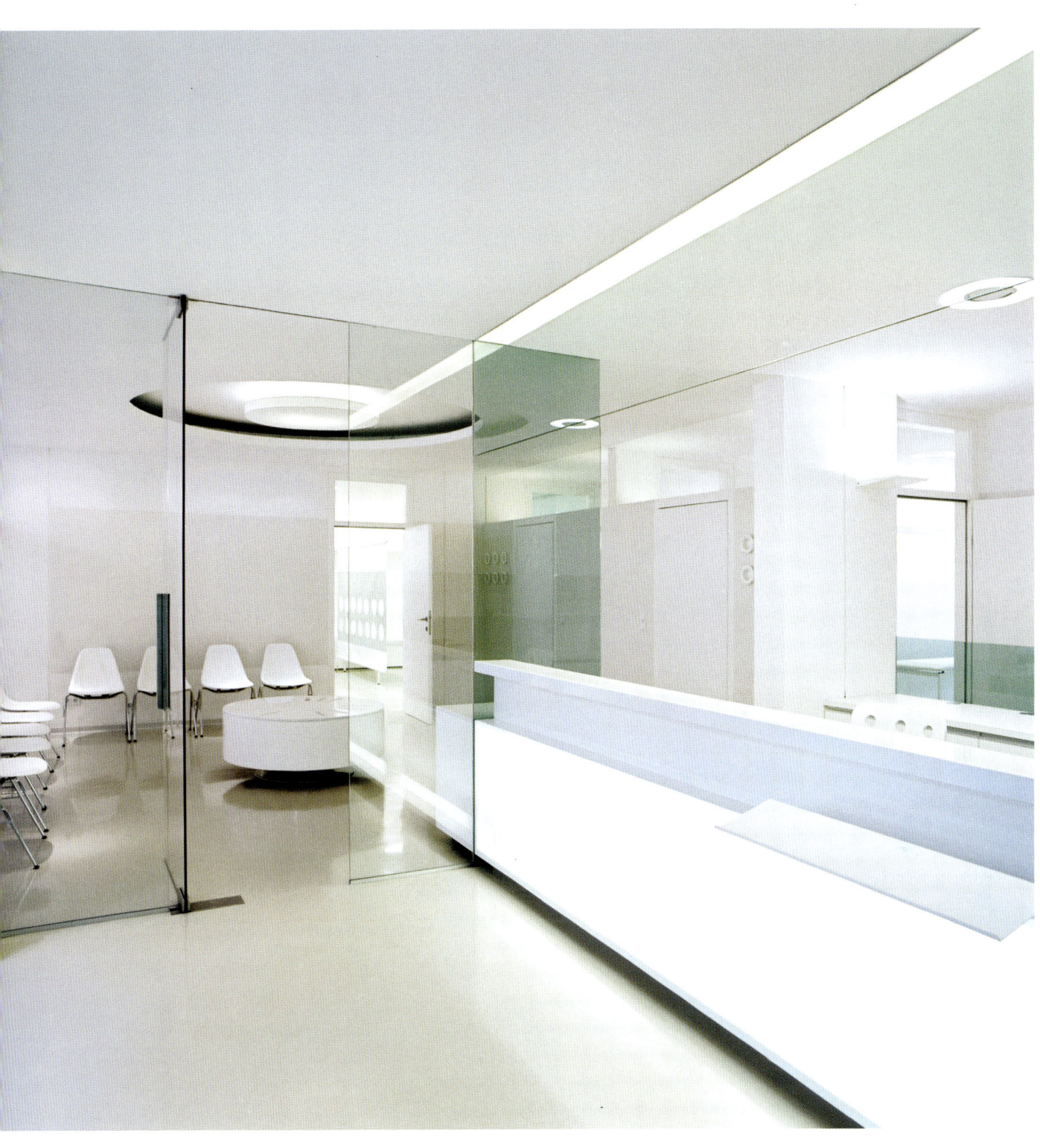

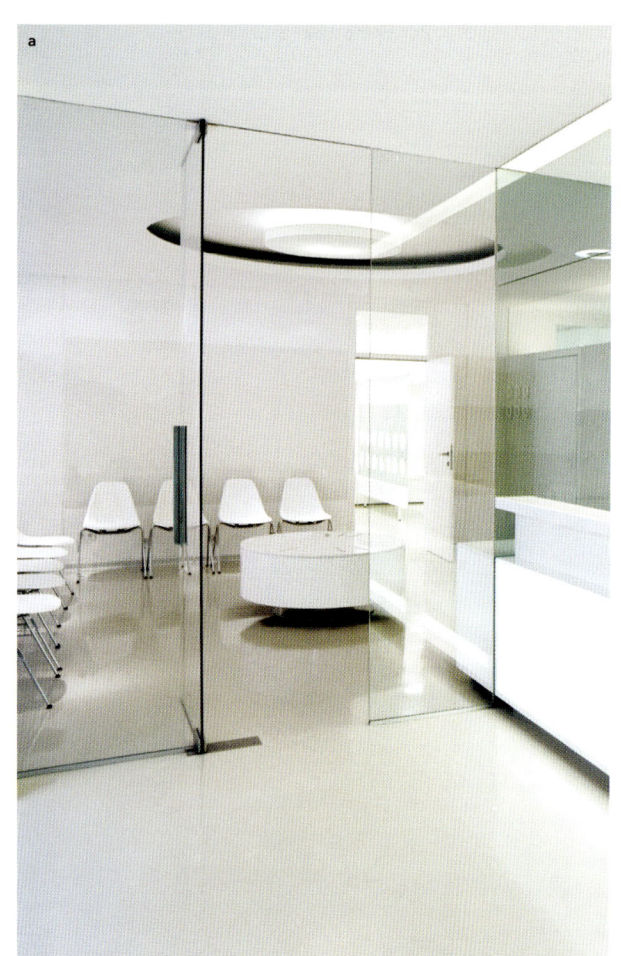

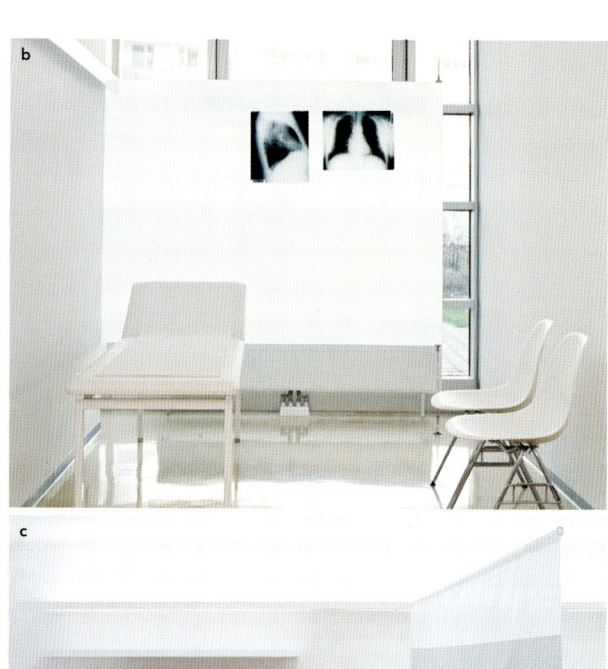

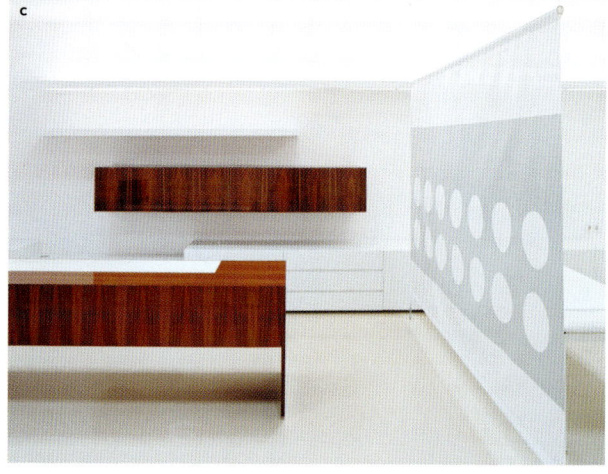

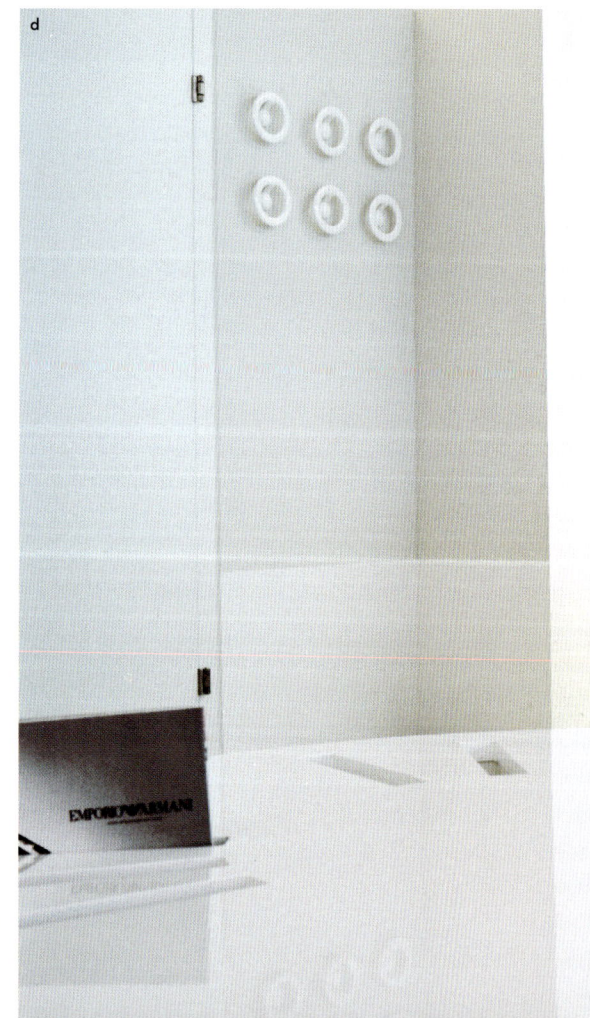

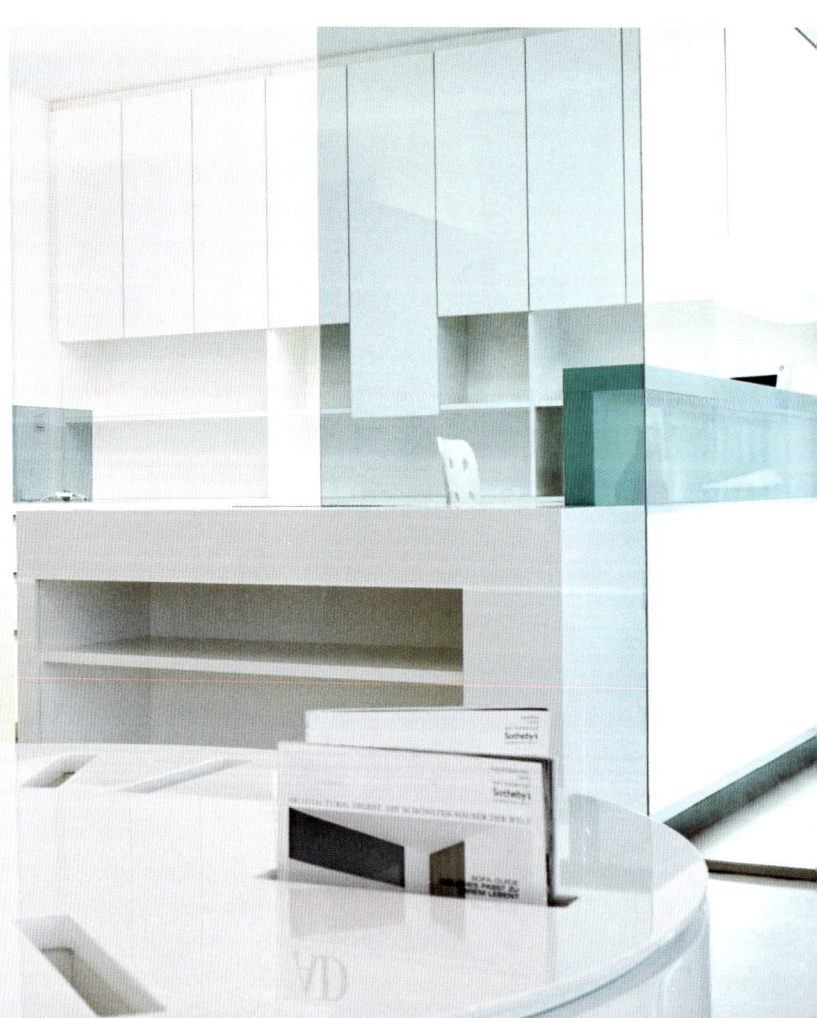

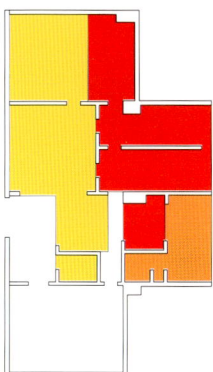

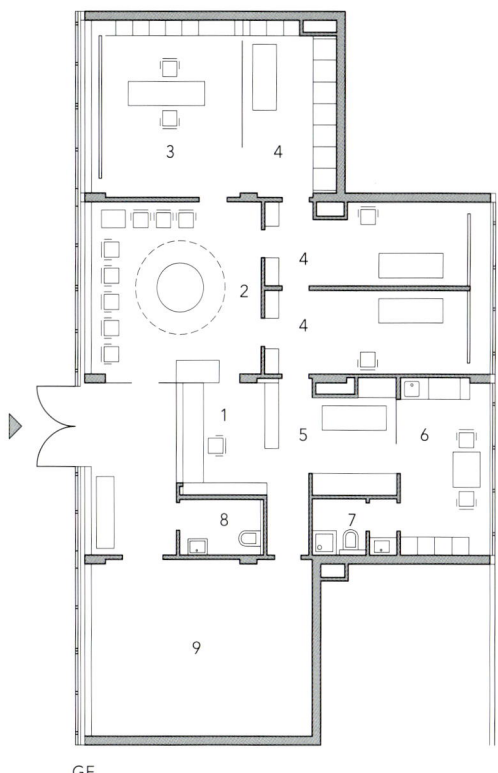

GF

**Client	Operator**	Dr. Wolfgang Supper
Planning time	08 2001 – 09 2001
Construction time	10 2001 – 01 2002
Usable floor space	132 sqm
Gross cubic capacity	483 cbm

a The consultation room and the three treatment rooms are directly connected to the central waiting area.
b The treatment room is protected from onlookers by a satinised glass pane.
c The use of bright colours, satinised glass and a sophisticated lighting system aid the desired transparency.
d One special feature is the "roulette", a so-called round rotating table in the waiting area, which acts as newspaper storage element.

Diagrammatic plans, to scale 1:400
Floor plans, to scale 1:200

Floor plan layout

1	Reception	**5**	Laboratory		and shower
2	Waiting area	**6**	Staff lounge	**8**	Patient toilet
3	Consultation room		and small kitchen	**9**	Multi-purpose room
4	Treatment room	**7**	Staff toilte		

In this multiple practice, patients access the reception and the adjacent waiting area directly from the entrance. The four consultation and treatment rooms are connected, so a corridor is not needed. In the adjacent room area, occupied by a laboratory and staff rooms, there is a short connecting corridor, which leads to an area where the practice could further expand, according to an existing proposal currently under consideration. All rooms requiring natural light have windows. There are no areas for adjoining rooms.

Usable floor spaces

Patient rooms	**yellow**	63 sqm	48 %
Examination			
Treatment rooms	**red**	52 sqm	39 %
Offices	Staff rooms	**orange**	17 sqm	13 %
Total		132 sqm	100 %

Performance data

Outpatients per year	30,000
Clinic opening hours	5 days	50 hours
Waiting time [with	without appointment]	5 min.	30 min.
Number of staff	5

The new outpatient department at the Frankenthal Municipal Clinic, a building dating from the 1970s, combines emergency treatment and elective care. Situated close to one another, all the individual outpatient departments are easily accessible. All consultations check-ups take place in this part of the clinic. Emergency admissions are brought straight into the emergency room, where they receive the necessary care, via a new approach for non-ambulant patients. A new bed-passenger lift goes directly up to the intensive care unit and to the operating theatres. Those patients able to walk are processed at a wooden desk and transferred for medical admission to examination rooms, which are designed to be used by physicians from all disciplines. Special examination rooms, functional diagnostics and radiology are nearby. Thus, each patient can be thoroughly examined without the need to cover long distances. The examination will determine whether the patient needs to receive further treatment as an inpatient, a part-inpatient or even as an outpatient. Patients whose diagnosis has not been fully determined are kept in the newly developed ten-bed admissions unit until final clarification. This unit also functions as a day clinic for chemotherapy patients and as a rest facility for those who have had operations.

The logical interior design concept helps the rooms exude freshness and tranquillity. Thanks to the elaborate lighting system, even inner areas are bright.

**SANDER.
HOFRICHTER
ARCHITEKTEN**

**MUNICIPAL CLINIC
OUTPATIENT DEPARTMENT**
FRANKENTHAL | G

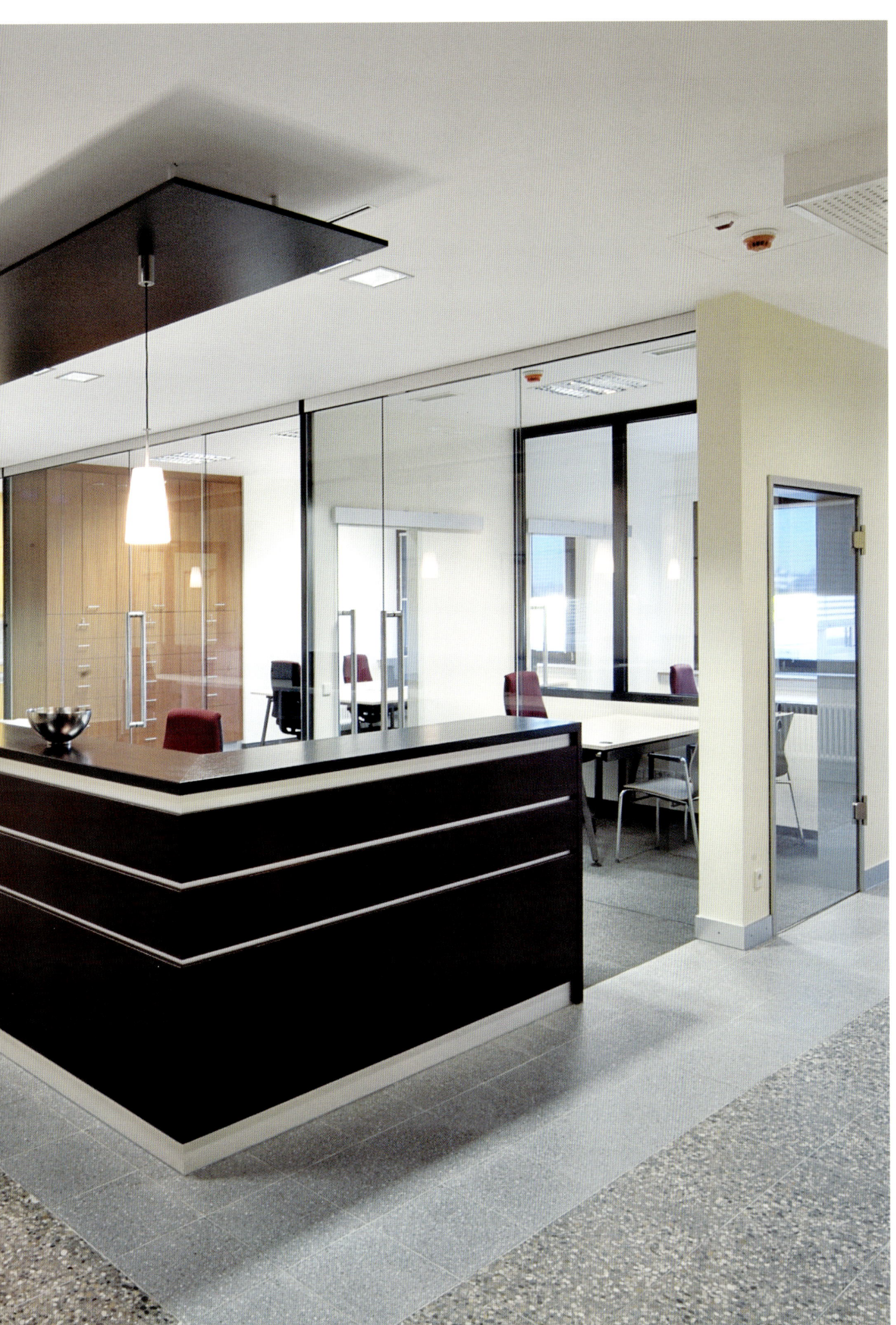

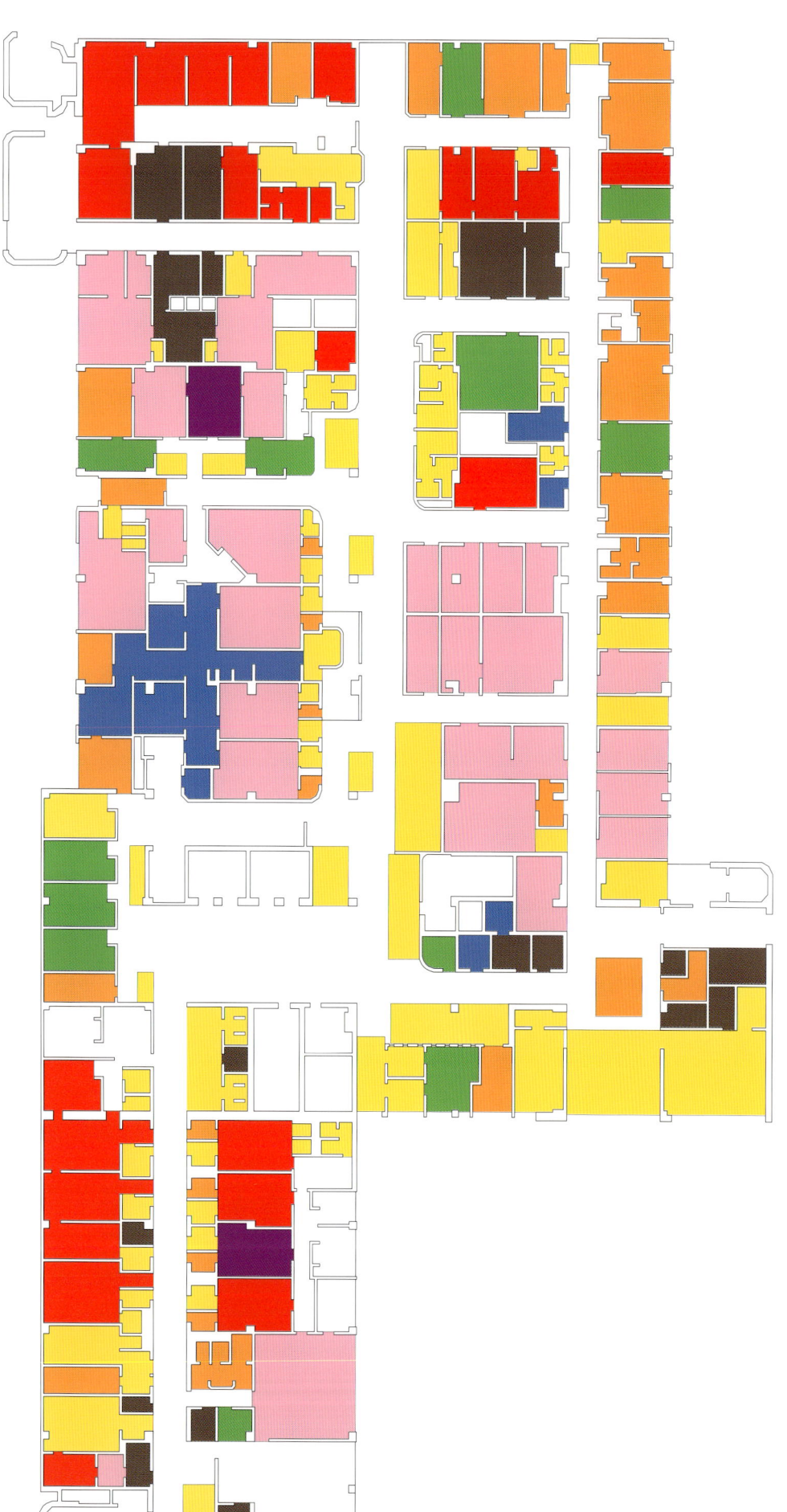

1 Waiting area
2 Patient toilet G
3 Store room
4 Patient toilet L
5 Staff changing cubicle
6 Patient changing cubicle
7 Treatment room
8 Patient shower
9 Patient toilet
10 Training room
11 Staff toilet
12 Staff shower
13 Washroom
14 Equipment room
15 Office
16 Fitness room
17 Store room
18 Inhalation room
19 Consultation room
20 Clean linen store room
21 Anteroom
22 Office
23 Reception
24 Dirty linen store room
25 Examination and treatment room
26 Admissions manager's office
27 Clerical services office
28 Coding office
29 Relatives' lounge
30 Assistant dietician's office
31 Film processing
32 Examination HRT
33 Patient transfer room
34 Examination mammography
35 Installations room
36 Examination X-ray
37 Admissions room
38 Examination CT
39 Computer room
40 Switch room
41 Darkroom
42 Doctor's office
43 Psychiatry office
44 Doctor's office
45 Examination endoscopy
46 Prep room endoscopy
47 Quiet room
48 Sterile goods store room
49 Equipment preparation
50 Samples laboratory
51 Outpatient lounge
52 Administrative office
53 Examination psychiatric outpatient
54 Library
55 Examination room psychiatry
56 Blood analysis laboratory

57 Washroom
58 Urine laboratory
59 Laboratory
60 Staff lounge
61 Laboratory monitoring
62 Laboratory reception
63 Specimen collection room
64 Gynaecology administrative office
65 Doctor's office [gynaecology]
66 Examination
67 Administrative office
68 Admissions consulting room
69 On duty office
70 Doctor's office [surgery]
71 Doctor's administrative office
72 Patient toilet and shower
73 IT room
74 AV Elektro
75 Consultation room
76 Staff toilet and shower
77 Emergency doctor on duty office
78 Functional diagnostics reception
79 Examination ECG
80 Examination pulmonary function
81 Procedure room
82 Plaster room
83 Examination admissions
84 Treatment room surgery
85 Examination ultrasound
86 Examination ergometry
87 Examination EEG
88 Patient room
89 Washroom
90 Patient sluice
91 Treatment room shock therapy
92 Examination gynaecology
93 Waste disposal room
94 Waste disposal room
95 Supply room
96 Filing room
97 Emergency room
98 Clean store room
99 Small kitchen
100 Bed store area
101 Workroom unsterile
102 Admissions room
103 Admissions room for short-term inpatients
104 Admissions room for emergencies
105 Reception control centre
106 Accounts office

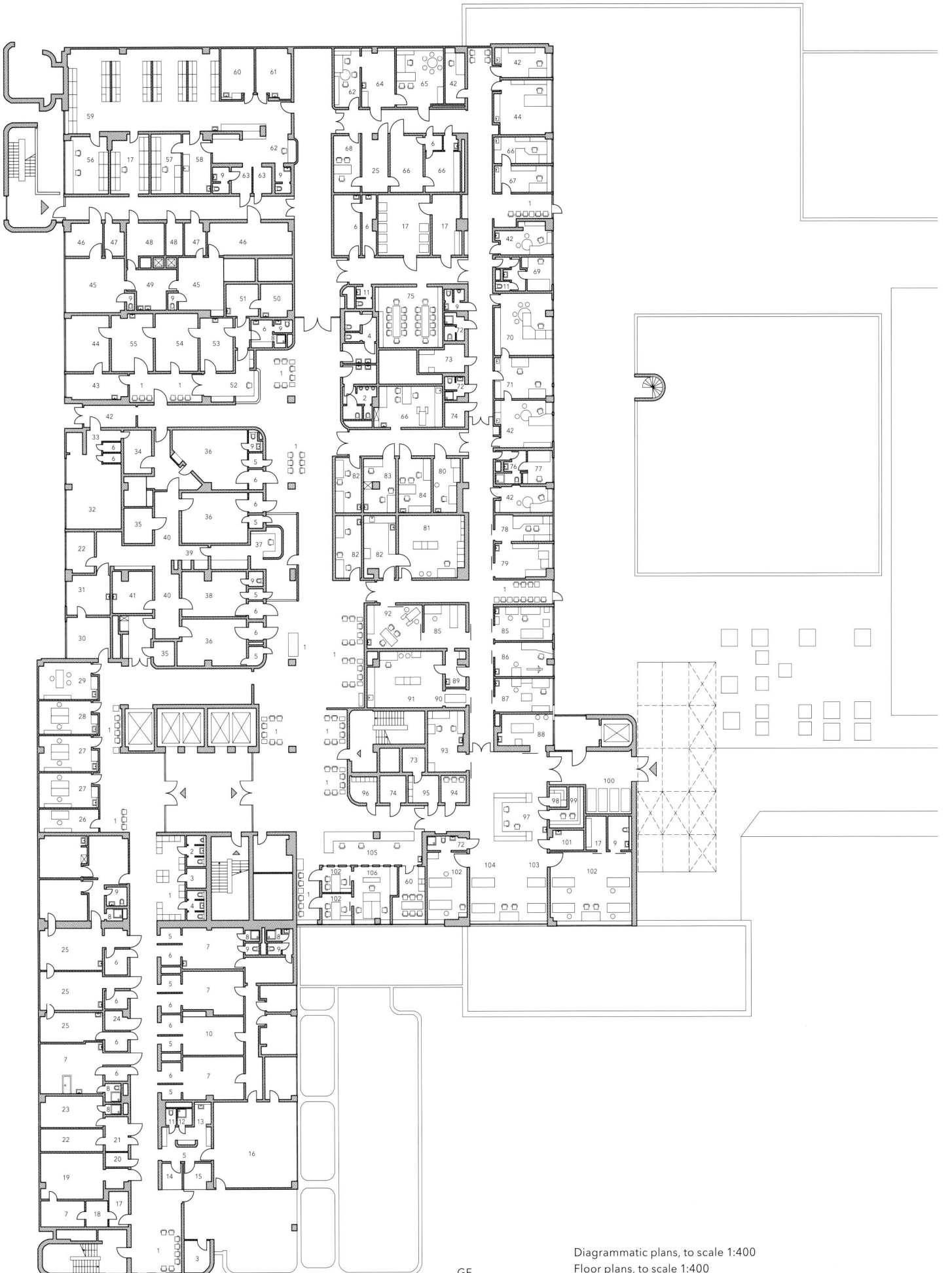

AMBULANCE IN HOSPITAL

GF

Diagrammatic plans, to scale 1:400
Floor plans, to scale 1:400

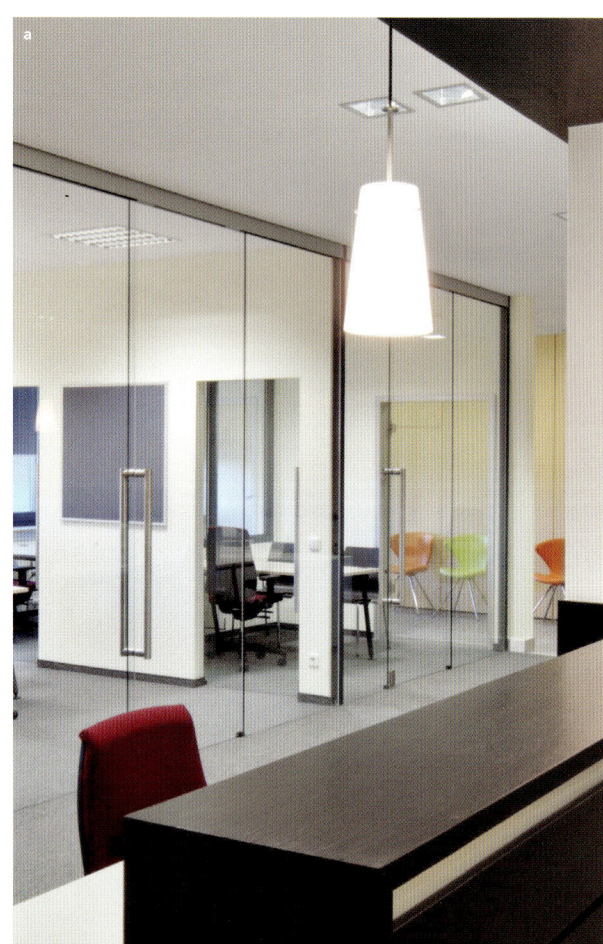

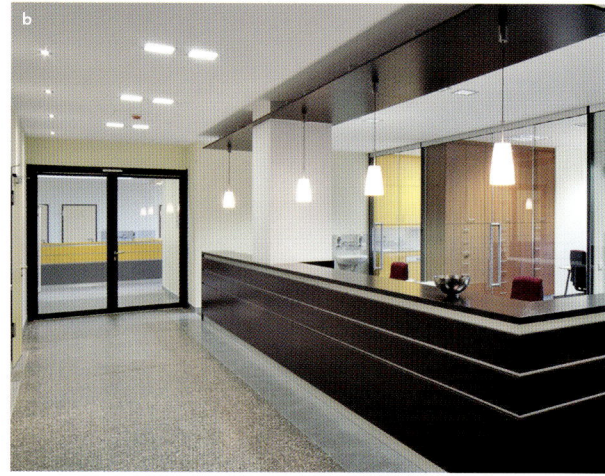

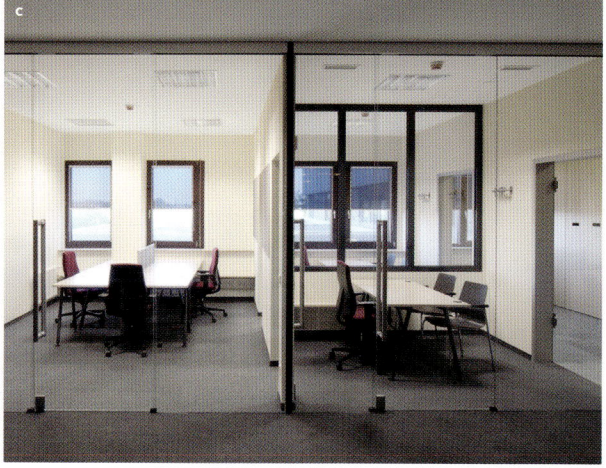

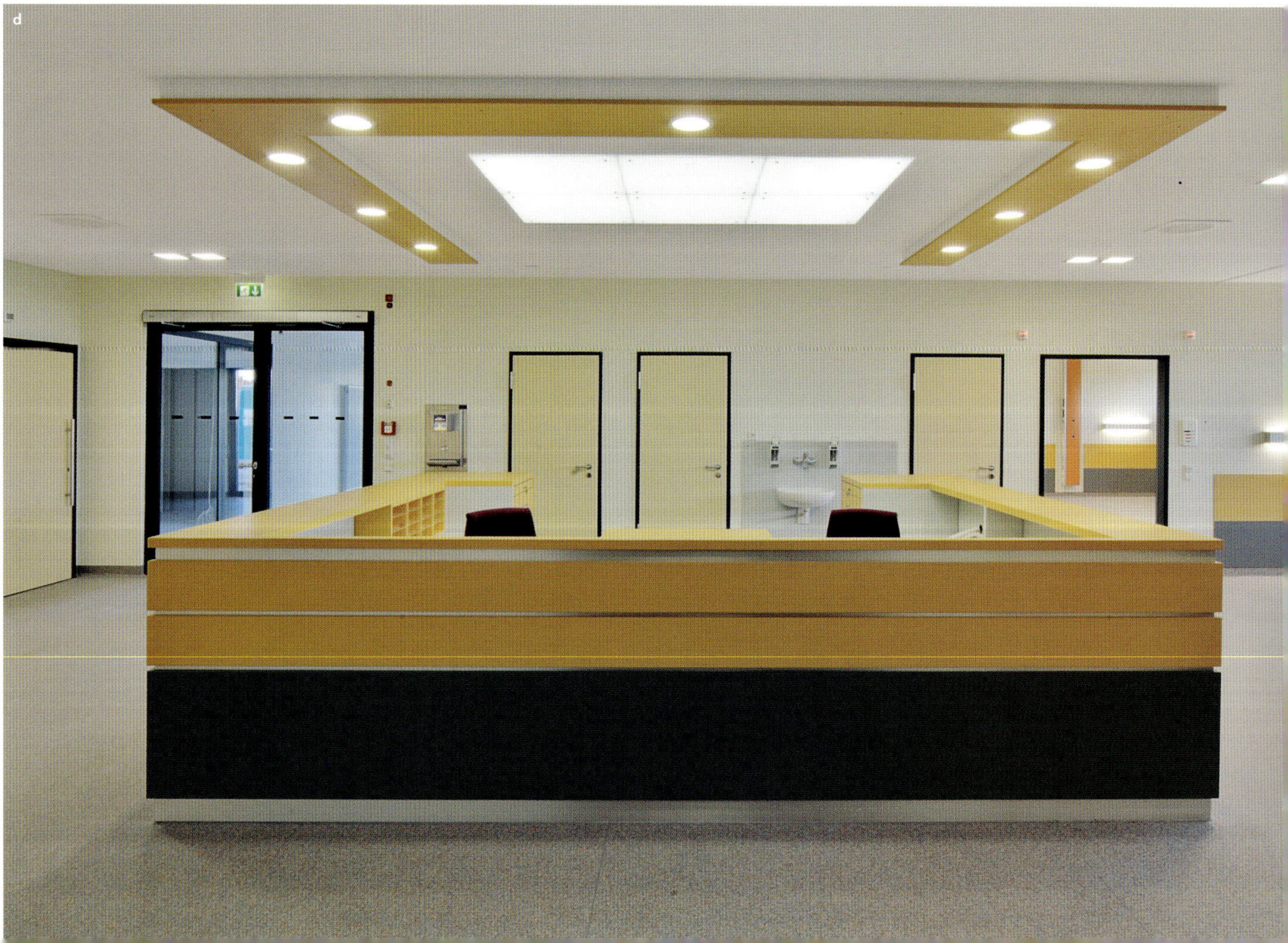

Client	Frankenthal
Operator	Municipal Clinic
	Frankenthal
Planning time	05 2005 – 05 2006
Construction time	05 2006 – 04 2009
Gross floor area	4,750 sqm
Usable floor space	2,330 sqm
Gross cubic capacity	18,335 cbm
Construction cost	2.1 million EUR
Total cost	2.9 million EUR

a   The use of a continuous colour and material
    concept creates a pleasant atmosphere in the
    bright, light rooms.
b   The sedate reception area for elective patients
    is situated right next to the bright yellow emer-
    gency room.
c   Behind the reception desk for elective patients
    are rooms that can be used interdisciplinarily
    for medical | administrative admission.
d   The patients' attention is drawn to the signalling
    colour at the emergency patient admission at
    the entrance of the new right of way for patients
    unable to walk.

Floor plan layout

The spatial concentration of numerous hospital outpatient departments offers much potential for thorough examination and for treatment. In addition,
with the convenient layout on one level, further extension of the floor plan is
inevitably associated with very long distances to walk and in particular with
many rooms that do not have natural light. The main corridors, accessible
from both sides of the central hub area, and the secondary corridor running
in parallel with the longer one, from which connecting corridors exit, prove
beneficial to the orientation system.

Usable floor spaces

Patient rooms	**yellow**	605 sqm	26 %
Examination				
Treatment rooms	**red**	370 sqm	16 %
Specialist rooms	**pink**	563 sqm	24 %
Administrative rooms	**green**	170 sqm	7 %
Offices	Staff rooms	**orange**	312 sqm	13 %
Supply	Waste disposal	**brown**	157 sqm	7 %
Training rooms	**violet**	38 sqm	2 %
Plant rooms	**blue**	115 sqm	5 %
Total		2.330 sqm	100 %

Performance data

Outpatients per year	13,000
	[entire hospital]
Inpatients per year	8,200
Clinic opening hours	7 days	168 hours
Waiting time [with	without appointment]	0 – 100 min.	0 – 160 min.
Type and number of staff	2 doctors
	2 nursing staff
	1 trainee
	2 – 3 administrative staff
	[daytime]
Clinic planning advice	Too far from the care
	support point, to the
	procedure rooms or to
	the plaster room.

A room on the ground floor, which was previously used as a hair salon, has been refashioned to extend the dental practice, based in a house in Frankfurt's West End dating from the turn of the 19th century. The required adjoining spaces, such as changing and store room, are located in the basement.

The contained current premises have benefited from a smooth, flattering and calming design concept. The three main design elements – an adjusted box intended for consultation purposes, a non-structural wall and a suspended ceiling – playfully break away from the axial alignment and the right-angled geometry of the existing walls and create a new perception of space. The bright, lime-yellow flooring stands out in the simple white rooms, adding to the general elated feeling created by the high-gloss surfaces. Light and shadows of the white silhouettes reflect on the floor, creating interesting spatial impressions. In the evenings, this vibrant room looks like a stage set in special lighting, the leading actor being the modern treatment chair, which is actually a small work of art in itself.

STENGELE + CIE.

DENTAL PRACTICE
FRANKFURT ON THE MAIN | G

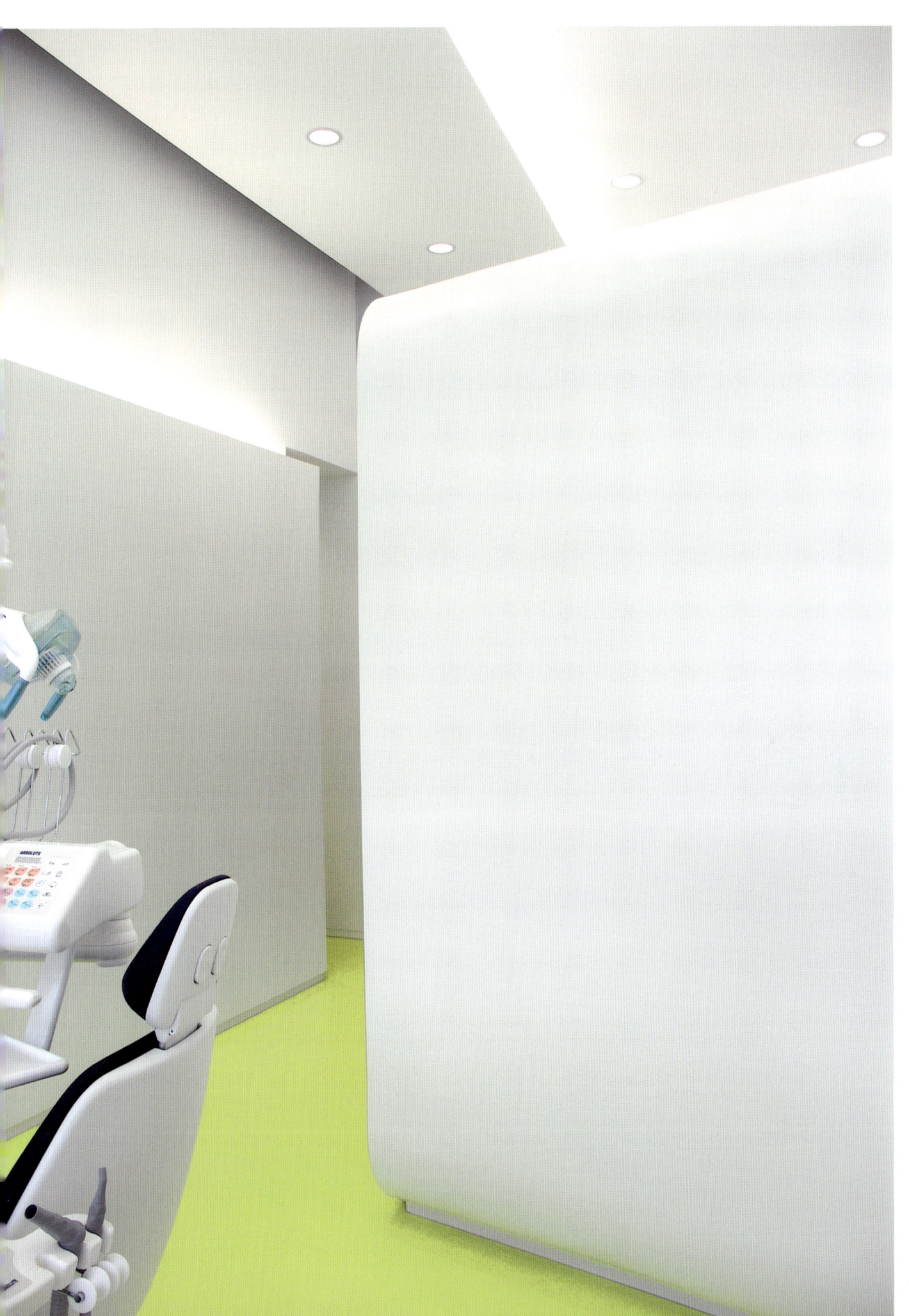

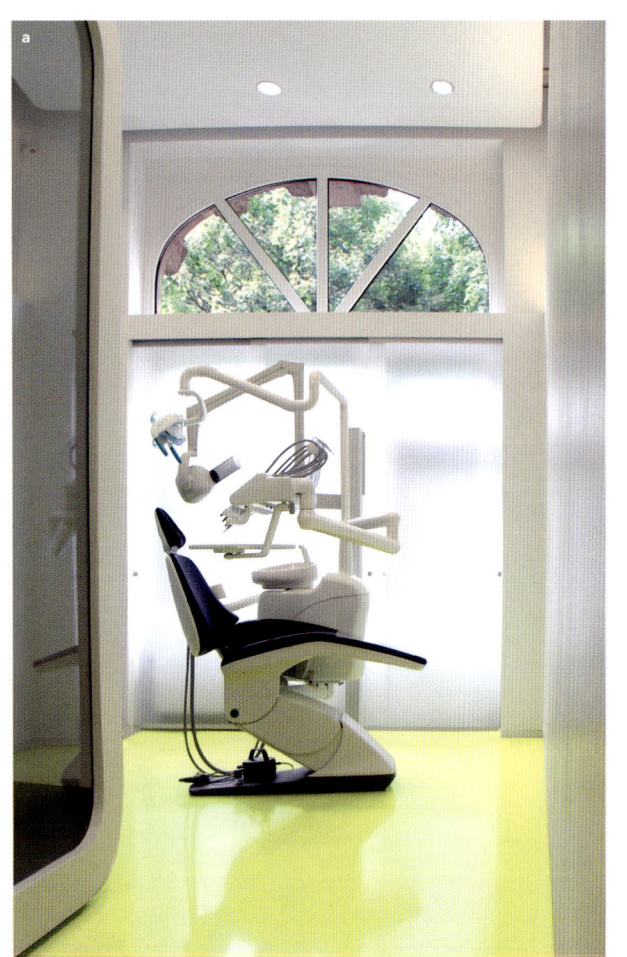

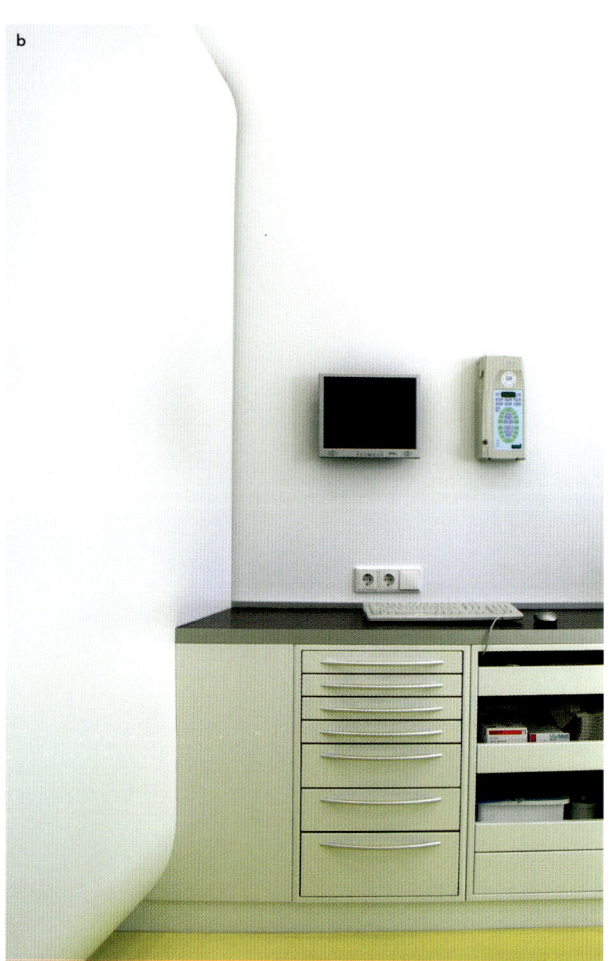

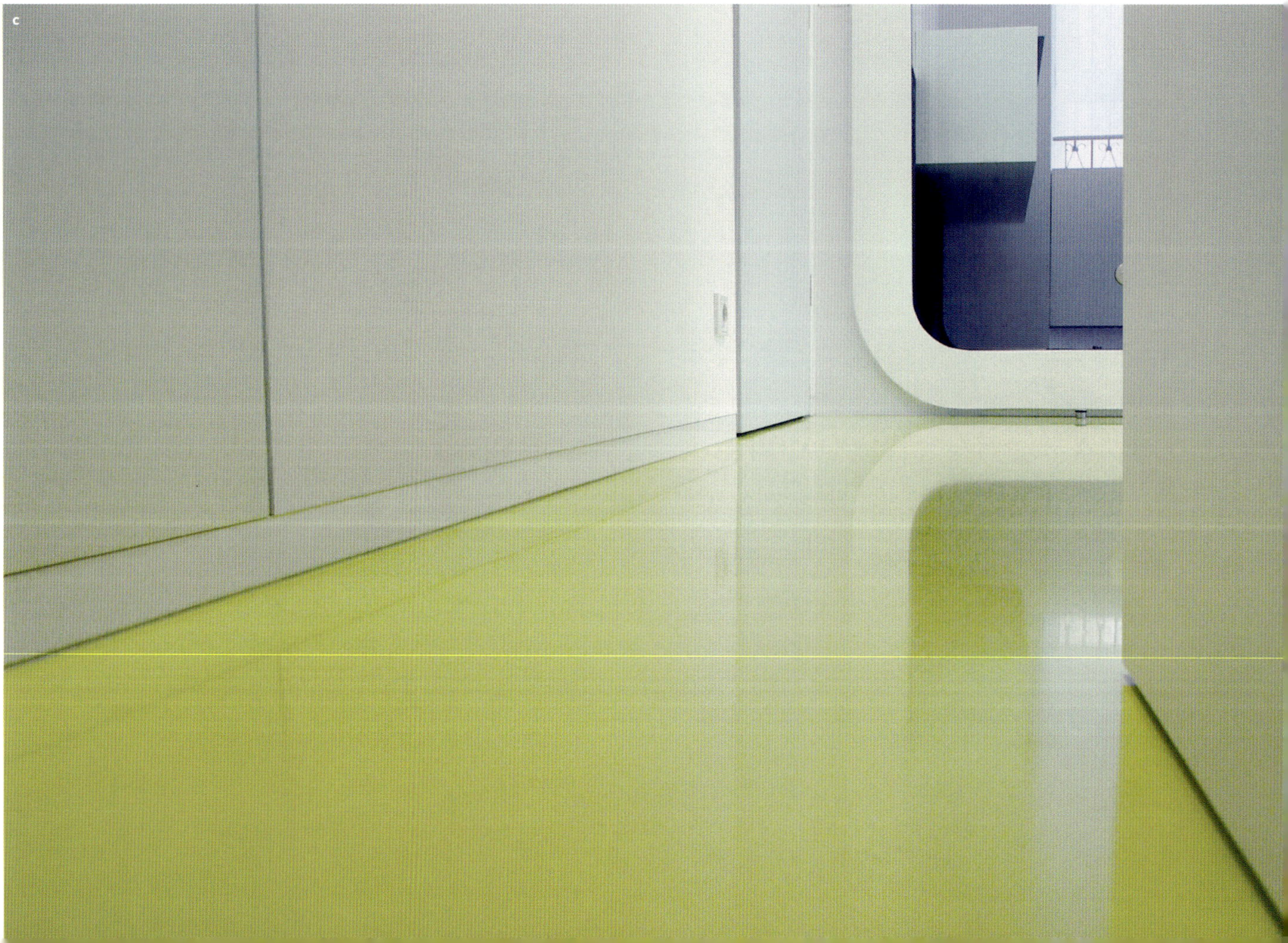

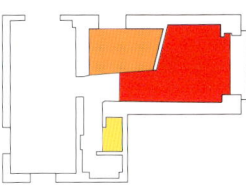

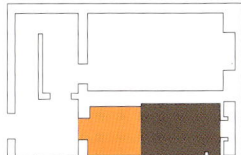

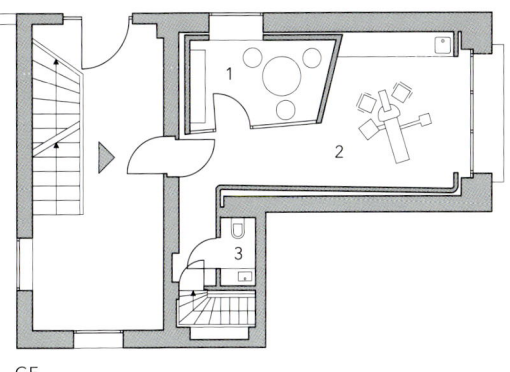

GF

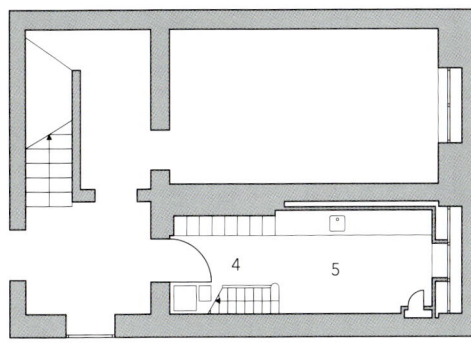

BSMT

Client	Operator	Dr. Dr. Frank Sanner
	Dr. Andreas Sanner
Planning time	04 2004 – 12 2004
Construction time	01 2005 – 03 2005
Gross floor area	72 sqm
Usable floor space	55 sqm
Gross cubic capacity	259 cbm

a An adjusted box, a non-structural wall and
  a suspended ceiling playfully break away
  from the alignments and right-angled
  geometry of the existing walls creating a
  new perception of space.
b The treatment room is furnished with functional facilities.
c The white silhouette of the consultation box
  is reflected in the high-gloss surface of the
  bright yellow flooring, which leads to interesting spatial impressions.

Diagrammatic plans, to scale 1:400
Floor plans, to scale 1:200

Floor plan layout

1	Consultation room	**3**	Patient toilet		cubicle
2	Treatment room	**4**	Staff changing	**5**	Store room

From the staircase on the ground floor, patients access the extension of
a partnership practice, which has its main rooms on the first floor. The
extension consists of a larger treatment room with a positioned consultation box and a toilet. A single-flight staircase leads to another room in the
basement, which houses the staff changing cubicle and a store room.

Usable floor spaces

Patient rooms	**yellow**	2 sqm	4 %
Examination |			
Treatment rooms	**red**	21 sqm	38 %
Offices | Staff rooms	**orange**	19 sqm	34 %
Supply | Waste disposal	**brown**	13 sqm	24 %
Total		55 sqm	100 %

The idea behind this practice is clearly expressed by its motto:

To create an environment that makes people forget their fears,
where people feel safe, where anything seems possible:
a place for relaxation, a space for exercise;
a place to distract and enthral the youngest;
a space that takes the older ones seriously and nurtures them.

Here an undeveloped and – apart from a few concrete pillars – entirely empty, attic was available to house this spacious practice building. By means of only a few carefully chosen features, this practice, furnished in warm shades and with white | green walls, has become a pleasant abode for both very young and older patients. The design is not confined, as it is often the case with this type of facility, to a form of expression aimed at two to eight-year-old children, but rather takes into account all age groups. On closer inspection, the playful aspect becomes apparent, achieved by means of toy rail track integrated into the floor and visible through a glass panel coloured light with its control switch, a subtle digital print wallpaper … The waiting area, situated behind a glass wall subtly decorated with a delicate pattern of see-through algae, is furnished with a large painting wall, where young patients can give free rein to their imagination. Important aspects of the room design are the visual relationships and visual axes which make the attic floor appear spacious.

BIRGIT STILETTO

**PAEDIATRIC AND
YOUTH MEDICINE CLINIC**
BAIERSBRONN | G

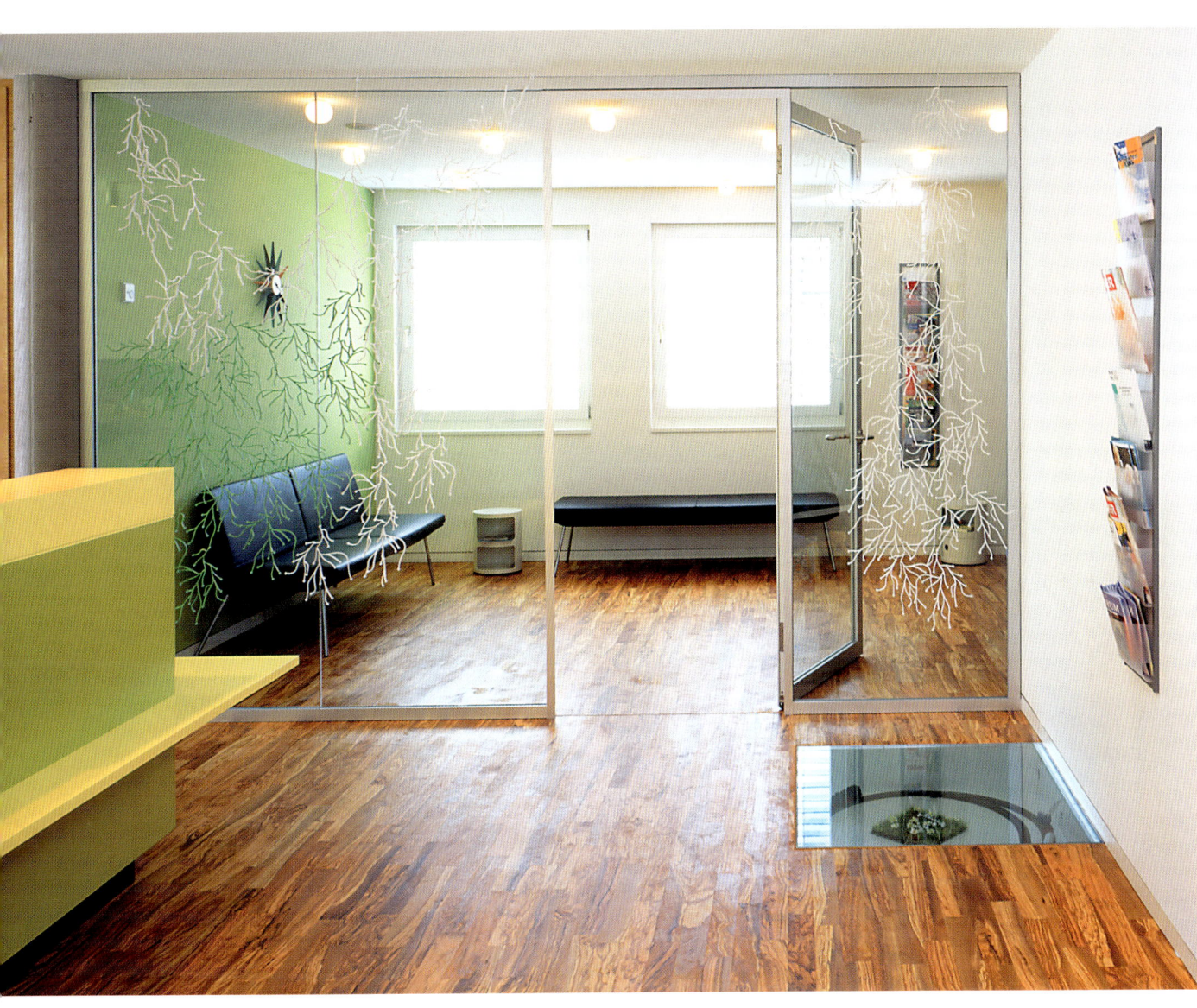

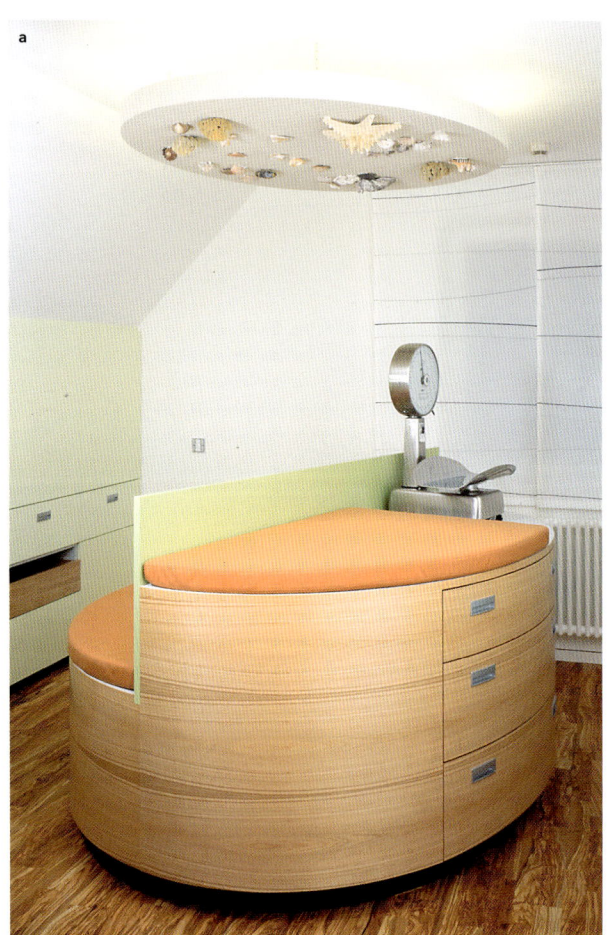

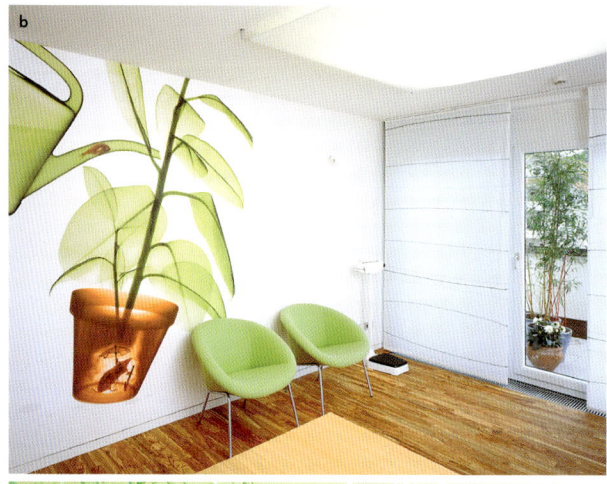

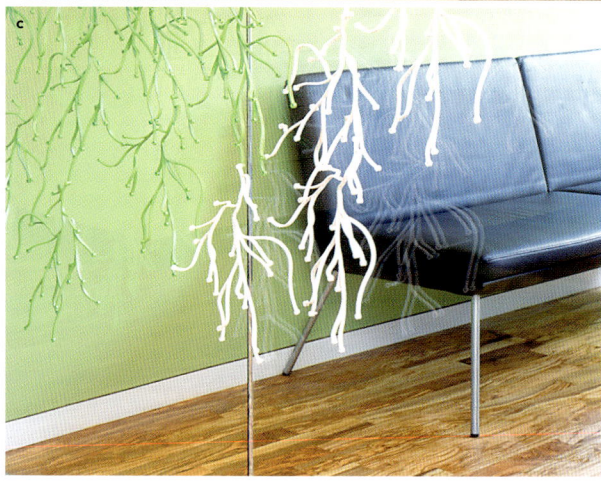

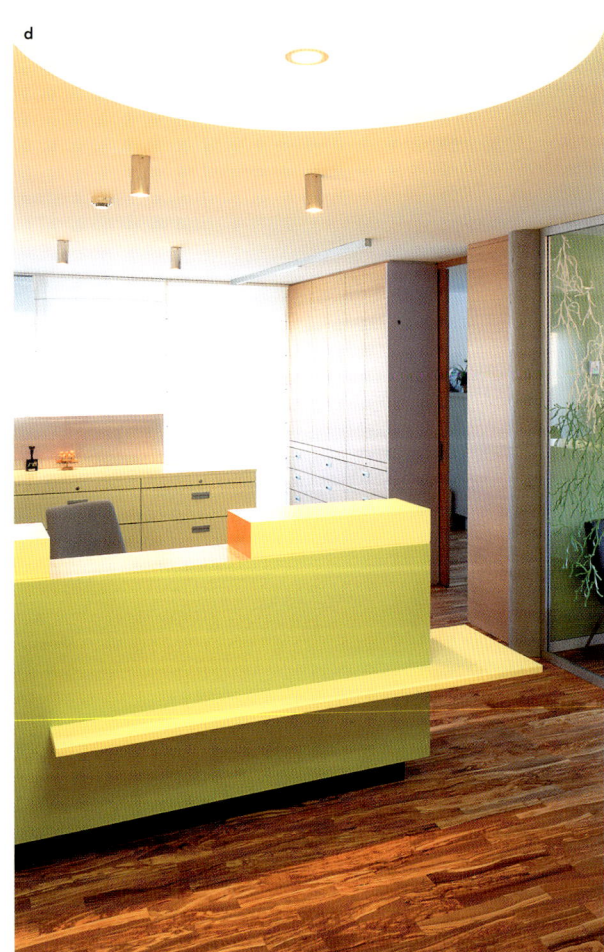

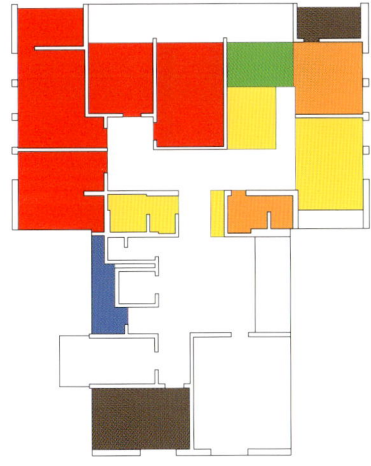

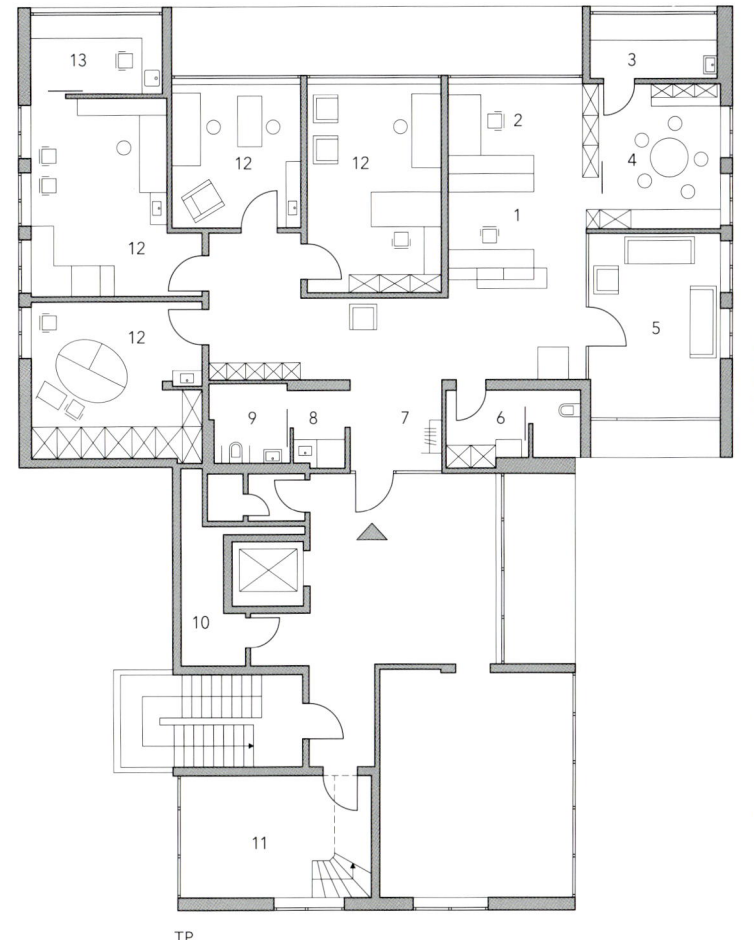

TP

Floor plan layout

1	Reception	**6**	Staff changing cubicle and toilet	**10**	Installations room
2	Office	**7**	Coat-rack	**11**	Store room
3	Cleaning room	**8**	Winding space	**12**	Treatment room
4	Staff lounge	**9**	Patient toilet	**13**	Laboratory
5	Waiting area				

The access point on the compact rectangular floor plan of the single-doctor practice is in the centre of one of the long sides. From there, via the somewhat eccentrically located reception and the directly adjacent waiting area in a short central corridor, patients access the practice rooms, which, with the exception of the sanitary facilities, are fully supplied with natural light.

Usable floor spaces

Patient rooms	**yellow**	40 sqm	20 %
Examination | Treatment rooms	**red**	94 sqm	47 %
Administrative rooms	**green**	10 sqm	5 %
Offices | Staff rooms	**orange**	24 sqm	12 %
Supply | Waste disposal	**brown**	26 sqm	13 %
Plant rooms	**blue**	7 sqm	3 %
Total		201 sqm	100 %

Performance data

Outpatients per year	5,000
Number and type of services per year	EEG, Sonography, ECG, Audiometry, ADHD diagnostics [200]
Services to other clinics	MRI, Consulting physicians [Orthopaedics, Surgery, Ophthalmology Psychology]
Clinic opening hours	5 days | 40 hours
Waiting time [with | without appointment]	5 – 30 min. | 30 – 60 min.
Type and number of staff	1 doctor 1 full-time staff 1 half-day staff 1 casual worker

Client | Operator	Dr. Markus Stiletto
Planning time	02 2005
Construction time	03 2005 – 07 2005
Gross floor area	231 sqm
Usable floor space	201 sqm
Gross cubic capacity	648 cbm
Construction cost	213,000 EUR
Total cost	343,000 EUR

a The elliptical shape of the treatment table, which stands freely in the room, enables use from both sides.

b In the treatment room, olive wood parquet flooring and digital print wallpaper create an atmosphere that appeals to all age-groups.

c The transparent waiting area is situated behind a glass wall, where delicate algae suggest a screen.

d The very clear structure of the practice is accentuated by interesting elements for example such as the toy railway integrated into the floor.

Diagrammatic plans, to scale 1:400
Floor plans, to scale 1:200

Hanging gardens as an eye-catching feature – this I-shaped ophthalmology practice is located with its very long glass frontage looking onto the courtyards of the Munich Perusapassage designed by Tita Giese. The challenge for the architects was to optimise the long narrow floor plan for the operational processes of the practice. Placing the individual rooms next to each other in a row preserves the "Passage" [arcade] character; an aisle to stroll alongside the hanging gardens has been left open up to the glass facade. In order to reinforce the impression of lingering a while, the longitudinal wall is broken into individual areas and has been set out in a buckled, linear progression.

Here it was possible to divide the practice into two reception areas thanks to the exceptional floor plan: The zone in the region of the entrances includes the general reception with waiting area and treatment rooms; the immediately adjacent zone includes the waiting area for patients undergoing treatment, the doctor's room and other examination cubicles. In order to reinforce the open, spacious character of the floor layout, predominantly white-lacquered built-in furniture has been used. The black pillars match the dark tubular steel chairs in the waiting area. Fine natural stone flooring encapsulates the public area and in the treatment rooms oak parquet flooring makes for a pleasant atmosphere.

**TOOLS OFF.
ARCHITECTURE**

FÜNF HÖFE OPHTHALMOLOGISTS
MUNICH | G

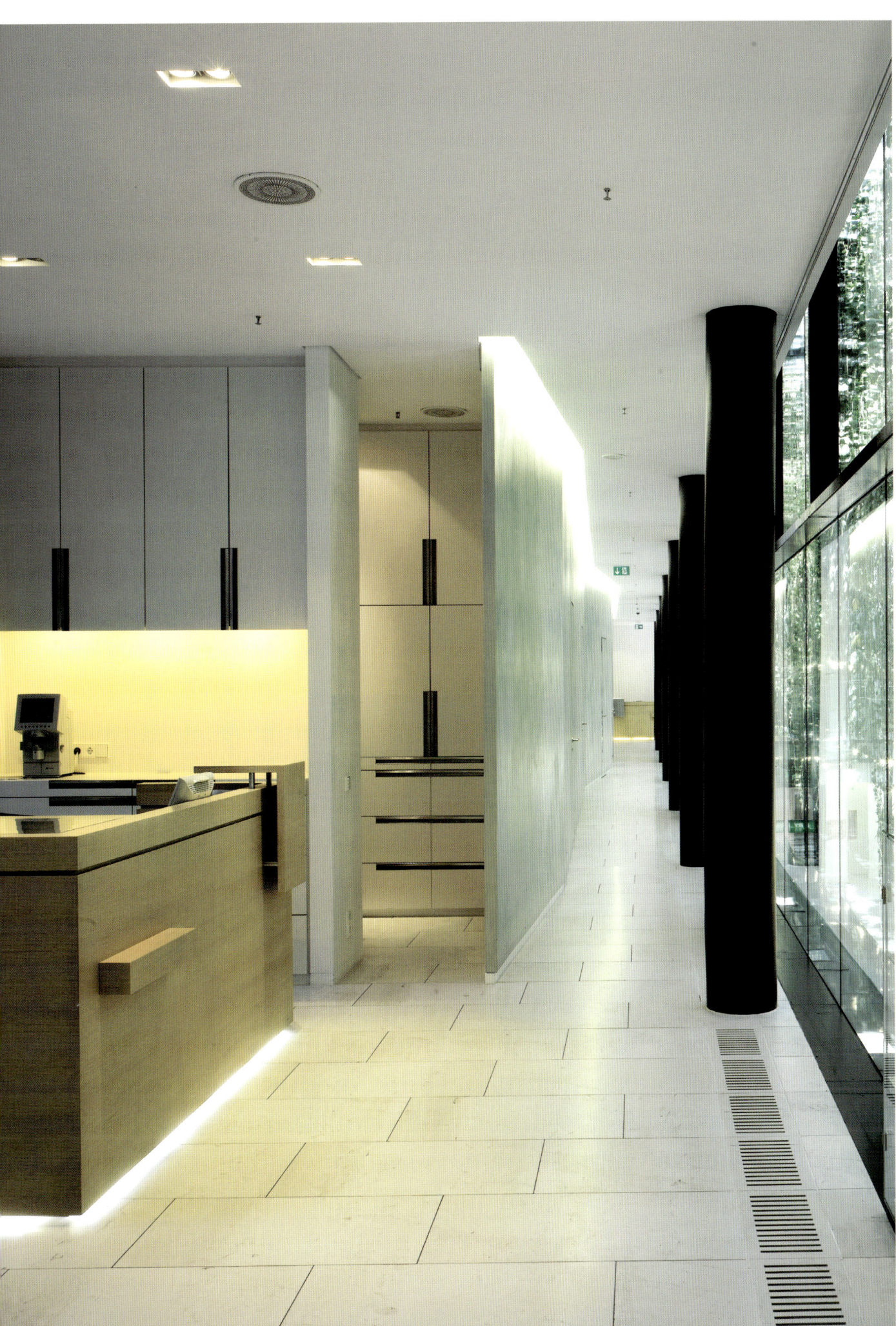

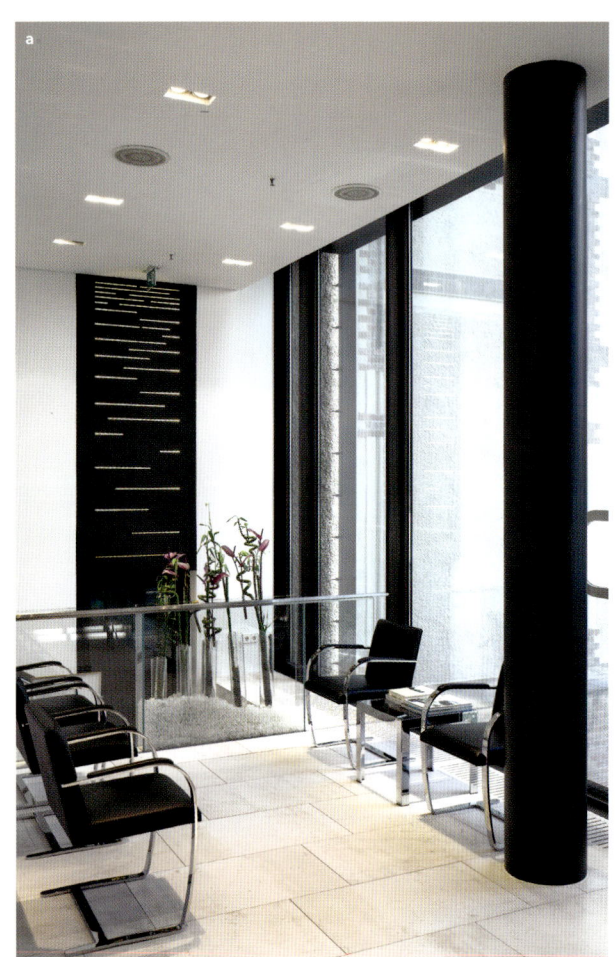
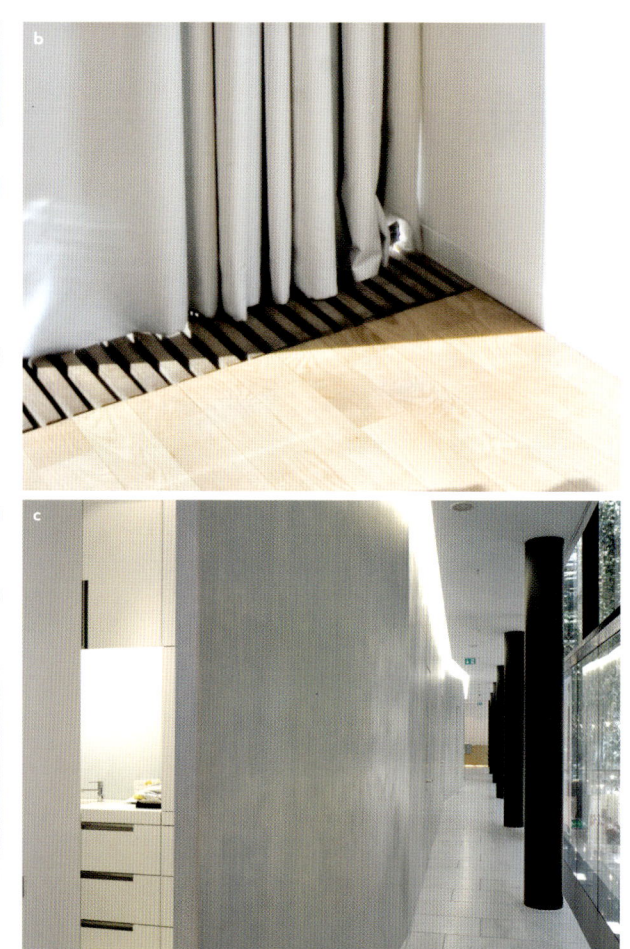

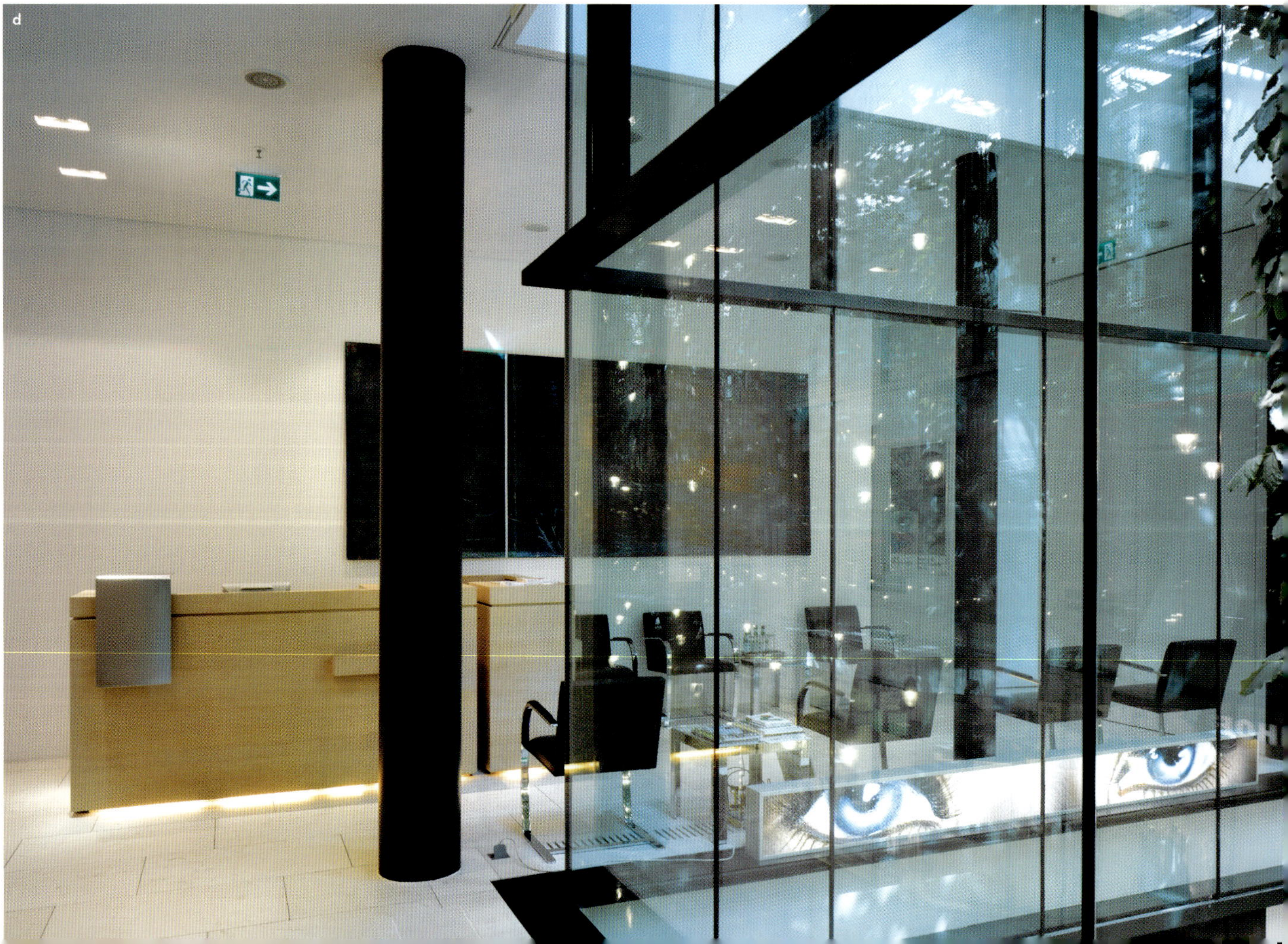

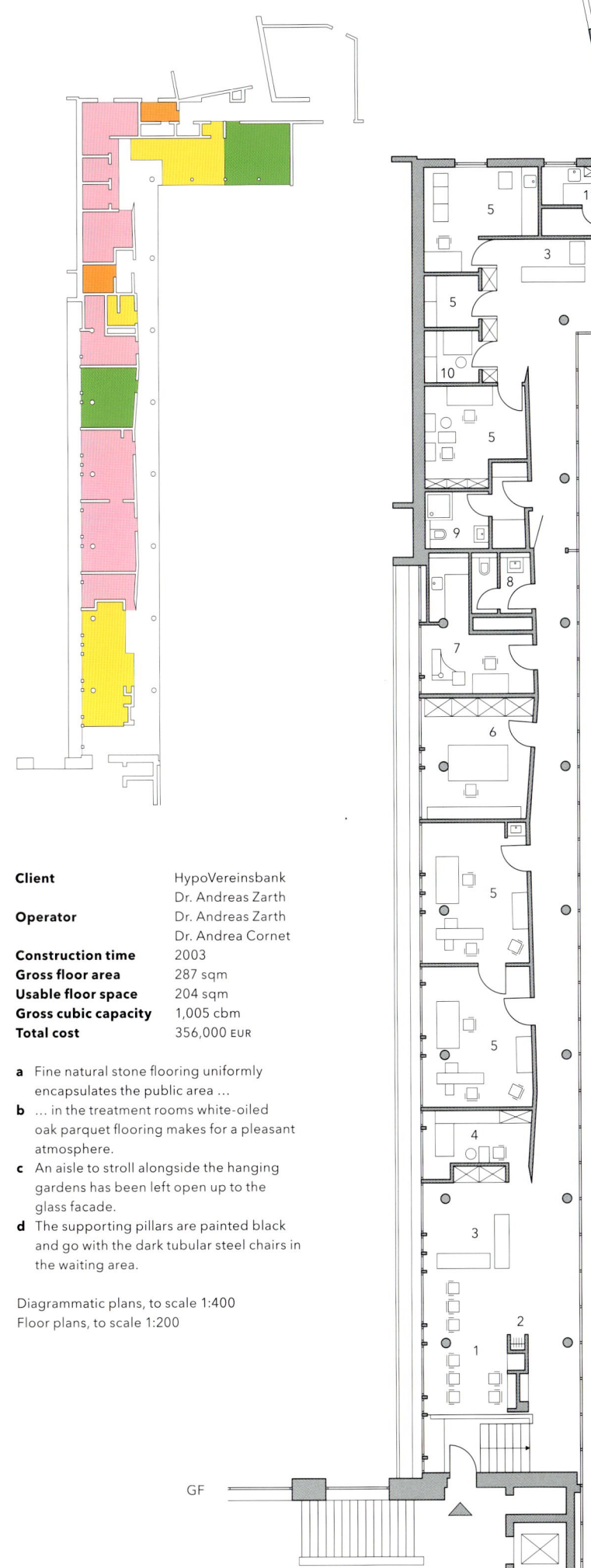

Client	HypoVereinsbank
	Dr. Andreas Zarth
Operator	Dr. Andreas Zarth
	Dr. Andrea Cornet
Construction time	2003
Gross floor area	287 sqm
Usable floor space	204 sqm
Gross cubic capacity	1,005 cbm
Total cost	356,000 EUR

a   Fine natural stone flooring uniformly
    encapsulates the public area …

b   … in the treatment rooms white-oiled
    oak parquet flooring makes for a pleasant
    atmosphere.

c   An aisle to stroll alongside the hanging
    gardens has been left open up to the
    glass facade.

d   The supporting pillars are painted black
    and go with the dark tubular steel chairs in
    the waiting area.

Diagrammatic plans, to scale 1:400
Floor plans, to scale 1:200

Floor plan layout

1	Waiting area	6	Office	10	Examination
2	Coat-rack	7	Treatment room	11	Small kitchen
3	Reception	8	Patient toilet	12	Office
4	Examination	9	Staff toilet		
5	Treatment room		and shower		

The floor plan, which is unusual for a multi-doctor practice, offers a top-quality experience. However, for the operation of the practice, the continuous add-on arrangement of the rooms, which for the most part have natural light, means that there are not only long distances to consider. Due to the entrances situated at the ends, each with reception and waiting area, staff and spatial synergetic effects have to be relinquished too. Areas for the staff lounge and for storage and cleaning are not shown.

Usable floor spaces

Patient rooms	yellow	57 sqm	28 %
Specialist rooms	pink	98 sqm	48 %
Administrative rooms	green	40 sqm	20 %
Offices	Staff rooms	orange	9 sqm	4 %
Total		204 sqm	100 %

Performance data

Clinic opening hours	5 days	55 hours
Type and number of staff	1 full-time doctor
	1 part-time doctor
	1 optician
	1 orthoptist
	7 additional staff

GF

The stately mansion in Rodenkirchen, Cologne, stood empty for a very long time, until it was given new life by means of its conversion into this Centre for Holistic Medicine. This imposing construction dating from the 1920s consists of a four-storey mansion and a two-storey coach house nestled in a 1,600 square metre park. Both buildings exhibit a colourful mixture of quite different styles adopted by successive conversions: Original stucco ceilings cohabit with suspended ceilings and carpets covering the old parquet flooring together with a staircase system typical of the 1970s.

The whole building needed to be restructured, while respecting previous interventions. The main focus of attention, however, was the foyer with its solid steel staircase. The granite covering of these stairs has been extended into the public area. Spacious room structures guide visitors entering by the backlit reception desk into the waiting area in the former garden hall. The examination and treatment rooms with newly-laid oak parquet flooring in herringbone bond, old wooden windows and restored doors and stucco ceilings guarantee a very intimate atmosphere. Here historical architecture forms a symbiotic relationship with modern features: This association symbolises, perhaps, the replacement of conventional medicine with alternative naturopathy, which is practised at the Villavita.

TRINT+KREUDER

VILLAVITA – CENTRE FOR HOLISTIC MEDICINE
COLOGNE | G

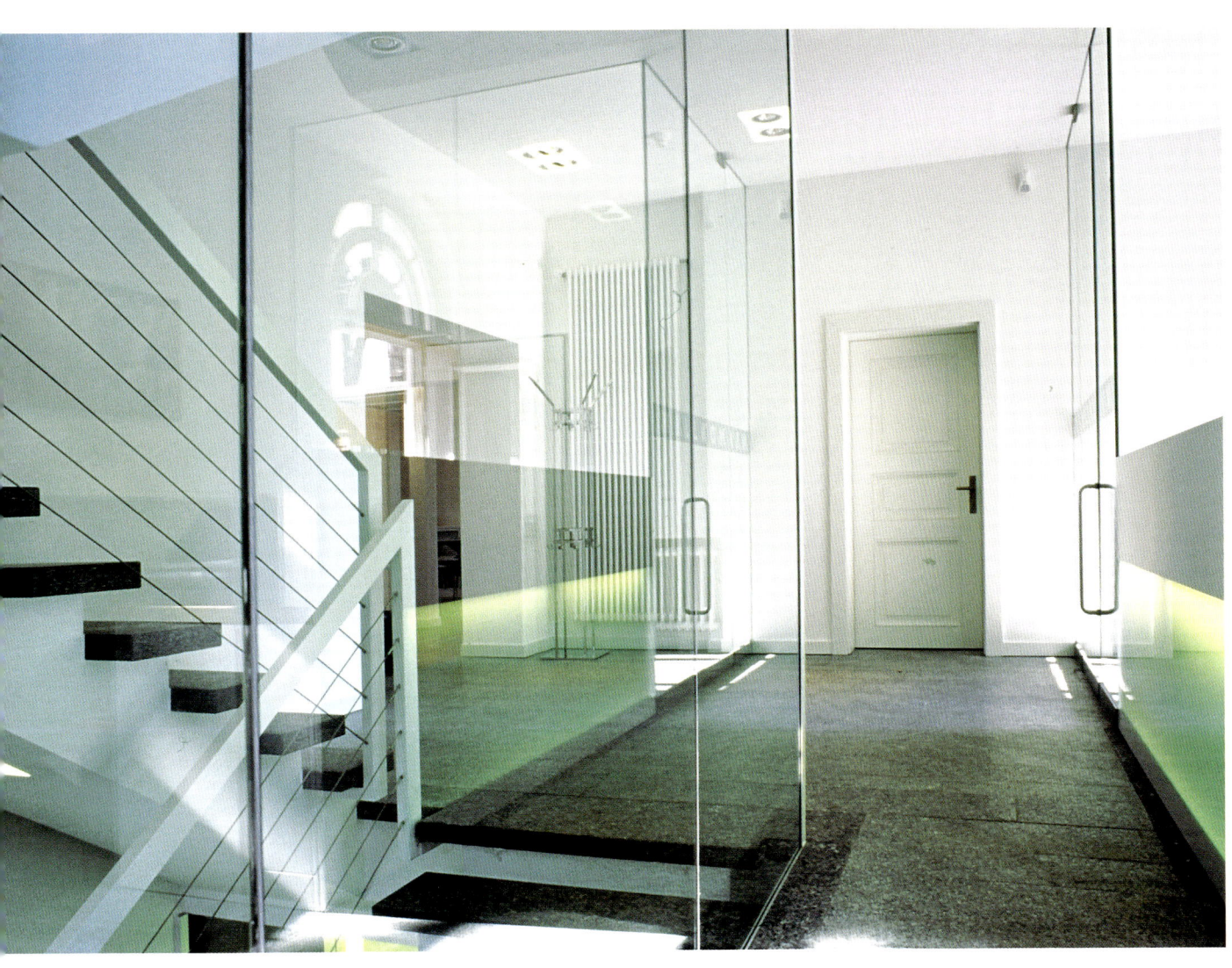

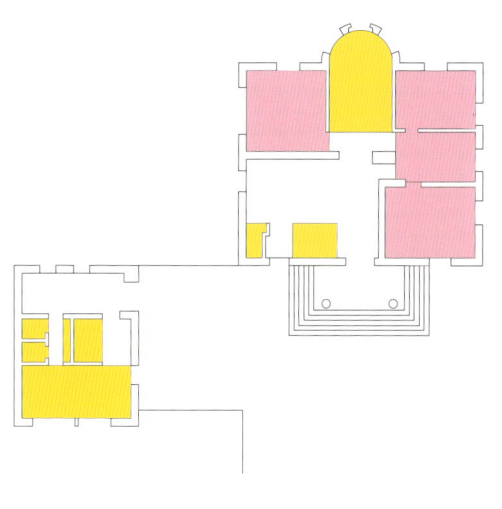

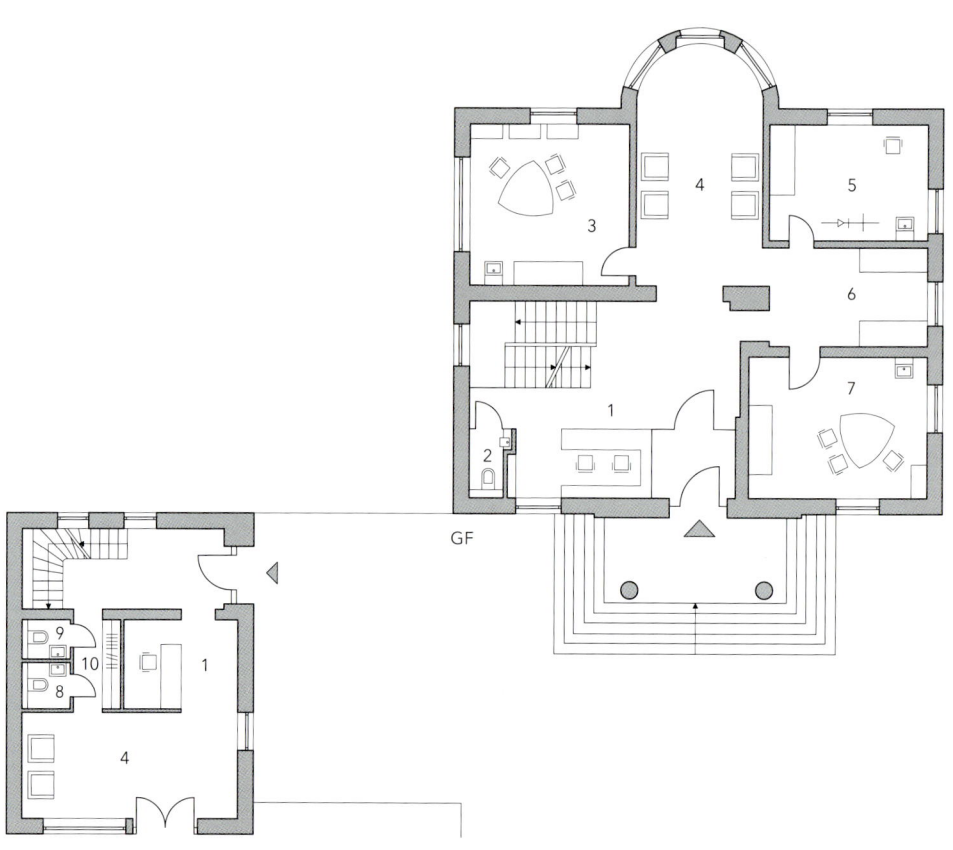

GF

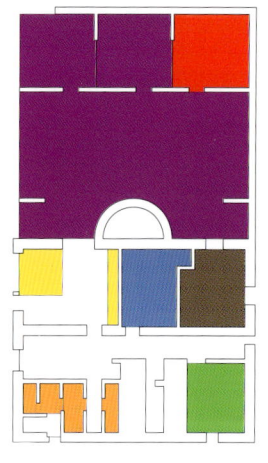

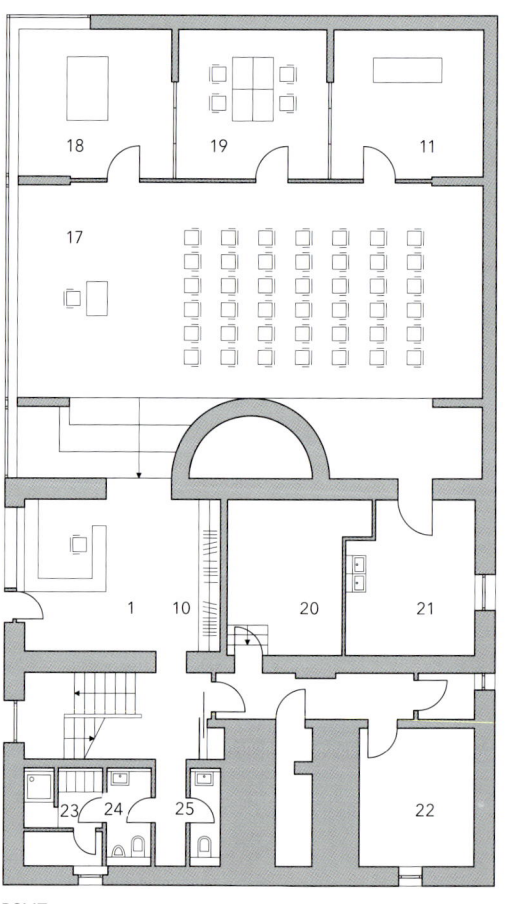

BSMT

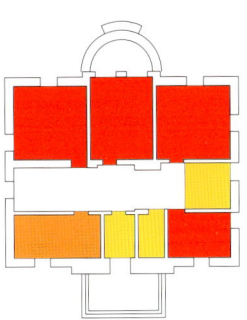

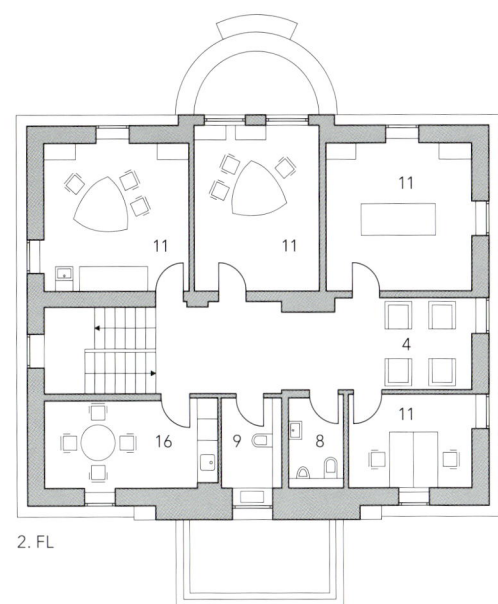

2. FL

1 Reception
2 Patient toilet
3 Examination and
   treatment room
   internal medicine
4 Waiting area
5 Examination
   ultrasound and ECG
6 Treatment room
   infusions
7 Examination and
   treatment room
   nuclear medicine
8 Patient toilet G
9 Patient toilet L
10 Coat-rack
11 Treatment room
12 Examination and
    treatment room TCM
13 Examination and
    treatment room
    gynaecology

14 Laboratory
15 Examination and
    treatment room
    for children
16 Staff lounge and
    small kitchen
17 Seminar room
    and occupational
    therapy room
18 Workroom
19 Computer room
20 Installations room
    for heating system
21 Store room chairs
22 Filing room
23 Staff changing
    cubicle
24 Staff toilet G
25 Staff toilet L

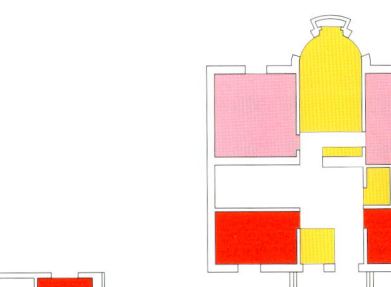

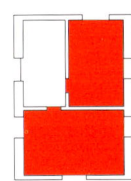

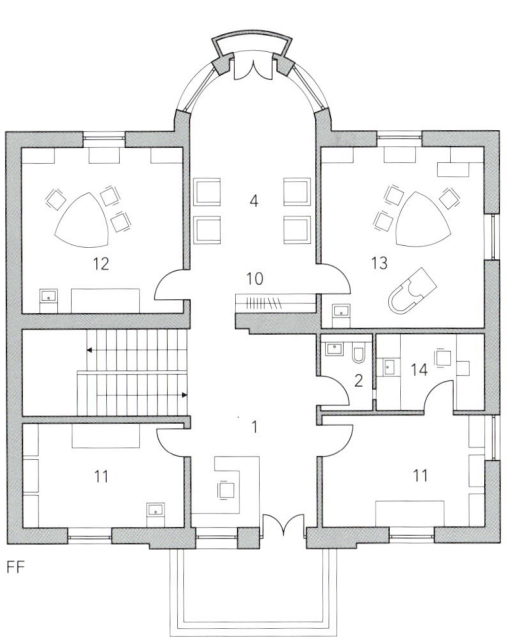

FF

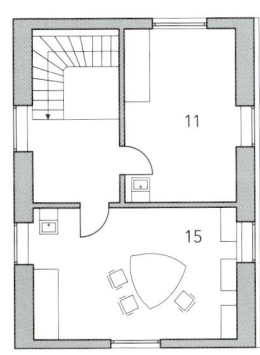

Diagrammatic plans, to scale 1:400
Floor plans, to scale 1:200

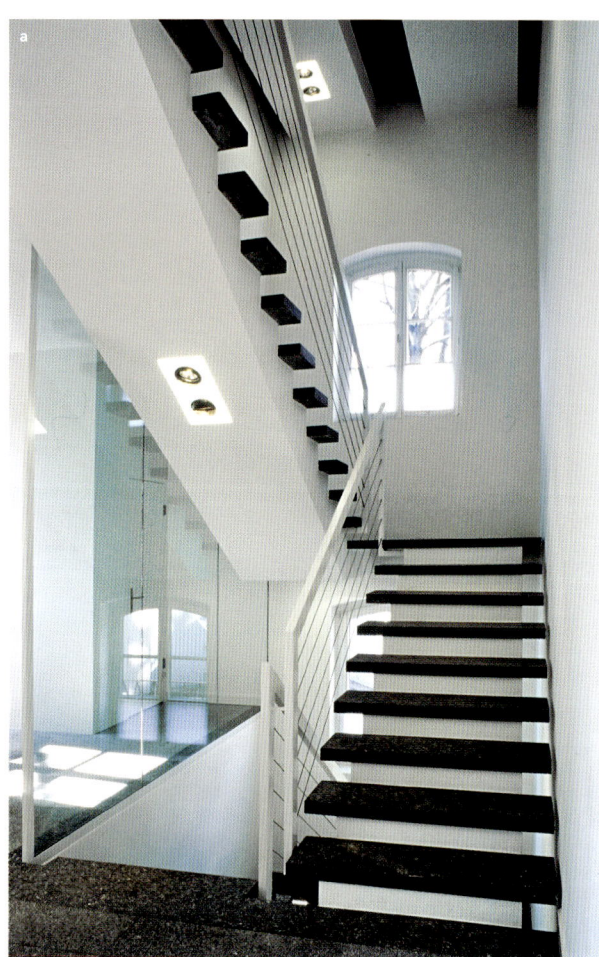

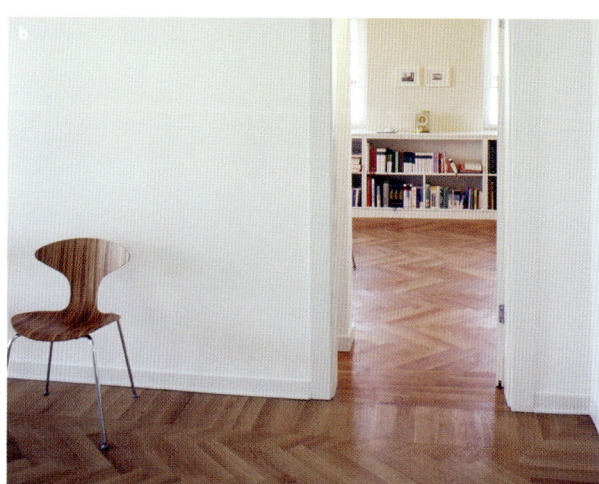

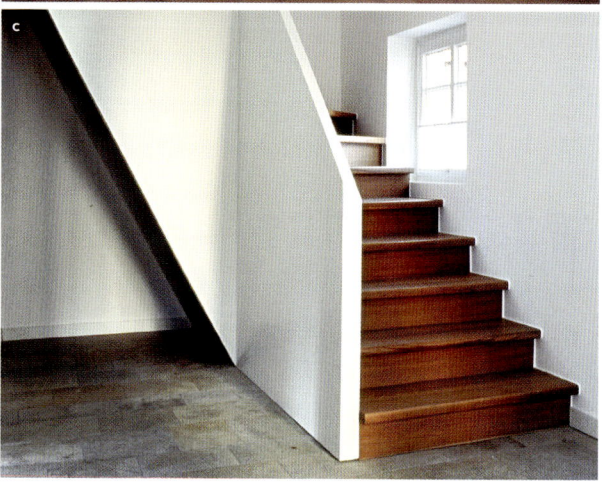

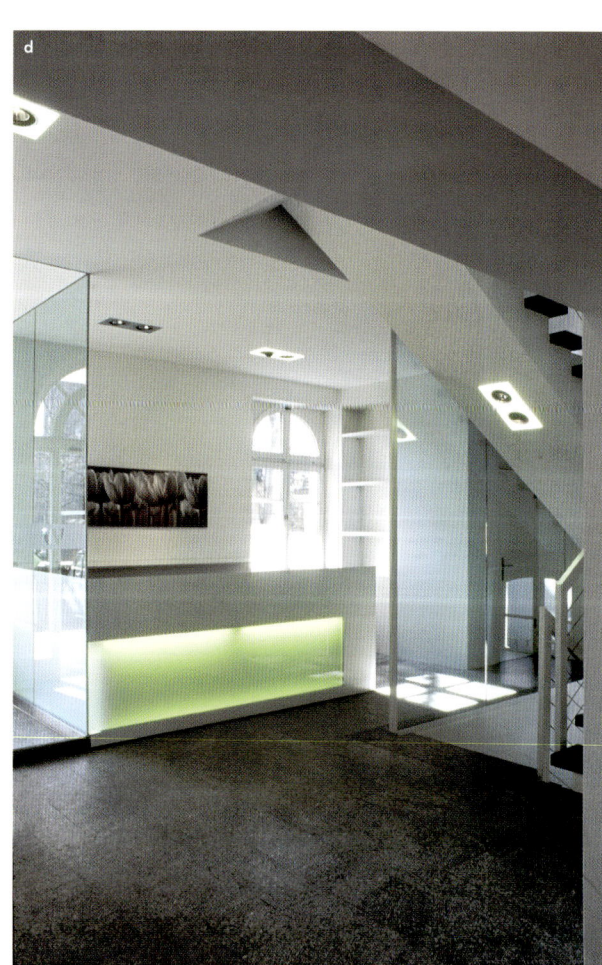

Client	Marita Müller GmbH
Operator	Villavita GmbH
Planning time	03 2004 – 12 2005
Construction time	02 2005 – 12 2005
Gross floor area	820 sqm
Usable floor space	599 sqm
Gross cubic capacity	3,500 cbm
Construction cost	500,000 EUR
Total cost	622,000 EUR

a The granite covering of the stairs in the foyer has been extended into the waiting area.

b The oak parquet flooring in herringbone bond in the examination and treatment rooms has been newly laid.

c The historical architecture of the four-storey large town house forms a harmonic symbiosis with modern features.

d Spacious room structures conduct visitors coming in from the backlit reception desk into the waiting area.

Floor plan layout

This operationally-elaborate multiple practice, located on four levels of the main building and on two levels of an adjoining building, is accessed by three entrances and has a total of four reception desks and four very spacious waiting areas, each provided with natural light, from which patients take a short walk to the examination and treatment rooms, which also have natural light. Unfortunately there is no lift.

Usable floor spaces

Patient rooms	**yellow**	115 sqm	19 %
Examination | Treatment rooms	**red**	155 sqm	26 %
Specialist rooms	**pink**	119 sqm	20 %
Administrative rooms	**green**	13 sqm	2 %
Offices | Staff rooms	**orange**	26 sqm	4 %
Supply | Waste disposal	**brown**	16 sqm	3 %
Training rooms	**violet**	140 sqm	23 %
Plant rooms	**blue**	15 sqm	3 %
Total		599 sqm	100 %

Performance data

Outpatients per year	15,000
Clinic opening hours	5 days | 42 hours
Waiting time [with appointment]	5 min.
Type and number of staff	2 doctors
	3 alternative practitioners
	1 full-time staff

Competence, precision and quality are what the Falkenried practice clinic strives for and these factors had to be reflected in the design of the premises.

The clinic is characterised by a design concept focused on material and not only limited to the essentials: exquisite materials and clear-cut architecture dominate the rooms. The colour palette ranges from warm shades [dark brown leather, cherrywood, sand-coloured cast iron base flooring] to cooler tones [aluminium, glass, anthracite-coloured Eternit]. Outside windows glazed down to floor level and translucent glass walls in the interior ensure that natural light penetrates deep into the rooms. Anthracite-coloured cubic functional boxes house the technical equipment of the practice and double up as design features at the same time. The centre-point of the clinic is the extremely spacious reception area, which opens up into a conically-tapering movement zone, which can also be used as a presentation and event area thanks to flexible boundary glass areas. Separated from the remaining treatment zones by automatic sliding glass doors, and situated next to two wards is the surgical wing, which boasts two operating theatres, sluice, sterilisation and recovery room. A bright, cast iron base flooring connects all spaces and puts patients and visitors at ease when entering the clinic.

WAGENKNECHT ARCHITEKTEN

FALKENRIED CLINIC
HAMBURG | G

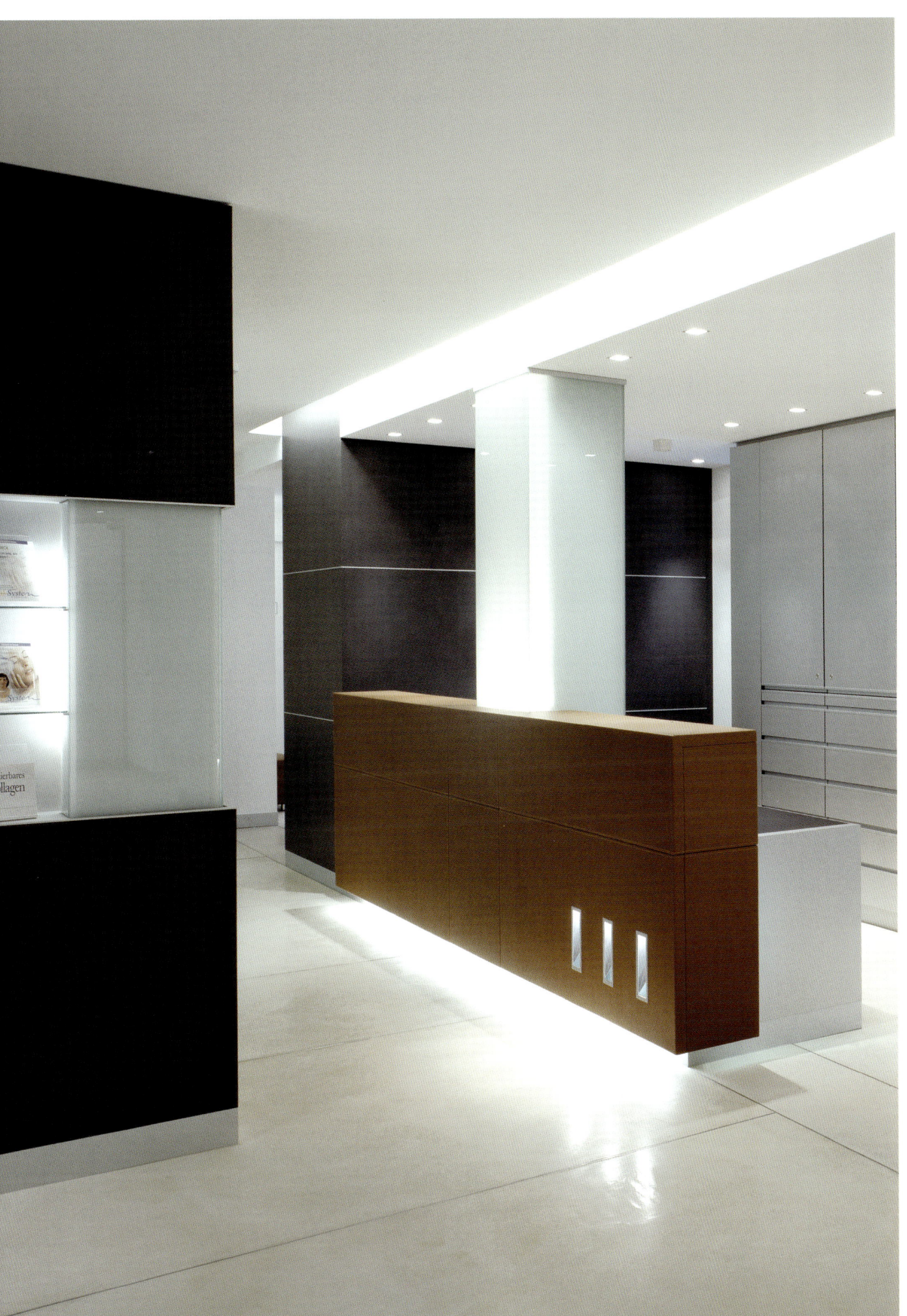

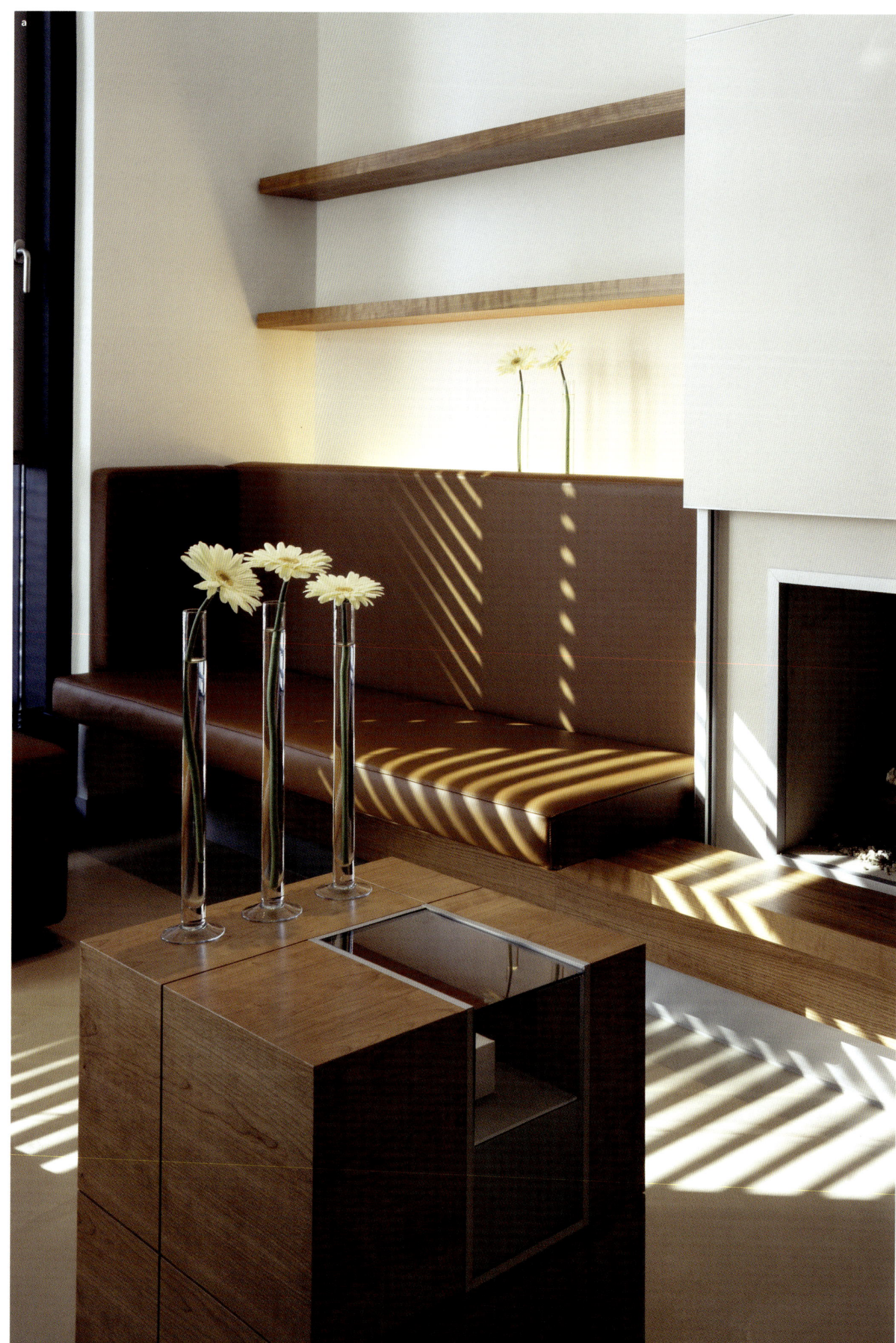

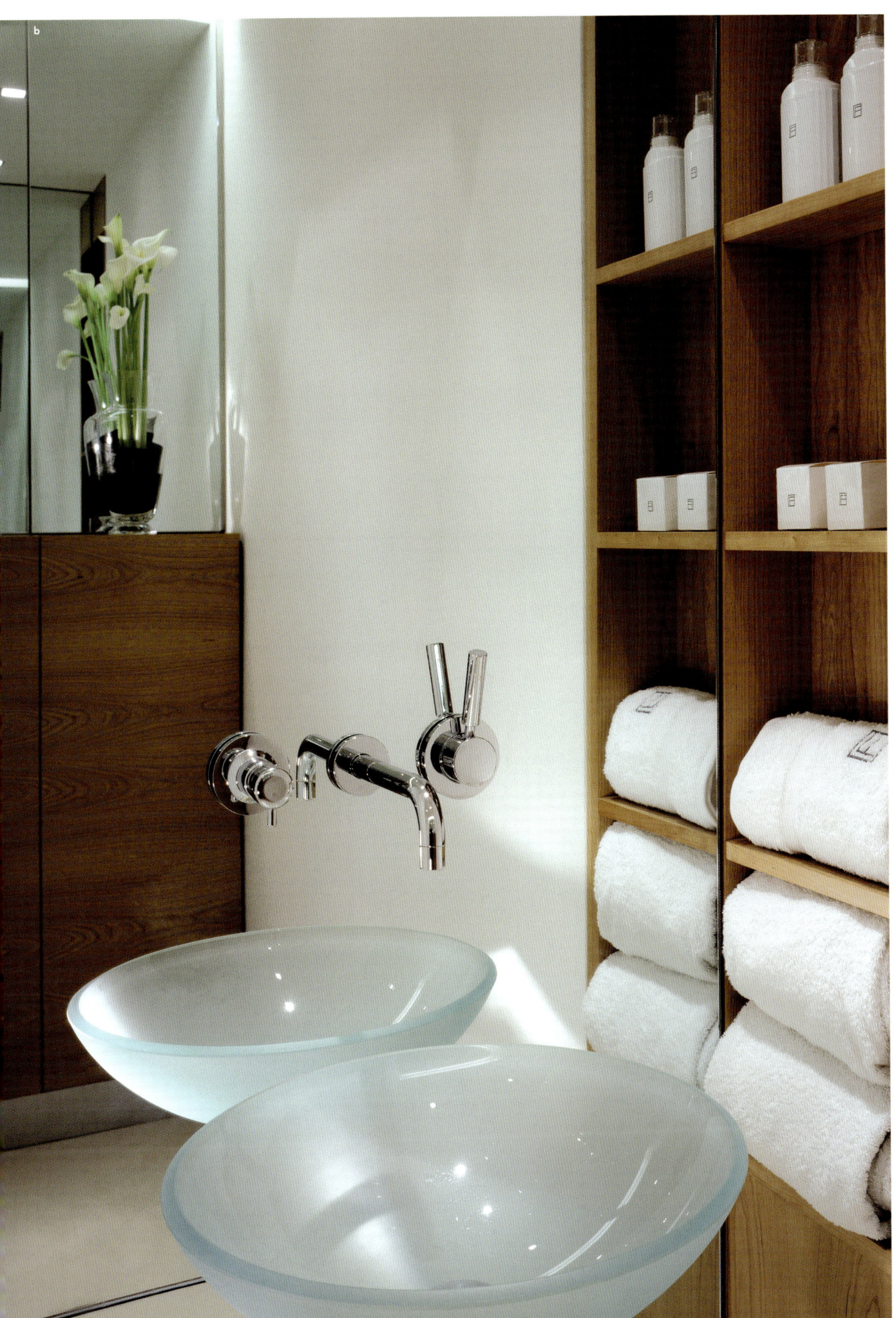

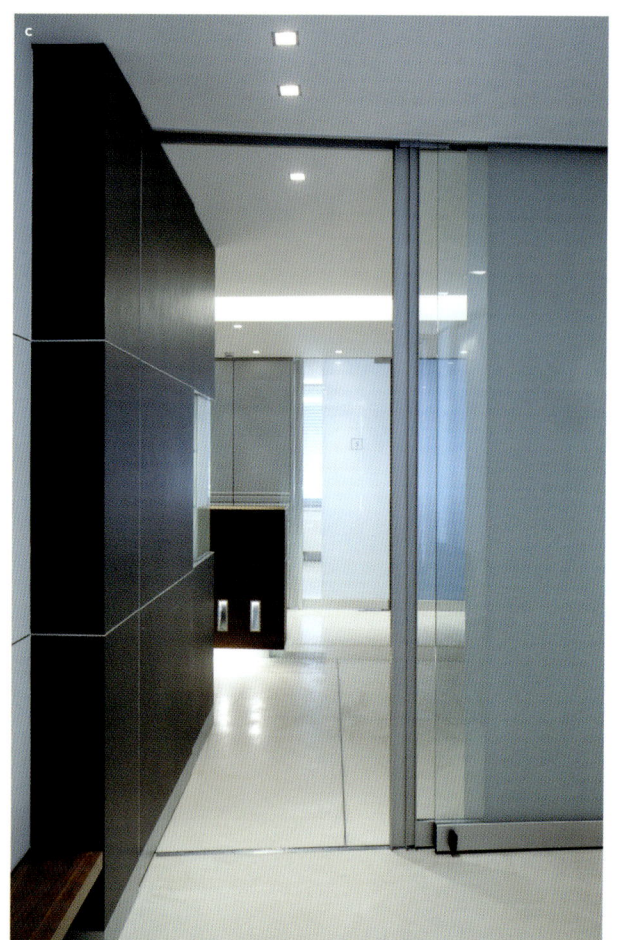

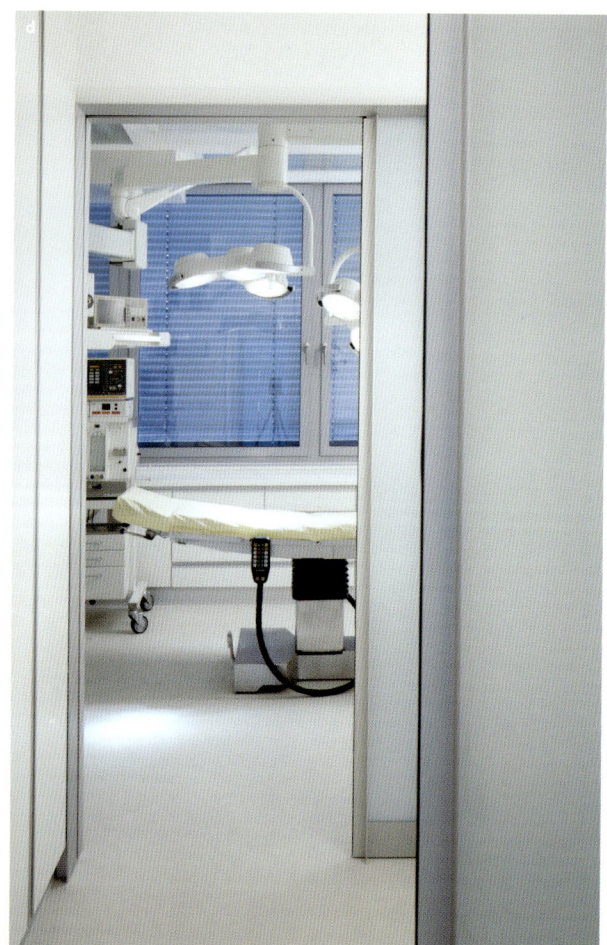

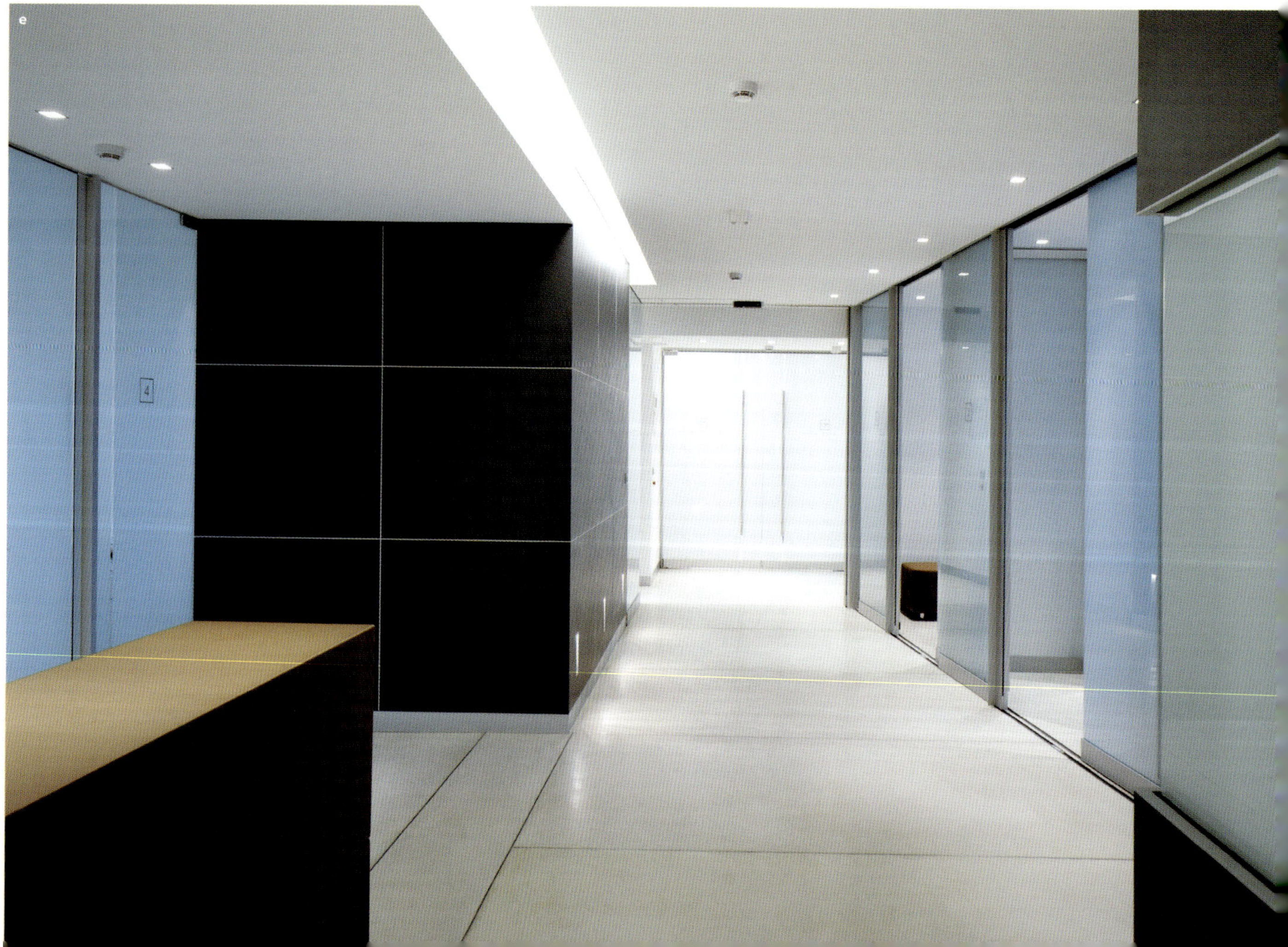

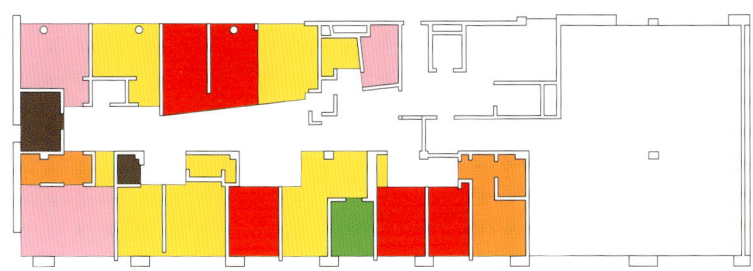

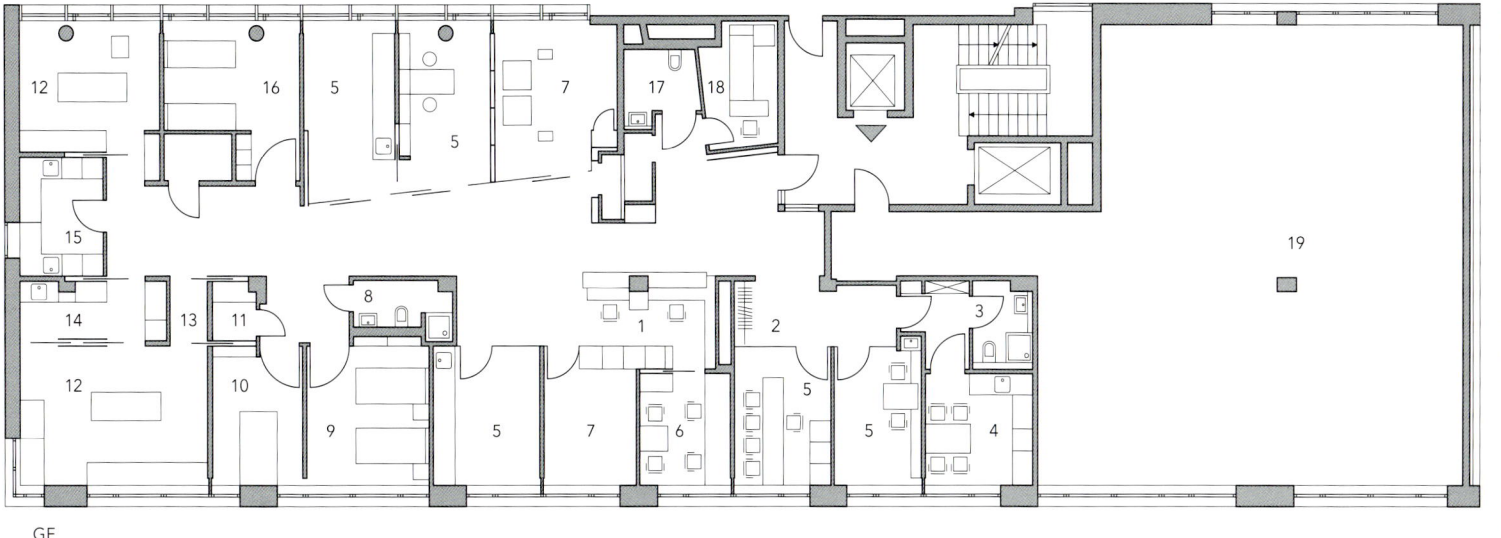

GF

Client | Operator   Dr. Wolfgang Friedrich
    Falkenried Clinic
Planning time   2003
Construction time   2004
Gross floor area   385 sqm
Usable floor space   237 sqm
Gross cubic capacity   1,155 cbm
Construction cost   350,000 EUR
Total cost   550,000 EUR

a In the waiting area dark brown leather, cherry-wood and sand-coloured cast iron base flooring create a homely atmosphere – there is even a fireplace.

b The high-quality furnishings in the patient toilet is reminiscent of those of a refined hotel.

c Translucent glass walls in the interior ensure that natural light penetrates into the depths of the rooms.

d The operating theatres are separated from the treatment area by means of automatic sliding glass doors.

e The spacious reception area, which opens up into a conically-tapered movement zone, can be used as a presentation and event space thanks to flexible boundary areas of glass.

Diagrammatic plans, to scale 1:400
Floor plans, to scale 1:200

Floor plan layout

1	Reception	**8**	Patient toilet	**15**	Sterilisation room
2	Coat-rack		and shower	**16**	Double room and
3	Staff toilet	**9**	Double room		recovery room
	and shower	**10**	Single room	**17**	Patient toilet
4	Staff lounge	**11**	Washroom	**18**	Examination
5	Treatment room	**12**	Operating theatre	**19**	Multi-purpose room
6	Office	**13**	Patient sluice		
7	Waiting area	**14**	Staff sluice		

Diagonally opposite the entrance of the multiple practice with clinic, situated on one of the narrow sides of the rectangular floor plan, is the reception with two waiting areas arranged at either side of the central corridor. From there patients go to the examination and treatment rooms, which are easy to locate. Almost all rooms in the practice have natural light. The planning of an expansion area is deemed far-sighted.

Usable floor spaces

Patient rooms	**yellow**	87 sqm	37 %
Examination | Treatment rooms	**red**	60 sqm	25 %
Specialist rooms	**pink**	46 sqm	19 %
Administrative rooms	**green**	8 sqm	3 %
Offices | Staff rooms	**orange**	26 sqm	11 %
Supply | Waste disposal	**brown**	10 sqm	5 %
Total		237 sqm	100 %

Performance data

Outpatients per year	4,000 – 5,000
Inpatients per year	500 – 700 day-patient
Clinic opening hours	7 days | 120 hours
Waiting time [with | without appointment]	15 min. | 20 – 30 min.
Number of staff	12 – 15

A blue glass wall greets visitors entering the spacious Lübeck multiple practice. It typifies the central aspect of the spatial floor plan design, which, at the request of the operator is based on the principles of Feng Shui. Opposite the "water element" in the form of the glass wall is the "earth element" in the shape of the desk and the back office in maple. The reception desk and the blue glass wall are arranged diagonally to form an inviting trapezoid. The guide wall, also clad with maple and horizontally-extending aluminium profiles, connects the reception desk to the surgery and treatment wing, whose units are accessible via a central distribution corridor. Light is a defining element in the design; the cove lighting running parallel to the corridor aids the guiding effect of the maple wall. Using illuminated ceiling panels and selectively-placed built-in lights, individual areas are accentuated. Ceiling-high glass elements, partly frosted, make the transitions appear as if they are floating and enable light to penetrate deep into the rooms.

Clear shapes, a few choice quality materials and clear-cut accessibility all have a calming effect on the patients and convey – in accordance with the ambitions of the practice – feelings of high standards and quality.

WAGENKNECHT ARCHITEKTEN

OMF SURGERY LINDENARCADEN
LÜBECK | G

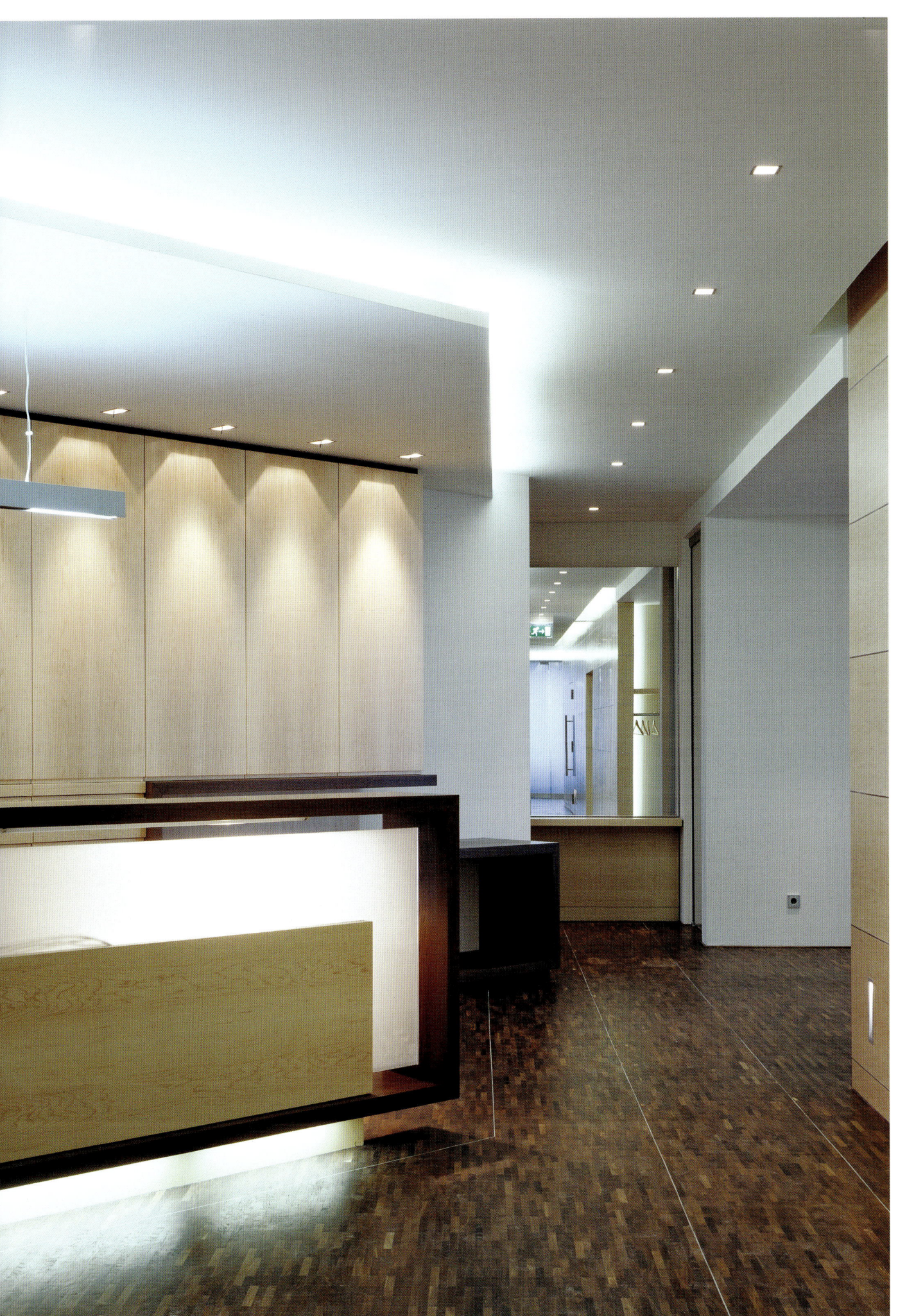

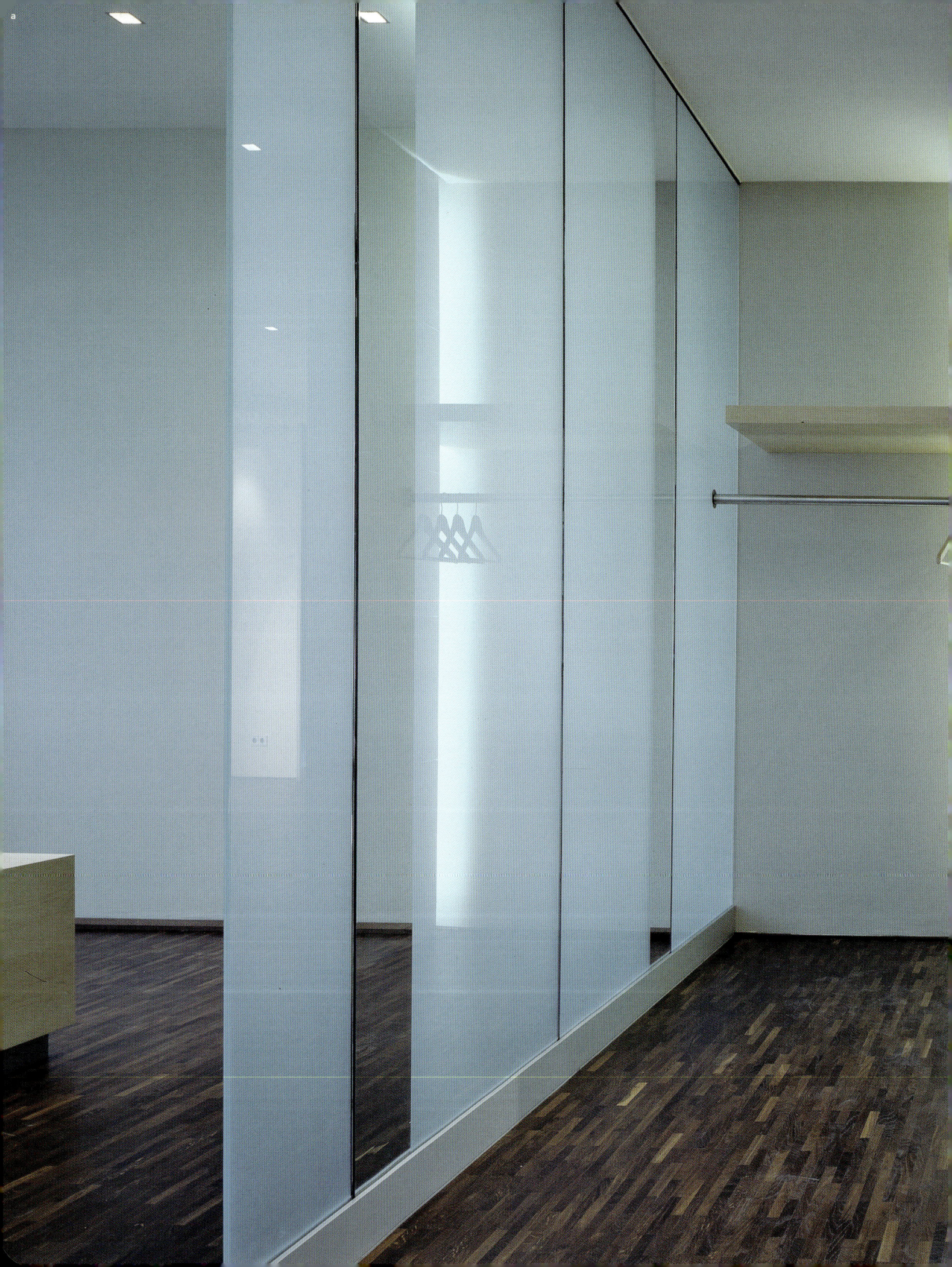

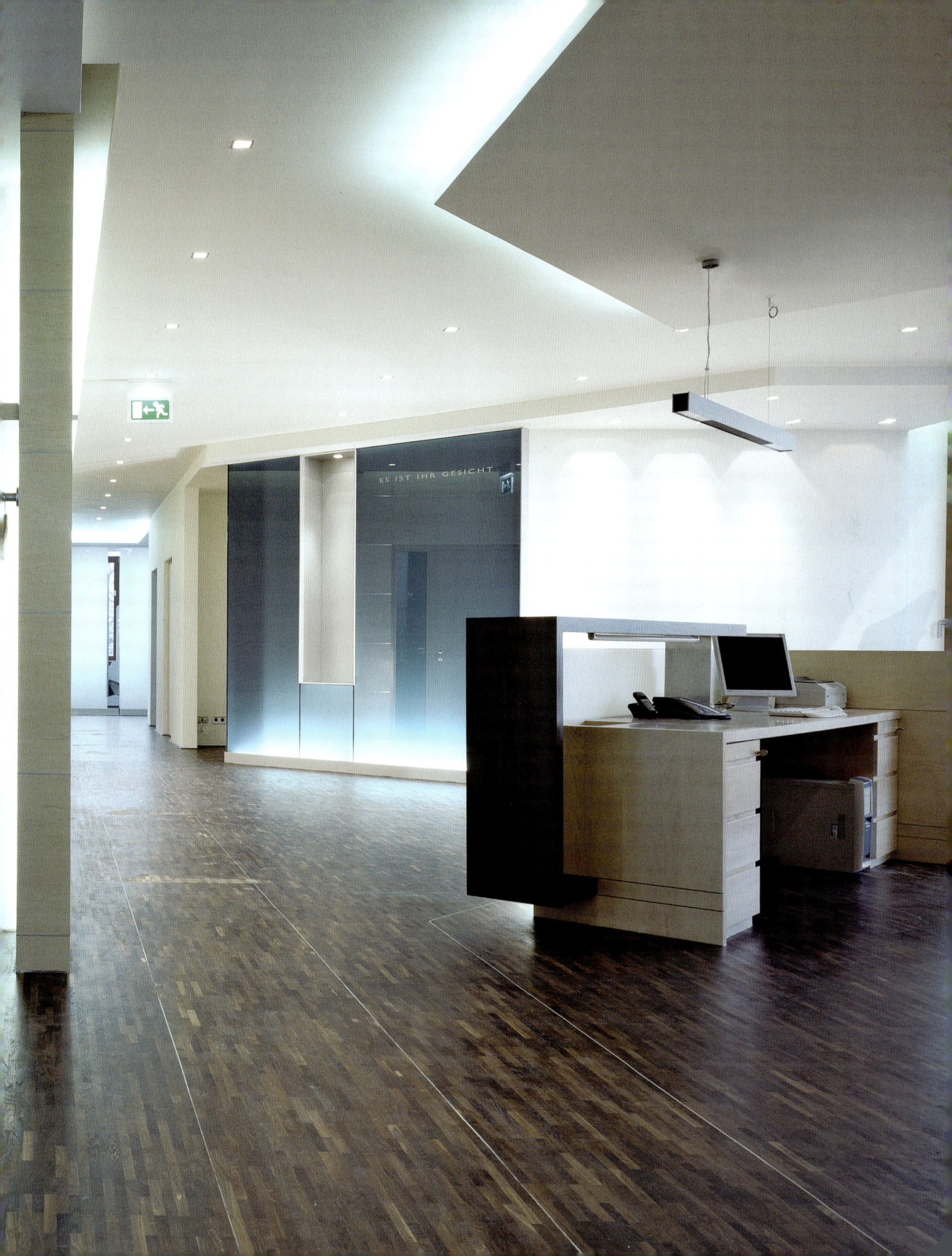

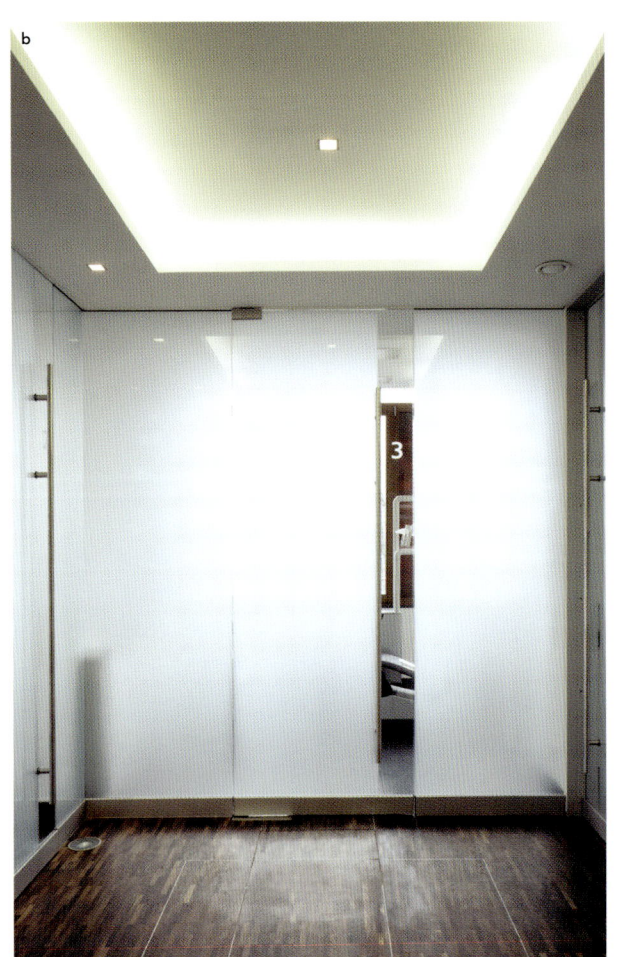

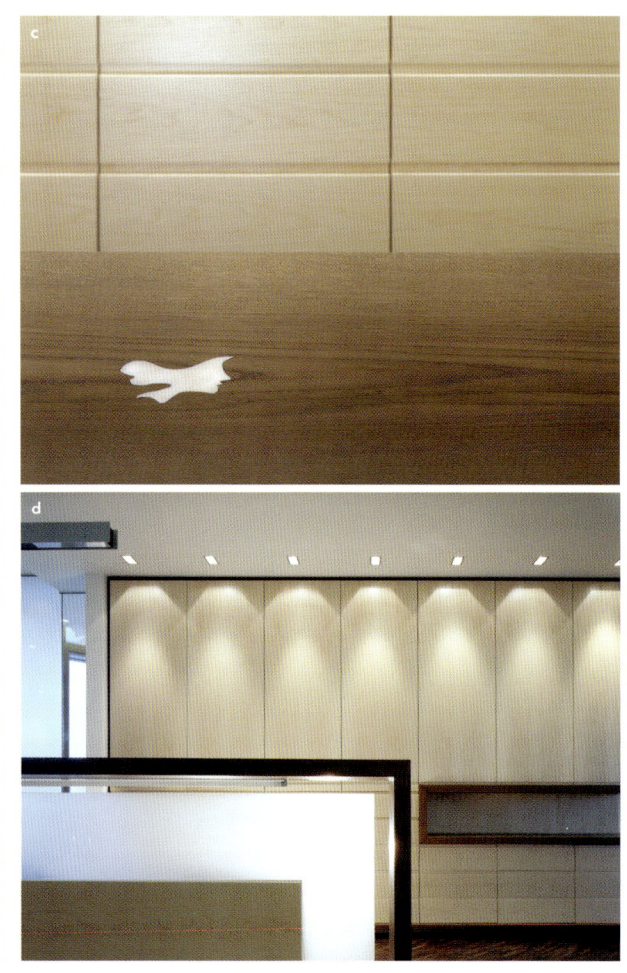

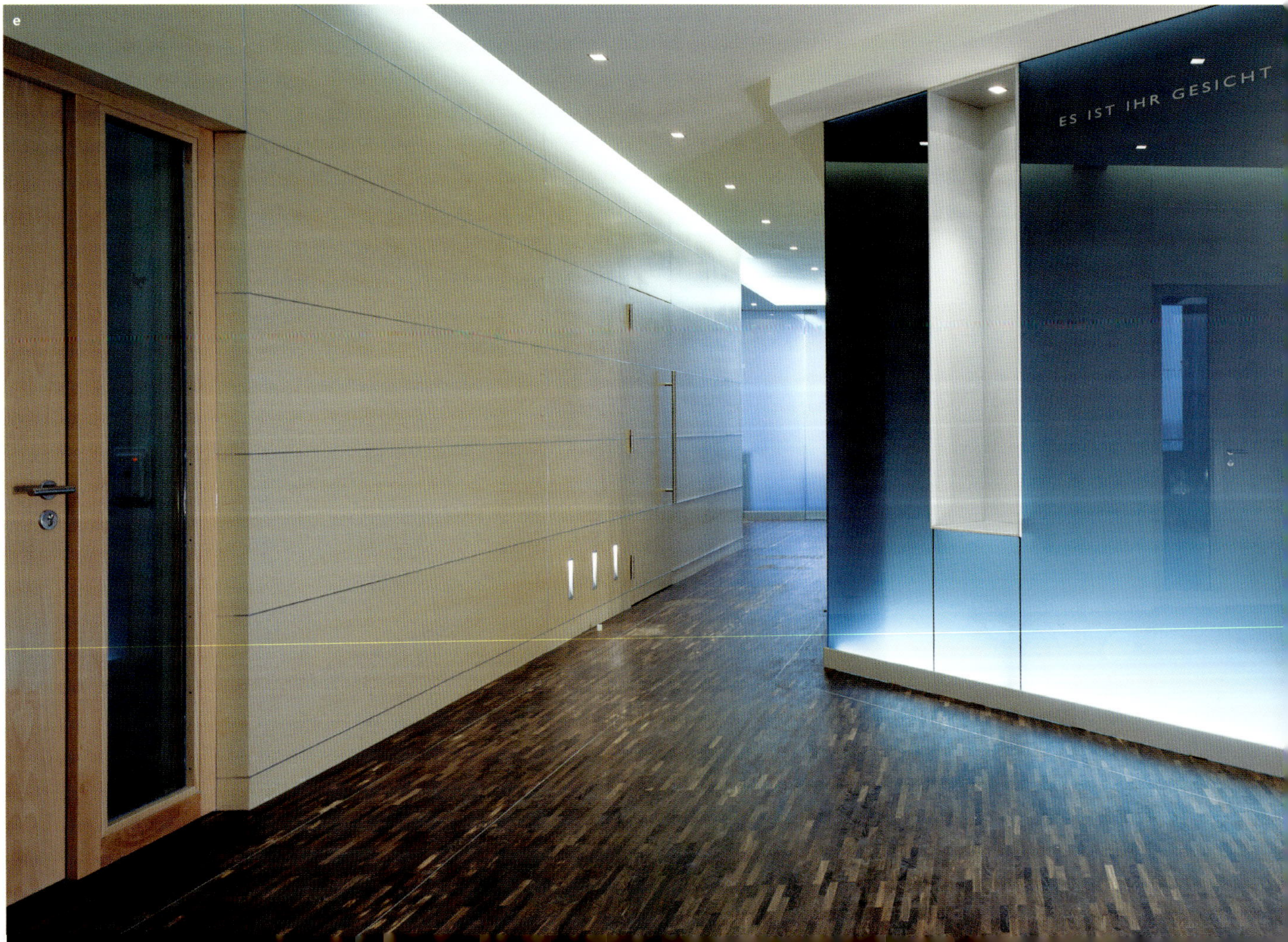

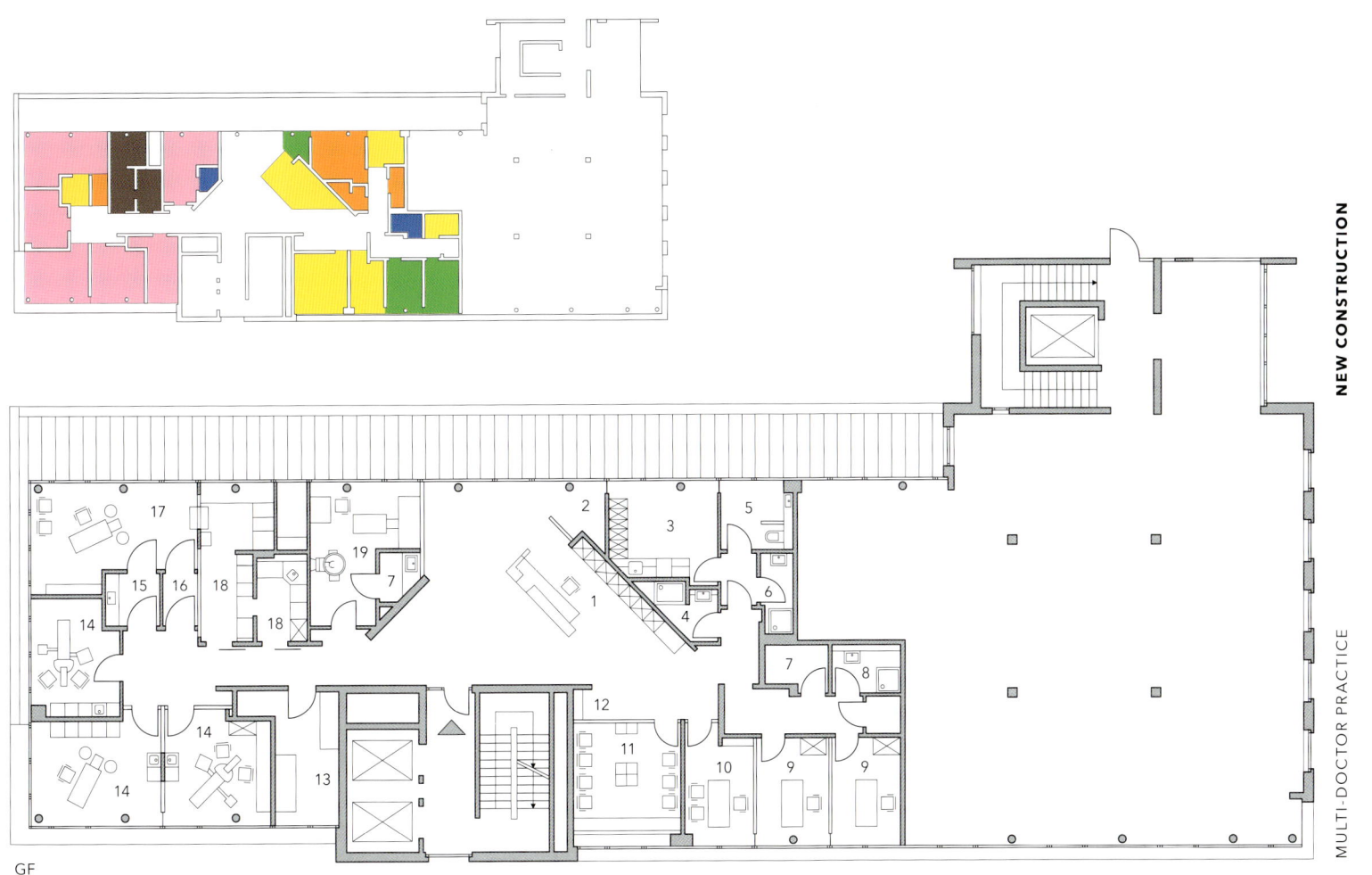

GF

Client	Dr. Dr. Hans-Peter Ulrich	
Operator	Dr. Dr. Hans-Peter Ulrich	
	Dr. Wilma Poeschel	
	Dr. Dr. Stephan Otten	
Planning time	2003	
Construction time	2004	
Gross floor area	378 sqm	
Usable floor space	179 sqm	
Gross cubic capacity	1,137 cbm	
Construction cost	350,000 EUR	
Total cost	490,000 EUR	

a Ceiling-high glass elements, only partly frosted, make the transitions appear as if they are float-ing and enable light to penetrate deep into the rooms.

b Illuminated ceiling panels and selectively-placed built-in lights accentuate individual areas in this practice.

c The practice logo is conspicuously emblazoned on the reception desk.

d Reception desk and blue glass wall opposite are arranged diagonally to one another to form an inviting trapezoid.

e The guide wall clad with maple and horizontally-extending aluminium profiles connects the reception desk to the treatment wing.

Diagrammatic plans, to scale 1:400
Floor plans, to scale 1:200

Floor plan layout

1	Reception	**8**	Patient shower	**15**	Patient sluice
2	Office	**9**	Office	**16**	Staff sluice
3	Staff lounge	**10**	Consultation room	**17**	Operating theatre
4	Staff shower L	**11**	Waiting area	**18**	Sterilisation
5	Toilet for the disabled	**12**	Coat-rack	**19**	Examination X-ray
6	Staff shower G	**13**	Recovery room		
7	Installations room EDV	**14**	Treatment room		

From the centre of this long rectangular floor plan, patients of the multiple practice access the reception and the visible waiting area situated to the right of the entrance. From there they have to find the examination and treatment rooms to the left of the entrance and the operating unit via a narrow central corridor. It is encouraging that all the important rooms receive natural light.

Usable floor spaces

Patient rooms	**yellow**	43 sqm	24 %
Specialist rooms	**pink**	76 sqm	42 %
Administrative rooms	**green**	19 sqm	11 %
Offices	Staff rooms	**orange**	19 sqm	11 %
Supply	Waste disposal	**brown**	17 sqm	9 %
Plant rooms	**blue**	5 sqm	3 %
Total		179 sqm	100 %

Performance data

Outpatients per year	4,000
Clinic opening hours	7 days	70 hours
Waiting time	according to urgency
Type and number of staff	3 doctors
	7 clerical staff

The rooms in this dental practice situated in a free-standing mansion dating from the turn of the 19th century in Berlin, were formerly used as an office. On entering, visitors find themselves in a bright, open-plan reception area. An attempt has been made to counteract the discomfort that a lot of patients feel when visiting a dentist, by using specific creative interventions. The central, unusually high reception desk made of walnut faces three large lattice windows, from whence the visitor's gaze is diverted through two open door apertures to the inviting red sofa in the waiting area. The brightness of this light-flooded, friendly room has a calming effect which is complemented by an open invitation to relax in the long seating area. Specifically-calming design features have been selected in the treatment rooms too, where large-scale nature photographs are a welcome antidote to the requisite medical devices. Despite the segmentation of the rooms – the former living area floor plan is still in evidence – an attractive sense of space has been generated with the help of visual effects and the omission of a few doors.

WALK |
ARCHITEKTEN

DENTAL PRACTICE
BERLIN | G

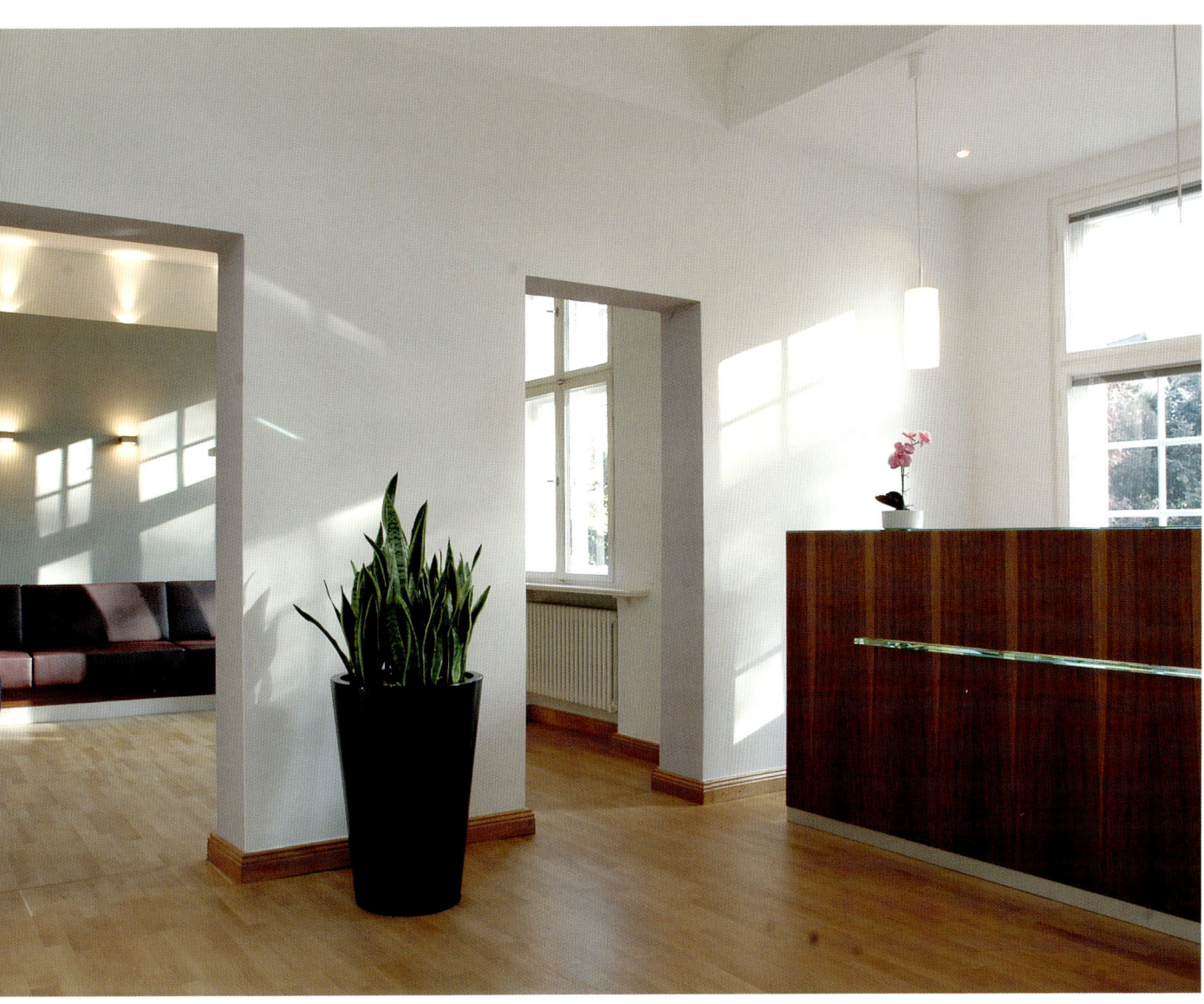

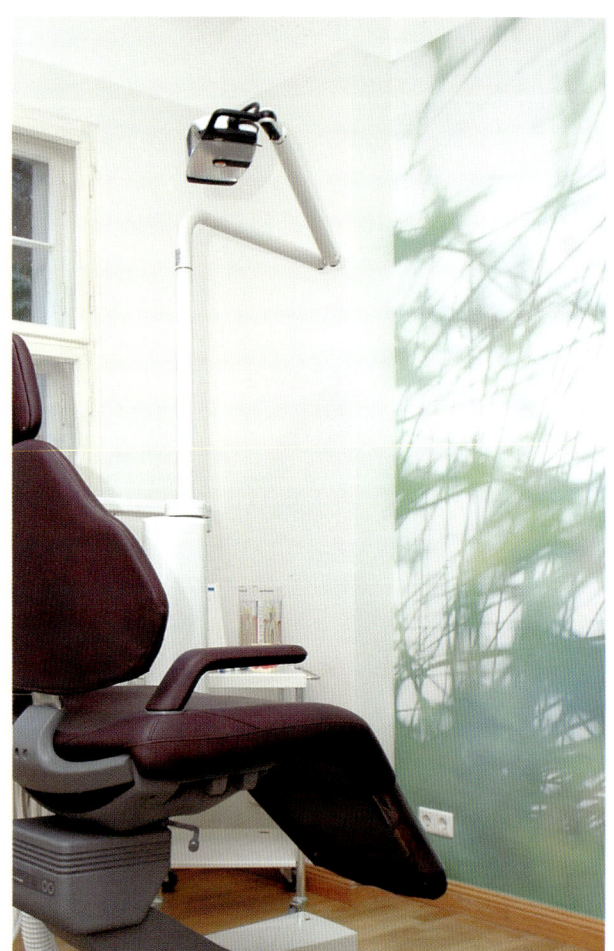

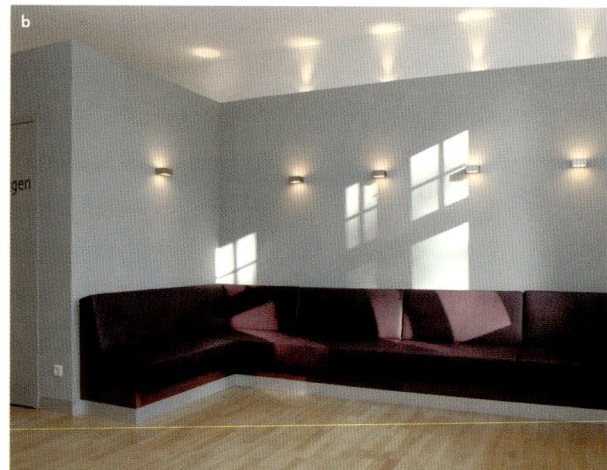

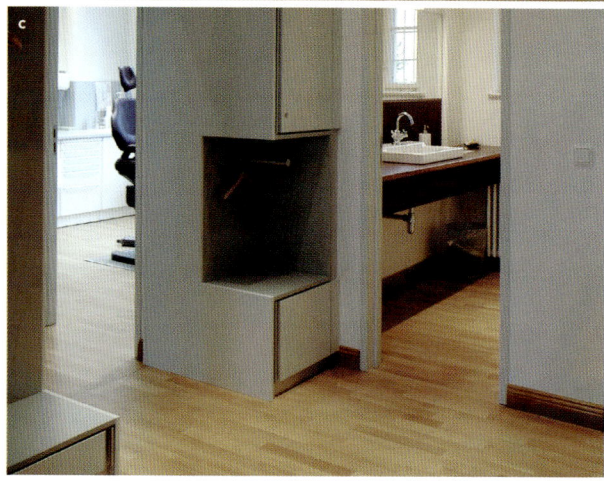

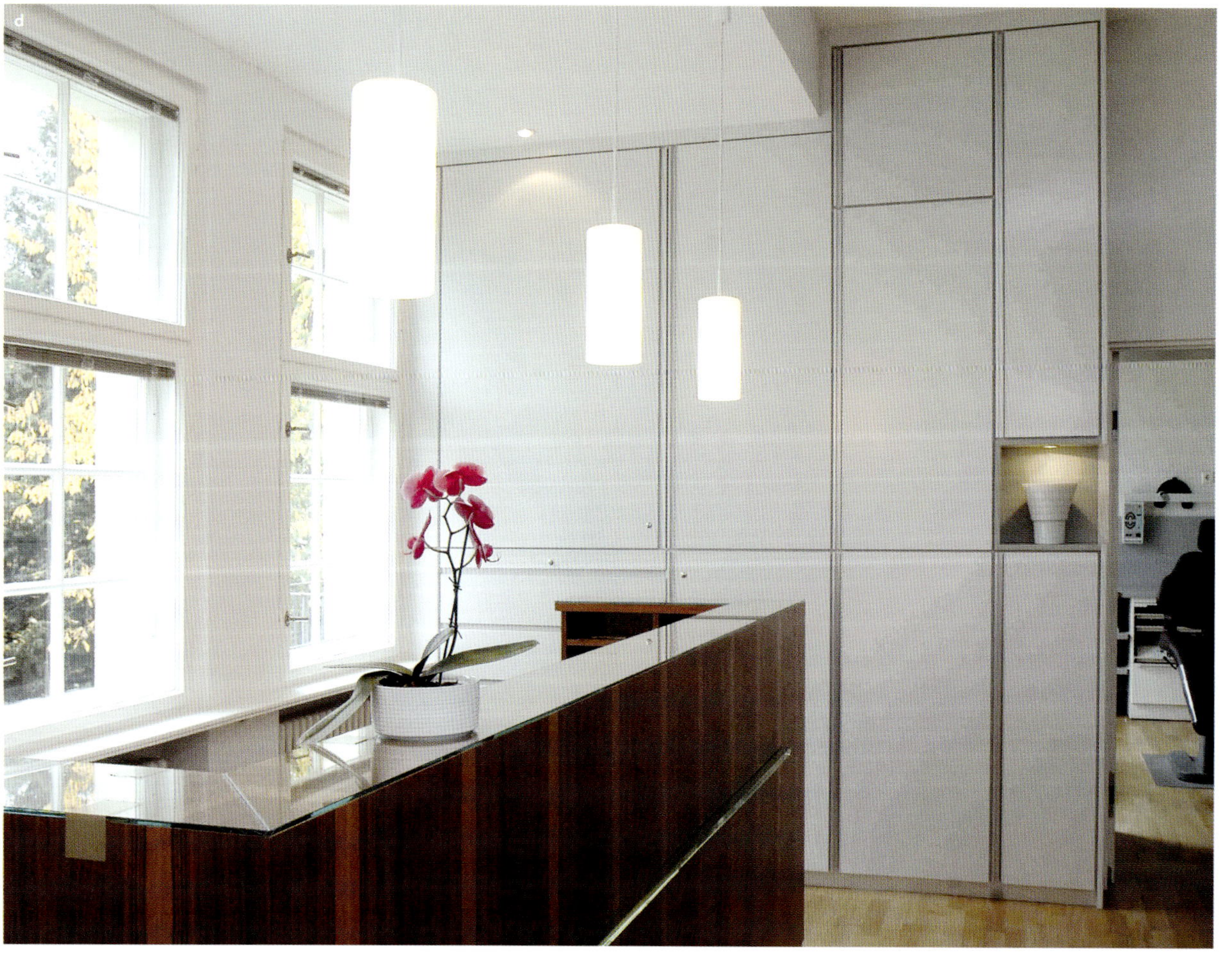

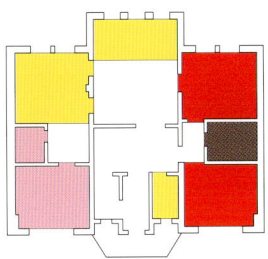

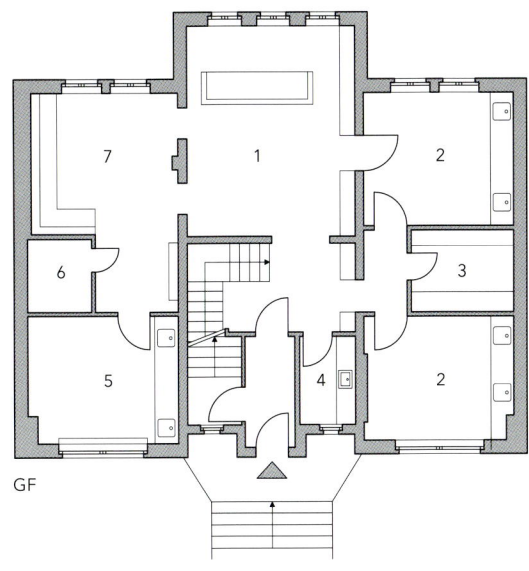

GF

Client | Operator   Dr. Kristina Hirsch
                        Dr. Helge Kohn
Planning time   02 2004 – 04 2004
Construction time   04 2004 – 07 2004
Gross floor area   206 sqm [GF + BSMT]
Usable floor space 91 sqm [GF]
Gross cubic capacity 618 cbm [GF + BSMT]
Construction cost   54,700 EUR
Total cost   84,000 EUR

a Large-scale nature photographs are a welcome antidote to the requisite medical devices in the treatment rooms.
b The long red sofa in the light-flooded waiting area has a positively inviting effect.
c Here the young patients have not been forgotten and have their own coat-rack integrated into the fittings in the corridor.
d Despite the segmentation of the rooms an attractive sense of space has been generated with the help of visual effects and the omission of a few doors.

Diagrammatic plans, to scale 1:400
Floor plans, to scale 1:200

Floor plan layout

1	Reception	**4**	Oral hygiene room	**6**	Examination X-ray
2	Treatment room	**5**	Treatment room	**7**	Waiting area
3	Sterilisation room		prevention		

From the entrance, situated in the centre of one of the long sides of the large town house, patients access the reception and waiting area of this partnership practice via a few steps. The examination and treatment stations can be reached from both rooms. A central staircase leads to the other rooms in the basement.

Usable floor spaces

Patient rooms	**yellow**	33 sqm	36 %
Examination |			
Treatment rooms	**red**	32 sqm	35 %
Specialist rooms	**pink**	19 sqm	21 %
Supply | Waste disposal	**brown**	7 sqm	8 %
Total		91 sqm	100 %

Performance data

Services to other clinics	Orthodontics
	Oral surgery
Number of staff	6 – 7

PROJECTS

ORTHOPAEDICS AT ROSENBERG, ST. GALLEN | CH
Architect: bhend.klammer
dipl. architekten eth siz, Christof Bhend,
Sergej Klammer, Zurich | CH
Collaboration: Roger Gerber
Construction management:
Huldi Schreiber, Novaron AG
Location of the building object: Silberturm,
Rorschacher Straße 150, 9000 St. Gallen | CH
Photos: Lucas Peters, Zurich | CH
Furniture: Swissfiber AG, Zurich | CH
Lighting: Zwicker Licht, St. Gallen | CH
Flooring: Swissfiber AG, Zurich | CH

PROPHYLAXIS CLINIC, COLOGNE | G
Architect: b-k-i brandherm + krumrey
innenarchitektur, Hamburg | Cologne | G
Location of the building object:
Kölner Straße 48, 51149 Cologne | G
Photos: Joachim Grothus, Bielefeld | G
Medical engineering:
Anton Gerl GmbH, Cologne | G
Lighting: Kreon, Opglabbeek | B

CENTRE FOR RADIO-ONCOLOGY, COLOGNE | G
Architect: b-k-i brandherm + krumrey
innenarchitektur, Hamburg | Cologne | G
Location of the building object:
Hohenstaufenring 28, 50674 Cologne | G
Photos: Uwe Spoering, Cologne | G

DENTAL CLINIC MARKTOBERDORF | G
Architect: Klaus R. Bürger,
Bürger Innenarchitektur, Krefeld | G
Location of the building object:
Marktplatz 8, 87616 Marktoberdorf | G
Graphic artist | artist: sicht-werk,
Dipl. Des. Carmen Schumacher, Krefeld | G
Photos: Uwe Spoering, Cologne | G
Lighting: Ansorg GmbH Lichttechnik,
Mühlheim | Ruhr | G

CARDIOVASCULAR CLINIC, ZURICH | CH
Architect: conex_ARCHITEKTEN, Bern | CH,
Thomas Fuhrer, Silvia Jenni; ueberwasser
architektur & projektmanagement,
Bern | CH, Lucius Ueberwasser
Location of the building object:
Seestraße 247, 8038 Zurich | CH
Photos: conex_ARCHITEKTEN, Bern | CH;
ueberwasser architektur &
projektmanagement, Bern | CH
Heating | airing: Meierhans + Partner,
Schwerzenbach | CH
Sanitary installations: Walter Müller
Partner AG, Zurich | CH
Furniture: zingg-lamprecht, Zurich | CH
Lighting: Zumtobel Licht GmbH,
Lemgo | CH
Sanitary: Keuco GmbH, Hemer; arwa AG,
Wallisellen | CH; Schär + Trojahn AG,
Niederwangen | CH

ENT AND PSYCHOTHERAPY CLINIC, DÜSSELDORF | G
Architect: Uta Cossmann,
Claudia de Bruyn, Düsseldorf | G
Location of the building object:
Dreherstraße 3 – 5, 40625 Düsseldorf | G
Photos: Nicole Zimmermann,
Düsseldorf | G; Uwe Spoering, Cologne | G

GASTROENTEROLOGY, REMSCHEID | G
Architect: Regina Dahmen-Ingenhoven,
Düsseldorf | G, Alexandra Zupanc
Realisation: Hennrich und Partner GbR
Architekten und Ingenieure, Remscheid | G
Location of the building object:
Rosenhügelerstraße 2, 42859
Remscheid | G
Graphic artist | artist:
Beate Steil, Düsseldorf | G
Photos: Holger Knauf, Düsseldorf | G
Interior: Koitka Innenausbau GmbH,
Düsseldorf | G

"LOUNGE DENTAL" DENTAL PRACTICE, DÜSSELDORF | G
Architect: Regina Dahmen-Ingenhoven,
Düsseldorf | G, Christiane Luiz
Location of the building object:
Königsallee 20, 40212 Düsseldorf | G
Photos: Holger Knauf, Düsseldorf | G
Interior:
Koitka Innenausbau GmbH, Düsseldorf | G

DENTAL PRACTICE, ANSBACH | G
Architect:
Etschmann Noack GmbH, Fürth | G,
Christine Etschmann, Johannes Noack
Realisation: Lammers GmbH, Ahaus | G
Location of the building object:
Draisstraße 2, 91522 Ansbach | G
Graphic artist | artist:
Peter Scheer, Munich | G
Photos: Johannes Noack, Fürth | G
Heating | airing:
Ingenieurbüro Terbrack, Ahaus | G
Furniture: Henry Schein Dental Depot
GmbH, Langen | G
Medical engineering:
Henry Schein Dental Depot GmbH,
Nürnberg | G
Sanitary:
Ceramica Catalano SRL, Rom | I

DENTAL PRACTICE, BREMEN | G
Architect:
GfG | Gruppe für Gestaltung, Bremen | G
Location of the building object:
Parkallee 301, 28213 Bremen | G
Graphic artist | artist: GfG | Gruppe für
Gestaltung, Bremen | G
Photos: Tom Kleiner, GfG, Bremen | G
Furniture: Vitra AG, Birsfelden | CH
Medical engineering:
Pluradent AG & Co. KG, Offenbach | G
Lighting: Artemide GmbH,
Fröndenberg | G; Modular Lighting
Instruments, Roeselare | B
Flooring: Forbo Flooring GmbH,
Paderborn | G

CLINIC AT OPERNPLATZ, HANOVER | G
Architect: gnosa architekten, Hamburg | G,
Lutz Gnosa, Mark Braunholz
Location of the building object:
Georgstraße 34, 30159 Hanover | G
Graphic artist | artist:
mylk* mediatektur GmbH, Hamburg | G
Photos: Klaus Frahm, Börnsen | G
Furniture: punct.object, Hamburg | G
Planning medical engineering:
Henry Schein Dental Depot GmbH,
Hanover | G
Facilities medical engineering:
Planmeca GmbH, Hamburg | G;
MEDIADENT Stahlmöbelwerk GmbH
Lighting: iGuzzini illuminazione
Deutschland GmbH, Planegg | G

CHILDREN'S DENTAL PRACTICE, BERLIN | G
Architect: GRAFT, Berlin | G
Location of the building object:
Kollwitzstraße 64, 10435 Berlin | G
Graphic artist | artist:
STRAUSS & HILLEGAART, Cottbus | G
Photos: Andi Albert, Würzburg | G
Airing: Climtech GmbH, Berlin | G
Sanitary installations:
Fa. Jürgen Urbach GmbH, Berlin | G
Statics: Ingenieurbüro Dr. Krämer GmbH,
Berlin | G
Furniture: Möbeltischlerei
Joachim Schmohl, Senzig | G
Lighting: GKW Lichtplanung, Berlin | G

"KU64" DENTAL PRACTICE, BERLIN | G
Architect: GRAFT, Berlin | G,
Lars Krückeberg, Wolfram Putz,
Thomas Willemeit
Project architect: Tobias Hein,
Karsten Sell
Location of the building object:
Kurfürstendamm 64, 10707 Berlin | G
Graphic artist | artist:
STRAUSS & HILLEGAART, Cottbus | G
Photos: hiepler, brunier, Berlin | G
Medical engineering:
Demedis Dental-Depot GmbH

DENTAL PRACTICE, GILCHING | G
Architect: günther & schabert, Munich | G,
Martina Günther, Jan Schabert
Location of the building object:
Römerstraße 43 A, 82205 Gilching | G
Photos: Monika Ribbe
Photodesign, Bad Aibling | G
Heating | airing | sanitary installations:
Karl Huber, Gilching | G
Furniture: günther & schabert, Munich | G;
Schreinerei Schaber, Haimhausen | G;
designfunktion GmbH, Munich | G
Medical engineering:
Schwavo Dentaltechnik, Rastede | G
Flooring: Freudenberg Noraplan

"EYE DO" EYE CLINIC, ROTTERDAM | NL
Architect: hell und freundlich, Cologne | G
Location of the building object: 's Graven-
weg 310,
3062 Rotterdam | NL
Photos: Ludger Einhoff

PRACTICE FOR ORAL AND MAXILLOFACIAL SURGERY, OBERHAUSEN | G
Architect: hell und freundlich, Cologne | G
Location of the building object: Friedrich-
List-Straße 18, 46045 Oberhausen | G
Photos: Ludger Einhoff
Flooring: Pandomo

EYE CENTRE, COLOGNE | G
Architect: hell und freundlich, Cologne | G
Location of the building object:
Wolfstraße 16, 50667 Cologne | G
Graphic artist | artist:
Bernd Fischer, Cologne | G
Photos: Ludger Einhoff

SPINAL COLUMN CENTRE, HANOVER | G
Architect: roland holz design,
Braunschweig | G
Location of the building object:
Arthur-Menge-Ufer 5, 30169 Hanover | G
Photos:
Andreas Borrmann, Braunschweig | G;
Roland Holz, Braunschweig | G
Heating | airing | sanitary installations:
Weymann GmbH, Lehrte | G
Furniture: Schawaller + Ulrich GmbH
Möbelwerkstätten, Braunschweig | G
Medical engineering: Siemens
Lighting: Fahlke & Dettmer.
Licht in der Architektur, Neustadt | G
Lighting: Regent Beleuchtungskörper AG,
Basel | CH
Sanitary: Keramag AG, Ratingen | G

WOMEN'S HEALTH CARE PRACTICE, BRAUNSCHWEIG | G
Architect: roland holz design,
Braunschweig | G in cooperation with
plan II Architekten, Braunschweig | G
Location of the building object:
Küchenstraße 10, 38100 Braunschweig | G
Photos:
Andreas Borrmann, Braunschweig | G;
Roland Holz, Braunschweig | G
Furniture: Pauli Tischlermeister GmbH,
Braunschweig | G; Claasen Einrichtungen
Medical engineering: GE – Health care
Lighting: Fahlke & Dettmer.
Licht in der Architektur, Neustadt
Lighting: RIDI Leuchten GmbH
Sanitary: Keramag AG, Ratingen | G;
Keuco GmbH, Hemer | G
Flooring: EGE Tapper, Noraplan

MKG-SURGERY AIRPORT CLINIC, FREISING | G
Architect: holzrausch GmbH, Forstern | G,
Sven Petzold, Tobias Petri, Gewerbering 14,
85659 Forstern | G, www.holzrausch.de
P: +49. 8124. 528282
F: +49. 8124. 528283
Location of the building object:
Clemensänger-Ring 9, 85356 Freising | G
Photos: K+W, Berlin | G
Drywall installation: Wendl GmbH
Furniture: holzrausch GmbH
Medical engineering:
Henry Schein Dental Depot GmbH,
Hanover | G
Lighting: holzrausch GmbH
Sanitary: Döhler, Freising | G
Flooring: Zementwerkstatt Weber

ZURICH WEST SCHOOL DENTAL CLINIC, ZURICH | CH
Architect: Hönig Architekten,
Patrick Hönig, Winterthur | CH,
Collaboration:
Tobias Deseyve, Marcel Schmid
Location of the building object:
Altstetterstraße 162, 8048 Zurich | CH
Photos: Walter Mair, Zurich | CH
Heating | airing | sanitary installations:
Reust, Marty & Beuchat AG, Zurich | CH,
HLKS-Ingenieure, Zurich | CH
Statics: Heyer, Kaufmann Partner,
Bauingenieure AG, Zurich | CH
Electrical engineering: Elara AG, Zurich | CH
Planning medical engineering: Peter Maag,
Dentalplanung, Bassersdorf | CH
Facilities medical engineering:
Kaladent, Urdorf | CH
Lighting: Zumtobel Licht GmbH, Zurich | CH

ZURICH CITY SCHOOL DENTAL CLINIC, ZURICH | CH
Architect: Hönig Architekten,
Patrick Hönig, Winterthur | CH,
Collaboration: Beat Stadelmann
Location of the building object:
Ulmbergstraße 1, 8002 Zurich | CH
Photos: Walter Mair, Zurich | CH
Heating | airing | sanitary installations:
Reust, Marty & Beuchat AG, Zurich | CH,
HLKS-Ingenieure, Zurich | CH
Statics:
Wolf, Kropf & Partner AG, Zurich | CH
Electrical engineering: Elara AG, Zurich | CH
Planning medical engineering: Peter Maag,
Dentalplanung, Bassersdorf | CH
Facilities medical engineering:
Kaladent AG, Urdorf | CH
Lighting: Zumtobel Licht GmbH, Zurich | CH

PRACTICE FOR ORAL AND MAXILLOFACIAL SURGERY, ST. GALLEN | CH
Architect: Hönig Architekten,
Patrick Hönig, Winterthur | CH
Location of the building object:
St. Leonhardstraße 78, 9000 St. Gallen | CH
Photos: Walter Mair, Zurich | CH
Planning medical engineering: Peter Maag,
Dentalplanung, Bassersdorf | CH
Facilities medical engineering:
Pluradent AG & Co. KG, Offenbach | G
Lighting: Zumtobel Licht GmbH, Lemgo | G

PRIVATE DENTAL PRACTICE, WUPPERTAL | G
Architect: INSTANTCONCEPT GMBH,
Wuppertal | G; Jörg Berghäuser,
Innenarchitekt [AdbK]
Location of the building object:
Falkenberg 57 a, 42113 Wuppertal | G
Photos: Gunnar Bäldle, Wuppertal | G
Furniture: Berghäuser und Sohn,
Wuppertal | G
Dentaltechnik: Kobert – Dental, Solingen
Lighting: Horstkamp, Wuppertal | G
Sanitary: Kuhl GmbH, Wuppertal | G

OTTO-SUHR-ALLEE DENTISTS, BERLIN | G
Architect: institut_feiner_dinge, Berlin | G,
Christian Thommes, Ralf Weißheimer
Location of the building object:
Otto-Suhr-Allee 90 | 92, 10585 Berlin | G
Graphic | logo:
institut_feiner_dinge, Berlin | G
Photos: photoartberlin.de, Jan Kulke
Furniture: Sedus, Waldshut-Tiengen | G;
Boecker GmbH Büro- und Objekt-
gestaltung, Berlin | G
Lighting: Belux AG, Birsfelden | CH;
Iris Hamelberg Porzellan, Berlin | G
Sanitary: Duravit AG, Hornberg | G; Keuco
GmbH, Hemer | G

DENTISTS IN KRONPRINZENKARREE, BERLIN | G
Architect: institut_feiner_dinge, Berlin | G,
Diana Hermann, Christian Thommes,
Ralf Weißheimer
Location of the building object:
Reinhardtstraße 50, 10117 Berlin | G
Graphic | logo: institut_feiner_dinge,
Berlin | G
Photos: Drama, Holger Foullois, Berlin | G
Furniture: Sedus, Waldshut-Tiengen | G;
Arper; MEDIADENT Stahlmöbelwerk GmbH
Lighting: Filumen. Interior Lighting,
Potsdam | G
Sanitary: Alape GmbH, Goslar | G;
Keuco GmbH, Hemer | G
Flooring: Forbo Flooring GmbH,
Paderborn | G

PRACTICE FOR NATUROPATHY AND GENERAL MEDICINE, COLOGNE | G
Architect: 100% interior, Sylvia Leydecker,
Cologne | G
Location of the building object:
Kaiser-Wilhelm-Ring 14 – 16,
50672 Cologne | G
Graphic artist | artist:
plankundplankdesign
Photos: Karin Hessmann, Dortmund | G
Furniture: Vitra AG, Birsfelden | CH; Bulo,
Mechelen | B; Signet Wohnmöbel,
Hochstadt | G
Lighting: Doctor Design Ltd., Helsinki | FIN;
Ansorg GmbH, Mülheim | Ruhr;
Belux AG, Birsfelden | CH

RADIOLOGY, SCHORNDORF | G
Architect: ippolito fleitz group,
Stuttgart | G, Peter Ippolito, Gunter Fleitz,
Collaboration: Hadi A.Tandawardaj,
Christian Kirschenmann, Monika Skrzypek
Location of the building object:
Schlichtener Straße 105,
73614 Schorndorf | G
Graphic | guidance system: Axel Knapp,
Stuttgart | G; Frank Faßmer, Stuttgart | G
Photos: Zooey Braun, Stuttgart | G
Furniture: Glock Holzinnenausbau, Murr | G
Lighting: Light Tech GmbH, Graz | A;
Viabizzuno SRL, Bologna | I; Systema 94
Flooring: Forbo Flooring GmbH,
Paderborn | G

KAISERPLATZ PRACTICE CLINIC, FRANKFURT ON THE MAIN | G

Architect: ippolito fleitz group, Stuttgart | G, Peter Ippolito, Gunter Fleitz,
Collaboration: Patrick Schmidt, Axel Knapp
Ground layout: g.u.t. Architekten, Gerhards und Thomé, Aachen | G
Location of the building object: Kaiserstraße 14, 60311 Frankfurt on the Main | G
Photos: Zooey Braun, Stuttgart | G
Furniture: Glock Holzinnenausbau GmbH, Murr | G
Lighting: Modular; Se'lux, Berlin | G
Sanitary: Duravit AG, Hornberg | G; Hansgrohe AG, Schiltach | G
Flooring: Kirchheimer Muschelkalk, DLW Linoleum

DENTAL CLINIC, ESCHENBACH | G

Architect: JURETZKA ARCHITEKTEN, Weiden | G, Armin Juretzka, Mirko Bertl, Melanie Danhof
Location of the building object: Friedhofweg 5, 92676 Eschenbach | G
Photos: Sommer Spahn GmbH, Amberg | G
Furniture: Vitra AG, Birsfelden | CH
Lighting: Modular Lighting Instruments, Wiesbaden | G
Sanitary: Duravit AG, Hornberg | G; Villeroy & Boch, Mettlach | G; Bisazza Mosaico | I
Flooring: Armstrong DLW, Bietigheim-Bissingen | G

ORTHOPAEDICS CENTRE, GRAZ | A

Architect: Andreas Kanzian, Graz | A
Location of the building object: Merangasse 12, 8010 Graz | A
Photos: Walter Luttenberger, Gratkorn | A
Heating | airing | sanitary installations: Neubauer GmbH, Eggersdorf | A
Medical engineering: Leupamed GmbH, Hausmannsstätten | A; Sensarama GmbH, Graz | A
Joineries: Tischlerei Spindler; Tischlerei Franz Hiebler KEG, Graz | A
Lighting: XAL Xenon Architectural Lighting GmbH, Graz | A

PRACTICE FOR GENERAL MEDICINE, PREDING | A

Architect: Andreas Kanzian, Graz | A
Location of the building object: Tobis 100, 8504 Preding | A
Photos: Walter Luttenberger, Gratkorn | A
Heating | airing | sanitary installations: Technisches Büro Bernhard Hammer GmbH, Graz | A
Furniture: Tischlerei Enderle, Graz | A; INSIDE Einrichtungen Gartner & Eisenberger, Graz | A; Kartell, Noviglio | I
Lighting: XAL, Graz | A
Flooring: Freudenberg Bausysteme KG

PRACTICE FOR INTERNAL MEDICINE, GRAZ | A

Architect: Andreas Kanzian, Graz | A
Location of the building object: Griesgasse 12, 8020 Graz | A
Photos: Walter Luttenberger, Gratkorn | A
Furniture: Tischlerei Enderle, Graz | A
Medical engineering: K. H. Dewert GmbH, Bielefeld | G
Lighting: ProdomoVienna, Vienna | A; XAL, Graz | A

"EDELWEISS" DENTAL PRACTICE, BERLIN | G

Design: klm architekten, Koeppen, Leder, Märker, Berlin | Leipzig | G
Realisation | planning | medical engineering: Henry Schein Dental Depot GmbH
Location of the building object: Joachimstaler Straße 34, 10719 Berlin | G
Graphic artist | artist: minigram – Studio für Markendesign; Heymann & Schnell
Photos: Olaf Koeppen, Leipzig | Berlin | G; Dirk Schaper, Berlin | G
Heating | airing | sanitary installations: Baukontor 2000
Furniture: Geilert & Kurth GmbH
Facilities medical engineering: Henry Schein Dental Depot GmbH, Langen | G
Lighting: Semperlux AG, Berlin | G; GKW-Lichtsysteme GmbH, Berlin | G
Flooring: Atala GmbH & Co., Berlin | G; JAB-Anstoetz KG, Bielefeld | G

"SANITAS" THERAPY CENTRE, WILDESHAUSEN | G

Architect: Ralf Krause, Innenarchitekt, Lübeck | G, Marc Brune, Architekt, Bremen | G
Location of the building object: Am Mühlendamm 3, 27793 Wildeshausen | G
Photos: greenbox, Bremen | G
Lighting: Hoffmeister Leuchten GmbH, Schalksmühle | G; Erco Leuchten GmbH, Lüdenscheid | G; Zumtobel Licht GmbH, Lemgo | G
Sanitary: Duravit AG, Hornberg | G; Hansgrohe AG, Schiltach | G; Alape GmbH, Goslar | G

ORTHODONTIC CLINIC, MINDELHEIM | G

Architect: landau + kindelbacher, Munich | G, Gerhard Landau, Ludwig Kindelbacher
Location of the building object: Maximilianstraße 71, 87719 Mindelheim | G
Photos: Christian Hacker, Munich | G

DENTAL PRACTICE, ALTENBURG | G

Architect: landau + kindelbacher, Munich | G, Gerhard Landau, Ludwig Kindelbacher,
Collaboration: Tina Allmeier
Location of the building object: Zeitzer Straße 21, 04600 Altenburg | G
Photos: Michael Heinrich, Munich | G

DENTAL CLINIC, SINDELFINGEN | G

Architect: Annette Lippmann, Stuttgart | G,
Engineer: JP Projektplanung, Jürgen Pfau, Ehningen | G
Location of the building object: Tilsiter Straße 8, 71065 Sindelfingen | G
Graphic: Annette Lippmann, Stuttgart | G
Photos: KD Busch, Fellbach | G; Annette Lippmann, Stuttgart | G
Interior: Schreinerei Nissler + Eder, Sindelfingen | G
Medical engineering: Wagner Dental, Stuttgart | G
Decorative lighting: Prandina | I; Regent Beleuchtungskörper AG, Basel | CH; Brumberg Leuchten GmbH, Sundern-Hellefeld | G
Technical lighting: Ridi Leuchten GmbH, Jungingen | G; RZB GmbH, Bamberg | G; Osram GmbH, Munich | G
Sanitary: Catalano, Rom | I; Keramag AG, Ratingen | G
Flooring: Ceramica Casalgrande Padana

CHILDREN'S EYE CENTRE, VIENNA | A

Architect: LOOPING ARCHITECTURE, Vienna | A, Eva Becker, Klaus Schober, Christa Stürzlinger, Ludwig Starz
Location of the building object: Albertgasse 41, 1080 Vienna | A
Photos: LOOPING ARCHITECTURE, Vienna | A
Furniture: Kohlmaier, Vienna | A

PRACTICE CLINIC AT THE OLD OPERA, FRANKFURT ON THE MAIN | G

Architect: eva lorey, Frankfurt on the Main | G,
Location of the building object: Kettenhofweg 1, 60325 Frankfurt on the Main | G
Photos: Sandra Hauer, Wiesbaden | G, www.nahdran.com
Furniture: Walter Knoll, Herrenberg | G
Lighting: TAL Lighting, Pittern | B; Modular Lighting Instruments, Roeselare | B; Doxis, Genk | B

DERMATOLOGICAL PRACTICE, STUTTGART | G

Architect: mikropolis, Prof. Ulrike Mansfeld, Bremen | G, Tilman Heller, Stuttgart | G
Location of the building object: Schwabstraße 91, 70193 Stuttgart | G
Photos: Peter Horn, Stuttgart | G
Interior: Baumgärtner Einrichtungen GmbH, Hassfurt | G; Strähle Raum-Systeme GmbH, Waiblingen | G
Lighting: Zumtobel Lighting, Dornbirn | A
Flooring: Armstrong DLW, Bietigheim-Bissingen | G

OTORHINOLARYNGOLOGY [ORL] CLINIC, STUTTGART | G

Architect: mikropolis, Prof. Ulrike Mansfeld, Bremen | G
Location of the building object: Haus der Gesundheit, Stuttgarter Straße 33–35, 70469 Stuttgart | G
Photos: Frank Bayh, Stefanie Rosenberger-Ochs
Interior: Seibold Innenausbau KG, Stuttgart | G
Flooring: Armstrong DLW, Bietigheim-Bissingen | G

ORTHOPAEDIC CLINIC IN ADLERSHOF HEALTH CENTRE, BERLIN | G

Architect: Mateja Mikulandra-Mackat, Berlin | G,
Construction management: Jörn Grünert, Berlin | G
Location of the building object: Gesundheitszentrum Adlershof, Albert-Einstein-Straße 2, 12489 Berlin | G
Photos: Werner Huthmacher, Berlin | G
Furniture: Vitra AG, Birsfelden | CH; Moroso, Cavalicco, Udine | I
Lighting: Mawa Design Licht- und Wohnideen, Michendorf | G
Sanitary: Duravit AG, Hornberg | G; Alape GmbH, Goslar | G

MATREI HEALTH CENTRE, MATREI | A

Architect: Gerhard Mitterberger, Graz | A,
Collaboration: Agnes Kassl, Mirjam Landl, Ingo Georg Gruber, Dagmar Herbst, Phillip Glanzl
Location of the building object: Eduard-Wallnöfer-Straße 3, 9971 Matrei | A
Graphic artist | artist: Peter Raneburger, Matrei | A
Photos: Zita Oberwalder, Graz | A
Statics: Johann Riebenbauer, Graz | A
Medical engineering: Dental Nagele GmbH, Völs | A

PAEDIATRIC PRACTICE, HAAN | G

Architect: null2elf, Düsseldorf | G, Birte Dischek, Barbara Lucas-Nülle
Location of the building object: Neuer Markt 27, 42781 Haan | G
Graphic artist | artist: null2elf, Düsseldorf | G
Photos: diebuilder, Sabrina & Niclas Kohl, Dortmund | G
Furniture: Johannes Droste GmbH, Gelsenkirchen | G
Flooring: objectflor GmbH, Cologne | G

DENTAL PRACTICE, KREFELD | G

Architect: null2elf, Düsseldorf | G, Birte Dischek, Barbara Lucas-Nülle
Location of the building object: Ostwall 165, 47798 Krefeld | G
Graphic artist | artist: Jörg Thomas Alvermann, null2elf, Düsseldorf | G
Photos: Jens Kirchner
Furniture: Johannes Droste GmbH, Gelsenkirchen | G
Flooring: Amtico, Coventry | GB

MEDICAL + DENTAL SUITE AT COLOGNE BONN AIRPORT, COLOGNE | G

Architect: Hubert Günther, pd raumplan, Cologne | G
Location of the building object: Flughafen Cologne Bonn, Terminal 1 A | B, 51147 Cologne | G
Photos: Ralf Baumgarten, Cologne | G
Furniture: Moroso, Cavalicco, Udine | I, Vitra AG, Birsfelden | CH
Lighting: TRILUX GmbH, Arnsberg | G; Molto Luce GmbH, Wels | A
Sanitary: Alape GmbH, Goslar | G; Dornbracht GmbH, Iserlohn | G; Duravit AG, Hornberg | G
Flooring: Pandomo

"GOETHE 10" PRACTICE CLINIC, FRANKFURT ON THE MAIN | G

Architect:
Hubert Günther, pd raumplan, Cologne | G
Location of the building object:
Goethestraße 10,
60313 Frankfurt on the Main | G
Photos: Ralf Baumgarten, Cologne | G
Furniture: Artifort, Schijndel | NL
Lighting: Modulor GmbH, Berlin | G
Sanitary: Catalano, Rom | I;
Duravit AG, Hornberg | G; Alape GmbH,
Goslar | G; Dornbracht GmbH, Iserlohn | G

VITALICUM, FRANKFURT ON THE MAIN | G

Architect:
Hubert Günther, pd raumplan, Cologne | G
Location of the building object:
Neue Mainzer Straße 84,
60311 Frankfurt on the Main | G
Photos: Ralf Baumgarten, Cologne | G
Furniture: Moroso, Cavalicco, Udine | I
Lighting: Modular Lighting, Zurich | CH;
Tobias Grau GmbH, Rellingen | G
Sanitary: Alape GmbH, Goslar | G;
Dornbracht GmbH, Iserlohn | G

"CENTRE D'ENDODONTIE" ENDODONTOLOGY CLINIC, PARIS | F

Architect:
Hubert Günther, pd raumplan, Cologne | G
Location of the building object:
1 Rue Margueritte, 75017 Paris | F
Photos: Ralf Baumgarten, Cologne | G
Furniture: B&B Italia, Novedrate | I
Lighting: Modular Lighting, Zurich | CH;
Prolicht GmbH, Neu-Götzens | A
Sanitary:
Grohe GmbH, Porta Westfalica | G;
Duravit AG, Hornberg | G

"A1" DENTAL PRACTICE AT OPERNPLATZ, FRANKFURT ON THE MAIN | G

Architect:
Hubert Günther, pd raumplan, Cologne | G
Location of the building object:
Neue Mainzer Straße 84,
60311 Frankfurt on the Main | G
Photos: Ralf Baumgarten, Cologne | G
Furniture: USM Haller – U. Schärer
Söhne AG, Münsingen | CH
Lighting: Modular GmbH, Berlin | G
Sanitary: Catalano, Rom | I;
Vola, Horsens | DK; Duravit AG, Hornberg | G

PRACTICE FOR GENERAL MEDICINE, REMSCHEID | G

Architect:
rischko architekten, Odenthal | G,
Oliver Rischko, Martina Rischko
Location of the building object:
Ringelstraße 17, 42897 Remscheid | G
Photos: Oliver Rischko, Odenthal | G
Furniture:
Schreinerei Leber, Kreuztal-Krombach | G;
KOINOR Polstermöbel, Michelau | G

SURGICAL CLINIC, MÖNCHENGLADBACH | G

Architect:
rischko architekten, Odenthal | G,
Oliver Rischko, Martina Rischko
Location of the building object:
Südwall 47, 41179 Mönchengladbach | G
Photos: Oliver Rischko, Odenthal | G
Furniture:
Schreinerei Leber, Kreuztal-Krombach | G
Medical engineering:
TECHNO-med-PLAN GmbH, Münster | G
Lighting: Delta Line + Light GmbH,
Übach-Palenberg | G
Schmitz-Leuchten GmbH, Arnsberg | G
Sanitary: Duravit AG, Hornberg | G;
Grohe GmbH, Porta Westfalica | G

PRACTICE FOR HOLISTIC MEDICINE, PULHEIM-BRAUWEILER | G

Architect:
rischko architekten, Odenthal | G,
Oliver Rischko, Martina Rischko
Location of the building object:
Bernhardstraße 33,
50259 Pulheim-Brauweiler | G
Photos: Oliver Rischko, Odenthal | G
Furniture:
Schreinerei Leber, Kreuztal-Krombach | G;
drabert by samas, Minden | G
Lighting: Troll, Canovelles | E
Sanitary: Duravit AG, Hornberg | G;
Hansgrohe AG, Schiltach | G

WIESENSTADT HEALTH CENTRE WIESENSTADT, VIENNA | A

Architect:
rochuskahrarchitektur, Vienna | A,
Rochus Kahr
Location of the building object:
Rösslergasse 1, 1230 Vienna | A
Photos: Klemens Horvath, Vienna | A
Furniture: Josef Göbel Tischlerwerk-
stätten, Fladnitz | A

MUNICIPAL CLINIC OUTPATIENT DEPARTMENT, FRANKENTHAL | G

Architect: sander.hofrichter architekten,
Ludwigshafen | G,
Klaus Gutschalk, Oliver Löwer, Ute Wiese
Location of the building object:
Elsa-Brändström-Straße 1,
67227 Frankenthal | G
Photos: Johannes Vogt, Mannheim | G
Heating | airing | sanitary installations:
PAV, Merzig | G
Statics:
Ackermann + Müller, Frankenthal | G
Electrical engineering:
EPL GmbH, Wiesbaden | G

DENTAL PRACTICE, FRANKFURT ON THE MAIN | G

Architect: stengele+cie.,
Frankfurt on the Main | G, Volker Stengele,
Nadine Aschenbrücker, Britta Damhuis,
Berthold Rank
Location of the building object:
Niedenau 50,
60325 Frankfurt on the Main | G
Photos: stengele+cie.,
Frankfurt on the Main | G
Medical engineering: Dental-Depot –
Medizinische Handels & Service GmbH,
Niedernberg | G
Facilities medical engineering: Eurodent,
Bologna | I; Rosso GmbH, Meerbusch | G
Lighting: Erco Leuchten, Lüdenscheid | G
Sanitary: Alape GmbH, Goslar | G;
Dornbracht GmbH, Iserlohn | G

PAEDIATRIC AND YOUTH MEDICINE CLINIC, BAIERSBRONN | G

Architect: Birgit Stiletto, Freudenstadt | G,
Matthias Jarcke
Location of the building object:
Rosenplatz 18, 72270 Baiersbronn | G
Graphic artist | artist: Fachhochschule
Wiesbaden | G, Fachbereich Gestaltung
Photos: Frank Schindler, Freudenstadt | G
Heating | airing: Liepelt Planungsbüro für
Haustechnik, Baiersbronn | G
Furniture: Vitra AG, Birsfelden | G,
Walter Knoll AG & Co. KG, Herrenberg | G
Lighting: Flos; Vanlux; Occhio
[AML Licht + Design GmbH], Munich | G;
Catellani | I; Targetti, Florenz | I
Sanitary: Duravit AG, Hornberg | G;
Catalano, Bologna | I;
Fratelli Fantini, Pella | I

FÜNF HÖFE OPHTHALMOLOGISTS, MUNICH | G

Architect: tools off.architeture, Munich | G
Location of the building object:
Theatinerstraße 14, Salvatorpassage |
Fünf Höfe, 80333 Munich | G
Graphic artist | artist: Manfred Fronske,
Landshut | G
Photos: Lothar Reichel, Munich | G
Heating | airing:
Kühn Bauer Partner, Munich | G
Lighting: Obermeyer Planen + Beraten
GmbH, Munich | G

VILLAVITA – CENTRE FOR HOLISTIC MEDICINE, COLOGNE | G

Architect: trint + kreuder d. n. a,
Cologne | G
Location of the building object:
Hauptstraße 24, 50996 Cologne | G
Photos: trint + kreuder d. n. a, Cologne | G
Furniture: Objektform GmbH, Bonn | G
Lighting:
Ose Franzen Lichtplanung, Sylt | G

FALKENRIED CLINIC, HAMBURG | G

Architect: Wagenknecht Architekten,
Hamburg | G, Tillmann Wagenknecht
Location of the building object:
Lehmweg 17, 20251 Hamburg | G
Photos: Klaus Frahm, Börnsen | G
Heating | airing | sanitary installations:
DJM Planung GmbH, Hamburg | G
Hygiene: BZH GmbH, Freiburg | G
Furniture: Tischlerei Steineker & Krall
GmbH, Hamburg | G
Medical engineering: Drägerwerk AG,
Lübeck | G
Lighting: DJM Planung GmbH,
Hamburg | G
Flooring: Scheer Surface Solutions GmbH,
Lorch | G

OMF SURGERY LINDENARCADEN, LÜBECK | G

Architect: Wagenknecht Architekten,
Hamburg | G, Tillmann Wagenknecht
Location of the building object:
Fackenburger Allee 1, 23554 Lübeck | G
Photos: Klaus Frahm, Börnsen | G
Heating | airing | sanitary installations:
DJM Planung GmbH, Hamburg | G
Furniture: Glasbau Wagenschein GmbH,
Bremen | G; Tischlerei Steineker & Krall
GmbH, Hamburg | G
Medical engineering:
Pluradent AG, Offenbach | G
Lighting: Kreon, Opglabbeek | B
Flooring: Bembé Parkett GmbH,
Bad Mergentheim | G

DENTAL PRACTICE, BERLIN | G

Architect: walk | architekten, Berlin | G,
Susann Walk
Location of the building object:
Altensteinstraße 44 a, 14195 Berlin | G
Graphic artist | artist:
extratapete GmbH, Berlin | G
Photos: Matthias Könsgen, Berlin | G
Heating | airing | sanitary installations:
K. u. A. Münster Sanitec GmbH, Berlin | G
Furniture: Vitra AG, Birsfelden | CH;
Ikea GmbH & Co. KG, Hofheim-Wallau | G
Medical engineering:
Fimet Oy, Monninkyla | FIN
Lighting: Zumtobel Lighting,
Dornbirn | A; Erco Leuchten GmbH,
Lüdenscheid | G
Sanitary installations:
Glashütte Limburg, Limburg | G

REGISTER
BUILDING WORK

REGISTER
CITIES

FRANZ LABRYGA
Born in 1929, professor of architecture, taught at TU Berlin 1974-1994. Many years director of the Institute of Hospital Construction, head of many committees, inclusive for Federal Health Agency and DIN. Member of Architects for Hospital Construction and Health (AKG). Numerous specialist publications.

PHILIPP MEUSER
Born in 1969, architect and journalist. Studied architecture in Berlin and Zurich. Author of books on public health building typologies. Architecture firm in Berlin together with Natascha Meuser.

AUTHORS

ARCHITECTS

SUBJECT INDEX

The *Deutsche Bibliothek* lists this publication
in the *Deutsche Nationalbibliografie*.
Detailed bibliographical data available on
the internet at http://dnb.ddb.de

ISBN 978-3-938666-54-8

© 2010 by DOM publishers, Berlin
www.dom-publishers.com

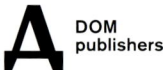

A DOM
publishers

Editor-in-chief
Philipp Meuser

Editing
Dörte Becker †

Final editing
Brigitta Hahn-Melcher
Mandy Kasek

Translation
archiTEXT s. a., Luxembourg

Proof reading
Mariangela Palazzi-Williams | MPW
Translations and Publishing Services

Design and composition
Torsten Köchlin

Book-cover design
Nicole Wolf

Engineering drawings
Kristin Egermann
Wera Pahl

Photo credits
Childs, Oliver: 16|11; iStockphoto: 18|17;
Jankowiak, Matthias: 12|4, 13|5; Jonsson,
Henrik: 22f.; Kaulitzki, Sebastian: 8f.; Knocke,
Karsten: 21|19; Körperwelten, Gunther von
Hagens, Institut für Plastination, www.
koerperwelten.de: 11|1–3; Leppert, Quirin:
18|18; Meuser, Philipp: 16|9, 16|12, 17|13, 17|15;
Scapinachis, Pablo Demetrio: 18|16; Schutz,
Bobby: 16|10; Tobolla, Jennifer: 17|14

Photo credits of the projects are stated in the
appendix on pages 374 to 377.

Also available:

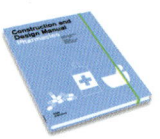

Dörte Becker | Philipp Meuser
Pharmacies
Construction and Design Manual.
ISBN 978-3-938666-55-5

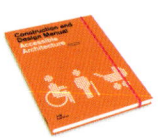

Joachim Fischer | Philipp Meuser
Accssible Architecture
Construction and Design Manual.
ISBN 978-3-938666-97-5